Life stage group	Potassium (g/d)	Chloride (g/d)	Calcium (mg/d)	Phosphorus (mg/d)	Magnesium (mg/d)	Iron (mg/d)	Zinc (mg/d)	Selenium (µg/d)	Iodine (µg/d)	Copper (µg/d)	Manganese (mg/d)	Fluoride (mg/d)	Chromium (µg/d)	Molybdenum (µg/d)	Total Water (L/d)[11]
Infants															
0-6 mo	0.4*	0.18*	210*	100*	30*	0.27*	2*	15*	110*	200*	0.003*	0.01*	0.2*	2*	0.7*
7-12 mo	0.7*	0.57*	270*	275*	75*	11	3	20*	130*	220*	0.6*	0.5*	5.5*	3*	0.8*
Children															
1-3 y	3.0*	1.5*	500*	460	80	7	3	20	90	340	1.2*	0.7*	11*	17	1.3*
4-8 y	3.8*	1.9*	800*	500	130	10	5	30	90	440	1.5*	1*	15*	22	1.7*
Males															
9-13 y	4.5*	2.3*	1,300*	1,250	240	8	8	40	120	700	1.9*	2*	25*	34	2.4*
14-18 y	4.7*	2.3*	1,300*	1,250	410	11	11	55	150	890	2.2*	3*	35*	43	3.3*
19-30 y	4.7*	2.3*	1,000*	700	400	8	11	55	150	900	2.3*	4*	35*	45	3.7*
31-50 y	4.7*	2.3*	1,000*	700	420	8	11	55	150	900	2.3*	4*	35*	45	3.7*
51-70 y	4.7*	2.0*	1,200*	700	420	8	11	55	150	900	2.3*	4*	30*	45	3.7*
>70 y	4.7*	1.8*	1,200*	700	420	8	11	55	150	900	2.3*	4*	30*	45	3.7*
Females															
9-13 y	4.5*	2.3*	1,300*	1,250	240	8	8	40	120	700	1.6*	2*	21*	34	2.1*
14-18 y	4.7*	2.3*	1,300*	1,250	360	15	9	55	150	890	1.6*	3*	24*	43	2.3*
19-30 y	4.7*	2.3*	1,000*	700	310	18	8	55	150	900	1.8*	3*	25*	45	2.7*
31-50 y	4.7*	2.3*	1,000*	700	320	18	8	55	150	900	1.8*	3*	25*	45	2.7*
51-70 y	4.7*	2.0*	1,200*	700	320	8	8	55	150	900	1.8*	3*	20*	45	2.7*
>70 y	4.7*	1.8*	1,200*	700	320	8	8	55	150	900	1.8*	3*	20*	45	2.7*
Pregnancy															
14-18 y	4.7*	2.3*	1,300*	1,250	400	27	12	60	220	1,000	2.0*	3*	29*	50	3.0*
19-30 y	4.7*	2.3*	1,000*	700	350	27	11	60	220	1,000	2.0*	3*	30*	50	3.0*
31-50 y	4.7*	2.3*	1,000*	700	360	27	11	60	220	1,000	2.0*	3*	30*	50	3.0*
Lactation															
14-18 y	5.1*	2.3*	1,300*	1,250	360	10	13	70	290	1,300	2.6*	3*	44*	50	3.8*
19-30 y	5.1*	2.3*	1,000*	700	310	9	12	70	290	1,300	2.6*	3*	45*	50	3.8*
31-50 y	5.1*	2.3*	1,000*	700	320	9	12	70	290	1,300	2.6*	3*	45*	50	3.8*

[11]The AI for water represents total water from drinking water, beverages, and moisture from food.

Sources: Data compiled from *Dietary Reference Intakes for Calcium, Phosphorus, Magnesium, Vitamin D, and Fluoride.* Washington, DC: National Academies Press; 1997. *Dietary Reference Intakes for Thiamin, Riboflavin, Niacin, Vitamin B6, Folate, Vitamin B12, Pantothenic Acid, Biotin, and Choline.* Washington, DC: National Academies Press; 1998. *Dietary Reference Intakes for Vitamin C, Vitamin E, Selenium, and Carotenoids.* Washington, DC: National Academies Press; 2000. *Dietary Reference Intakes for Vitamin A, Vitamin K, Arsenic, Boron, Chromium, Copper, Iron, Manganese, Molybdenum, Nickel, Silicon, Vanadium, and Zinc.* Washington, DC: National Academies Press; 2001. *Dietary Reference Intakes for Water, Potassium, Sodium, Chloride, and Sulfate.* Food and Nutrition Board. Washington, DC: National Academies Press; 2005. These reports may be accessed via http://nap.edu. Reprinted with permission by the National Academy of Sciences, courtesy of the National Academies Press, Washington, DC.

Community
Nutrition

Community Nutrition

Planning Health Promotion and Disease Prevention

Nweze Eunice Nnakwe, PhD, RD, LD, CFCS

Professor, Department of Family and Consumer Science
Illinois State University

JONES AND BARTLETT PUBLISHERS
Sudbury, Massachusetts
BOSTON   TORONTO   LONDON   SINGAPORE

World Headquarters
Jones and Bartlett Publishers
40 Tall Pine Drive
Sudbury, MA 01776
978-443-5000
info@jbpub.com
www.jbpub.com

Jones and Bartlett Publishers Canada
6339 Ormindale Way
Mississauga, Ontario L5V 1J2
Canada

Jones and Bartlett Publishers International
Barb House, Barb Mews
London W6 7PA
United Kingdom

Jones and Bartlett's books and products are available through most bookstores and online booksellers. To contact Jones and Bartlett Publishers directly, call 800-832-0034, fax 978-443-8000, or visit our website www.jbpub.com.

Substantial discounts on bulk quantities of Jones and Bartlett's publications are available to corporations, professional associations, and other qualified organizations. For details and specific discount information, contact the special sales department at Jones and Bartlett via the above contact information or send an email to specialsales@jbpub.com.

Production Credits
Publisher: Cathleen Sether
Acquisitions Editor: Shoshanna Goldberg
Associate Editor: Amy L. Flagg
Editorial Assistant: Kyle Hoover
Production Manager: Julie Champagne Bolduc
Production Assistant: Jessica Steele Newfell
Marketing Manager: Jessica Faucher
V.P., Manufacturing and Inventory Control: Therese Connell
Composition: Publishers' Design and Production Services, Inc.
Cover Design: Kristin E. Parker
Senior Photo Researcher and Photographer: Christine McKeen
Cover Image: © Tonis Valing/ShutterStock, Inc.
Printing and Binding: Courier Stoughton
Cover Printing: Courier Stoughton

Library of Congress Cataloging-in-Publication Data
Nnakwe, Nweze Eunice.
    Community nutrition : planning health promotion and disease prevention / Nweze Eunice Nnakwe.
        p. ; cm.
    Includes bibliographical references.
    ISBN-13: 978-0-7637-4760-2 (pbk.)
    ISBN-10: 0-7637-4760-2
    1. Nutrition. 2. Community health services. I. Title.
    [DNLM: 1. Community Health Services. 2. Nutrition Physiology.   QU 145 N738n 2008]
    TX354.N63 2008
    363.8'5610973—dc22
                                                                    2007049472

6048

Printed in the United States of America
12 11 10 09 08   10 9 8 7 6 5 4 3 2 1

This book is dedicated to God, who makes all things possible;
to my parents, who taught me the value of life;
to my husband for his support and patience;
to my daughters, Ify, Chimma, and Chinonye;
to my sons, Chiemeka and Ikechi, for their love and support; and
to my grandchildren with love, Nonye, Ayanna, Omari, and Varleine.

Brief Contents

Contents

Successful Community Strategies Contents

Preface

The goal of *Community Nutrition: Planning Health Promotion and Disease Prevention* is to provide community nutrition students, community nurses, and health educators with the knowledge, skills, tools, and evidence-based approaches they need to promote health, prevent disease, and meet the changing face of community and public health. This textbook reinforces core nutrition concepts and presents the tools and skills needed to enter the health professions. It presents a community-based care perspective—instead of the hospital-based care perspective used by most other books in this area—to reflect the increased emphasis of practitioners on providing community-based services that emphasize primary, secondary, and tertiary prevention.

The book is divided into three parts. Part I provides an overview of community and public health nutrition landscapes and lays the groundwork for primary, secondary, and tertiary prevention. This section begins with a discussion of various community approaches to health promotion and disease prevention in Chapter 1. Chapter 2 discusses nutrition screening and assessment methods, including diet assessment methods. Chapter 3 describes the nuts and bolts of nutrition epidemiology and research methods and provides community nutritionists with a step-by-step method of implementing different stages of the research process. In Chapter 4, U.S. nutrition monitoring and food assistance programs for at-risk populations are discussed. This chapter also provides a detailed description of the "working poor" and explains how to evaluate food insecurity. Chapter 5 discusses the U.S. healthcare system. Chapter 6 provides strategies that can be used to develop public policy and discusses how dietitians can become involved in the policy process. In addition, it discusses bioterrorism preparedness. Chapter 7 provides an overview of world hunger and food insecurity and discusses the role of women in the prevention of food insecurity and current nutrition issues. It also discusses "Millennial Morbidities" in developing and developed countries, and equips nutritionists with the tools to provide nutrition intervention during emergency relief periods.

Part II focuses on the knowledge and intervention skills needed to promote health and prevent disease throughout the life cycle. Chapter 8 discusses nutrition during pregnancy and infancy and provides community nutritionists with information regarding nutrition care during these stages of life. Chapter 9 describes current nutrition trends and the factors that contribute to overweight and obesity in childhood and adolescence. Chapter 10 focuses on special health issues in adulthood and challenges community and public health nutritionists to integrate evidence-based intervention strategies into their nutrition programs. It also addresses "Millennial Morbidities" and equips community nutritionists with the knowledge and tools to address such chronic health conditions as cardiovascular disease, obesity, cancer, and osteoporosis. Chapter 11 discusses health promotion and disease prevention in older persons and provides multiple nutrition screening initiative tools for community and public health nutritionists to use in the nutrition care process.

Part III focuses on the skills, knowledge, and tools community nutritionists need to design effective nutrition and health promotion programs. This section applies the information presented in Parts I and II while discussing the principles of planning successful community nutrition programs. Chapter 12 presents several research-based theoretical frameworks that can guide nutrition education. It discusses steps for translating theory into research–oriented educational strategies and presents practical activities that nutritionists can use to conduct nutrition education. Chapter 13 addresses the process of grantsmanship, nutrition, and ethics and lays the foundation for writing and implementing grant proposals. Chapter 14 discusses the principles of nutrition education. It presents the procedural model for designing research-based educational programs and strategies that provide valuable nutrition education throughout the life span. Chapter 15 focuses on marketing nutrition programs and the role of the food industry on food choice, including how advertising affects childhood obesity. Chapter 16 addresses cultural influences and public health nutrition. It provides community nutritionists with multiple ways of acquiring cultural competency and identifies barriers to effective multicultural health promotion and disease prevention programs. It also discusses cultural differences and possible reasons for health disparities in the United States.

This book's comprehensive coverage makes it an essential resource for community nutrition courses and a useful reference tool. It provides pertinent statistics on the national health objectives for 2010 and discusses traditional concepts as well as current and emerging nutrition issues. Real-world examples throughout the text explain nutritional concepts and present the reader with an application of these important topics. The book presents concise information and provides helpful activities so that the reader can consider important issues without receiving a great deal of unnecessary information.

This book includes a variety of features that help students and other health professionals prepare and provide effective nutrition intervention to different groups in the community:

- **Learning Objectives** emphasize key concepts to help students focus on what they need to learn.

- **Boxes** highlight important points in each chapter.
- **Successful Community Strategies** discuss effective intervention programs and provide examples of best research-based practices for each chapter.
- **Chapter Summaries** highlight important concepts for each chapter.
- **Critical Thinking Activities** incorporate a variety of cognitive skills such as synthesizing, analyzing, applying, and evaluating information. The activities help students develop expertise and provide them with the opportunity to understand and evaluate health information and then apply the concepts in community settings.
- **Case Studies** provide students the opportunity to apply what they have learned in each chapter.
- **References** offer students resources for future study.

Companion Website:
http://nutrition.jbpub.com/communitynutrition

The companion website for this book offers tools for both students and instructors.

For Students
- Animated Flashcards
- BMI Calculator

- Chemistry Review
- Crossword Puzzles
- Eating Great in College
- Health and Nutrition Directory
- Interactive Glossary
- Nutrition Journals
- Nutrition Links
- Nutrition Science Animations
- Practice Quizzes
- Share Healthy Recipes
- Web Links

For Instructors
Comprehensive online teaching resources are available to adopters of the book and are cross-platform for Windows and Macintosh systems.

- **Instructor's Manual** includes annotated lecture outlines and ready-to-use lesson plans that outline all of the topics covered in the text. They are provided in an electronic format that can be easily modified.
- **PowerPoint Presentation Slides** present a template for each chapter that includes the chapter outline for building lecture presentations.
- **TestBank** helps the instructor choose a variety of situational questions organized by chapter.

Acknowledgments

The author's writing is one small part of the work that is involved in the development and production of a textbook. Many people worked dexterously with a shared goal to produce a visually appealing, error-free, up-to-date, high-quality textbook. I would like to acknowledge the dedication and hard work of these individuals; without them this project would never have been realized.

A heartfelt thanks to Jacqueline Geraci for her unwavering support and significant contributions. I also extend my thanks to the Jones and Bartlett editorial team, both past and present, for their hard work on this project: Shoshanna Goldberg, Amy Flagg, Kyle Hoover, Nicole Quinn, and Patrice Andrews. Julie Bolduc and Jess Newfell managed the production of this text, performing an astonishing job of keeping a very complex procedure progressing smoothly. Thank you also to Jessica Faucher, who maintains a strong focus on the goal of this text and the needs of its audience.

Jones and Bartlett is a company that is progressive in integrating technology with print materials for learning. The excellent web-based materials that are a part of *Community Nutrition* could not have been developed without this type of technical support.

A special thanks to my graduate students and the administrative assistants for their contributions to the preparation of this textbook and to my undergraduate students for their constructive feedback.

Lastly, many community and public health instructors and researchers contributed significantly to the development of this book. I am very grateful to the following reviewers who contributed their expertise and valuable direction to the development of this text:

Melanie Tracy Burns, PhD, RD, Eastern Illinois University

Katherine L. Cason, PhD, RD, Clemson University

Nancy Cotugna, PhD, RD, University of Delaware

Lynn Duerr, PhD, RD, CD, Indiana State University

Erin Francort, RD, Idaho State University

Jeanne Florini, MS, RD, LD, St. Louis Community College at Florissant Valley

Carol Friesen, PhD, RD, Ball State University

Nancy Harris, MS, RD, LDN, FADA, East Carolina University

Mary Mitchell, PhD, RD, Ohio State University

Martha L. Rew, MS, RD, LD, Texas Woman's University

Thanks to all of you.

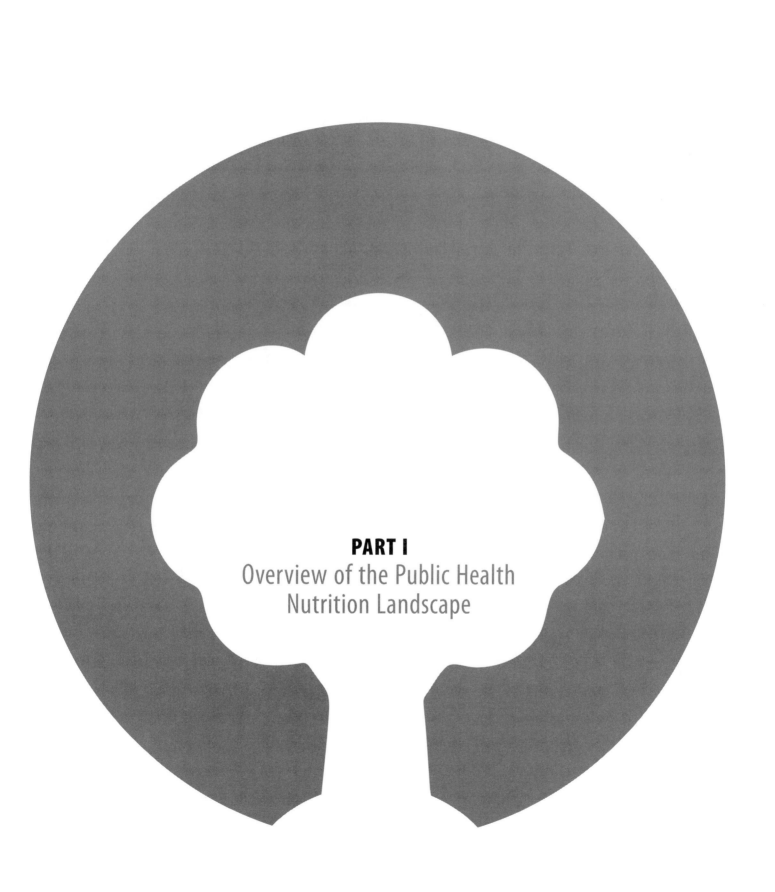

PART I
Overview of the Public Health
Nutrition Landscape

Community Nutrition and Public Health

LEARNING OBJECTIVES

- Define public health and community nutrition.
- Discuss the relationship between diet and diseases.
- List current nutrition- and diet-related public health problems.
- Explain primary, secondary, and tertiary prevention.
- Outline the educational requirements, practice settings, roles, and responsibilities of community and public health nutritionists.
- Define the terms *Registered Dietitian (RD)* and *public health nutrition*.

Introduction

Community nutrition is a modern and comprehensive profession that includes, but is not limited to, public health nutrition, dietetics/nutrition education, and medical nutrition therapy.[1] Community nutrition deals with a variety of food and nutrition issues related to individuals, families, and special groups that have a common link such as place of residence, language, culture, or health issues.[2] There is an increasing need to focus on community in **health promotion** and disease prevention because behavior is highly influenced by the environment in which people live. Local values, norms, and behavior patterns have a significant effect on shaping an individual's attitudes and behaviors.[3,4] The increasing movement toward using a community approach requires community **nutritionists** to become more visible and vocal leaders of community health. However, before community nutrition-

ists can participate in nutrition and healthcare planning, they must be knowledgeable about the concept of community as client.

The Concept of Community

The concept of community varies widely. The World Health Organization (WHO) defines **community** as "a social group determined by geographic boundaries and/or common values and interests."[5] Community members know and interact with one another; function within a particular social structure; and show and create norms, values, and social institutions.[6] Suburbs and other areas surrounding the legal limits of a city are also an integral part of that city's total community.[7]

A second definition of community is demographic and involves viewing the community as a subgroup of the population, such as people of a particular age, gender, social class, or race.[8] A community can also be defined on the basis of a common interest or goal. A collection of people, even if they are scattered geographically, can have a common interest that binds its members. This is called a common-interest community.[9] Many successful prevention and health promotion efforts, including improved services and increased community awareness of specific problems, have resulted from the work of common-interest communities. The following are some examples of common-interest communities:[9]

- Members of a national professional organization (e.g., American Dietetic Association, American Medical Association, Federation of American Societies for Experimental Biology, African American Career Women, National Association of Asian American Professionals, American Public Health Association)
- Members of churches
- Disabled individuals scattered throughout a large city
- Individuals with specific health condition (e.g., diabetes, hypertension, breast cancer, mental illness)
- Teenage mothers
- Homebound elderly persons

Community nutrition and dietetics professionals are also members of a community and are public health agency professionals who provide nutrition services that emphasize community health promotion and disease prevention. They deal with the needs of individuals through primary, secondary, and tertiary preventions (which will be discussed in more detail later in this chapter).

- *Primary prevention* involves designing activities to prevent a problem or disease before it occurs.
- *Secondary prevention* involves planning activities related to early diagnosis and treatment, including screening for diseases.
- *Tertiary prevention* consists of designing activities to treat a disease state or injury and to prevent it from progressing further.[10]

community nutrition An area of nutrition that addresses the entire range of food and nutrition issues related to preventing disease and improving the health of individuals, families, and the community.

health promotion The process of enabling people to increase control of and improve their health.

nutritionist A professional with academic credentials in nutrition; may also be a registered dietitian.

community A group of people who share a common geographical location, values, culture, or languages.

primary prevention Activities designed to prevent a problem or disease before it occurs.

secondary prevention Activities related to early diagnosis and treatment, including screening for diseases.

tertiary prevention Designing activities to treat a disease state or injury and to prevent it from further progression.

public health The science and art of preventing disease, prolonging life, developing policy, and promoting health and efficiency through organized community effort.

public health nutrition Focuses on the community and society as a whole and aims at optimal nutrition and health status. Public health nutritionist positions require dietetic registration by the Commission on Dietetic Registration and a graduate-level science degree that includes study of environmental sciences, health promotion, and disease prevention programs.

These professionals establish links with other professionals involved in a wide range of education and human services, such as child care agencies; social work agencies; services to older persons; high schools; colleges and universities; and community-based epidemiological research.

Public Health and Nutrition

Public health is defined as "the science and art of preventing disease, prolonging life, and promoting health and efficiency through organized community efforts, so organizing these benefits as to enable every citizen to realize his/her birthright of health and longevity."[11] It has been viewed as the scientific diagnosis and treatment of the community. In this vision, the community, instead of the individual, is seen as the patient. When the focus is on the community, patterns and processes begin to emerge and combine to form a unified whole.[12] Using this approach avoids focusing on risks and diseases; instead, the focus is on the community's strengths and resilience. Community strengths can be physiological, psychological, social, or spiritual. They include such factors as education, coping skills, support systems, knowledge, communication skills, nutrition, coherent belief systems, fitness, ability to develop a supportive environment, and self-care skills.[3]

Increasing nutrition knowledge can reduce medical care costs and improve the quality of life.[13-16] The negative consequences of nutrition-related problems include malnutrition and chronic health conditions such as obesity, cardiovascular disease, cancer, and diabetes mellitus.[17,18] In addition, these conditions contribute significantly to the world's burden of morbidity, incapacity, and mortality, despite the tremendous amount of biological knowledge accumulated over the years.[18] The WHO estimated that prevention of the major nutrition-related risk factors (cigarette smoking, inactivity, poor dietary habits, and alcohol abuse) could translate into a gain of 5 years of disability-free life expectancy.[19, 20]

A community and public health nutrition approach will make it possible to reverse the course of major nutrition problems.[21,22] Dietetic professionals can take the lead in prevention programming because their training as counselors and educators provides skills that make them important members of a public health profession.

Public health nutrition was developed in the United States in response to societal events and changes to the following situations:[1,23,24]

- Infant mortality
- Access to healthcare
- Epidemics of communicable disease
- Poor hygiene and sanitation
- Malnutrition
- Agriculture and food production (in response to changes in food production)
- Economic depression, wars, and civil rights
- Aging of the population
- Behavior-related problems/lifestyle (poor dietary practices, alcohol abuse, inactivity, and cigarette smoking)
- Chronic diseases (obesity, heart disease, diabetes mellitus, mental health, cancer, osteoporosis, and hypertension)
- Poverty and immigration
- Preschool/after-school child care and school-based meals

The Relationship Between Eating Behaviors and Chronic Diseases

As evidenced by an introductory review of literature and research in the area of eating behavior and chronic disease, the relationship between

TABLE 1.1 Some Possible Health Problems Linked with Poor Dietary Habits								
Behavior	Risk of Heart Disease	Risk of Some Cancers	Risk of Diabetes	Risk of Obesity	Risk of Osteoporosis	Risk of Birth Defects	Risk of High Blood Pressure	Risk of Anemia
Eat foods lower in total fat, saturated fat, and cholesterol	✔	✔	✔	✔			✔	
Eat foods lower in calories; balance caloric intake with physical activity	✔	✔	✔	✔			✔	
Drink alcohol in moderation	✔	✔						
Eat less cured and smoked foods		✔						
Prepare foods with less salt	✔						✔	
Eat foods high in calcium and vitamin D	✔				✔		✔	
Eat foods high in iron								✔
Eat foods high in folic acid	✔	✔				✔		✔
Eat foods high in antioxidants	✔	✔	✔			✔	✔	
Eat foods high in soluble and insoluble fiber	✔	✔	✔	✔		✔	✔	✔
Eat foods high in omega-3 fatty acids	✔	✔	✔			✔		
Breastfeed infants			✔	✔				

eating behaviors and chronic diseases is significant and impacts individuals and communities greatly.[25] **Table 1.1** shows dietary factors that are linked to some of the most common chronic diseases. It is important to note that dietary factors overlap with other problems and are applicable to many of the health conditions listed.

The *Surgeon General's Report on Nutrition and Health*, government agencies, and nonprofit health and scientific organizations have provided comprehensive analyses of the relationship among diet, lifestyle, and major chronic diseases.[26–28] Health conditions such as coronary heart disease, stroke, cancer, and diabetes are still the leading causes of death and disability in the United States, and changes in Americans' current dietary practices could produce substantial health gains.

There have been concerns about the eating patterns of the U.S. population since the 1980s. Health policy makers have linked several dietary-related factors to chronic diseases, such as heart disease, cancer, birth defects, and osteoporosis, among the U.S. population and that of other industrialized countries.[25,29] This link between diet and disease has led to the publication of guidelines to promote healthier eating habits. The National Academy of Sciences, the U.S. Department of Health and Human Services, and the U.S. Surgeon General have published the majority of these guidelines.[11,12,26]

In addition to dietary intake, many other factors contribute to chronic diseases, such as genetic factors and lifestyle factors (e.g., cigarette smoking).[30] Medical geneticists working on the Human Genome Project, a major international initiative to decipher the 3-billion-unit code of DNA in the 80,000 to 100,000 genes found in humans, have already identified genes associated with many chronic diseases, such as breast, colon, and prostate cancers; severe obesity; and diabetes.[31–34]

Programs to promote health and longevity start with examining the major causes of death and disability. The top causes of death from

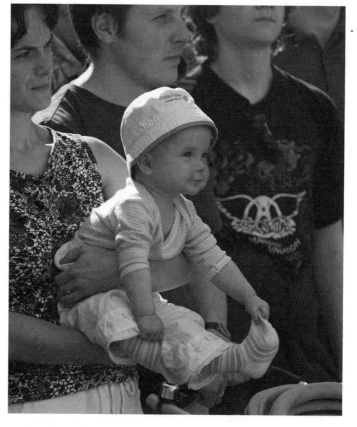

Public speaking is a great way to pass along nutrition information.

Box 1-1 The 10 Leading Causes of Death in the United States

1. Heart disease
2. Cancer
3. Stroke
4. Chronic lower respiratory disease
5. Accidents
6. Diabetes
7. Pneumonia/influenza
8. Alzheimer's disease
9. Nephritis, nephritic syndrome, and nephrosis
10. Septicemia

Source: National Center for Health Statistics. www.cdc.gov/nchs/data/dis/2003. Accessed July 11, 2006.

---

the National Center for Health Statistics and Global Statistics and the WHO's 2003 and 2004 data are presented in Boxes 1-1 and 1-2.[35,36]

The public health approach to prevention understands that the reduction of risk for individuals with average risk profiles might be small or negligible. However, high-risk persons need special attention through primary, secondary, and tertiary preventions. Although it may not eliminate a disease for people who are genetically inclined to it, good primary prevention strategies could reduce the severity of the disease.[37]

Reducing Risk Through Prevention

Prevention is important in public health as well as community nutrition practice. The three important parts of prevention are personal, community-based, and systems-based.[6] Each part has a different role

---

Box 1-2 The 10 Leading Causes of Death Worldwide

1. Ischemic heart disease
2. Stroke
3. Acute lower respiratory infections
4. HIV/AIDS
5. Chronic obstructive pulmonary disease
6. Perinatal conditions
7. Diarrheal diseases
8. Tuberculosis
9. Malaria
10. Cancer of the lung/bronchus/trachea

Source: World Health Organization. www.who.int/features/qa/. Accessed July 11, 2006.

---

and focus. Establishing an overall effective community nutrition practice involves correctly using and combining each part.

- *Personal prevention* involves people at the individual level; for instance, educating and supporting a breastfeeding mother to promote the health of her infant.
- *Community-based prevention* targets groups; for example, public campaigns for low-fat diets to decrease the incidences of obesity and/or heart disease.[38,39]
- *Systems-based prevention* deals with changing policies and laws in order to achieve the objectives of prevention practice; for example, laws regarding childhood immunization, food labels, food safety, and sanitation.

One part of systems-based prevention deals with socioeconomic status, which affects health through environmental or behavioral factors. The socioeconomic model hypothesizes that poor families do not have the economic, social, or community resources needed to be in good health. For instance, poverty affects children's well-being by influencing health and nutrition, the home environment, and neighborhood conditions.[40a,40b] The combined effects of poverty provide the foundation for a cycle of poverty and hopelessness among family members, who in turn engage in risky health behaviors, such as substance abuse, smoking, and poor dietary habits, that can result in obesity and nutrition-related chronic diseases.

Socioeconomic models have been used to develop policies and disease prevention strategies, such as the Mackenbach model, which can be used as a basis for developing policies and intervention strategies. The Mackenbach model is presented in **Figure 1-1**. Mackenbach proposed that the link between socioeconomic status and health-related problems is triggered and maintained by two processes (selective and causative) that are active during different periods of life.[41] The selective

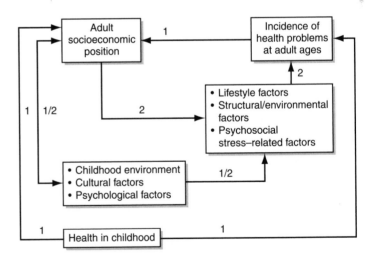

1: Selective processes.
2: Causative processes.
Note: The different arrows between socioeconomic factors represent potential entry points for policies and interventions to reduce health inequalities.

FIGURE 1-1 Selective and Causative Factors Involved in the Development of Health Inequalities in Society

Source: Mackenbach J, Bakker M. *Reducing Inequalities in Health: A European Perspective.* London: Routledge; 2002:18. Reprinted with permission.

Primary Prevention	Personal Approach
Health Promotion • Nutrition education • Water fluoridation to prevent dental decay • Provision of nutritious foods • Physical activity education • Genetic screening • Food intake analysis • Food safety education • Prenatal care **Specific Protection** • Use of specific immunizations • Attention to personal hygiene • Use of 24-hour recall and food frequency list • Use of environmental sanitation • Protection against obesity • Protection from foodborne illness • Use of specific nutrients • Protection from carcinogens • Avoidance of food allergens	• Breastfeeding support • Wellness education for an individual/physical activity • Stress management education for an individual to reduce blood pressure **Community Approach** • "Fruits & Veggies—More Matters" campaign • School health education • Community campaign for wellness (Heart Healthy for women) **System Approach** • Congregate dining meals for older persons • School breakfast required to meet the Dietary Guidelines • Calcium-fortified foods • Folic acid fortification of foods • Advocating for support of fruits in the school vending machine • Advocating for recreational activities at schools and daycares

Secondary Prevention	Personal Approach

Early Diagnosis and Prompt Treatment
• Screening surveys
• Selective examinations to:
  • Prevent disease process
  • Prevent the spread of communicable disease
  • Identify and intervene for individuals at risk of obesity, diabetes, and iron deficiency anemia
Disability Limitations
• Adequate food intake to arrest disease process and prevent further complications
• Provision of exercise facilities to limit disability and prevent death from obesity, heart disease, and cancer
	• Nutrition education for high-risk pregnant teenagers
	• Bone density screening for individuals at risk
	• Blood pressure screening for individuals at risk
	
	Community Approach
	• Cholesterol screenings
	• Blood pressure screening at the community center
	
	System Approach
	• "Shape up America"
	• Fat and calorie labels
	• Pasteurization of dairy products
	• Fortification of milk with vitamin D

Tertiary Prevention	Personal Approach
Restoration and Rehabilitation • Provision of medical nutrition therapy for individuals with nutrition-related problems • Education for the public and industry to produce low-fat foods	• Medical nutrition therapy for individuals with special healthcare conditions (e.g., heart disease) **Community Approach** • Advocating for special diets to be provided with diabetic nutrition education in the community **System Approach** • Passing legislation mandating that low-fat diets be provided in schools • New regulations for folate fortification of certain foods • Legislation to mandate payment of nutrition services for diabetes and obesity services • Advocating for fast-food restaurants to provide information on the fat content of meals

FIGURE 1-2 The Three Levels of Prevention and Intervention Approaches

Modified from: Mandle CL. *Health Promotion Throughout the Lifespan*. 5th ed. St. Louis: Mosby; 2002. Public Health Nutrition Practice Group, 1995. Also Owen AL, Splett PL, Owen GM. *Nutrition in the Community*. 4th ed. New York: McGraw-Hill; 1999. Reprinted with permission.

process is represented by childhood health, which determines adult health as well as socioeconomic position. The causative process represents three groups of risk factors (lifestyle, structural/environmental, and psychosocial stress-related factors), which are intermediaries between socioeconomic position and health problems. The model also acknowledges that childhood environment and cultural and psychological factors contribute to inequalities in health through both selection and causation. Health inequalities become self-perpetuating through a cycle of inadequate childhood health, adult socioeconomic position, and incidence of health problems at adult ages.[41]

Levels of Prevention

Each part of prevention itself has three levels. *Primary prevention* is an early intervention focused on controlling risk factors or preventing diseases before they happen, thus reducing their incidence. Examples of primary prevention include fortifying milk with vitamin D to prevent rickets in children, fortifying infant formula with iron to prevent anemia, and fluoridating public water supplies to prevent dental decay. *Secondary prevention* includes identifying disease early (before clinical signs and symptoms manifest) through screening. Timely intervention is provided to deter the disease process and prevent disability that may be caused by the disease. For instance, providing nutrition education on the importance of reducing dietary cholesterol, saturated fat, and caloric intake and increasing dietary fiber to individuals with high blood cholesterol is a secondary intervention to prevent the complications of heart disease.[42–45] *Tertiary prevention* is intervention to reduce the severity of diagnosed health conditions in order to prevent or delay disability and death. For example, providing education programs for persons recently diagnosed with hypertension is an intervention to prevent disability and additional health problems.[46] **Figure 1-2** presents the three levels of prevention and intervention approaches.

interdisciplinary team
Collaborating personnel representing different disciplines (e.g., nurses, social workers, physicians, daycare workers, dietitians, and dietetic technicians).

Figure 1-3 shows that a natural progression of a disease starts at the induction or initiation period. It also shows the relationship between disease progression and level of intervention. Early intervention (primary prevention) can reduce disease progression in its early stages. For example, for bacterial infections (such as *E. coli*), the incubation period is an early stage of disease development when individuals are not yet feeling the infection's effects. Also, an intervention such as a structured daily physical activity can slow weight gain and prevent obesity. Latency or dormancy is a similar early period when a disease (such as cardiovascular disease) has the potential of being expressed. Secondary prevention, such as blood pressure screening, will detect clinical symptoms and can help prevent the progression of a disease. The expression period is when the disease has occurred. At this point an intervention (tertiary prevention) is provided to reduce the severity of the disease or to prevent death; for example, a person could reduce their dietary fat intake to manage heart disease.[1]

Health Promotion

Health promotion is another major concept that is important to community and public health nutrition. Health promotion can be defined as the process of enabling people to increase control over the determinants of good health and subsequently improve their health. Two strategies that can be used to design a health promotion campaign in order to reduce risk are presented in **Table 1.2,** and the advantages and disadvantages of these strategies are presented in Box 1-3.

Knowledge and Skills of Public Health and Community Nutritionists

In most instances a community or public health nutritionist must be a member of an interdisciplinary team in order to provide an effective nutrition program. An ***interdisciplinary team*** is a collaboration among personnel representing different disciplines of public health workers (nurses, social workers, physicians, daycare workers, dietitians, and dietetic technicians). They use various approaches to diagnose and address public or community issues, including:[47]

FIGURE 1-3 Levels of Epidemiologic Research: A Conceptual Elaboration

Source: Copyright 1982, Kleinbaum DG, Kupper LL. *Epidemiologic Research: Principles and Quantitative Methods Solution Manual*, p. 22. New York: Van Nostrand Reinhold. Reprinted with permission of John Wiley & Sons, Inc.

	Concept	Benefit	Example
TABLE 1.2			**Strategies for Designing a Health Promotion Campaign**
Population	Instruction is directed at the entire population (national, local community, schools, and neighborhoods) with messages and programs aimed at reducing behavioral risk factors, such as poor eating habits or physical inactivity.	Members of the community may lower their risk by a small percentage, thereby reducing new cases of chronic health conditions and mortality.	A nutritionist changing the eating patterns of families and advocating for fluoridation of the water supply—rather than screening all postmenopausal women for bone loss or hiring dentists to treat every child and adolescent—may reduce the risk of osteoporosis and dental decay. Instruction about reducing sodium intake may reduce a population's mean systolic blood pressure by 3 percent, which will decrease the number of people in the high-risk group by 25 percent if high risk for systolic blood pressure is considered to begin at 140 mm Hg. If excess body weight is 92kg/202 pounds, reducing the population's mean weight by 1kg/2.2 pounds (about 1 percent) will cut the number of overweight people by 25 percent. Instruction could be provided to engage in regular physical activity and reduce excess calorie consumption. If everyone is encouraged to consume high calcium and/or low-fat food products and then food industries develop and market these food products, this will subsequently prevent osteoporosis and obesity. The Fruits & Veggies—More Matters campaign is an example of a population approach to health promotion.
Individual	The nutritionist focuses on identifying individuals at risk, and the intervention is directed specifically at these "high-risk" individuals.	This method may be more beneficial when the risk conditions are highly restricted, such as with preschool children who were exposed to foods containing lead.	Intervention could be limited to persons with family histories of heart disease, and these people could be taught about reducing fat intake and increasing physical activities to reduce the potential of experiencing heart disease. Nutrition intervention could be limited to the children of adult alcoholics, individuals with a family history of diabetes, and low-income pregnant women participating in the Special Supplemental Nutrition Program for Women, Infants, and Children (WIC), which may translate to risk reduction.

Data from: Webb G. *Nutrition: A Health Promotion Approach*. 2nd ed. New York: Arnold; 2002.

Box 1-3 Advantages and Disadvantages of Population and Individual Health Promotion Strategies

Advantages

Population Approach
- The population approach may instigate a behavior change that may become the norm and create conditions that make it easier for any individual to change. For example, if everyone is urged to reduce their fat and saturated fat intake, this increases the incentive for the food industry to develop and market products that are low in fat and/or saturated fat, such as low-fat milk, which makes it easier to adopt a low-fat diet.
- The population approach is likely to save more lives and prevent more illness than the individual approach when the risk factors are widely diffused throughout the community.

Individual Approach
- Using the individual approach, people at high risk are specifically targeted, and the intervention is provided on

time. More attention is given to ensuring that individuals with chronic disease are following necessary, strict dietary programs.
- Using the individual approach reduces the costs associated with screening an entire population and releases health professionals to attend to the community's other healthcare needs.

Disadvantages

Population Approach
- This approach requires mass change and may not be needed by the entire population.
- It may not be cost effective and may inconvenience people.

Individual Approach
- With the individual approach, screening may not be universal and thus some high-risk individuals may not be identified.

Data from: Webb G. *Nutrition: A Health Promotion Approach*. 2nd ed. New York: Arnold; 2002.

- Utilizing interventions that promote health and prevent communicable or chronic diseases by managing or controlling the community's environment.
- Channeling funds and energy to problems that affect the lives of the largest numbers of people in a community.
- Seeking out unserved or underserved populations (due to income, age, ethnicity, heredity, or lifestyle) and those who are vulnerable to disease, hunger, or malnutrition.
- Collaborating with the public, consumers, community leaders, legislators, policy makers, administrators, and health and human service professionals to assess and respond to community needs and consumer demands.
- Monitoring the public or community's health in relation to public health objectives, and continuously addressing current and future needs.
- Planning, organizing, managing, directing, coordinating, and evaluating the nutrition component of health agency services.

For community nutritionists to accomplish these actions, they need to acquire normal and clinical nutrition knowledge and be skilled in educating the public regarding changes in eating behavior. The minimum education requirements for a community nutritionist include a bachelor's degree in foods and nutrition or dietetics from an accredited college or university and a Master of Public Health degree with a major in nutrition or a Master of Science degree in applied human nutrition with a minor in public health or community health.[47] Some community nutrition positions require certification as a *Registered Dietitian (RD)* and/or an advanced degree in nutrition. Academic training includes knowledge of biostatistics and skill in collecting, analyzing, and reporting demographic, health, and food nutrition data.[48,49]

The community nutritionist must understand the epidemiology of health and disease patterns in the population as well as trends of diseases over a long period of time. She or he must be knowledgeable about the principles of health education, program planning, program evaluation, community organization, management, and marketing and policy formation.[50] Marketing skills are very important because they help nutritionists know how to convey effective nutrition messages using a variety of media formats for their audiences. Community nutritionists must keep current with advances in research and food and nutrition sciences, and changing practices in public health service.[48]

In some situations, Dietetic Technicians, Registered (DTRs) are employed in the food service area, clinical settings, and community settings. They may assist the community nutritionist/Registered Dietitian in determining the community's nutritional needs and in providing community nutrition programs and services. At a minimum, DTRs must have an associate's degree from an approved educational program. After that, they must successfully complete a national examination administered by the Commission on Dietetic Registration (CDR).

Both community and public health nutritionists provide a wide variety of nutrition services through government and non-government agencies at the local, state, national, and international levels.[47] In most cases, the activities require multitasking roles such as blood pressure screening, diet counseling, and medical nutrition therapy. At the international level, duties may include education on sanitation, water purification, and gardening.

Places of Employment for Public Health and Community Nutritionists

Community and public health nutritionists work in official community settings or voluntary agencies to promote health, prevent disease, conduct epidemiologic research, and provide both primary and secondary preventive care. The agencies include city, county, state,

Successful Community Strategies 🏠🏠🏠

The National Cancer Institute's Health Promotion Intervention

Community and public health nutritionists can also target worksites as a priority location for intervention efforts. An effective worksite nutrition program must include how to effectively communicate to clients how to choose and prepare foods that follow established dietary guidelines. One example of an effective worksite program is Working Well, which was a randomized worksite intervention trial. This 5-year study funded by the National Cancer Institute (NCI) tested the effectiveness of health promotion interventions directed at individual and organizational changes to reduce employee cancer risk in 57 matched pairs of worksites. Workers and worksites from a variety of geographic and industrial settings were utilized. Four project study centers, a coordinating center,

and the NCI collaborated on common elements of design, data collection and analysis, and intervention standards for the common risk factor areas. All Working Well study centers targeted nutrition and at least one other prevention component (e.g., smoking, cancer screening, occupational health, or physical activity). The study centers were Brown University School of Medicine and The Miriam Hospital (Rhode Island); the University of Florida; the University of Massachusetts Medical School and Dana-Farber Cancer Institute; and the University of Texas M.D. Anderson Cancer Center.

The Working Well intervention was based on a conceptual model that incorporated three important elements:

- The use of participatory strategies operated through a primary worksite contact and an employee advisory board
- An ecological approach targeting both individual behavior change and change in environmental and organizational structures
- The use of adult education and behavior change strategies in all aspects of intervention planning and delivery

The nutrition intervention messages are available in a summarized format at http://nutrition.jbpub.com/communitynutrition. The messages were translated from nutrient terms into food terminology. They addressed groups of foods that contribute the highest amount of fat and fiber to the U.S. diet. All groups of foods were stated in positive terms.

federal, and international agencies.[47] The following are examples of places where community and public health nutritionists may be employed:

State/City/County Level

- Cooperative extension services
- Home healthcare agencies
- Hospital outpatient nutrition education departments
- Local public health agencies
- Migrant worker health centers
- Native American health services
- Neighborhood or community health centers
- Nonprofit and for-profit private health agencies
- Universities, colleges, and medical schools
- Wellness programs

National/Regional Level

- Food and Drug Administration (FDA)
- U.S. Department of Agriculture (USDA)
- U.S. Department of Health and Human Services (USDHHS)

International Level

- Food and Agriculture Organization of the United Nations (FAO)
- Pan American Health Organization (PAHO)
- United Nations (UN)
- United Nations Children's Emergency Fund (UNICEF)
- World Food Agency (WFA)
- World Health Organization (WHO)

Preventive Nutrition

Preventive nutrition can be defined as dietary practices and interventions directed toward a reduction in disease risk and/or improvement in health outcomes.[51] Preventive nutrition is an important strategy that works to prevent disease instead of treating the condition after it materializes.

The U.S. government and other health agencies have taken actions to reduce the incidences of chronic diseases, such as recommending a reduction in saturated fat intake for cardiovascular disease prevention and inclusion of B vitamins, vitamins A and D, iron, and calcium in staple foods such as grain products, milk, and cereals to prevent nutrient-related health conditions.[52,53] These preventive nutrition strategies have been part of public health policy for many years and have been effective in preventing nutrition-related health conditions.[54,55] For example, there has been a decrease in cardiovascular disease mortality in the past 25 years due to the massive campaign to reduce fat intake and increase physical activity in the United States and most industrialized countries.[28,56]

Other concerns have prompted policy change regarding prevention of chronic diseases. The high costs of medical care put economic pressure on both individuals and nations to prevent chronic diseases.

> **Registered Dietitian (RD)**
> A dietitian meeting eligibility requirements (education, experience, and a credentialing examination) of the Commission on Dietetic Registration. Some RDs possess additional certifications in specialized areas of practice, such as diabetes, pediatrics, geriatrics, or renal nutrition.
>
> **preventive nutrition** Dietary practices and interventions directed toward reducing disease risk and/or improving health outcomes.

The intervention was implemented in 114 worksites employing 37,291 workers who were engaged in a variety of businesses. In the fall of 1990, 20,801 respondents completed and returned a self-administered baseline survey. The worksite mean response rate was 71.6 percent. Responses to behavioral items regarding meat were used to measure meat preparation behaviors that could not be obtained from the food frequency questionnaire (FFQ).

The intervention outcome showed that the average servings of fruits and vegetables per day were less than three in all study centers—2.7 in Florida, Massachusetts, and Rhode Island and 2.4 in Texas. Less than 30 percent of workers in Rhode Island and Massachusetts reported eating beans and lentils at least once a week while 42 percent in Florida and 56 percent in Texas reported frequent bean and lentil consumption. Fifty-six to 64 percent of workers reported eating high-fiber cereal at least half of the time that they ate cereal, and 34 to 46 percent reported eating dark bread at least half of the time that they ate bread.

The majority of workers reported eating chicken and fish that were not fried (55 to 84 percent), rarely eating visible meat fat (57 to 69 percent), and choosing lean meat (68 to 81 percent). On the other hand, avoiding the skin on chicken was reported less frequently (33 to 47 percent). Avoidance of meat fat was lower in Texas than in the other study sites for all four measures.

With regard to fat in dairy products, 65 to 71 percent drank low-fat or skim milk more than half of the time that they drank milk. Also, a smaller percentage, 42 to 64 percent, used low-fat cheese or low-fat frozen dairy products. The percentage that used low-fat dairy products other than milk was much higher in the Florida worksite than in worksites at the other study centers. Finally, 46 to 53 percent of subjects used low-fat salad dressing.

Modified from: Hunt MK, Stoddard, A.M. et al. Measures of food choice behavior related to intervention messages in worksite health promotion. *J Nutr Educ* 1997; 29:3–11. Copyright by Elsevier. Reprinted with permission.

The cost of cardiovascular diseases and stroke in the United States for 2006 was estimated at $403.1 billion.[57] Estimates show that $22 billion per year could be saved in this disease category if preventive nutrition measures were fully implemented.[51]

Another disease category that could be significantly impacted if prevention were emphasized more strongly is that of birth defects. Birth defects are the number one cause of hospitalizations.[58] The possibility of reducing infant morbidity and mortality by nutritional interventions becomes a tangible outcome when research shows that women who take a folic acid–containing multivitamin daily for at least 1 month before conception and during their pregnancies have about a 50 percent decrease in neural tube defects.[57,58] This outcome alone is expected to save about $70 million annually.[59]

In addition, a decrease in medical care for breastfed infants is the primary socioeconomic benefit of breastfeeding. Medicaid costs for infants breastfed by low-income mothers in Colorado were $175 lower than for infants who were fed formula.[60] However, breastfed infants are less likely to have any illness during the first year of life. It is reported that infants who were never breastfed required more care for lower respiratory tract illness, otitis media (ear infection), and gastrointestinal disease than infants breastfed for at least 3 months.[61]

The Cooperative Extension System

The Cooperative Extension System (CES) is an agency under the U.S. Department of Agriculture. It provides educational programs that help individuals and families acquire life skills. The CES's mission is to empower people through education using scientific, research-based information.[1] Typically, land grant universities or colleges help carry out the CES's mission by providing their expertise to county and regional extension offices, which administer these programs. The colleges and universities help the public through nonformal, noncredit programs. The federal government provides support for the programs through the Cooperative State Research, Education, and Extension Service (CSREES). CSREES supports both the universities and their local offices by annually distributing federal funding to supplement state and county programs.[62]

The Morrill Act of 1862 established land-grant universities to educate citizens in agriculture, home economics, mechanical arts, and other practical professions. In 1914 the Smith-Lever Act established a partnership between the USDA and land-grant universities. Currently, CES works in six major areas:[62]

- *4-H youth development:* Helps youth make life and career choices. At-risk youth participate in school retention and enrichment programs. They learn science, math, and social skills using hands-on projects and activities.
- *Agriculture:* Helps individuals learn new ways to improve their agricultural income through research-based management skills, resource management, controlling crop pests, soil testing, livestock production practices, and marketing.
- *Leadership development:* Trains extension professionals and volunteers to serve in leadership roles in the community and deliver

Successful Community Strategies 🏠🏠🏠

The Clemson University Cooperative Extension Nutrition Program on Low-Fat Products and Fat Intake[64–69]

The percentage of calories from saturated and polyunsaturated fat and the amount of cholesterol in the diet are important determinants of the level of plasma cholesterol, a major contributor to heart disease risk. It is estimated on average that a 1 percent decrease in the intake of saturated fat results in a 2-mg/dl decrease in plasma cholesterol. This, in turn, can bring about a reduction in heart disease risk. High intake of dietary fat is also associated with an increased risk for developing cancer of the colon, prostate, and breast.

Programs that have demonstrated effective community interventions for a decrease in dietary fat include a program from Clemson University in South Carolina, which incorporated community nutrition classes, grocery store tours, speakers' bureaus, professional education classes, home study courses, and worksite nutrition education programs. This program focused on the impact of low-fat diets on serum cholesterol. The intervention community, compared with a control community, had a significant decrease in the intake of dietary fat (9 percent vs. 4 percent) and an increase in awareness of restaurant information (33 percent vs. 19 percent).

In South Carolina, 61 percent of adults were overweight or obese. From 1990 to 2002, the obesity rate among adults in South Carolina increased by 90 percent. The African American, Hispanic, and Native American populations in South Carolina had significantly high prevalence rates of obesity. About 15 percent of South Carolina's high school students were at risk of becoming overweight and approximately 11 percent were overweight. Data showed that less than 25 percent of all South Carolina's adults and only 18 percent of South Carolina high school students ate the recommended five or more servings of fruits and vegetables each day. Obesity is associated with many health conditions, some of which include heart disease, stroke, and diabetes. These also make up the three major causes of death and disability in South Carolina. In South Carolina, medical expenditure due to obesity per year was $1.06 billion.

Clemson's Extension agent provided low-fat programs at regional volunteer leader training, an assisted living facility, three community groups, and a summer youth camp. A low-fat nutrition education program was presented to 38 family and community project leaders at regional programs in gardening, health and safety, and family and consumer issues.

- *Natural resources:* Provides educational programs in water quality, timber management, composting, lawn and waste management, and recycling to landowners and homeowners.
- *Family and consumer sciences:* Teaches families and individuals about nutrition, food preparation, positive child care, family communication, financial management, and healthcare strategies so they can become healthy.
- *Community and economic development:* Helps local governments improve job creation and retention, small and medium-sized business development, effective and coordinated emergency response, solid waste disposal, tourism development, workforce education, and land use planning.

In addition, the Expanded Food and Nutrition Education Program (EFNEP) is a federally funded program designed specifically for nutrition education. The county extension home economists provide on-the-job training and supervise paraprofessionals and volunteers who teach EFNEP to low-income families and individuals.[63] The Successful Community Strategies features in this chapter discuss the successful Clemson University Cooperative Extension Nutrition Program on low-fat products and fat intake as well as a National Cancer Institute health promotion intervention program.

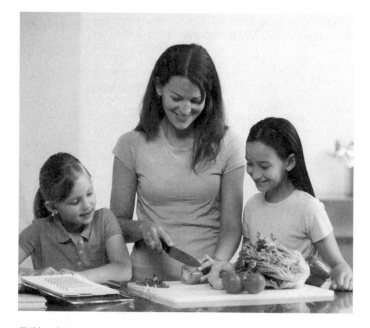

Children learn more about nutritious foods when they are involved in meal preparation.

leader training. These project leaders taught the program to over 400 adult members in their four counties. In addition, the agent taught four 1-hour lessons emphasizing dietary guidelines to a senior group, two adult groups, and a group of young mothers of preschoolers. Also, a 3-hour workshop on nutritious snacks and nutrition facts labels was provided to 10 middle school youth. Thirty-two articles on low-fat ideas and nutrition tips were sent to 18 print media outlets in a three-county area (Richland, Lexington, and Fairfield). These print media outlets reached a circulation of 473,000. The local Fairfield County newspaper (*Herald Independent*) published the nutrition articles 21 times from June 2004 to January 2005. Two Lexington County papers (*The Twin City News* and *The Chronicle and Dispatch News*) published the nutrition articles 16 times from April 2004

to January 2005. These three newspapers had a circulation of 19,600 weekly. The state newspaper published three special interviews with the Extension agent concerning nutrition information on a vegetable featured in their Life and Style food section. The newspaper had a circulation of 150,000 daily. The *Focus on Family Matters* quarterly newsletter published nine articles providing research-based nutrition information. The newsletter had a circulation of 1,000 in Lexington, Richland, and Fairfield counties. Nutrition recipe analyses on calories, carbohydrates, dietary fiber, sugar, fat, cholesterol, and sodium were published in the Cook's Corner column of *Living in South Carolina* magazine. The agent analyzed 45 recipes for 11 monthly columns. The magazine had a circulation statewide of 523,000 homes and businesses with a readership of 1.2 million monthly.

At the end of the Extension programs, 89 percent of participants surveyed said that the program increased their nutrition knowledge. About 72 percent said they would read the Nutrition Facts Label on packaged foods. Seventy-five percent said they would reduce their intake of refined sugars. About 78 percent said that they planned to control portion sizes and servings for each food group. Seventy percent said they would include 30 minutes of exercise per day. Sixty-five percent said they would include more whole grain breads and cereals in their diet. Eighty-seven percent said they would make one positive change as a result of the low-fat and healthy ideas programs.

Chapter Summary

- Community nutrition is a modern and comprehensive profession that includes, among other disciplines, public health, dietetics/nutrition education, and medical nutrition therapy.
- The World Health Organization (WHO) defined community as "a social group determined by geographic boundaries and/or common values and interests." Community members know and interact with one another, function within a particular social structure, and create norms, values, and social institutions.
- A community can also be defined on the basis of a common interest or goal. A collection of people, even if they are scattered geographically, can have a common interest that binds the members together.
- Community strengths can be physiological, psychological, social, or spiritual.
- Community nutrition and dietetics professionals are community and public health agency professionals who provide nutrition services that emphasize community health promotion and disease prevention.
- Public health has been viewed as the scientific diagnosis and treatment of the community. In this vision, the community, instead of the individual, is seen as the patient.
- In addition to dietary factors, two primary determinants of health status are genetics and lifestyle.
- Prevention is important in public health as well as in community nutrition practice. The three aspects of prevention are personal, community-based, and systems-based health.
- The three levels of prevention are primary, secondary, and tertiary prevention.
- Population and individual approaches are the two important strategies to choose from when designing a health promotion campaign aimed at risk reduction. The population approach directs instruction at the whole population or large sections of it whereas the individual approach identifies those most at risk from the risk factor, and intervention is targeted specifically at these "high-risk" individuals.
- Health promotion can be defined as the process of enabling people to increase control over the determinants of good health and subsequently improve their health.
- The negative consequences of nutrition-related problems include malnutrition and chronic health conditions such as obesity, cardiovascular diseases, cancer, diabetes mellitus, and childhood deaths.
- Public health and community nutritionists carry out a wide variety of nutrition activities through various agencies at the local, state, national, and international levels. In most cases, the activities require multitasking roles such as blood pressure screening, diet counseling, and medical nutrition therapy.
- Preventive nutrition can be defined as dietary practices and interventions directed toward the reduction in disease risk and/or improvement in health outcomes.
- The Cooperative Extension (CE) System is an agency under the U.S. Department of Agriculture. It provides educational programs that help individuals and families acquire life skills.

working poor Families whose earnings are less than twice the federal poverty level and in which the adults work an average of half time or more during the year.

Critical Thinking Activities

The **working poor** (defined as families whose earnings are less than twice the federal poverty level and in which the adults work an average of half time or more during the year[71]) are increasing in the current economy. Many public health programs may be eliminated or minimized, such as immunizations for all children and flu shots on demand for all people. Additionally, eligibility criteria for the Special Supplemental Nutrition Program for Women, Infants, and Children (WIC) program may be altered.

- Divide into groups and provide each group a certain amount of money, for instance, $100,000. Then distribute the funds among the three levels of prevention (primary, secondary, and tertiary) and discuss the rationale behind the decisions. The table below presents examples of programs.
- Select four health issues from Table 1.1 and discuss the types of early intervention programs that can prevent the health conditions.

Primary Prevention	Secondary Prevention	Tertiary Prevention
Local Fruits & Veggies—More Matters campaign to schools	Worksite nutrition education for high-risk employees	Medical nutrition therapy for individuals with nutrition-related problems (e.g., heart disease)
School breakfast and lunch	Health fair screening and referrals to primary care providers	
Breastfeeding support		
Immunizations for all children		
Prenatal care		

Case Study 1-1

Beatrice is a community nutritionist (RD) who was employed to provide nutrition education programs to a group of pregnant teenagers attending high school in a Midwestern city of 200,000 people. The teenagers eat most of their meals on campus. Some participate in the school lunch program; others prefer purchasing foods from the vending machine located a few feet away from the cafeteria. Beatrice was asked to help improve the teenagers' nutrition and fitness status. Meetings with the teenagers revealed their opinions about food and physical activity. A 3-day dietary record and food frequency questionnaire were administered to the teenagers, and body measurements, such as height and weight for determining body mass index (BMI), were collected. She uncovered the following information:

- Analysis of the teenagers' food choices revealed a high fat intake of 39 percent of total calories.
- Thirty percent of the teen mothers surveyed were obese and anemic, 40 percent were overweight, and 30 percent were underweight and anemic.
- In the vending machines in and around the high school, 80 percent of snacks were sugary or high fat, such as chips, and the machines contained soft drinks or other items with empty calories.

- Further analysis showed that the teen mothers' physical activity levels were inadequate.

The following plans reflect the program Beatrice devised after several meetings with the pregnant teenagers:

- Included fresh fruits and vegetables on every cafeteria menu. (These foods can offer vitamins, minerals, and fiber as well as decrease the number of high-fat items available.)
- Evaluated and found a place where they can perform physical activity and campaigned for needed changes.
- Established a place for physical activity around the teens' homes. (Inactivity is a major contributor to obesity.)
- Collaborated with the school food service director and the vending machine vendors to stock the vending machines with snacks low in fat and sugar and replace sugary soft drinks with fruit juices.

Activities

- Divide into groups and determine the locations for the WIC and Food Stamp Programs in your community. Then, encourage the teen mothers to enroll in these programs to obtain adequate prenatal care and nutrition counseling by giving them the addresses of the Food Stamp and WIC Programs and the name of the WIC nutritionist.
- Collect and analyze a 3-day food record from a female high school student and compare the results with a female college student.
- Analyze a school lunch meal and determine the fat, protein, calcium, vitamin D, folic acid, iron, and fiber content.
- Provide a list of foods that are high in iron, calcium, and vitamin D.
- Provide a list of foods fortified with folic acid.
- Provide a list of foods low in saturated fat and cholesterol.

References

1. Frank-Spohrer G. *Community Nutrition: Applying Epidemiology to Contemporary Practice.* 2nd ed. Sudbury, MA: Jones and Bartlett; 2008.

2. Winterfeldt EA, Ebro LL. *Dietetics: Practice and Future Trends.* Sudbury, MA: Jones and Bartlett; 2005.

3. Goodman R, Wandersman A, Chinman M, Imm P, Morrissey E. An ecological assessment of community-based interventions for prevention and health promotion: approaches to measuring community coalitions. *J Community Psychol.* 1996; 24:1–9.

4. Merzel C, D'Afflitti J. Reconsidering community-based health promotion: promise, performance, and potential. *Am J Public Health.* 2003; 93(4):557–574.

5. World Health Organization. *Diet, Nutrition and the Prevention of Chronic Diseases.* Geneva: Author; 1990.

6. Hawe P. Capturing the meaning of community in community intervention evaluation: some contributions from community psychology. *Health Promotion Int.* 1994; 9(3):199–210.

7. Denver A. *Community Health Analysis: Global Awareness at the Local Level.* 2nd ed. Gaithersburg, MD: Aspen; 1991.

8. McKenzie JF, Pinger RR, Kotecki JE. *An Introduction to Community Health.* 4th ed. Sudbury, MA: Jones and Bartlett; 2002.

9. Allender JA, Spradley BW. *Community Health Nursing: Promoting and Protecting the Public's Health.* 6th ed. New York: Lippincott Williams and Wilkins; 2005.

10. Lancaster SA. *Community and Public Health Nursing.* 5th ed. New York: Mosby; 2000.

11. Winslow C. *The Untitled Field of Public Health.* Vol 2. Chicago: Modern Medicine; 1920: 183.

12. Keegan DBA. *Holistic Nursing Practice.* Sudbury, MA: Jones and Bartlett; 2005.

13. Finkelstein EA, Ruhm CJ, Kosa KM. Economic causes and consequences of obesity. *Ann Rev Public Health.* 2005; 26:239–257.

14. Nedra K, Williams P, Pfister R. Cost savings and clinical effectiveness of an extension service diabetes program. *Diabetes Spectrum.* 2004; 17:171–175.

15. Qureshi AI, Suri MF, Kirmani JF. The relative impact of inadequate primary and secondary prevention on cardiovascular mortality in the United States. *Stroke.* 2004; 35(10):2346–2350.

16. Guthrie JJ, Smallwood DM. Evaluating the effects of the Dietary Guidelines for Americans on consumer behavior and health: methodological challenges. *J Am Diet Assoc.* 2003; 103(12):S42–S49.

17. Richardson RA, Cotton JW, Mark OR. Diet and colorectal cancer risk. Impact of a nutrition education leaflet. *J Hum Nutr Diet.* 2004; 17(6):576.

18. Beaudry M, Hamelin AM, Delisle H. Public nutrition: an emerging paradigm. *Can J Public Health.* 2004; 95(5):375–377.

19. World Health Organization. *Health and Welfare Canada and Canadian Public Health Association Ottawa Charter for Health Promotion.* Ottawa, Ontario: Author; 1986.

20. Pena M, Bacallao J, eds. *Obesity and Poverty: A New Public Health Challenge.* Washington, DC: World Health Organization; 2000.

21. U.S. Department of Health and Human Services, Healthy People 2010, 2nd ed. *With understanding and improving health and objectives for improving health, 2 vols.* Washington, DC: U.S. Government Printing Office; November 2000.

22. Centers for Disease Control and Prevention. The Surgeon General's call to action to prevent and decrease overweight and obesity, 2007. Available at: http://www.cdc.gov/nccdphp/dnpa/obesity/consequences.htm. Accessed April 10, 2006.

23. Kaufman M. *Nutrition in Public Health: A Handbook for Developing Programs and Services.* Sudbury, MA: Jones and Bartlett; 2007.

24. Webb G. *Nutrition: A Health Promotion Approach.* 2nd ed. New York: Arnold; 2002.

25. Millen BE, Quatromoni PA, Nam BH, et al. Dietary patterns, smoking, and subclinical heart disease in women: opportunities for primary prevention from the Framingham Nutrition Studies. *J Am Diet Assoc.* 2004; 104(2):208–214.

26. U.S. Department of Health and Human Services. *The Surgeon General's Report on Nutrition and Health.* PHS Publication No. 88-50210. Washington, DC: Author; 1988.

27. U.S. Department of Health and Human Services. Nutrition and Your Health: Dietary Guidelines for Americans, 2004. Available at: http://www.health.gov/dietaryguidelines. Accessed April 10, 2006.

28. American Heart Association. Healthy Lifestyle Diet and Nutrition, 2004. Available at: http://www.americanheart.org. Accessed May 5, 2006.

29. Tulchinsky TH, Kaluski DN, Berry EM. Food fortification and risk group supplementation are vital parts of a comprehensive nutrition policy for prevention of chronic diseases. *Eur J Public Health.* 2004; 14(3):226–228.

30. Bauman AE. Updating the evidence that physical activity is good for health: an epidemiological review 2000–2003. *J Sci Med Sport.* 2004; 7(1):6–19.

31. Mullen B, Cupples A, Franz M, Gagnon D. Diet and Heart Disease Risk Factors in Adult American Men and Women: The Framingham Offspring-Spouse Nutrition Studies. *Int J Epidemiol.* 2006; 22(6):1014–1025.

32. William M. *Nutrition for Health, Fitness and Sport.* 6th ed. St. Louis, MO: McGraw-Hill; 2002.

33. Berdanier C, Feldman E, Flatt W, Sachiko J. *Handbook of Nutrition and Food.* New York: CRC Press; 2007.

34. Roche HM. Dietary lipids and gene expression. *Transactions.* 2004; 32(Pt 6):999–1002.

35. National Center for Health Statistics. Death-leading causes. Available at: http://www.cdc.gov/nchs/fastats/lcod.htm. Accessed January 30, 2008.

36. World Health Organization. The top ten causes of death. Available at: http://www.who.int/mediacentre/factsheets/fs310/en/index.html. Accessed January 30, 2008.

37. Vanden Heuvel JP. Diet, fatty acids, and regulation of genes important for heart disease. *Curr Atherosclerosis Rep.* 2004; 6(6):432–440.

38. Skidmore PM, Yarnell JW. The obesity epidemic: prospects for prevention. *QJM.* 2004; 97(12):817–825.

39. Bautista-Castaño I, Doreste J, Serra-Majem L. Effectiveness of interventions in the prevention of childhood obesity. *Eur J Epidemiol.* 2004; 19(7):617–622.

40a. Nies MA, McEwen M. *Community Health Nursing: Promoting the Health of Populations.* 3rd ed. London: Saunders; 2001.

40b. Gakidou E, Oza S, Vidal Fuertes C, Li A, Lee D. Improving child survival through environmental and nutritional interventions. *JAMA.* 2007; 298:1876-1887.

41. Mackenbach J, Bakker M. *Reducing Inequalities in Health. A European Perspective.* London: Routledge; 2002.

42. Qureshi AI, Suri MF, Kirmani JF, Divani AA. The relative impact of inadequate primary and secondary prevention on cardiovascular mortality in the United States. *Stroke.* 2004; 35(10):2346–2350.

43. Stoddard AM, Palombo R, Troped PJ, Sorensen G, Will JC. Cardiovascular disease risk reduction: the Massachusetts WISEWOMAN project. *J Women's Health.* 2004; 13(5):539–546.

44. Cheng C, Graziani C, Diamond JJ. Cholesterol-lowering effect of the Food for Heart Nutrition Education Program. *J Am Diet Assoc.* 2004; 104(12):1868–1872.

45. Pereira M, O'Reilly E, Augustsson K, Fraser G, Goldbourt U. Dietary fiber and risk of coronary heart disease. A pooled analysis of cohort studies. *Arch Intern Med.* 2004; 164:370–376.

46. Bemelmans WJ, Broer J, Hulshof KF, Siero FW, May JF, Meyboom-de Jong B. Long-term effects of nutritional group education for persons at high cardiovascular risk. *Eur J Public Health.* 2004; 14(3):240–245.

47. Kaufman M. *Nutrition in Promoting the Public's Health: Strategies, Principles, and Practice.* 2nd ed. Sudbury, MA: Jones and Bartlett; 2007.

48. Dodds JM, Laraia BA, Carbone ET. Development of a master's in public health nutrition degree program using distance education. *J Am Diet Assoc.* 2003; 103:602–607.

49. Winterfeldt EA, Ebro LL. *Dietetics: Practice and Future Trends.* Sudbury, MA: Jones and Bartlett; 2005.

50. Johnson DB, Eaton DL, Wahl PW, Gleason C. Public health nutrition practice in the United Sates. *J Am Diet Assoc.* 2001; 101(5):529–534.

51. Bendich A, Richard J. *Preventive Nutrition: The Comprehensive Guide for Health Professionals.* Totowa, NJ: Humana Press; 2001.

52. Reddy K, Katan M. Diet, nutrition and the prevention of hypertension and cardiovascular diseases. *Health Nutrition.* 2007; 7(1A):167–186.

53. Dietrich M, Brown, C, Block G. The effect of folate fortification of cereal-grain products on blood folate status, dietary folate intake, and dietary folate sources among adult non-supplement users in the United States. *JACN.* 2005; 24(4):266–274.

54. Shepherd SK. Consumer information gap on behavioral aspects of dietary change. *J Nutr Educ Behav.* 2004; 36(3):113.

55. Cohen SJ, Meister JS, deZapien JG. Special action groups for policy change and infrastructure support to foster healthier communities on the Arizona-Mexico border. *Public Health Rep.* 2004; 119(1):40–47.

56. Thomas HN, Wayne R. Heart disease and stroke statistics—2006 update: a report from the American Heart Association Statistics Committee and Stroke Statistics Subcommittee. *Circ.* 2006; 113:e85–e151.

57. Canfield MA, Anderson JL, Waller DK, Palmer SE, Kaye CI. Folic acid awareness and use among women with a history of a neural tube defect pregnancy—Texas, 2000–2001. *MMWR Recommend Rep.* 2002; 51(RR-13):16–19.

58. Mosley BB. Folic acid and the decline in neural tube defects in Arkansas. *J Arkansas Med Soc.* 2007; 103(10):247–250.

59. Bendich A. *Preventive Nutrition: The Comprehensive Guide for Health Professionals.* Totowa, NJ: Humana Press; 2005.

60. Splett PL, Montgomery DL. *The Economic Benefits of Breastfeeding an Infant in the WIC Program: Twelve-Month Follow-Up Study.* Washington, DC: Food and Consumer Service, U.S. Department of Agriculture; 1998.

61. Cattaneo A, Ronfani L, Burmaz T, Quintero-Romero S, Macaluso A, Di Mario S. Infant feeding and cost of health care: a cohort study. *Pædiatrica.* 2006; 95:540–546.

62. U.S. Department of Agriculture. Extension. Available at: http://www.csrees.usda.gov/qlinks/extension.html. Accessed April 1, 2005.

63. U.S. Department of Agriculture. Expanded Food and Nutrition Education Program. Available at: http://www.csrees.usda.gov/nea/food/efnep/about.html. Accessed April 1, 2005.

64. Lupo BH. Low-fat products and nutrition success story, 2005. Available at: http://www.clemson.edu/lexington/Accomp133.htm. Accessed January, 26, 2008.

65. Pieterse Z, Jerling JC, Oosthuizen W, et al. Substitution of high monounsaturated fatty acid avocado for mixed dietary fats during an energy-restricted diet: effects on weight loss, serum lipids, fibrinogen, and vascular function. *Nutr.* 2005; 21(1):67–75.

66. Constant J. The role of eggs, margarines and fish oils in the nutritional management of coronary artery disease and strokes. *Keio J Med.* 2004; 53(3):131–136.

67. Washington State. Washington State Risk and Protective Factors: Nutrition. Available at: http://depts.washington.edu/commnutr/wadocs/wadocs-nutrition.htm. Accessed April 10, 2006.

68. Newman VA, Thomson CA, Rock CL, et al. Achieving substantial changes in eating behavior among women previously treated for breast cancer—an overview of the intervention. *J Am Diet Assoc.* 2005; 105(3):382–391.

69. Bemelmans WJ, Broer J, Hulshof KF, Siero FW, May JF, Meyboom-de Jong B. Long-term effects of nutritional group education for persons at high cardiovascular risk. *Eur J Public Health.* 2004; 14(3):240–245.

70. Kazis R, Miller MS. *Low-Wage Workers in the New Economy.* Washington, DC: The Urban Institute Press; 2001.

CHAPTER 2

Nutrition Screening and Assessment

LEARNING OBJECTIVES

- Define screening and assessment.
- Discuss the historical perspective of nutritional assessment.
- Define community nutrition assessment.
- List the needs assessment techniques.
- Explain the different methods of assessing nutritional status.
- Describe the various methods of dietary assessment and their advantages and disadvantages.
- Identify the appropriate dietary assessment tool for research purposes.

Introduction

Community *assessment* is the process of critically thinking about a community by getting to know and understanding the community as a client.[1] Community assessment helps identify community needs, clarify problems, and identify strengths and resources. *Community nutrition assessment* is an attempt to evaluate the *nutritional status* of individuals or populations through measurement of food and nutrient intake and evaluation of nutrition-related health indicators.[2] The U.S. Department of Health and Human Services defines nutritional assessment as "the measurement of indicators of dietary status and nutrition-related health status to identify the possible occurrence, nature, and

extent of impaired nutritional status," which can range from deficiency to toxicity.[3]

The type of information that can be collected during the community health assessment process includes statistical community profiles, qualitative data on the experiences of the community or population, and local resources and assets.[4] There are groups in every community that are interested in nutrition, including churches; healthcare institutions; government agencies; breastfeeding support groups; Head Start; schools and universities; parents; wellness programs; hospitals; doctors, nurses, and other healthcare professionals; the elderly; and international agencies.[5] A thoughtful compilation of assets prevents the assessment from becoming a log of morbidity and mortality statistics.

The Purpose of Community Nutrition Assessment

Community assessment is a very important component of community nutrition practice. The purpose of a broad community nutrition assessment is to reveal the important nutrition-related needs in the community while finding opportunities for intervention. In order to accomplish this goal, data on the problems and their determinants are needed. A nutritional assessment of the community uses nutritional status measures acquired from **anthropometric**, biochemical, clinical, and dietary intake data as well as epidemiological information.[6]

Community assessment is recognized as an important function of public health because it plays a primary role in promoting the health of communities.[7,8] Therefore, a comprehensive community assessment is needed to identify the health problems in the community and to address the cause of the problems. A community nutrition assessment needs to do the following:[1]

- Identify the health of individuals within the community
- Identify the health of the community itself
- Determine the characteristics, resources, and needs of the community
- Work with community members on those issues that arise
- Address not only individuals' behaviors, but also applicable environmental variables

Community assessment is used by many health and human service agencies, public and private agency planners, and businesses (market research).[5] It is the most cost-effective way to collect data because it uses existing vital statistics that are accessible, seeks the opinions of targeted group members and local health experts, and makes observations. Most of these data may not be specific to nutrition and diet, hence, the community or public health nutritionist needs to relate the available data to nutrition and diet issues. The nutritionist can focus on data associated with conditions that relate to nutrition, such as the number of infants with low birth weights, the number of low-income families that cannot purchase adequate food, or the number of elderly individuals who cannot participate in the Peace Meal Program (a senior nutrition program that offers midday meals to people ages 60 and above). Also, the rates of infant mortality, heart disease, and cancer can reveal whether the incidence of these problems is abnormally high in the community.[9]

assessment Determining nutritional status by analyzing clinical, dietary, and social history; anthropometric data; biochemical data; and drug–nutrient interactions.

community nutrition assessment An attempt to evaluate the nutritional status of individuals or populations through measurements of food and nutrient intake and evaluation of nutrition-related health indicators.

nutritional status A measurement of the extent to which an individual's physiologic needs for nutrients are being met.

anthropometry The measurement of human body size, weight, and proportions.

body mass index (BMI) Weight (kg)/height (m²); an index calculated by a ratio of height to weight, used as a measure of obesity.

In addition, the nutritionist can use his or her knowledge of average household incomes; of the proportion of families participating in the Food Stamp Program, soup kitchens, school breakfasts, school lunches, and food banks; and of the age distribution of the group to identify important nutrition concerns and issues.

Historical Development of Nutritional Assessment

Nutrition assessment is a constant and evolving process. In 1932, the Health Organization of the League of Nations (HOLN) held its first conference to discuss the physical, clinical, and physiological aspects of nutrition assessment. This conference motivated the publication of the procedures needed for conducting nutrition surveys.[10] Subsequently, the monograph published by the Technical Commission of Nutrition of the Health Organization (TCNHO) was the first organized dietary standards. About the same time, Bigwood's *Guiding Principles for Studies on the Nutrition of Populations* provided detailed procedures for conducting nutrition surveys.[11] The basic philosophy of nutrition assessment has remained the same over the years, but these initial methods have been revised.[12]

In the 1940s under the auspices of the United Nations, the Food and Agriculture Organization (FAO) and the World Health Organization (WHO) were established. Representatives from each organization were selected to form a Joint Expert Committee on Nutrition. In 1949, these representatives compiled information on nutritional status, dietary patterns, food supplies, and the economics of particular populations and recommended the establishment of nutrition policies for each nation. In 1951, the Joint Commission of the WHO published a report that emphasized anthropometric, clinical, and dietary data, but it did not make recommendations or set standards.[12,13]

Nutrition Assessment in the United States

Despite these international organizations' attention to nutritional assessment, the United States did not recognize malnutrition as a health problem until fairly recently. Before the 1960s, the incidence of malnutrition in the United States was not noticed because little or no attention was given to nutritional health. This changed after the National Center for Health Statistics (NCHS) conducted the Ten-State Nutrition Survey (TSNS) between 1968 and 1970, and the first National Health and Nutrition Examination Survey (NHANES) between 1971 and 1974. These surveys discovered evidence of clinical and subclinical malnutrition in individuals in different areas of the country.[12,14] Results showed that population groups that were at nutritional risk were also socially, economically, educationally, or medically deprived. Malnutrition was associated with poor growth, developmental disability, poor pregnancy outcomes, susceptibility to infectious diseases, delayed recovery from illness, and reduced life expectancy.

These studies' dietary, clinical, and biochemical data have been reexamined by factor analysis, which analyzed eating habits as a means of relating food intake to health. The data also were analyzed to see the relationship between the combination of foods the participants ate and the condition of their nutritional health, for both samples in total and for various age, sex, race, regional, and income groups. Results showed significant associations between certain eating patterns and the lack of clinical symptoms and biochemical deficiencies. The factor analysis showed that some eating patterns were evidently better or worse than others.[15] The authors concluded that this food eating pattern model is a useful tool for: 1) examining the association between food consumption and the incidence of disease states, such as obesity, hypertension, cardiovascular disease, cancer, and periodontal disease, for various large scale dietary-health surveys; 2) establishing food regulatory policies; 3) setting national dietary goals; and 4) educating the public on nutrition and health issues.[15]

NHANES II was conducted between 1976 and 1980, and it targeted non-institutionalized persons from 6 months to 74 years old. It used a similar data collection method as NHANES I. The Hispanic Health and Nutrition Examination Survey (HHANES) was conducted between 1982 and 1984. It was designed to obtain data from physical examinations, anthropometric measurements, laboratory analyses, and diagnostic tests of Mexican Americans, Puerto Rican Americans, and Cuban Americans. Dietary intake was analyzed using a 24-hour recall and a food frequency questionnaire. The targeted population was individuals aged 6 months through 74 years.[16,17]

The third NHANES survey was conducted between 1988 and 1994 using nationwide samples of about 40,000 non-institutionalized persons, ages 2 months and older. To obtain reliable estimates, infants and young children (1 to 5 years) and older persons (60+ years) were sampled at a higher rate. Dietary intake was assessed by a 24-hour recall and food frequency questionnaire. The examination parts of the study were varied based on age. Infants 2 to 11 months old received a physician's examination, body measurements, and other assessments. A dietary interview was conducted with the child's caregiver or parent. Between the ages of 1 and 19 years, additional assessments were included, such as a dental exam, vision test, cognitive test, allergy skin test, and spirometry (a measurement of lung capacity). Individuals over the age of 20 years received these assessments in addition to an oral glucose tolerance test, bone density test, fitness test, electrocardiogram, and other tests.[18]

Growth Charts

In 1977, the NCHS developed growth charts as a clinical tool for health professionals to determine whether a child's level of growth was adequate. The WHO also adopted the 1977 charts for international use. With more recent and comprehensive national data available, along with improved statistical procedures, the 1977 growth charts were revised and updated in 2000 by the Centers for Disease Control and Prevention (CDC) to make them a more valuable clinical tool for health professionals. Most of the data used to construct these charts came from the NHANES surveys, which has periodically collected height, weight, and other health information on the U.S. population.[19] The revised growth charts provide an improved tool for evaluating the growth of children in community, clinical, and research settings.

The *body mass index (BMI)* is a significant new feature of the revised growth charts. These BMI-for-age charts were created for use in place of the 1977 weight-for-stature charts. Body Mass Index, also called the quetelet index, is the most commonly used approach to determine whether adults are overweight or obese and is also the recommended measure to determine whether children are overweight or underweight. The BMI growth charts can be used clinically beginning at 2 years of age, when an accurate stature can be obtained.[19] To establish the BMI of a client, measure his or her height without shoes and his or her weight with minimal clothing. Then use the following equation to calculate the BMI:[20]

$$BMI = \frac{Weight\ (kg)}{Height\ (m)^2}$$

or

$$BMI = \frac{Weight\ (lb)}{Height\ (in)^2}$$

For example, BMI for an adult would be:

- Divide the individual's weight (in pounds) by his or her height (in inches)
- Divide the result again by the individual's height
- Multiply the result by 703

Weight = 170 lb ÷ 2.2 = 77.3 kg
Height = 5'11" (71 in) × 2.54 = 180.3 cm (1.83 m)
BMI = 77.3 ÷ 1.83² = 23.1

Community Needs Assessment

A needs assessment measures the current situation of a particular group or community.[21] Conducting a needs assessment involves completing a series of tasks and clearly identifying the priority health-related needs of a well-defined target population. A survey must be designed to ask about the needs of the community or group. This can include a variety of issues such as food stores moving out of the area, food assistance agencies, ethnic or racial needs, the number of healthcare professionals in the area, access to healthcare, and so on. Assessing community members' initial awareness about nutrition and then supporting community nutrition needs and services is essential if changes in behavior, norms, and public policy are to be evaluated.[8,9,22] In addition, a community needs assessment survey can be conducted when community groups want to take action, influence policy, or make changes.[4]

Table 2.1 presents a subjective data assessment grid that can be used to evaluate healthcare professionals' and other important community members' knowledge of nutrition, the perceived proper nutrition needs, and attitudes toward nutrition and health. It is used as a starting point for program planning that involves the stakeholders (community leaders), and as a basis for developing programs that respond to their perceived needs that they will adopt. These data, along with data that characterize the community's nutrition and health status, are needed to develop programs for healthier living conditions.[5,23]

Community needs assessment studies are an effective way to find out what people are thinking and how they feel. Although information from a needs assessment study is valuable and useful, the process of gathering the information is also valuable. Needs assessment studies allow community groups or sponsoring agencies to:[24]

- Collect information about community attitudes and opinions regarding specific nutrition, health, and other issues
- Determine how the community prioritizes the issues
- Provide the community the opportunity to determine policies, goals, methods, and procedures for solving the problem
- Evaluate current programs and policies and available resources

Tables 2.2 and **2.3** present examples of secondary and demographic datasets that could be sources for a community needs assessment.

Methods of Performing a Community Needs Assessment

There are various methods of effectively assessing a community's needs. Selecting the best method is essential because the community group or organization may use the information gathered to make decisions about allocating public or private resources, determining program elimination or addition, and the like. Needs assessments can reveal and

TABLE
2.1   **Subjective Data: Community Nutrition Assessment**

	Perceived Nutrition Needs in the Community	Attitude Toward Nutrition Services			Knowledge of Nutrition		
	List	+	0	−	+	0	−
Clients/patients							
Public							
Media							
Government officials							
Agency administrators							
Physicians/dentists							
Hospital administrators							
Nurses							
Health educators							
Nutritionists/dietitians							
Agency board members							
Principals/teachers							
Social workers							
Clergy							

Key: + = positive, supportive attitude toward nutrition and health services; 0 = neutral or apathetic attitude toward nutrition; − = negative attitude toward nutrition.

Adapted from: Kaufman M. *Nutrition in Public Health: A Handbook for Developing Programs and Services*. Rockville, MD: Aspen; 1990:52.

TABLE
2.2   **Secondary Datasets That Could Be Sources for a Community Needs Assessment**

Description	Sources/Websites
2000 Census datasets	http://www.census.gov/main/www/cen2000.html
Data warehouse for NCHS public use data files for: • National Health and Nutrition Examination Survey • National Health Care Survey • National Health Interview Survey • National Immunization Survey • Longitudinal Studies on Aging	http://www.cdc.gov/nchs/datawh/ftpserv/ftpdata/ftpdata.htm
Youth Risk Behavior Surveillance System: • Monitors priority health risk behaviors that contribute markedly to the leading causes of death, disability, and social problems among youth and adults in the United States • Data files and documentation	http://www.cdc.gov/healthyYouth/yrbs
DataFerrett System: • Collaboration between NCHS and the Bureau of the Census to provide NCHS datasets in the Census's DataFerrett system • A unique data mining and extraction tool that allows you to select a data basket full of variables, recode those variables as needed, and then develop and customize tables and charts	http://www.cdc.gov/nchs/datawh/ferret/ferret.htm
U.S. Department of Agriculture (Economic Research Service): • Early Childhood Longitudinal Survey's Food Security in the United States	http://ers.usda.gov/data/foodsecurity/eclsk

Source: Edelstein S. *Nutrition in Public Health: A Handbook for Developing Programs and Services*. 2nd ed. Sudbury, MA: Jones and Bartlett; 2006.

TABLE 2.3	Sources of Demographic and Health Statistics for the Community Needs Assessment	

Description/Type of Data	Website with Link to Statistical Information
Census data: Statistical Abstract of the United States, 2007–2008	http://www.census.gov/prod/www/statistical-abstract.html
Census data: American Community Survey: • Includes state and county data	http://www.census.gov/acs/www/
National health statistics produced in report format by NCHS (2004) • Comprehensive report drawing from a variety of data sources	http://www.cdc.gov/nchs/data/hus/hus04.pdf
FastStats A to Z: • Provides state-specific fertility and natality information (e.g., age and parity of mother, duration of pregnancy, percentage of mothers who get prenatal care, number of unmarried mothers, infant's birth weight, type of birth [i.e., single, twin]), infant morbidity and mortality statistics, and health and health risk behavior data	http://www.cdc.gov/nchs/fastats/map_page.htm
NHANES results	http://www.cdc.gov/nchs/about/major/nhanes/survey_results_and_products.htm
Links to NCHS surveys related to health and healthcare	http://www.cdc.gov/nchs/default.htm
National Vital Statistics system: • Annual reports that present detailed vital statistics data, including natality, mortality, marriage, and divorce	http://www.cdc.gov/nchs/products/pubs/pubd/vsus/vsus.htm
The Behavioral Risk Factor Surveillance System (BRFSS): • The world's largest telephone survey; tracks health risks in the United States • Includes national and state statistics as well as statistics on selected metropolitan areas	http://www.cdc.gov/brfss
Youth Risk Behavior Surveillance System (YRBSS): • Developed in 1990 to monitor priority health risk behaviors that contribute markedly to the leading causes of death, disability, and social problems among youth and adults in the United States	http://www.cdc.gov/healthyYouth/yrbs
The Pediatric Nutrition Surveillance System (PedNSS) and the Pregnancy Nutrition Surveillance System (PNSS): • Program-based surveillance systems that monitor the nutritional status of low-income infants, children, and women in federally funded maternal and child health programs	http://www.cdc.gov/pednss
Data warehouse for NCHS data: • Includes links to detailed statistical tables on a variety of health topics	http://www.cdc.gov/nchs/datawh.htm
U.S. Department of Agriculture: • International food consumption patterns	http://www.ers.usda.gov
U.S. Department of Agriculture: Economic Research Service	http://www.ers.usda.gov/data/internationalFoodDemand
U.S. Department of Agriculture: Food Stamp Program statistics	http://www.fns.usda.gov/pd/fspmain.htm
U. S. Department of Agriculture: WIC Program statistics	http://www.fns.usda.gov/pd/wicmain.htm
U.S. Department of Agriculture: Food Security in the United States: • Links to a variety of statistics on food security	http://www.ers.usda.gov/data/foodsecurity

Source: Edelstein S. *Nutrition in Public Health: A Handbook for Developing Programs and Services.* 2nd ed. Sudbury, MA: Jones and Bartlett; 2006.

document a community need and have the added benefit of involving the public in problem solving and goal setting.[25]

Five different approaches are used frequently for collecting new information on the needs of community. Different approaches are appropriate for different needs. To determine which approach is appropriate, examine the situation and the purpose of the needs assessment, and review the advantages and disadvantages of the various approaches. Sometimes, an assessment may need a combination of two or more techniques to obtain an accurate result or a good picture of the community's needs. The following are the five needs assessment techniques that community nutritionists can use to assess the community:[21,26]

- *Existing data approach:* The nutritionist can use existing statistical data, such as national vital statistics, to obtain information about the well-being of people. This approach uses descriptive statistics such as census data, labor surveys, income data, NHANES data for food consumption patterns, USDA data from the Food Stamp Program, and school and hospital information to prepare an assessment report for the community. The advantage of this approach is that:
  - The data are available, are relatively inexpensive, and are faster to use than conducting an original study.
  - The nutritionist can benefit from the research of top experts in the field, which ensures quality data.
  - The nutritionist will benefit from utilizing samples from larger populations.

  The disadvantage is that:
  - The nutritionist must relate the data to a particular community's nutrition issues.
  - Since many surveys deal with national populations, the nutritionist may experience difficulty finding data for a well-defined minority subgroup.
  - There is the potential of manipulating the data in such a way that the validity and reliability of the original research is lessened.
  - Some research may involve very large samples and difficult statistical packages.
- *Survey approach:* This approach requires some training or experience on how to create and administer survey questionnaires (e.g., writing clear and precise questions). In this approach, data are collected through personal interviews, telephone surveys, hand-delivered questionnaires, or mailed questionnaires. The data are collected from a wide range of representative community residents about issues pertaining to their well-being and needs. Responses are generally representative of the whole community. The nutritionist should consider the following before deciding to use this approach for the needs assessment: 1) cost of implementation, 2) time needed for completion, 3) individuals' rate of refusal, and 4) the magnitude and type of training the supporting staff need to carry out the survey. Some of the advantages to this approach are that:
  - The entire population may be surveyed.
  - It provides an opportunity for many people to feel involved in the decision-making process.
  - It works well in combination with other systematic needs assessment techniques.

  Some of the disadvantages to this approach are that:
  - It may be expensive.

- It requires a great deal of time and expertise to develop the survey, train interviewers or staff, conduct interviews, and analyze and interpret the results.
- *Key informant approach:* This approach requires the nutritionist to first identify the key leaders, decision makers, and professionals in the community (e.g., school faculty and administrators, hospital administrators, church leaders, mayors, commissioners, physicians) who can identify accurately the priority needs and concerns of the community. The nutritionist needs to compile a list of the key informants' names and decide how to collect data from them. As with the survey approach, you'll need to create a questionnaire for gathering the information. Key informants would complete the questionnaire or be interviewed to obtain their perception of the community's needs. The information is then analyzed and presented to the community. Some of the advantages of this approach are:
  - This technique can be combined effectively with other techniques.
  - It is inexpensive.
  - It allows continuous clarification of ideas and information.

  Some of the disadvantages include:
  - An additional approach is needed because these results do not represent the total community perspective.
  - The information obtained from this technique may be biased.
- *Community forum:* One or more public meetings are held and the participants discuss the needs of the community. The nutritionist should create a list of questions to be used for the group discussion. All members of the community, including key informants, should be encouraged to attend and express their concerns about their well-being and perceived needs. Some of the advantages of this technique are:
  - It allows input from many individuals with different perspectives on the needs of the community.
  - It provides an opportunity for all the community members to participate in the needs assessment.
  - In-depth information can be collected.
  - It can be combined effectively with other techniques.

  Some of the disadvantages include:
  - The information collected may be limited to those who agree to participate.
  - Only those who are more vocal will be heard if the forum is not well conducted.
  - It may generate more questions than answers.
- *Focus group interview:* This approach involves selecting and interviewing people for their particular skills, experiences, or positions. Group discussions are then used to obtain detailed information about a particular issue. The participants are asked to respond to a series of questions about a topic or an issue. It is more effective to divide the participants into groups of 8, 10, or 20 if a large number of participants are involved. Each group member is asked to write his or her ideas on a piece of paper; all of the ideas are then listed on a chart or board. Each idea is discussed, clarified, and evaluated by the group, and then each person assigns a priority to each idea, or ranks the ideas by silent ballot. All the prioritized ideas are tallied and the final group ideas are listed and discussed. Some of the advantages of this approach are:
  - It can be used to expand the data obtained from surveys or existing data.

- The data can be used to create surveys for future use.
- It provides an opportunity to clarify ideas.
- It stimulates critical thinking.

Some of the disadvantages include:

- It does not give everybody in the community the opportunity to provide ideas.
- It must be combined with another technique because data from this approach may not be enough to get a complete picture of the issues.

A Framework for Performing an Assessment

One person can carry out a needs assessment survey, but generally, the survey will be more useful if it is designed and carried out by a group of individuals. This is particularly true if no one working on it has special experience in the field. The WHO and other authors suggested the following nine-step framework that provides a useful guide for planning and conducting a needs assessment.[24,27,28]

1. Decide when to conduct the needs assessment and set up a committee that will motivate community members to become involved in the needs assessment. Then, develop a plan of action.
2. List important issues or needs of the community. Decide what information needs to be collected after reviewing available information.
3. Determine the target population to be surveyed and how the data will be collected.
4. Determine the availability of existing data, and what information will need to be gathered using a survey. Determine the cost estimates and the time frame.
5. Identify and train the assessment team. Develop and pretest the questionnaire, and then randomly select a sample of the individuals to survey.
6. Collect the data.
7. Analyze the data.
8. Interpret the results to identify priority needs, possible intervention strategies, and resources.
9. Present the results of the needs assessment to all the stakeholders and the community members.

Nutritional Needs Assessment

Dietary assessment is the first step in identifying nutritional deficiency. Nutritional needs assessments are conducted using different methods to determine the nutritional status of individuals or the entire population, dietary intake, and possible dietary inadequacies. The main methods of assessing individuals' food consumption (discussed later in the chapter) are a 24-hour recall, a food diary or record, a dietary history, and a food frequency questionnaire. These methods are based on the dietary, laboratory, anthropometric, and clinical measures presented in **Table 2.4**. They can be used either alone or combined with other methods for more effective results.

Other factors, sometimes called *ecological factors*, that may influence the nutrition status of individuals or populations include socioeconomic and demographic data, such as:[28,29]

- Household composition (e.g., single parent head of household, number of children)
- Education (e.g., literacy)
- Ethnicity
- Religion

- Cultural practices
- Income
- Employment status
- Material and community resources (e.g., access to health and agricultural services, land ownership)
- Ready access to a good source of drinking water
- Household sanitation

Additional factors including the cost of foods, the adequacy of food preparation equipment, the availability of food reserves, and the percentage of household income spent on certain foods such as meats, fruits and vegetables, and grains also may be collected.[29] Data on health and vital statistics also may be obtained, such as the following:[29]

- The proportion of children immunized against measles and other infectious diseases
- The proportion of infants born with a low birth weight
- The percentage of mothers who are breastfeeding
- The proportion of mothers who used drugs or other substances while pregnant
- Mortality and morbidity rates

The story of the Delta Nutrition Intervention Research Initiative is discussed in this chapter as a Successful Community Strategy.

Different Methods and Tools for Assessing Nutrition Status

Nutrients play many roles in the body, so measures of nutritional status must include many factors. Often these factors are termed the ABCDs of nutrition assessment: anthropometric measurements, biochemical tests, clinical observations, and dietary intake (see Table 2.4).[37]

Anthropometric Measurements and Body Composition

Anthropometric measurements are physical measurements of the body, such as height and weight, head circumference, or skinfold measurement.

TABLE 2.4	The ABCDs of Nutrition Assessment
Assessment Method	**Reasons for Use**
Anthropometric measures	Measures growth in children; shows changes in weight that can reflect diseases (e.g., obesity, cancer, or thyroid problems); monitors progress in fat loss
Biochemical tests	Measures blood, and/or urine, and/or feces for nutrients or metabolites that indicate deficiencies, infection, or disease
Clinical/physical observations	Assesses change in skin color, health, hair texture, fingernail shape, eyes, etc.
Dietary intake	Evaluates diet for nutrient intake (e.g., fat; calcium; iron; vitamins D, A, and C; protein) or food eaten (e.g., number of servings of fruits and vegetables), as well as eating patterns

Source: Insel P, Turner RE, Ross D. *Nutrition*. 3rd ed. Sudbury, MA: Jones and Bartlett; 2007.

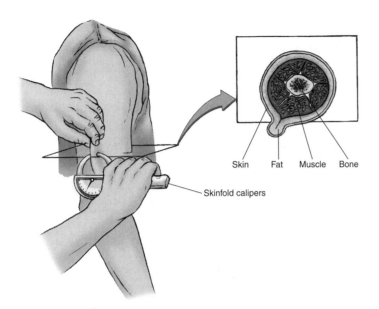

Skin   Fat   Muscle   Bone

Skinfold calipers

FIGURE 2-1 Skinfold Measurements

Height and Weight

Weight is a critical measurement in nutrition assessment. It is used to assess children's growth, predict energy expenditure and protein needs, and determine body composition. Weight should be measured using a calibrated scale.

Head Circumference

The anthropometric assessment of infants and young children also includes head circumference. It is measured using a flexible tape measure, placed snugly around the head of the child. Head circumference measures are useful indicators of normal growth and development during the rapid growth period from birth to age 3.[38] Most assessments in the scientific and research communities use metric measurements.

Skinfold Measurement

Skinfold measurements around different parts of the body can provide information about a person's percentage of body fat. The information obtained using this method can help determine the physical fitness of an individual or that person's risk of obesity. Skinfold data are collected using skinfold calipers (see **Figure 2-1**). The measurements can be compared to percentile tables for specific sex and age categories.

National Center for Health Statistics' Percentiles for Physical Growth

The National Center for Health Statistics (NCHS) creates percentiles for physical growth charts that are standard for evaluating the physical growth of males and females from birth to age 20 years. The standards are based on anthropometric measurements made on large, nationally representative samples of children in the United States. A single measurement is plotted on the percentile graph to determine how the child ranks in comparison to other children of the same age and sex in the United States. If the measurement is less than the 10th percentile, it should be checked for accuracy and compared with other types of assessment. Length-for-age less than the fifth percentile indicates chronic undernutrition. Weight-for-length less than the fifth percentile may reveal acute malnutrition.[19,39,40] Excessive weight-for-length (above the 95th percentile) indicates obesity. Infants whose weight-for-length falls below the 5th percentile are classified as failure-to-thrive, and those below the 10th percentile are suspected for failure-

Successful Community Strategies 🏠🏠🏠

The Delta Nutrition Intervention Research Initiative (NIRI)[30–36]

Information gathered from community-level nutritional assessment can be used to develop community-wide programs addressing specific problem areas, such as childhood obesity or iron-deficiency anemia. Nutrition programs should be integrated into community-based health programs.

The Lower Mississippi Delta Nutrition Intervention Research Initiative (Delta NIRI) provides an excellent example of how community assessment can be utilized to address important community nutrition problems. In response to the nutrition-related health problems in this region, the U.S. Congress directed the U.S. Department of Agriculture (USDA) Research Service to establish Delta NIRI. The purpose was to conduct a comprehensive assessment of rural communities, examine perceptions of community key informants regarding nutrition and health problems, evaluate

the contributors to the problems, and assess the resources in Lower Mississippi Delta (LMD) counties. An additional purpose was to promote capacity-building and sustainability at the community level.

The LMD area of Arkansas, Louisiana, and Mississippi is characterized by high rates of poverty, low education attainment, and food insecurity. Food insecurity, when people live with hunger and the fear of starvation, is two and a half times the national average in each of these states. There is a high prevalence of hypertension, diabetes, obesity, anemia, and heart disease, all of which are influenced by nutrition.

The participation of the key informants allowed scientists to evaluate and generate knowledge about nutrition and health needs, food habits,

and food consumption in 36 counties in the LMD. An adult food questionnaire developed by Tufts Human Nutrition Research Center was used to determine the composition of the diet and nutritional needs of the diverse population. In addition, a food frequency questionnaire developed by Baylor University scientists was used to survey children. Based on existing literature on disease prevalence in the region, it was assumed that key informants would report hypertension, obesity, and diabetes as among the most important health problems in their counties.

Key informants were individuals who, by virtue of their role or position, have knowledge of and access to the community. The assessment used a modified key informant approach to conduct in-person interviews with 490 key informants in 36 selected counties and parishes.

to-thrive.[19,40,41] **Box 2-1** provides instructions on how to plot the measures on a growth chart. The physical growth charts for girls and boys from birth to 20 years can be found at http://www.cdc.gov/growthcharts.

Biochemical Tests/Data

Biochemical tests measure body fluids such as blood, urine, or feces. They are used mainly to detect subclinical deficiencies such as iron-deficiency anemia. They provide an objective means of determining nutritional status. They are also used to measure nutrients or the urinary excretion rate of nutrients or metabolites. **Table 2.5** presents examples of types of standard biochemical tests used in community and public health settings.

Clinical Observations/Physical Examinations

Physical examinations are used to determine physical signs of nutrient deficiency or excess that developed over a long period of time (advanced stage of nutrient deficiency). A clinical nutrition examination would observe a person's hair, nails, skin, eyes, lips, mouth, muscles, and joints for specific signs.[2] For example, changes in hair color would suggest a protein deficiency. **Table 2.6** presents examples of generally used physical examination tests that use appearance as an indicator of nutrition status.

Dietary Assessment Methods

Dietary information may confirm a lack or excess of a dietary constituent detected by anthropometric, biochemical, or clinical evaluations. There are primarily four ways to gather data on dietary intake: diet history, food frequency questionnaire (FFQ), food record or diaries, and 24-hour recall.

A **diet history** is any dietary assessment that asks clients to report about their past diet. It refers to the collection of the detailed make-up of meals (including preparation methods and foods eaten in combination), the intake frequency of various foods, and other risk factors such as the economic status of the client.[43] A trained interviewer typically completes this assessment. Many investigators now use the term *dietary history* to refer to the food frequency method of dietary assessment.

> *Box* **2-1 How to Plot Measurements on a Growth Chart**
>
> 1. Choose the percentile chart based on age and gender.
> 2. Find the infant's weight in pounds or kilograms along the vertical axis of the chart.
> 3. Find the infant's age along the horizontal axis of the chart.
> 4. Ascertain and mark the chart where the age and weight lines intersect and record the percentile.

diet history A detailed dietary assessment, which may include a 24-hour recall, food frequency questionnaire, and additional information such as weight history, previous diet changes, use of supplements, and food intolerances.

The Delta NIRI conducted a comprehensive rural community assessment through five surveys: key informant survey, food of our Delta survey (FOODS 2000), food store survey, focus groups, and a community resources assessment. In one of the surveys (FOODS 2000), more than 1,500 people were followed by an in-store survey conducted in 174 stores, supermarkets, small to medium grocery stores, and convenience stores that identified the problems of access to and quality of foods in this high health risk, low-income region. A series of three focus groups were held in nine counties and parishes to identify barriers to improving food choices, food security, and shopping practices. In addition, a questionnaire developed to obtain perceptions of nutrition and health problems was pretested, revised, and administered to key informants by personal interviews.

Preliminary results show that key informants identified resources available in their counties to address food and nutrition problems. Ninety percent or more of key informants identified food stamps, school lunches, Head Start, Elderly Nutrition Programs, and the Special Supplemental Nutrition Program for Women, Infants, and Children (WIC) as available resources. Key informants identified hypertension as the most important health problem in their counties. They also saw multiple factors as contributing to the problems, but rated individual-level factors (food choices, education, willingness to change, and health behavior) as more important than community-level factors (food and healthcare access and resources).

Results showed that 97 percent identified consumption of high-fat foods and 94 percent identified consumption of too much fast food as nutrition concerns in their counties. Poverty, a lack of education, and an unwillingness to change were seen as major contributors to these problems by 92 percent, 94 percent, and 94 percent of key informants, respectively. The informants ranked hypertension, teen pregnancy, drug addiction, and heart disease, in that order, as the most significant health problems. Lack of exercise, poor food choices, and inadequate health insurance were seen as major factors contributing to health problems by 98 percent, 95 percent, and 91 percent of key informants, respectively. Data from this key informant survey demonstrated that perceptions of nutrition and health problems reflected the values and concerns of the local community. These results will help guide future planning for interventions to improve the nutrition and health status of the Delta community.

TABLE
2.5

Biochemical Tests Used in Community and Public Health Settings

Nutritional Indicators	Reference Range	Applications
Body protein status	Serum albumin: 3.5–5.0 g/dl (represents 50–60 percent total serum protein) Other serum protein	• High prevalence of children and pregnant women with abnormal blood protein levels is likely to be a public health problem of severe malnutrition. • Prevalence of stunting. • Prevalence of wasting. • Prevalence of kwashiorkor.
Iron status	Hemoglobin: male, 13–118 g/dl; female, 12–16 g/dl Hematocrit: male, 45–62 percent; female, 37–48 percent Others are serum ferritin, erythrocyte, protoporphyrin, and transferring saturation	• Prevalence of iron-deficiency anemia is likely to be a public health problem. • Proportion of children (of defined age and sex) and pregnant women with two or more abnormal iron indices (serum ferritin, erythrocyte, protoporphyrin, transferring saturation, and hemoglobin) plus abnormal hemoglobin.
Serum retinol	≤ 0.70 μmol/L in children 6–71 months	• Vitamin A deficiency is a severe public health problem in developing countries. • Clinical indicators: prevalence of maternal blindness more than 5 percent.
Iodine status	Median urinary iodine: ≤ 20 μg/L based on ≥ 300 casual urine samples	• Severe risk of iodine deficiency disorders is likely to be a public health problem. • Clinical indicators: proportion of children with total goiter rate more than 30 percent.
Blood lipids and lipoproteins status	Cholesterol: less than 225 mg/dl (for ages 40–49 years; increases with age) and lipoprotein levels	• Proportion of men and women with abnormal blood cholesterol and lipoprotein levels (very low density lipoprotein [VLDL], low density lipoprotein [LDL], and high density lipoprotein [LDL]). • Coronary heart disease risk is likely to be a public health problem.
Lead status	40 μg/L (normally much lower in children)	• Prevalence of abnormal blood lead levels is likely to be a public health problem. • A high proportion of children with abnormal levels is a severe public health problem.
Blood glucose	70–110 mg/dl (tested after fasting)	• Diabetes mellitus is likely to be a public health problem.

Modified from: Gibson RS. *Principles of Nutritional Assessment*. 2nd ed. New York: Oxford University Press; 2005.

TABLE
2.6

Physical Examination Tests That Use General Appearance as an Indicator of Nutrition Status[29,37,42,48]

Physical Appearance	Normal	Abnormal	Nutrient Deficiencies	Could Indicate
Demeanor	Alert, responsive Positive outlook	Lethargic Negative attitude (irritable, etc.) Sleep disturbances Impaired coordination	Calories, protein, iron, fat, pantothenic acid	Poverty, malnutrition, hunger, and food insecurity
Weight	Reasonable for build Appropriate weight for height and height for age	Underweight Overweight, obese	Calories, fat, protein Excessive intake of calories, lack of physical activity	Malnutrition Overnutrition
Hair	Glossy, full, firmly rooted Uniform color	Dull, sparse Easily or painlessly plucked Thin, lack luster, dyspigmentation	Protein, vitamin C, calories, biotin, vitamin A-toxicity	Socioeconomic factors (poverty, and hunger)

TABLE 2.6 (*Continued*)

Physical Appearance	Normal	Abnormal	Nutrient Deficiencies	Could Indicate
Eyes	Bright, clear, shiny	Pale conjuctiva (dryness, thickening, and lack of luster of the bulbar conjunctiva of the exposed part of the eye ball) Redness, dryness Bitot's spots (well-demarcated, superficially dry, white-grey foamy plaques usually located lateral to the cornea in both eyes) Keratomalacia (softening of cornea)	Vitamin A, thiamin, vitamin E, vitamin B_{12}, vitamin A copper, toxicity	Lack of adequate fruit, vegetable, and grain products intakes
Lips	Smooth	Chapped, red, swollen Angular stomatitis (lesions and fissuring at the corners of the mouth)	Riboflavin, niacin, biotin, vitamins B_1, B_2, B_6, and B_{12}, vitamin C	Inadequate fruit and vegetable intakes
Tongue	Deep red Slightly rough	Bright red or purple Swollen (edema) or shrunken Geographic tongue (irregularly distributed patchy areas of atrophy of epithelium, etiology unknown)	Vitamin C, protein, riboflavin, and niacin	Lack of protein, fruits, and vegetables
Teeth	Bright, painless	Cavities Painful, mottled, chipped, or missing	Calcium, vitamin D, fluoride	Inadequate intake of dairy product, fortified milk, fruits, and vegetables
Gums	Pink, firm	Spongy, bleeding, receding Swelling of gingival tissue between teeth, which may bleed with slight pressure	Vitamin C	Lack of citrus fruits intake and cigarette smoking
Skin	Clear, smooth, firm Slightly moist	Rashes, swelling Light or dark spots Dry, follicular hyperkeratosis (hypertrophy of the corneous layer of skin surrounding the hair follicles with formation of plaques) Petachiae (small hemorrhagic spots in skin or mucous membranes) Pellagrous dermatosis (symmetrical, clearly demarcated, hyperpigmented areas of skin most commonly exposed to sunlight)	Zinc, vitamins B, and B_{12}, protein, vitamin C, essential fatty acids, vitamin A, folate, B-carotene, carotenoids, vitamin A toxicity	Inadequate protein, fruit, and vegetable intakes
Nails	Pink, firm	Koilonychia (spoon-shaped deformity of finger nails of both hands in older children and adults), ridged spongy bases	Iron or selenium toxicity	Inadequate intake of meat, leafy vegetables, and grains products
Face	Smooth, clear of spots	Diffuse depigmentation (this occurs in people of African descent) Pallor (anemia may exaggerate the appearance of the condition)	Severe protein-calorie malnutrition and iron deficiency	Inadequate intake of meat, nuts, and legumes
Mobility/weak joints	Erect posture Good muscle tone Walks without pain or difficulty	Muscle wasting Skeletal deformities Loss of balance	Calcium, vitamins D, & A, protein and B_1, B_2, Beading of ribs (symmetrical nodular enlargement of costochondral junctions in ribs)	Inadequate intake meat, legumes, nuts, dairy products, fruits, and vegetables

food frequency questionnaire A method of dietary assessment in which the questions relate to how often foods are consumed.

food record A written record of the amounts of all foods and liquids consumed during a time period, usually 3 to 7 days; often includes information on time, place, and situation of eating.

The *Food Frequency Questionnaire (FFQ)* asks how often the respondent consumed specific foods or groups of foods for a specific period, instead of specific foods the respondents consumed daily.[44] Sometimes information about portion size, methods of cooking, or the combinations of foods eaten at meals is collected. **Table 2.7** presents a sample FFQ.

In *food records* or diaries, the respondent provides detailed information about daily eating habits. The respondent is usually asked to record all foods and beverages consumed during a defined period, typically over 3 to 7 consecutive days. The amount consumed may be measured using a scale or household measures (such as cups and tablespoons) or estimated using models, pictures, or no particular aid. The respondents normally become fatigued after several days of recording.[45] One of the disadvantages of dietary records includes incomplete records in the final days of a 7-day recording period. It may be more difficult for individuals with low socioeconomic status, recent immigrants, children, the poorly educated, and some elderly groups if they are required to respond on paper. Dictaphones, computer recording, and self-recording scales have been used to help respondents track their intake.[46]

TABLE 2.7 **Food Frequency Questionnaire**

Below is a list of food items. Please indicate how often/frequently you consume each.

Foods	Examples	Serving Size	Day	Week	Month	Year	*Seldom	Never
Dark green vegetables / Dark yellow vegetables / Other green vegetables / Other vegetables	Spinach, pumpkin, broccoli, squash, carrots, sweet potatoes, kale, peas, corn, vegetable juice	1 cup of raw romaine lettuce and spinach / ½ cup of other vegetables / ¾ cup vegetable juice						
Wheat germ / Cereal / Pasta / Potato / Other grain / Pancakes	Whole wheat bread, bagel, cereals, rice, spaghetti, macaroni, crackers	1 slice of bread / 1 cup of ready-to-eat cereal / ½ cup of cooked cereal / 6 whole crackers						
Citrus fruit or juice / Other fruits / Tomatoes / Dried fruits	Apple, banana, grape, kiwi, blueberry, date, peach, pear, orange, apricot, fig, tomato, canned fruit juice	1 medium piece of whole fruit / ½ cup of berries / ½ cup of chopped, cooked, or canned fruit / ¾ cup of fruit juice						
Milk and milk products	Milk, yogurt, frozen yogurt, cheese, cottage cheese	1 cup of milk or yogurt / ½ cup frozen yogurt / ⅓ cup cottage cheese						
Oil / Margarine / Butter / Salad dressing / Bacon and sausage / Fried foods / Salt pork / Cream, sweet / Cream, sour	Canola oil, corn oil, cottonseed oil, olive oil, safflower oil, soybean oil, sunflower oil, shortening, stick margarine, tub margarine, mayonnaise	Most Americans consume enough oil in the foods they eat, such as: nuts / fish / cooking oil / salad dressings						

TABLE 2.7 **(Continued)**

Below is a list of food items. Please indicate how often/frequently you consume each.

Foods	Examples	Serving Size	How Many Times					
			Day	Week	Month	Year	*Seldom	Never
Beef, hamburger Pork, ham Liver Fish Lunch meat Franks Pizza Poultry Eggs Peanut butter Dried peas/beans	Duck, goose, turkey, ground chicken and turkey, beef, lamb, pork, veal, black-eyed peas, chickpeas (garbanzo beans), lima beans (mature), navy beans, pinto beans, soy beans, split peas, tofu (bean curd made from soy beans), white beans, catfish, cod, flounder, haddock, halibut, herring, mackerel, pollock, salmon	2 to 3 ounces of meat or fish 2 tablespoons peanut butter ½ cup dried peas/beans						
Nuts Seeds Sprouts	Almonds, cashews, hazelnuts (filberts), mixed nuts, pecans, pistachios, pumpkin seeds, sesame seeds, sunflower seeds, walnuts	⅓ cup						
Candy Pie, cake, cookies Potato chips, pretzels, popcorn, etc. Teas/sugar Soda pop Kool-aid Wine Beer Hard liquor Ice milk Sherbet	Regular soft drinks, fruit drinks (such as fruit punch), brown sugar, corn syrup, high-fructose corn syrup, honey fructose, fruit juice concentrates, candy	Calorie allowance is part of total estimated calorie needs, not in addition to total calorie needs						
Other foods not listed								

*Seldom (less than six times per year)

Use These Tips for Estimating Serving Sizes:	
Four dice	= 1 ounce of cheese
One deck of playing cards or the palm of a woman's hand	= 3 ounces of cooked meat
One golf ball	= 2 tablespoons
A computer mouse	= 1 small baked potato
A baseball	= 1 cup

Modified from: Simko MD, Cowell C, Gilbride JA. *Nutrition Assessment: A Comprehensive Guide for Planning Intervention*. Rockville, MD: Aspen; 1984. Reprinted with permission.

24-hour recall A method of dietary assessment in which the individual is asked to remember everything eaten during the past 24 hours.

As its name implies, a **24-hour recall** typically is administered for a 24-hour period. The respondents are asked to remember all foods and beverages they consumed in the past 24 hours (usually midnight to midnight). A trained staff or a nutritionist typically collects this data either by interview, self-administered questionnaire, or telephone.[47] Comprehensive population surveys normally use 24-hour recall as the main method of data collection. **Table 2.8** presents a sample of a 24-hour recall form, and **Table 2.9** shows advantages and disadvantages of dietary assessment instruments.

TABLE 2.8   **Sample 24-Hour Recall Form**

Name: _____   Date: _____

Day of Week of Recall: _____

| | | | | | | Office Use Only | | |
Place	Time*	Food Items	Type and Preparation**	Amount	Place Eaten***	Food Code	Amount	Code
	*A.M.	Breakfast	**Fried, baked, boiled		***Home			
	A.M.	Snack	Toasted		Restaurant			
	Midday	Lunch	Whole wheat		Carried Lunch			
	Afternoon	Snack	Fresh, frozen, canned		School			
	P.M.	Supper	Creamed		Senior center			
					Child care center, etc.			

Additional Questions:

Was intake unusual in any way? Yes _____ No _____

If yes, why (in what way)? _____

_____

Do you take vitamin or mineral supplements? Yes _____ No _____

If yes, how many per day? _____ per week? _____

If yes, what kind (give brand name if known)?

Multivitamin _____

Iron _____

Ascorbic Acid _____

Other (list) _____

Do you exercise:

If yes, how many times per week? _____ For how long? _____

Source: Simko MD, Cowell C, Gilbride JA. *Nutrition Assessment: A Comprehensive Guide for Planning Intervention.* Rockville, MD: Aspen; 1984. Peprinted with permission.

TABLE 2.9	Advantages and Disadvantages of Dietary Assessment Instruments	
Instrument	**Advantages**	**Disadvantages**
Food record	Intake quantified	High investigator cost
	Could enhance self-monitoring for weight control	High respondent burden
		Extensive respondent training and motivation required
		Many days needed to capture individual's usual intake
		Affects eating behavior
		Intake often underreported
		Reports of intake decrease with time
		Number of days reported decreases with time
		May lead to substantial sample bias
24-hour dietary recall	Intake quantified	High investigator cost
	Appropriate for most populations: low sample bias	Many days needed to capture an individual's usual intake
	Relatively low respondent burden	
	Does not affect eating behavior	Intake often underreported
Food frequency questionnaire	Usual individual intake asked about	Not quantifiably precise
	Information on total diet obtained	Difficult cognitive task for respondent
	Low investigator cost	Intake often misreported
	Does not affect eating behavior	
Diet history	Usual individual intake asked about	Not quantifiably precise
	Information on total diet obtained	Difficult cognitive task for respondent
	Information often available on foods consumed by meal	Intake often misreported
	Can have low investigator cost	Can have high investigator burden
	Does not affect eating behavior	

Source: Coulston AM, Rock CL, Monsen ER. *Nutrition in the Prevention and Treatment of Disease.* New York: Academic Press; 2001. Copyright Academic Press (2001). Reprinted with permission.

How to Analyze Dietary Intake Data

After the data have been collected, they should be reviewed to ensure completion. Then, analyze the data to determine the nutrient content and compare the results using dietary standards or other reference points. This can be completed using a nutrient analysis software program or online program, such as http://www.mypyramidtracker.gov.

Computer programs automatically perform the math using large databases and do not require the nutritionist to look up foods in nutrient composition tables.[37]

Comparison to Dietary Standards

The respondent's nutrient intake can be compared to dietary standards using the Recommended Dietary Allowances (RDA) or Adequate Intake (AI) values. A comparison of individual diets to RDA or AI values needs to be interpreted with caution because the RDAs are the nutrient intakes that are sufficient to meet the needs of nearly all individuals (about 97 percent) in an age and gender group. Also, it is important to know that AI is not a standard, but can be used as a guide for the

nutrient intake of individuals and groups in situations where no RDA for a nutrient has been established. AIs are based on observed or experimentally determined estimates of the average nutrient intake that appears to maintain a defined nutritional state in certain populations (for example, normal circulating nutrient values or bone health).[49]

Comparison to MyPyramid

The respondent's food intake can be compared to MyPyramid, a guide created by the USDA to help individuals plan healthy diets. (See Appendix E for the USDA MyPyramid food guidance system and Appendix F for Canada's Food Guide for Healthy Eating.) A nutritionist can categorize the listed foods into the different groups on the pyramid to determine the number of servings or amounts the respondents ate.

Comparison to *Dietary Guidelines for Americans*

A nutritionist also can compare the respondent's diet to the *Dietary Guidelines for Americans*, a guide about lifestyle behaviors that relate to nutritional health, such as choosing nutrient-dense foods and

TABLE 2.10	Scheme for Determining Nutritional Deficiency	
Depletion Stage		**Method(s) Used**
1. Dietary inadequacy		Dietary
2. Decreased level in reserve tissue store		Biochemical
3. Decreased level in body fluids		Biochemical
4. Decreased functional level in tissues		Anthropometric/biochemical
5. Decreased activity of nutrient-dependent enzyme or mRNA for some proteins		Biochemical/molecular/genetic
6. Functional change		Behavioral/physiological/biochemical
7. Clinical symptoms		Clinical/observation
8. Anatomical sign		Clinical/physical/observation

From: Sahn DE, Lockwood R, Scrimshaw NS. *Methods for the Evaluation of the Impact of Food and Nutrition Programmes.* Tokyo: United Nations University Press; 1984. Reprinted with permission.

being more physically active. This evaluation shows whether the respondent's diet is high or low in saturated fat and sodium, whether they are consuming adequate amounts of fruits and vegetables, and whether they perform regular physical activity. It is most effective to use a combination of these three methods to determine dietary inadequacies. The Dietary Guidelines are available at http://www.health.gov/dietaryguidelines. **Table 2.10** presents a generalized scheme for determining nutrient deficiency.

Screening for Community Health

So far, this chapter has focused on different methods of studying community nutritional problems and assessing health risks for communities and their populations. The nutritional assessment process includes screening and assessment, and the major purpose of both is to screen for nutritional risks and apply specific assessment techniques to determine an action plan.[7,9] *Screening* is an attempt to detect unrecognized or subclinical health conditions among individuals. Community screening tests are not intended to be diagnostic.[25] Their purpose is to identify individuals who have a high risk of having or developing a specific health condition so they can be referred for definitive diagnosis and treatment. It also identifies individuals who may actually have an illness.[50,51] Screening carries an ethical commitment to continue working with these individuals and to provide them with access to diagnostic and treatment services.

Reliability and Validity of Screening for Community Health

One major concern about screening methods is the accuracy of the information gathered. *Reliability* is the consistency or repeatability and reproducibility of test results or whether a testing instrument will measure nutrient intake the same way twice on the same client.[51,52] A

screening instrument that produces the same result on two or more different occasions, even when administered by different investigators, is considered reliable. *Validity* is the ability of a test instrument to measure accurately what it is supposed to measure. For example, a validity study may compare the results from a food frequency questionnaire to a more accurate but difficult method such as food record.[52]

The Purpose of Assessment

All persons should receive nutritional status assessments throughout their life cycle as well as during illness. Assessment determines nutritional status by analyzing clinical, dietary, and social history; anthropometric data; biochemical data; and drug-nutrient interactions. Different approaches, such as calculating an individual's BMI and anthropometric measurements, can be used to assess both the healthy population's and the critically ill's nutritional status.

Assessment of dietary intake is very important to the work of improving the health of individuals, communities, and populations. Berdanier et al. stated that dietary intake data are used for three major purposes:[7]

1. Dietary assessment at the individual level can be used to determine the individual's dietary adequacy and dietary patterns, and for educating and counseling the individual.
2. Dietary assessment is an essential component of research studies that determine the health of individuals and populations. For example, etiologic studies assess dietary intake as an exposure for association with disease outcomes. Behavioral research assesses dietary intake in order to develop and test strategies that encourage adoption of healthful eating patterns.
3. Dietary assessment also is important in identifying national health priorities, identifying population subgroups at risk or in need of special assistance, determining the success of public health interventions in improving dietary patterns, and developing public health dietary recommendations at the population/national level.[7]

Dietitians and nutritionists are responsible for nutrition assessment in community, population, and clinical settings. Several factors must be considered when conducting a nutritional assessment of the population. These factors include, but are not limited to, cost, convenience, and invasiveness. However, it is important to use the most convenient assessment method that can correlate findings with clinical, anthropometric, dietary, biochemical, and ecological factors.[12]

Reliability and Validity

Test results may yield invalid or unreliable results due to inconsistent administration of the instrument. To reduce the possibility of human error, it is very important to train all the personnel who will administer the testing instrument. Additional strategies that can be used to enhance accuracy include making precise measurements and calibrating the instruments before administering the test. The validity and reliability of the test instruments also depend on the responses of the participants.[51] It is important to modify the instrument for a specific population. For instance, one study found that although FFQ assessments were useful for ranking adults' consumption of fruits and vegetables, as compared to dietary recall they underestimated the prevalence of fruit and vegetable consumption among high school students.[52]

In addition, two major theoretical perspectives (cognitive and situational) have been proposed to explain the source of validity problems that may occur with some self-reported data. The cognitive perspective focuses on the mental processes associated with validity problems, with inaccuracies originating from comprehension, recall, and other cognitive operations present in self-reported data.[53] The situational perspective focuses on validity problems that arise from factors related to social desirability and interviewing conditions (e.g., the presence of others while responding to questions, respondents' perceptions of the level of privacy or confidentiality provided).[54] Many other factors affect the reliability and validity of dietary assessment questionnaires. These include, but are not limited to:[54,55]

- Degree of variability permitted by the instrument (convenience of recording food intake, external environment, portion size used, types of foods listed, etc.)
- Quality control of coding and keying
- Real dietary change in the time between the two administrations of the questionnaire
- Respondent characteristics (level of education, cultural background, age, etc.)
- Questionnaire design
- The qualifications of the interviewer
- Adequacy of the reference data

Thus, to improve the reliability and validity of the diet recall, it is important to use a standardized protocol that specifies exact techniques for interviewing, recording, and calculating results. The instrument should use standardized graduated food models to quantify foods and beverages consumed. Similarly, use probing questions to determine foods and beverages most commonly forgotten. It is also important to use a culturally appropriate survey instrument.

Sensitivity and Specificity

Two other measurements of a test are its sensitivity and specificity. A screening method with high *sensitivity* means there are few false negatives. A sensitivity test is able to correctly identify and classify individuals within the population who are truly malnourished as confirmed by a test (a true positive). For example, screening individuals who are at risk for poor nutrition (such as those with low hemoglobin levels) and who qualify for a nutrition assistance program will yield a high sensitivity rate.[50,51] A screening method with high sensitivity means there are few false negatives. For example, if a sensitive mammogram finds a suspicious lump in a woman's breast, the test is usually followed up with a biopsy to determine whether the lump is indeed cancerous.

A screening method with high *specificity* has few false positives. A specificity test is able to, for example, correctly identify individuals who are not malnourished within a population (true negative). For instance, when screening well-nourished individuals without risk factors for poor nutrition, the method identifies those who do not need the nutrition service.

TABLE 2.11	**Sensitivity and Specificity of a Screening Test**	

	The Real Situation	
Screening Test Results	Malnourished	No Malnutrition
Positive	True positive (TP)	False positive (FP)
Negative	False negative (FN)	True negative (TN)
Total	Total diseased (TD)	Total not diseased (TND)

Sensitivity rate = TP (TP ÷ TD) × 100

Specificity rate = TN (TN ÷ TND) × 100

False negative rate = FN (FN ÷ TD) × 100

False positive rate = FP (FP ÷ TND) × 100

Modified from: Habicht J. Some characteristics of indicators of nutritional status for use in screening and surveillance. *Am J Clin Nutr.* 1980; 33:531–535. Reprinted with permission from the American Society for Nutrition.

Preferably, a screening test's sensitivity and specificity should be 100 percent. As shown in **Table 2.11**, sensitivity, or the true positive rate, is the complement of the false negative rate, and specificity, or the true negative rate, is the complement of the false positive rate. Therefore, as sensitivity increases, specificity decreases.

In practice, nutritionists must strive to seek a balance between sensitivity and specificity. Both sensitivity and specificity can be improved by adjusting the screening process (such as adding another test). An example of this might be to include a screening test that uses oral glucose tolerance to determine the body's ability to utilize glucose instead of a urinary glucose test, or performing a screening test that uses phlebotomy to detect high blood cholesterol concentrations instead of just a finger prick cholesterol test.

screening An effort to detect unrecognized health conditions among individuals.

reliability The consistency or repeatability and reproducibility of test results.

validity The ability of the test instrument to measure what it is supposed to measure accurately.

sensitivity The ability to correctly identify individuals or a proportion of persons with a disease or condition.

specificity The ability to correctly identify individuals or a proportion of persons without a disease or condition, as confirmed by a test.

Chapter Summary

- The ABCDs of nutrition assessment are anthropometric measurements, biochemical tests, clinical/physical observations, and dietary intake.
- The goals of screening are to identify individuals who are at nutritional risk and those who need further assessment.
- It is important to use the most convenient screening method, and it is also advisable to maintain accuracy and to correlate findings with clinical, anthropometric, dietary, biochemical, and ecological factors.
- Preferably, all persons should have nutritional status assessments throughout their life cycle as well as during illness. Different approaches can be applied to the healthy population and to the critically ill.
- At the population level, assessment of dietary intake is necessary to identify national health priorities and to develop public health dietary recommendations. These assessments are used to determine the success of public health interventions in improving dietary patterns and to identify population subgroups at risk or in need of special assistance.
- One major concern about screening methods is the accuracy of the information gathered.
- Reliability refers to the consistency or repeatability of test results; validity refers to the ability of the test to measure what it is supposed to measure.
- A sensitivity test is able to correctly identify and classify individuals within the population who are truly malnourished as confirmed by the test (a true positive).
- A screening method with high specificity has few false positives.

Critical Thinking Activities

- With the consent of the participants (e.g., women, older persons, college students, high school students) in a week-long health fair in the community, collect a 24-hour recall. Analyze the subjects' dietary intake using computer software. Immediately review a printout of the data collected, including nutrient totals if the system being used permits.
  - Query the participants on whether the amount they consumed was typical; if not, identify the reason the amount consumed was unusually low or high.
  - Make a form like the example shown below to list the foods and amounts eaten from the 24-hour recall. Next to each food, list the MyPyramid food group to which it belongs. In the next column, list the number of MyPyramid servings or fractions of servings it provides. For mixed foods, list all ingredients separately and identify the food groups and serving sizes that apply.

Food	Amount	MyPyramid Group	Number of Servings

- Are foods represented from each food group?
- Does the diet follow the *Dietary Guidelines for Americans*?
- Examine your own nutritional risk factors:
  - What do you eat?
  - How do you eat?
  - What factors would affect the absorption and utilization of the nutrients you consume?
- Use your height and weight and determine if your Body Mass Index (BMI) is in the healthy range.

Case Study 2-1

Ayanna, a community nutritionist consulting at local grade schools, was asked to provide nutrition screening to the fifth-, sixth-, and seventh-grade students in a low-income and ethnically diverse school district as well as in a district with more European American students. The overall objective was to screen students from the five lower and middle socioeconomic and culturally diverse schools who may not have access to nutrition screening and to evaluate the rate of obesity in these age groups. The nutritionist sent flyers to the parents or guardians through the students and posted flyers at the school cafeteria and at different bulletin boards within the schools. In addition, a total of five announcements were made over the intercom before class periods in all the schools. Information about the event was also included in the school's newsletter. Screenings were conducted after school hours on different days of the week for 2 weeks to accommodate the target group. Despite all recruiting efforts, the results indicated that the targeted group did not use the service as hoped, and the predominant individuals who accessed the service were European American middle-class, insured students. Results also showed that 13 percent of the students screened were overweight, 20 percent were obese, and 5 percent of non-Caucasian students were underweight.

Activities

- Use the food frequency questionnaire form provided in this chapter to assess the dietary adequacy of both men and women participating in a Peace Meal Program (which provides a hot, midday meal to people ages 60 and over), high school students, or pregnant teenagers.
- Use the National Vital Statistics System to find the applicable annual reports to determine the rates of natality, mortality, marriage, and divorce in your state and county.
- Use the Pediatric Nutrition Surveillance System and the Pregnancy Nutrition Surveillance System to determine the nutritional status of low-income infants, children, and women in federally funded maternal and child health programs.
- Use a skinfold caliper to determine the percentage of body fat for a group of female athletes.

References

1. Lancaster SA. *Community and Public Health Nursing.* 5th ed. New York: Mosby; 2000.

2. Lee RD, Nieman DC. *Nutritional Assessment.* St. Louis, MO: Brown & Benchmark; 1996.

3. U.S. Department of Health and Human Services. *Nutrition Monitoring in the United States—An Updated Report on Nutrition Monitoring.* Washington, DC: U.S. Government Printing Office; 1989.

4. Washington State. The Washington State Community Nutrition Assessment Education Project. An Introduction to Community Nutrition Assessment. April 1999. Available at: http://depts.washington.edu/commnutr/assess/cna-intro.htm. Accessed October 12, 2006.

5. Kaufman M. *Nutrition in Public Health: A Handbook for Developing Programs and Services*. Rockville, Maryland: Aspen; 1990.

6. Kaufman M. *Nutrition in Promoting the Public's Health: Strategies, Principles, and Practice*. Sudbury, MA: Jones and Bartlett; 2007.

7. Berdanier CD, Feldman E, Flatt W. *Handbook of Nutrition and Food*. New York: CRC Press; 2002.

8. Washington State. Washington State Risk and Protective Factors: Nutrition. April 1999. Available at: http://depts.washington.edu/commnutr/wadocs/wadocs-nutrition.htm. Accessed October 12, 2006.

9. Council on Practice Quality Management Committee. ADA's definitions for nutrition screening and nutrition assessment. *J Am Diet Assoc*. 1994; 94:838–839.

10. Caliendo MA. *Nutrition and the Food Crisis*. New York: MacMillan; 1979.

11. Bigwood EJ. *Guiding Principles for Studies on the Nutrition of Populations*. Technical Committee on Nutrition. Geneva, Switzerland: League of Nations, Health Organization; 1939; Vol. 3, Nr 1.

12. Simko MD, Gilbride JA, Cowell C. *Nutrition Assessment. A Comprehensive Guide for Planning Intervention*. Rockville, Maryland: Aspen; 1984.

13. Frankle RT, Owen AY. *Nutrition in the Community*. St. Louis, MO: Mosby; 1978.

14. Interdepartmental Committee on Nutrition for National Development. *Manual for Nutrition Surveys*. Washington DC: U.S. Government Printing Office; 1957.

15. Schwerin HS, Stanton JL, Riley AM, et al. Food eating patterns and health: A reexamination of the Ten-State and HANES I surveys. *Am J Clin Nutr*. 1981; 34(4):568–580.

16. Ford EE, Giles WH. Changes in prevalence of nonfatal coronary heart disease in the United States from 1971–1994. *Ethnicity Dis*. 2003; 13(1):85–93.

17. Murphy SS. Use of national survey data bases for nutrition research. *Clin Nutr*. 1987; 6(5):208–218.

18. National Center for Health Statistics. National Health and Nutrition Examination Survey History. Available at: http://www.cdc.gov/nchs/about/major/nhanes/history.htm. Accessed November 4, 2006.

19. Centers for Disease Control and Prevention. Growth Chart: National Center for Health Statistics in Collaboration with the National Center for Chronic Disease Prevention and Health Promotion; 2000. Available at: http://www.cdc.gov/growthcharts. Accessed February 6, 2008.

20. Insel P, Turner E, Ross D. *Nutrition 2002 Update*. Sudbury, MA: Jones and Bartlett; 2002.

21. Carter KA, Lionel J. *Conducting a Community Needs Assessment: Primary Data Collection Technique*. Gainesville, FL: Cooperative Extension Service, Institute of Food and Agricultural Sciences (IFAS), University of Florida; 1992.

22. Sanders CG, Aycockn N, Samuel-Hodge CD, Garcia BA, Kelsey K, Garner U, Ammerman A. Extending the reach of public health nutrition: training community practitioners in multilevel approaches. *J Womens Health*. 2004; 13(5):589–597.

23. Frank-Spohrer G. *Community Nutrition: Applying Epidemiology to Contemporary Practice*. Gaithersburg, Maryland: Aspen; 1996.

24. Kettering C. Community Needs Assessment: Taking the Pulse of Your Community. Available at: http://www.communitydevelopment.uiuc.edu/resources/factsheets/needpuls.html. Accessed March 20, 2005.

25. Todorovic V. Nutritional screening in the community: developing strategies. *Br J Community Nurs*. 2004; 9(11):464–470.

26. Iowa State University Extension. Needs Assessment Strategies for Community Groups And Organizations. Available at: http://www.extension.iastate.edu/communities/tools/assess. Accessed March 18, 2005.

27. World Health Organization. *Reproductive Health During Conflict and Displacement: A Guide for Programme Managers*. Geneva, Switzerland: 2000.

28. Hodges BC, Videto DM. *Assessment and Planning in Health Programs*. Sudbury, MA: Jones and Bartlett; 2005.

29. Gibson RS. *Principles of Nutritional Assessment*. 2nd ed. Dunedin, New Zealand: Oxford University Press; 2005.

30. Bogle M. Assessment of Community Nutrition and Health Needs in the Delta Nutrition Intervention Research Initiative. Available at: http://www.ars.usda.gov/research/publications/publications.htm?SEQ-NO_115=107940. Accessed March 20, 2005.

31. Yadrick K, Horton J, Stuff J, McGee B, et al. Perceptions of community nutrition and health needs in the lower Mississippi Delta: a key informant approach. *J Nutr Educ*. 2001; 33(5):266–277.

32. Bogle M. 2007 Annual Report. Available at: http://www.ars.usda.gov/research/projects/projects.htm?ACCN_NO=407644&showpars=true&fy=2007. Accessed April 4, 2008.

33. Thornton A. Demographic, social, and economic characteristics. In: Harrison G, ed. *Nutrition and Health Status in the Lower Mississippi Delta of Arkansas, Louisiana, and Mississippi: A Review of Existing Data*. Rockville, MD: Westat; 1997:9–23.

34. Smith J, Lensing S, Horton JA. Prevalence of self-reported nutrition-related health problems in the Lower Mississippi Delta. *Am J Public Health*. 1999; 89:1418–1421.

35. Berdanier CD, Feldman E, Flatt W. *Handbook of Nutrition and Food*. New York: CRC Press; 2002.

36. National Research Council Food and Nutrition Board. *Diet and Health: Implications for Reducing Chronic Disease Risk*. Washington, DC: National Academy Press; 1989.

37. Insel P, Turner RE, Ross D. *Nutrition*. 3rd ed. Sudbury, MA: Jones and Bartlett; 2007.

38. Centers for Disease Control and Prevention, National Center on Health Statistics. CDC Growth Charts: United States. Available at: http://www.cdc.gov/nchs/about/major/nhanes/growthcharts/charts.htm. Accessed September 2003.

39. Aziz S, Asim D, Kehkashan P. Anthropometric indices of middle socio-economic class school children in Karachi compared with NCHS standards—a pilot study. *J Pak Med Ass*. 2006; 56:264–267.

40. Boyle M. *Community Nutrition in Action: An Entrepreneurial Approach*. 4th ed. Belmont, CA: Thomson Wadsworth; 2005.

41. Bassali RW, Benjamin J. Failure to thrive. *eMedicine*. 2006. Available at: http://www.emedicine.com/PED/topic738.htm#section~author_information. Accessed February 6, 2008.

42. Lutz C, Przytulski K. *Nutrition and Diet Therapy*. 3rd ed. Philadelphia: F.A. Davis; 2001.

43. Burke BS. The dietary history as a tool in research. *J Am Diet Assoc*. 1947; 23:1041–1046.

44. Zulkifli SN, Yu SM. The food frequency method for dietary assessment. *J Am Diet Assoc*. 1992; 92:681–685.

45. Kretsch MJ, Fong AK. Validity and reproducibility of a new computerized dietary assessment method: effects of gender and educational level. *Nutr Res*. 1993; 13:133–146.

46. Lindquist CH, Cummings T, Goran MI. Use of tape-recorded food records in assessing children's dietary intake. *Obes Res*. 2000; 8:2–11.

47. Casey PH, Goolsby SL, Lensing SY, Perloff BP, Bogle ML. The use of telephone interview methodology to obtain 24-hour dietary recalls. *J Am Diet Assoc*. 1999; 99:1406–1411.

48. Institute of Medicine of the National Academies. *Dietary Reference Intakes*. Washington, DC: National Academies Press; 2003.

49. MacIntyre UE, Venter CS, Vorster HH. A culture-sensitive quantitative food frequency questionnaire used in an African population: Relative validation by 7-day weighted records and biomarkers. *Pub Health Nutr*. 2001; 4(1):63–71.

50. Anderson E, McFarlane J. *Community as Partner: Theory and Practice in Nursing*. 3rd ed. Philadelphia: Lippincott; 2000.

51. Coulston A, Rock C, Monsen E. *Nutrition in the Prevention and Treatment of Disease*. New York: Academic Press; 2001.

52. Field AE, Colditz GA, Fox MK, et al. Comparison of 4 questionnaires for assessment of fruit and vegetable intake. *Am J Pub Health* 1998; 88:1216–1218.

53. Means B, Habina K, Swan GE, et al. Cognitive research on response error in survey questions on smoking. *Vital Health Statistics.* DHHS Pub. No. PHS 92-1080. Washington, DC: Government Printing Office; 1992.

54. Block G, Hartman AM. Issues in reproducibility and validity of dietary studies. *Am J Clin Nutr.* 1989; 50:1133S–1138S.

55. Brener ND, Billy JO, Grady MA. Assessment of factors affecting the validity of self-reported health-risk behavior among adolescents: evidence from the scientific literature. *J Adolesc Health.* 2003; 33:436–457.

Nutrition Epidemiology and Research Methods

LEARNING OBJECTIVES

- Describe the stages of the research process.
- Explain ways in which community and public health nutritionists can participate in the research process.
- Define nutrition epidemiology.
- Discuss the different data collection methods.

Introduction

Community and public health nutrition research has increased over the years, but nutritionists must continue to increase the scientific knowledge base that is unique to their practice to provide high quality, scientifically oriented, evidence-based services and solutions to today's nutrition-related health conditions. *Community nutrition research* is defined as the "organized study of a trend at both the basic and more applied levels that focuses on social, structural, and physical environmental inequities through active involvement of community members, organizational representatives, and researchers in all aspects of the research process with the specific topics varying between investigators and the public."[1] Learning to conduct successful research and epidemiological studies is crucial to community nutrition.

Epidemiology is the study of the determinants, occurrence, and distribution of health and disease in a defined population.[2,3] It studies scien-tifically the factors that affect the health of individuals in the community and the public. It also serves as the foundation for intervention programs that use evidence-based information to address the prevention of health conditions.[2-4] Today, epidemiologists employ a range of study designs, from observational to experimental, with the purpose of revealing unbiased relationships between exposures (such as nutrition, biological agents, stress, or chemicals) to outcomes (such as diseases, wellness, and health indicators). Epidemiologic studies are usually categorized as:[3,5]

- Descriptive (organizing data by time, place, and person)
- Analytic (aiming to examine associations or commonly hypothesized causal relationships, and incorporating a case-control or cohort study)
- Experimental (clinical or community trials of treatments and other interventions)

community nutrition research
Organized study of a trend at both the basic and more applied levels that focuses on social, structural, and physical environmental inequities through active involvement of community members.

dependent variables Outcomes that are measured in an experiment.

independent variables Conditions of an experiment that are systematically manipulated by the investigator.

This chapter discusses the research process and epidemiologic studies in dietetic practice.

The Research Process

In community and public health nutrition, research, nutrition, and epidemiologic processes are used to solve health-related problems. These processes involve assessment, planning, implementation, evaluation, and action. The action stage involves a continuous assessment of the community's needs coupled with planning, implementation, and evaluation. The epidemiologic and research processes develop knowledge.[5] The nutrition process uses nutrition knowledge to provide nutrition-related services to individuals, families, groups, communities, and the public. The community nutritionist must consider several stages when planning or conducting nutrition research. These stages are presented in **Box 3-1**.

The research process requires a great deal of time and patience. Therefore, the researcher must first select the health problem that is important to the community and apply the problem to each stage of the research process. The researcher can start from the first stage (assessment/conceptual) and progress from stage to stage. Each stage must be consistent with the objective of the research project and all must reflect the total study. Sometimes the researcher may go back and forth among the different stages of the research process, but it is important to start with the first stage.

Assessment/Conceptual Stage

During the conceptual stage the researcher must translate the abstract concept into a measurable outcome. This stage is driven by the nutritionist's curiosity, interest, or the results of the community's needs assessment. It also stimulates or generates research questions that typically narrow the problem down to a more specific issue that must be

---

Box 3-1 Stages of the Research Process

Assessment/Conceptual Stage
- Identify and choose the problem/issue that is important to the community.
- Review related literature.
- Contact people in the field and discuss the problem with them.
- Identify available resources (personnel, equipment, data process capabilities, nutrient database, and other collaborative opportunities).
- Identify the purpose of the research (*what*, such as body weight, iron levels, calcium levels, or sodium intake).
- Determine the direct and indirect costs for conducting the research.
- Choose the population to be studied.

Planning/Designing Stage
- State the research problem (*who*, such as gender, age, or ethnicity).
- Continue the review of related literature.
- Select an appropriate theoretical framework.
- Select a research design and appropriate methodology (*how*, such as alterations in food selection, physical activity level, or eating habits).
- Design the data collection plan (*when*, such as the starting and ending of the research).
- Select appropriate statistical methods and data analysis methods.
- Finalize and review the research plan.

- Implement the human subject approval process obtained from the local institutional review board, or boards can be included to support the research study.
- Implement pilot studies and revisions in design. (The results from the pilot studies may be used to support an application for funding for the study.)

Implementation/Empirical Stage
- Invite/select community members to participate (key informants, focus group, community forum, etc.).
- Implement the data collection plan (collected by questionnaire using 24-hour recall or food frequency checklist, interviews, physical examination such as anthropometric measurements, and laboratory evaluation such as blood for iron status, bone density measurement, and blood pressure measurement).
- Prepare data for analysis. (If unavoidable, only minimal necessary individually identifiable information should be used.)

Evaluation/Analytical Stage
- Analyze the data using the appropriate statistical method.
- Interpret the results. (Consider limitations to the study methodology such as low response rate.)
- Draw conclusions.

Action/Dissemination Stage
- Present the research findings to the target community.
- Use the results in practice (nutrition education programs).
- Present the results to the funding agency, if applicable.

Modified from: Stanhope M, Lancaster J. *Community and Public Health Nursing.* 5th ed. New York: Mosby; 2000. Reprinted with permission.

addressed.[6] For example, a nutritionist may wonder why some African American older persons experience high rates of hypertension. The nutritionist would then critically review related research literature to gain more knowledge of the nutrition problem and how the results from the various studies relate to the nutrition problem. It is important for the nutritionist to evaluate the quality of the literature being reviewed—for example, the appropriateness of the methodology used. It is also important to note that in some situations the concept for the research study may not have been tested in published literature.

This initial literature review helps the nutritionist select a hypothesis/purpose and scope for the study. In the example given, the nutritionist would have learned from the review of literature that high sodium intake and obesity are linked to hypertension in some individuals.[7] The hypothesis then could be stated in this way: There will be a significant decrease in the sodium, fat, and caloric intake of those African American older persons in a particular community who participate in a nutrition intervention program. Another example of a community-based research study might be to increase bone density in postmenopausal women. The hypothesis could be that there will be a significant increase in the level of physical activity and the intake of calcium and vitamin D for postmenopausal women employees in 10 worksites who received a nutrition intervention program, compared with postmenopausal women employees in 10 (control) worksites who did not receive the intervention program.

Once the research question (hypothesis) has been developed, the next step is to clearly define the characteristics of the study population. For example, the study population may include older African American people in a particular community, or postmenopausal women of different ethnic backgrounds within a specific age range who live in a specified geographic area served by a particular community or public health agency. Strategies for collecting the data will vary with the community and the health issues to be addressed. Some suggested strategies that have been successfully used include community surveys (both self-administered and assisted questionnaires), focus groups, direct interviews, community forums, and collection of health services data.[8,9]

Planning/Designing Stage

After the researcher has reviewed the related literature and determined the purpose, scope, and characteristics of the study, he or she needs to plan/design the study. Planning is a logical, organized process that proceeds step by step. It involves determining the procedure for collecting the data, and making the concept of the study clear to the community, staff, and funding agency. In the planning stage, the specific research focus is stated and important terms are defined.[5,10]

Designing a research project for the community is a problem-solving process. After the nutritionist has conducted the community needs assessment, he or she selects the most pressing nutrition problem for the study and decides on a methodology consistent with the research question. The researcher can use the information obtained from the literature review to define terms and to develop a scientific body of knowledge for the research study.

The nutritionist must also select a theoretical framework that is appropriate for the problem to be investigated. In the fictitious examples provided earlier, the nutritionist could select the Health Belief Model, which can be used for an intervention for persons with clinical nutrition–related risk factors, such as cardiovascular disease, hypertension, or osteoporosis.[11-13] Such individuals are faced with important and often overriding concerns about health. However, the Health Belief Model is of limited use for studies on subjects such as the primary prevention of cancer.[14] See Chapter 12 for details on the Health Belief Model and other models.

After selecting the theoretical framework, the nutritionist determines the important variables of the study, such as the **dependent** and **independent variables**. A variable is a characteristic of a person, object, or phenomenon that can take on different values.[15] These may be in the form of numbers (e.g., age, weight, height, income) or non-numerical characteristics (e.g., gender, ethnicity, religion, and geographical location). Dependent variables are the outcomes that are measured in an experiment. They are expected to change as a result of an experimental manipulation of the independent variable(s). Independent variables are the conditions of an experiment that are methodically manipulated by the investigator. The state of the problem and the objective of the study determine whether a variable is dependent or independent. Therefore, when designing a research study, it is important to state which variable is the dependent and which is the independent.

Another variable to consider is the confounding variable. A variable that is associated with a health problem and with a possible cause of the problem (e.g., cigarette smoking causes cancer) may be a confounding variable.[16] Confounding variables may strengthen or weaken the relationship between the health problem being studied and the potential cause. For example, a confounding variable may influence the outcome of a research study. **Figure 3-1** presents dependent, independent, and confounding variables. The figure shows the relationship between bottle-feeding and diarrhea in infants, but a confounding variable (such as the mother's level of education, income, or age) may be related to bottle-feeding and diarrhea. Therefore, the mother's education level, income, and age should be considered in determining the cause of diarrhea. The researcher may consider this variable in the research design (for example, selecting only mothers with a specific level of education, income, and age) or separate mothers according to education level, income, and age during data analysis to determine the relationship between bottle-feeding and the incidence of diarrhea.[16,17]

After determining the variables for the study, the nutritionist next selects a research procedure that is appropriate to the incident being investigated. The technique may be historical, observational, surveys, or experimental. The researcher must consider the different requirements a research design creates, determine whether the data will be collected at one point in time or longitudinally, and whether the data will be collected from a single group or across various groups in the population. The nutritionist may decide that a survey is the most appropriate procedure for investigating the dietary habits and intervention studies because it permits collecting data during one time period.

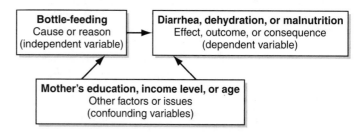

FIGURE 3-1 Examples of Dependent, Independent, and Confounding Variables

Source: Varkevisser CM, Brownlee B. *Designing and Conducting Health System Research*. International Development Research Center. Ottawa, Canada: World Health Organization; 2003. Reprinted with permission.

Considering Methodologies

The researcher also should consider the methodologies appropriate to the research question. Quantitative methods have been the standard methodology used in nutrition research because they depend on isolation of one or more variables that can be measured and analyzed statistically. In quantitative (objective) research, random sample surveys and structured interviews are used to collect mostly quantifiable data that are analyzed using statistical techniques. This method promotes gathering data that can be verified by another researcher and generalized to other populations. Deductive reasoning, objectivity, quasi-experiments, statistical techniques, and control characterize these methods.[10]

Although many nutrition research questions are open to traditional methodologies, others require a different approach. There is a growing acceptance of nutrition science as a composite of different viewpoints and varied research methodologies.[10,18] Although recognition of qualitative (subjective) methods for scientific study is relatively recent in nutrition literature, they began to be used in the United States during the late 1800s.[5] Qualitative strategies were used to reveal the rapidly developing social problems in cities at that time caused by industrialization, urbanization, and mass immigration. Munhall and Boyd stated that qualitative descriptions encouraged social change by making urban problems visible to the public.[19]

Qualitative methods may be more beneficial for a particular incident being studied. For example, qualitative approaches are rarely appropriate in genetic engineering but may be appropriate when analyzing a social behavior, such as food choice and dieting. They use semistructured or interactive interviews to collect data relating to people's judgments, attitudes, preferences, priorities, and/or a perception about the nutrition issue; the data are then analyzed through sociological or anthropological research techniques. Inductive reasoning, subjectivity, discovery, description, and the meaning of an experience to an individual or groups typify qualitative methods.[20]

Both quantitative and qualitative data collection methods can be combined in a single research study. For example, adding subjective and open-ended questions to a standard household survey could provide a better approach to defining and measuring poverty.[21] The use of mixed methods will increase as the ability to acquire and analyze large amounts of quantitative data improves along with improvements in electronic technologies. For example, it is now possible to measure and record in an accessible database every step and movement made by an individual, as well as every word he or she speaks and hears.[18]

Selecting a Data-Gathering Method

Once the researcher has considered the preferred methodology, the next stage involves selecting a data-gathering method, such as observing, measuring, or interviewing. The researcher should identify specific techniques or instruments that are consistent with the research design. For example, if a questionnaire is considered for data collection, a specific instrument can be selected, such as a food frequency questionnaire, 24-hour recall, or 3-day food record (see Chapter 2).

Because decisions need to be made about a data-gathering method for each of the major variables in the research study, the researcher may decide to use more than one instrument. In the examples described previously about investigating Afri-

random sampling When every case or participant has an equal opportunity to be included in a study.

deliberate sampling Inviting specific people to participate in a study.

can American sodium and caloric intake and increasing postmenopausal women's calcium and vitamin D intake, the researcher may decide to use both focus groups and interviewing methods. An interview (using 24-hour recall or a food frequency checklist) may be used to determine the nutrient intake and eating habits of these individuals.

The research questions and methodologies chosen must guide the plan for data analysis. It is helpful to identify the computer software that will assist with data analysis and decide how results will be presented. For example, the researcher may want to prepare tables for the data once they are collected. These tables will help ensure that all the data necessary for answering the research questions have been collected.

The research questions and plan for data analysis will guide sample selection and size. There are many methods of sample selection, but two will be considered here: random and deliberate sampling. **Random sampling** means that every case or participant has an equal opportunity to be included in the study.[5] For example, first the target group or community is informed about the research study's purpose/aim as well as its risks, and is asked to participate. Then, individuals consenting to participate in the study are assigned randomly to one, two, or more treatment or intervention groups. The individuals randomized to receive the standard intervention treatment serve as the control group. The main factor is random assignment; that is, chance determines the intervention assignment. **Deliberate sampling** means that specific target groups or communities are invited to participate in the study.[5] The choice of research methodologies will determine the characteristics of the sample population.

After consultation with a statistician, the researcher determines the factors, such as the sample size, gender, and age range. The researcher may use power analysis software that can help determine sample size. Most of the time, it is impossible to know the exact number of people living in the community being studied, so the nutritionist may estimate the total population based on census data.

Protecting the Subjects and Researcher

An important aspect of the design phase is research approval by the institutional review board (IRB). IRBs are groups of representatives of various related disciplines or departments organized to review research proposals. Their major concerns are protecting human research participants from physical or mental harm and protecting the researcher from unnecessary complaints. This process also satisfies a number of funding agencies and federal, state, and institutional regulations. If the research is being conducted in a university setting, every university has a committee that reviews research proposals involving health services.

The nutritionist must obtain approval from the committee before the research begins. The first step is to communicate clearly to the review committee, in writing, what is planned, how participants will be involved in the research, and whether their participation will put them at risk for physical or mental harm. The researcher is ethically responsible for carrying out these plans as directed or approved by the committee. Changes that occur in the plans need to be reported to the committee for further authorization. In situations where there is no existing institutional review board, a committee should be organized, consisting of experts in the area of the research study who will review and approve the research design before data collection begins.

Performing a Pilot Study

Pilot studies can be used to test data-gathering methods and to verify the data analysis plan. A pilot study is very important when the data-gathering technique is unfamiliar to the researcher or has not been used by other researchers. It is also necessary when the instrument is new or has not been used with the population that is being studied, or when the study is being conducted in an unfamiliar environment.[5] In addition, the data and results obtained from the pilot study can be used to increase support and funding for a major research project.

In the fictitious example using African American older persons, the researcher might decide to pilot test the study with 20 older African Americans from a neighboring county, after obtaining permission from both the IRB and the participants.

Next, the assumptions and limitations of research need to be identified. *Assumptions* are characteristics of the research situation that will not be explored in the study.[5] The assumption may be determined from the findings in the literature the researcher reviewed. For example, in the fictitious scenario, it is assumed that some older African Americans are consuming foods high in sodium. *Limitations* are unmanageable elements of the research study. These elements limit the certainty of the findings or their applicability to the population in general. In the fictitious examples, a limitation is that deliberate sampling does not ensure that all older African American persons or postmenopausal women are equally represented. As a result, the study findings may not be applicable beyond the study sample.

Implementation/Empirical Stage

The implementation phase of the research plan is when the researcher actually carries out the research procedures. The researcher must comply with the objectives or the hypothesis of the project and must invest enough time to obtain longitudinal data and breadth of information. The implementation stage includes carrying out the following activities:[5,22]

- Inviting the sample group or community members to participate in the project/research
- Obtaining informed consent from the participants
- Collecting and verifying the data
- Analyzing the data

The researcher may recruit participants by sending a letter of invitation to potential participants, composing a radio announcement, or providing information to churches, local community centers, schools, men's and women's associations, and so on. Many factors can affect the recruitment process, such as the sample size, exclusion criteria for participation, perceived benefits, length of the study, and location of the study.[10,23]

After the participants have been recruited, the next step is to obtain informed consent for participation in the study. The researcher and the participants must sign consent forms after a detailed explanation of the research protocol.

The nutritionist then collects data using focus groups and interviews or any other appropriate method. Information collected in qualitative studies is validated with participants by analyzing the results for completeness. If the method is qualitative, the nutritionist may carry out the data analysis concomitantly with data collection. If the method is quantitative, analysis would be performed at the conclusion of the data collection phase.

Regardless of the type of method utilized for the study, the researcher must consider several data collection and analysis guidelines that must be observed throughout the study period. These include, but are not limited to:[19,23,24]

- *Awareness:* The researcher and the staff must understand the guidelines of all methodologies used.
- *Management plan:* This should include the responsibilities of each staff member, contingency plans, a written work plan that includes specific objectives, action plan, and a time line. A regular meeting schedule also must be established.
- *Recruitment and retention goal:* The researcher must make a significant effort to meet the targeted sample size, and must have a retention strategy in place (such as follow-up telephone calls, continuous social support, conducting raffles, paying attention to details, making the study area comfortable, etc.).
- *Data collection:* The researcher needs to gather data from all the participants at the appropriate times.
- *Re-examining the procedures:* The researcher needs to make sure the data collection procedure corresponded with the research objective(s).

Evaluation/Analytical Stage

In the evaluation stage, the researcher analyzes the data collected during the implementation stage. The researcher must familiarize him- or herself with the data through repeated reading and listening to the staff and study participants. Evaluation methods can vary greatly depending on the theoretical focus (i.e., qualitative or quantitative research) and methods. This stage includes:[23,24]

- Coordinating and coding the collected data
- Transcribing interviews and other material
- Choosing a data entry and analysis program (e.g., the Statistical Package for the Social Sciences [SPSS] available at http://www.spss.com)
- Reviewing data (e.g., surveys, questionnaires) for completeness
- Entering the data into a secured computer for statistical analysis
- Controlling access to the data to ensure confidentiality
- Storing the data in a secured area using a consistent method for storage

The last step of data analysis consists of interpreting and comparing the results with previous research, seeing whether the findings support the research study's hypotheses, theory, or research questions, and then drawing conclusions. The researcher then writes a report to present the findings. A research report is a carefully structured piece that clearly states the purpose, findings, relevance, and implications of the research activity.[24] Research reports should provide clear documentation of what, how, why, and when the study was conducted. A combination of visual and literary description will help make the information presented precise. The researcher must include all the findings. Hypotheses that were not supported also need to be reported. Within the report, the researcher should make recommendations for further research that is consistent with the findings of the research study. The researcher also may indicate whether there is a need to replicate the study with other populations or communities.

Action/Dissemination Stage

The results of nutrition research should be used in practice. The research findings must be presented to as wide a range of people as possible, such as in professional journals and to professional colleagues at their annual meeting; to persons in decision-making positions such as administrators, policy makers, and legislators; and even to reporters for articles in a local newspaper. Consistent with primary healthcare and health promotion approaches, relevant research findings must also be reported to community groups. This information can become part of the community's educational experience and can help the community make appropriate decisions based on local needs.[5,24] The nutritionist must make specific recommendations for improving the health of the community based on the research findings.

Reporting the results of research outcomes in professional journals and at professional meetings facilitates the growth and use of nutrition knowledge. By applying research results, nutritionists can institute social change. Policy makers, other professionals, and the community would learn that the research findings are relevant and applicable. The results of a study involving the community could support the expansion of community or public health nutrition services. The nutrition profession is in urgent need of research documenting the cost effectiveness of nutrition care. Effectiveness, however, can be measured in many ways beyond cost, including quality of care, client satisfaction, and the ability for a person to maintain independence.[25]

Concepts of Collaborative Research

Collaboration involves mutual participation in decision making and working with others toward a common goal. It is a process of joint decision making in an atmosphere of shared respect and cooperation.[26] Collaboration should always involve interaction among community nutritionists, clients, and other healthcare practitioners. Nutrition professionals work as members of a team in all healthcare settings. In community nutrition settings, the nutritionist is part of a multidisciplinary team that includes other healthcare workers as well as community organizations, social service agencies, and the judicial system. The multidisciplinary team can conduct research studies that can benefit the public. The need for collaborative research is especially strong now due to the prevalence of health disparities in the United States. In addition, there is a belief that partnerships between researchers and community members can contribute not only to the ability of communities to effectively address local issues, but also to the development of new knowledge.[27–29]

Successful collaboration requires that the multidisciplinary team develop a common purpose, communicate to coordinate efforts, and recognize the unique and complementary skills possessed by each team member. Each team member brings special abilities and expertise to the collaborative process. Collaboration does not work when one team member designs a research project or nutrition program and then "coordinates" by informing others of the plan. For a nutrition program or research to be successful, collaboration must be a joint effort on the part of the clients and all team members in order to identify mutual goals and acceptable means for meeting those goals.[30]

collaboration Working with others toward a common goal.

coordination Efficient management of services without gaps or overlaps.

demography An analytic tool used to measure a population by recording births, deaths, age distribution, and other vital statistics.

Although they do share some similarities, collaboration and *coordination* are different. Coordination is the act of managing interdependencies between activities. It is the ability to manage services without gaps or overlaps.[31] The nutritionist, as coordinator, may or may not consult others when carrying out a management function. Collaboration, on the other hand, involves joint decision making between two or more people.

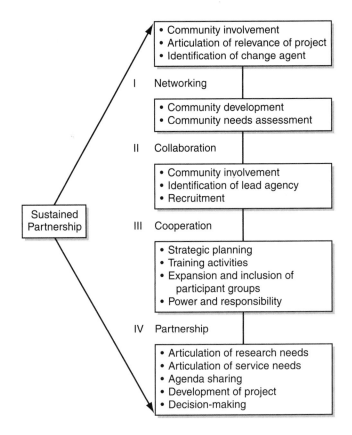

FIGURE 3-2 The Four Phases of Collaborative Development

Source: Amuwo S, Jenkins E. True partnership evolves over time. In: Sullivan M, James K (eds.). *Collaborative Research: University and Community Partnership.* Washington, DC: American Public Health Association; 2001: 25–43. Reprinted with permission.

Collaboration also can enhance the opportunity for obtaining grant money. Some granting agencies encourage collaborative efforts. A community nutritionist can collaborate with statisticians, epidemiologists, nurses, social workers, physicians, and colleagues to complement his or her nutrition expertise.[10] Collaboration is especially helpful for a new university faculty member, first-time grant seeker, or a nutritionist who wants to change his or her focus area of research. Community nutritionists can find collaborators by networking with colleagues and community members, and communicating with other professionals or experts in the area of interest.

Amuwo and Jenkins outlined four distinct phases necessary for successful partnership building in community-based research, based on their experiences with collaborative work: networking, cooperation, collaboration, and partnership (see **Figure 3-2**).[32] Within these four phases, they identified 12 concrete, systematic steps that a partnership-building effort must complete in a rather sequential order:[32]

1. Involve the community early so they can see the importance of the program.
2. Be aware that partnership building is a nonlinear procedure.
3. Recruit and empower important community-based personnel.
4. Conduct a community needs assessment (both human and capital resources).
5. Recognize that other grassroots community organizations are potential partners.

6. Recruit community-based staff.
7. Engage in strategic planning.
8. Meet training needs.
9. Involve other relevant community members, public institutions, and organizations.
10. Communicate and pursue research and service agendas at the community level.
11. Facilitate the transfer of knowledge.
12. Maintain trusting and collaborative relationships.

Epidemiology in Community Health

Epidemiologic and demographic measures and research methods are used to study health-related conditions. For example, they are used to investigate outbreaks of food poisoning, chickenpox, measles, and acquired immunodeficiency syndrome (AIDS). They are also used to investigate environmental conditions, lifestyles, health-promotion strategies, and other factors that affect health.[15]

The science of epidemiology is important to community and public health nutritionists because it can be utilized to assess and understand health, diseases, and injury in a community or target population. Epidemiology is a population-focused applied science that uses research and a statistical data collection methodology to determine the following:[33]

- The population that is affected by a disease or disorder
- The incidence or prevalence of a health problem in the community
- The likelihood the causes and risk factors contributing to the health problem may or may not be determined

Descriptive Measures of Community Health

Descriptive epidemiologic studies explain the occurrence of disease and are collected using various methods. The data are then assembled based on time (e.g., changes of eating habits over a long period of time), place (geographic areas), and person (e.g., age, gender, ethnicity, lifestyle).[5,34] These data can be used to quantify the extent and location of nutrition problems within a population and to suggest associations between diet and disease that can be evaluated in analytic research.[10]

Demographic Measures

Demography is an analytic tool used to measure a population by recording births, deaths, age distribution, and other vital statistics.[15,33] Some human characteristics, or demographics, may be associated with wellness or illness. Age, race, gender, ethnicity, income, and educational level are important demographics that may affect health outcomes. For example, men are more likely than women to develop certain heart diseases, and African Americans are more likely than European Americans to experience hypertension.[35–37] Community nutritionists must be familiar with the demographic characteristics of the community they serve and with the health problems associated with that community before developing a health promotion program.

Morbidity and Mortality

Epidemiology studies both wellness and illness. Wellness is hard to measure; therefore, the measures of health are expressed in terms of morbidity (illness) and mortality (death).[15] The Centers for Disease Control and Prevention (CDC)'s website (http://ww.cdc.gov) is an excellent source of morbidity and mortality data organized by states and for select cities.[38]

Incidence and Prevalence

Two types of disease frequency measures are used to determine the morbidity rate in a defined population—incidence and prevalence. *Incidence* is the rate of acquisition of a new health condition or the number of persons in a defined population who developed the condition during a specified period of time.[15] The calculation of incidence, therefore, requires that a population be followed over a period of time in what is called a prospective or cohort (forward-looking) study.[34]

On the other hand, *prevalence* is the total number of persons in the defined population who are affected by a certain disease or condition at a specified time. This includes both new and existing cases.[10] Therefore, prevalence may be calculated in a "one-shot" cross-sectional ("slice of time") or retrospective (backward-looking) study.[15]

Interpretation of Incidence and Prevalence

In both incidence and prevalence, it is important to clearly define the condition being studied; otherwise, scientists may make a mistake in differentiating between incidence (new cases) and prevalence.[39,40] Scientists must allow enough time to identify new cases to determine incidence and prevalence. This period of time must be long enough to adequately detect the condition, especially in the case of rare diseases or diseases with a low rate of diagnosis. However, the time period cannot be so long that it will be affected by mortality and other follow-up losses.[41]

Measures of incidence and prevalence provide different information and have different implications. For example, an increase in the prevalence of diabetes or endometrial cancer means that there are more persons with these health conditions in the population. This may be due to more new cases (in other words, increased incidence) or because individuals with these health conditions are living longer. In either case, the community may need to direct resources toward treating the problem. However, if knowledge of incidence is lacking, it will be difficult to decide whether to target the resources toward primary prevention or toward secondary and tertiary treatment services.

Here is a specific example of differentiating incidence from prevalence. In a community health center, 120 infants free from measles are followed for 3 weeks. In this period of time, 45 developed measles. Remember, incidence gives an approximation of the likelihood (or risk) that a client will develop a particular health condition during a specified period of time. Therefore, there is an incidence rate of 45 per 120 (or 37.5 percent) during the 3-week period. However, prevalence computes the proportion of a given population with the problem. So at the same community health center, 150 infants were screened for the presence of measles and 30 infants were affected. This results in a prevalence of measles of 20 percent (30 ÷ 150). In this case, prevalence means the proportion of infants with the problem (for example, measles) at the specified period.[42] The formulas for calculating both are in **Box 3-2**.

Rates

The mathematical measures that are used to articulate incidence and prevalence are known as *rates*. Epidemiologic studies must relate the occurrence of a health condition to the population base. Rates express a mathematical relationship in which the numerator is the number of persons experiencing the condition and the denominator is the population at risk, or the total number of persons who have the possibility of experiencing the condition. The formula for calculating rate is shown in the following section.[15] Epidemiologists use rates to examine the experience of particular groups of people at specified times, in different cities or countries. Another important use of rates is in calculating

---

Box 3-2 The Formulas for Both Prevalence and Incidence

Incidence: Number of new cases during a specified period _____
              Total number of a defined population at risk at the time _____

Prevalence: Number of both existing and new cases during a specified period _____
              Total number of a defined population at risk _____

---

the risks to individuals and groups of experiencing an event such as a heart attack or an occurrence such as cancer or obesity.

Example of a Rate

In the United States, an acceptable definition for infant mortality rate (IMR) is the number of deaths during the first year of life (i.e., the number of both neonatal and postneonatal deaths) per 1,000 live births. To calculate IMR, add the number of neonatal (the first 28 days of life) and postneonatal (between the 28th and 365th days of life) deaths and divide by the number of live births; then, multiply the result by 1,000. The numerator represents the number of infants experiencing the "condition" of dying in the first year of life, and the denominator represents the population of infants at risk of dying in that year.[15,43]

If 500,000 live births and 10,000 infant deaths were reported in the United States for a given year, the rate can be calculated as follows:[15]

1. Infant mortality rate = $\dfrac{\text{Number of infant deaths (age} < 1 \text{ year) during time interval}}{\text{Total live births during time interval}} \times 1,000$

2. Divide 10,000 by 500,000 = 0.020 of the infants died during the first year of life.

3. Because it is difficult to relate to 0.020 infants, multiply 0.020 by a constant, in this case 1,000, resulting in 20 infants who died during the first year of life per 1,000 live births. This means that the infant mortality rate was 20 infant deaths per 1,000 live births for that year.

Interpretation of Rates

International comparisons and rankings of infant mortality should be interpreted with caution. For example, a study investigated how infant mortality rates are reported in the United States, Norway, and Israel. Results showed that the United States reported live births less than 750 g while other countries did not report live births less than 750 g. Disparities among countries resulted from differences in birth and death registration practices.[44]

Also, to determine if the population in a specific community is at greater or lesser risk for a condition, the research must compare the rates for the community with rates from similar communities, the state,

or the country. Most often rates are based on data from a calendar year, which may create some problems. When calculating an infant mortality rate, it is important to recognize that some of the infants who die during a given calendar year may not be a part of the demographics, such as those who died in 2005 but who were actually born in 2004 and thus were not part of the 2005 population at risk. Also, some of the infants who were born in 2005 might die in 2006 and not be reflected in the 2005 infant mortality rate.[15] A cohort research study (discussed below) can help overcome the limitations of the conventionally calculated calendar year rate.[45]

The Epidemiologic Methods

Epidemiologic research methods can be descriptive, analytic, or experimental. Although all can be used in studying the occurrence of disease, the method used most often is descriptive epidemiology. Once the basic epidemiology of disease has been described, analytic methods can be used to study the disease further, and an experimental approach can be developed to test a hypothesis.[3]

In epidemiologic studies, the investigator attempts to identify risk factors for particular diseases, conditions, behaviors, or risks that result from particular causes, such as environmental or industrial agents.[46,47] Epidemiology uses different methods—such as statistical, pathological, clinical, demographic, microbiological, and sociological—to study disease processes. These are not exclusive to epidemiology; however, the ways in which they are used distinctively define the epidemiologic method.[10] The following example uses the investigation of the diet-disease hypothesis to show the scientific approach of epidemiologists.

Observation

There are many instances of disease control based on epidemiologic observations. In an observational study (descriptive method), the investigators observe the behaviors of participants without interfering. For example, epidemiologic researchers observed consistently that vegetarian groups in the United States and overseas have lower blood pressure than nonvegetarians in most of the studies. The term *vegetarian* includes several heterogeneous groups, but in general, vegetarian diets are usually high in whole grains, beans, fruits, and vegetables, and sometimes fish, dairy products, and eggs. The aspects of the vegetarian diet that have been observed to be protective against hypertension include low intake of animal products and high intake of potassium, magnesium, fiber, and (sometimes) calcium.[48]

Counting Cases or Events

Counting cases is a descriptive epidemiologic method that is sometimes useful for health policy. It can be used to know the number of people with a particular characteristic or number of events that occurred in a given region or community. For example, the migration studies of indigenous populations showed that the prevalence of hypertension increased because of urbanization. With urbanization, people consumed more processed foods and less fresh foods (that were previously available). In addition, researchers observed lifestyle changes (e.g., lack of physical activity, overeating) that caused increases in body weight, sodium intake, and dietary fat during the process of acculturation.[49]

Relating Cases or Events to Population at Risk

Inherent in the epidemiological method is the need for measuring the number of disease cases or events in a population and relating the number of cases to a population base. Cases that fit the case description are identified, counted, and correlated to time, place, and individuals. In reviewing 53 observational studies of calcium and hypertension, 5 studies were prospective and 48 were cross-sectional, of which 4 also contained a longitudinal component. Various dietary methodologies were used; the most common was the 24-hour dietary recall. Most studies controlled for age, sex, and body mass index, with variable control for other confounding variables.[50] All together, these studies showed only modest associations between calcium and blood pressure. But in the beginning, the higher calcium and magnesium content of "hard" water, and its relation to cardiovascular mortality, triggered epidemiologic inquiry into the relationship of both minerals to blood pressure.[51]

Making Comparisons

Another scientific approach epidemiologists use is making comparisons. The Dietary Approaches to Stop Hypertension (DASH) sodium multicenter trial, for example, was created to resolve the controversy surrounding sodium intake and blood pressure.[52] The effect of dietary composition on blood pressure is an important public health topic. The National Heart Lung and Blood Institute funded the DASH study, which compared the effects of three sodium levels on blood pressure versus a control. The subjects were asked to eat either a control diet typical of intake in the United States or the DASH diet, a diet rich in fruits, vegetables, and low-fat dairy foods; low in saturated fat, total fat, and cholesterol; high in dietary fiber, potassium, calcium, and magnesium; and moderately high in protein. Within each diet (control and DASH), subjects ate foods with high, intermediate, and low levels of sodium. The investigators found that reducing the sodium intake from the high to the intermediate level reduced systolic blood pressure by 2.1 mm Hg.[52,53] Reducing the sodium intake from the intermediate to the low level caused additional reductions of 4.6 mm Hg on the control diet and 1.7 mm Hg on the DASH diet. The effects of sodium intake were observed in those subjects with and without hypertension, all races, and both women and men. Compared to the control diet with the highest sodium level, the DASH diet with the lowest sodium level reduced systolic blood pressure by 8.9 mm Hg in subjects with hypertension and 7.1 mm Hg in those without hypertension.[52]

In another comparative study, the European Prospective Investigation into Cancer and Nutrition (EPIC) study recruited 20,343 participants for a cohort study. The participants had no hypertension. The investigators examined whether the Mediterranean diet (see the feature in this chapter Successful Community Strategies), and olive oil in particular, can reduce blood pressure. Results showed that intakes of olive oil, vegetables, and fruit were associated with a reduction in blood pressure whereas intakes of cereals, meat and meat products, and alcohol were associated with higher blood pressure.[54]

Developing the Hypothesis

The hypothesis or research question is an assumption written in a clear, concise manner about what the investigator thinks will happen in the research project. For example, after reviewing the results of the migration studies and the vegetarian group's studies in the United States, researchers developed the hypothesis that diets low in sodium and high in fruits, vegetables, and fiber can reduce blood pressure.

Testing the Hypothesis

In testing the hypothesis, research observations have shown a direct relationship between higher sodium intake and higher blood pressure

across population groups.[55-58] The INTERSALT study (International Study of Salt) measured the relationship between 24-hour urinary sodium excretion and blood pressure in 10,079 men and women from 52 centers around the world.[55] Results showed a positive relationship between mean urinary sodium excretion and blood pressure; that is, the participant's blood pressure increased with an increase in sodium excretion. A slight positive relationship also was observed when the researchers adjusted for alcohol and body mass index. The researchers also reported a strong positive relationship between sodium intake and the slope of blood pressure increase with age across populations, indicating a role for sodium in age-related blood pressure increase.

In a recent reanalysis of the original INTERSALT data, corrected for measurement error due to the use of single 24-hour urine collections, results were stronger: a 100 mmol/day (2,300 mg sodium) increase in urinary sodium was associated with an increase of 3–6 mm Hg in systolic blood pressure and of 0–3 mm Hg diastolic blood pressure.[55,58] In a meta-analysis of observational studies, Law et al.[59] reported stronger results than INTERSALT, especially in the elderly and those with higher baseline blood pressures, but diet and other variables were not assessed in a standard manner across studies.[56]

Drawing Scientific Inferences

The data showing that diet modification can prevent and lower blood pressure is significant. The intervention approaches and methods involved in some data collection are still being clarified. Because of a variety of research design limitations, inadequate statistical power, and measurement issues, studies of single nutrients (except for potassium) have mainly been inconsistent.[60] However, when several nutrients, lifestyle, or dietary factors are combined in the same intervention studies, as in the DASH study, blood pressure was effectively reduced.[61] It has been shown that nutrients have interactive effects when they are consumed together in a diet.[62] In addition to the DASH dietary pattern, other factors such as reduced sodium intake, weight loss, and moderate alcohol intake have been shown to reduce blood pressure. Simultaneous observance of several recommendations (as with the DASH diet) is likely to be the best strategy for preventing and lowering blood pressure. Future research should center on methods to motivate and maintain dietary changes for controlling blood pressure, plus address the unanswered nutritional hypotheses.

The implication of these findings is that the success of dietary intervention depends on support from clinicians, government agencies, private institutes, and industries at both the population and individual levels. In particular, industries can improve the nutritional value of the food supply, such as reducing the sodium and fat content of processed foods; this is a very critical role in implementing dietary changes. Dietetic and other healthcare professionals must also play a significant role in educating the public and promoting adherence to nutritional guidelines for the prevention of hypertension and other health conditions.[56,63]

Conducting Experimental Studies

Another scientific approach that epidemiologists use is conducting experimental studies. One such study examined the effects on blood pressure of long-term substitution of dietary sucrose for cornstarch in semisynthetic diets containing 60 percent carbohydrate in spontaneously hypertensive rats (SHR). Four diets were initiated when the SHR were 8–9 weeks of age. A total of 32 SHR were placed on normal (0.08

percent NaCl) or high-sodium diets (0.2 percent NaCl). Each sodium group was further subdivided into two groups—one group ingested 60 percent sucrose and the other 0 percent sucrose (60 percent cornstarch). Blood pressure and weight were measured at 1- to 2-month intervals for 17 weeks. No differences were found in blood pressure between either sodium group.[63]

In an analytical research design, the aim is to evaluate hypotheses based on existing knowledge or findings. The DASH trial, discussed earlier, was a randomized, multicenter, controlled feeding study to compare the effects of three dietary patterns on blood pressure. The control group consumed fruits and vegetables and a combination diet (having less total fat, less saturated fat, and less cholesterol than the fruit and vegetable diet or the control diet). The dietary patterns differed in selected nutrients hypothesized to alter blood pressure. This study examined the food-group structure and nutrient composition of the study diets and participants' nutrient consumption during the intervention. Participants consumed the control dietary pattern during a 3-week start-up period. They were then randomized either to continue on the control diet or to change to the fruits and vegetables or the combination diet for 8 weeks. Sodium intake and body weight were constant during the entire feeding period. Analysis of variance models compared the nutrient content of the three diets.

Targeting a few nutrients thought to influence blood pressure resulted in diets that were very different in their food-group and nutrient composition. The control and fruits and vegetables diets contained more oils, table fats, salad dressings, and red meats and were higher in saturated fat, total fat, and cholesterol than was the combination diet. The fruits and vegetables and combination diets contained relatively more servings of fruits, juices, vegetables, and nuts/seeds, and were higher in magnesium, potassium, and fiber than was the control diet. Both the fruits and vegetables and combination diets were low in sweets and sugar-containing drinks. The combination diet contained a greater variety of fruits, and its high calcium content was obtained by increasing low-fat dairy products. In addition, the distinct food-grouping pattern across the three diets resulted in substantial differences in the levels of vitamins A, B_6, C, and E; folate; and zinc.[64]

Figure 3-3 presents examples of the scientific method used by epidemiologists.

Epidemiologic Approaches to Community Health Assessment

The changing disease patterns throughout the world are linked to changing lifestyles. One of the functions of epidemiologic approaches is to determine the etiology or cause of the disease or risk factors for the disease. One way that epidemiologists study the cause and effect of disease is through a three-sided conceptual model known as the epidemiologic triangle.[5] This model explains how changes in one element can influence the occurrence of a disease by increasing or decreasing an individual's risk for the health condition.

The Epidemiologic Triangle

The epidemiologic triangle explores health and disease using three elements: an agent, a host, and an environment (each of which is discussed below). All three of the components of this model are of equal strength. **Figure 3-4** shows the model in its normal state of equilibrium. Equilibrium does not mean optimal health, but it does signal the usual patterns of illness and health in a population. Any change in one of the components (agent, host, or environment) will result in disequilibrium (i.e., a change in the usual patterns).[15]

The nutritionist using the epidemiologic triangle in a situation such as teenage obesity might focus on diet as the *agent* causing teenage obesity. However, behavior could also be a factor. An example of a behavioral factor is a sedentary lifestyle that promotes weight gain. The nutritionist would strive to determine whether there has been a change in any of the possible agents.

The *host* factors are personal characteristics of the teenage population who are at risk of obesity and other health-related conditions, such as diabetes. The personal characteristics include age, ethnicity, gender, socioeconomic status, eating patterns, exercise behavior, and lifestyle. Some personal characteristics, such as gender, age, and ethnicity, are not modifiable, but others are. Characteristics that can be changed include nutritional status, physical activity, and income level. By evaluating these factors, it may be possible to identify groups of teenagers who are at an increased risk of dying from obesity-related health conditions.

Finally, the *environment* must be assessed. Environmental factors are external factors that encompass an agent and a host. They may be exclusively physical, such as climate or surroundings (e.g., an urban housing area in the Midwestern United States). An environmental factor also may have multiple levels, such as low, middle, and high socioeconomic status. Low socioeconomic status is associated with the reduced availability of health and social services.[65] High socioeconomic status is associated with excessive behaviors, such as heavy drinking, overeating, and risk taking.[2,66]

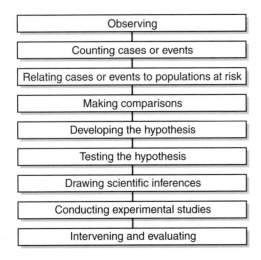

| Observing |
| Counting cases or events |
| Relating cases or events to populations at risk |
| Making comparisons |
| Developing the hypothesis |
| Testing the hypothesis |
| Drawing scientific inferences |
| Conducting experimental studies |
| Intervening and evaluating |

FIGURE 3-3 Examples of the Scientific Method of Epidemiologists

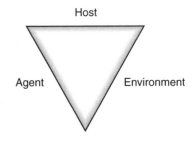

FIGURE 3-4 Epidemiologic Triangle Mode

Modified from: Stanhope M, Lancaster J. *Community and Public Health Nursing.* 5th ed. New York: Mosby; 2000. Reprinted with permission.

The analysis of these three areas, agent, host, and environment, should provide information regarding groups at risk for increased rates of obesity and may provide direction toward a program aimed at reducing the risks. Therefore, the epidemiologic triangle can provide a useful guide for investigating different health problems of teenage obesity, as well as other health problems.

Nutritional Epidemiology

Nutritional epidemiology is the study of dietary intake and the occurrence of disease in human populations.[56] In nutritional epidemiology, accurate quantification of nutritional *exposure* is critical. Exposure is the characteristics or agents (e.g., food, medications, time in the sun) that a person comes in contact with that may be related to disease risk (see **Table 3.1**).[67] It is complicated and challenging to evaluate and associate dietary intake with a disease risk. For instance, cigarette smoking can be accurately assessed as an activity with a simple yes or no question. It has been reported that cigarette smoking is addictive, and smokers seem to be consistent in their habits, instead of stopping and starting. Most smokers seem to smoke about the same number of cigarettes per day, and because of the expense, most people know how many cigarettes they smoke per day.[68]

In comparison, it is difficult for clients to report accurately the food consumed for more than one week because they may consume hundreds, even thousands of different foods during that time period. In addition, the difficulty may be due to:[56]

- Other people preparing the meals (e.g., restaurant, friends, spouse, prepackaged foods) so that the client does not know what, or how much, he or she has consumed
- Seasonal variations in food intake
- Life events (e.g., weekends, holidays, vacations, birthdays)

Indeed, the daily variability in food intake makes it difficult to identify any critically consistent pattern.[55] This means that researchers must depend on food composition databases to calculate the exposure variable. These issues have made it difficult to obtain consistent and strong evidence about how diet affects disease risk.

In the past 20 years, nutritional epidemiologic research has focused on nutrient-based analyses to help guide the search for underlying causes of disease risk. However, food-based hypotheses and analyses have been shown to complement this philosophy and can be an effective method to link food intake to a health condition. For example, Ness and Powles conducted a systematic review of the reported associations between the consumption of fruits and vegetables and the risk of cardiovascular diseases.[69] Results showed that 9 of 10 ecological studies, 2 of 3 case-control studies, and 6 of 16 cohort studies found a significant protective association between the consumption of fruits and vegetables and coronary heart disease. For stroke, 3 of 5 ecological studies and 6 of 8 cohort studies found a significant protective association with consumption of fruits and vegetables. For total circulatory disease, one of two cohort studies reported a significant protective association.[69] Hence, the tools and methods of nutritional epidemiology can be developed to deal with scientific issues unique to the biology of chronic diseases. Specifically, epidemiologic methods were designed to address the following:[56]

- The length of time for disease development
- The multifactorial nature of chronic diseases
- The fact that research using human beings prevents direct observations of cause and effect

> **nutritional epidemiology**
> Study of dietary intake and the occurrence of disease in human populations.
>
> **exposure** Characteristics or agents (e.g., food, medications, sunlight) that the participant comes in contact with that may be related to disease risk.

TABLE 3.1	Examples of Exposures Relevant to Nutritional Epidemiologic Studies	
Exposure	**Diet-Related Example**	**Other Example**
Agent that may cause or protect from disease	Fruit and vegetable consumption may provide protection against colon cancer, heart disease, and stroke.	Physical activity may provide protection against colon cancer, obesity, and heart disease.
Constitutional host factors	Persons can have a genetic predisposition to nutrition-related diseases (e.g., diabetes, heart disease, cancer).	Older adults and low-income individuals are more predisposed to chronic disease.
Other host factors	Food preferences learned during childhood can determine food choices.	More educated adults may have better disease screening.
Agents that may confound the association between another agent and disease	Correlation between dietary constituents (e.g., a diet high in fruits and vegetables is usually low in calories and fat and high in antioxidants).	Alcohol and substance abusers and smokers are less likely to engage in physical activity.
Agents that may modify the effects of other agents	Fruits and vegetables may protect against lung cancer among smokers.	Smoking causes an increased risk of lung cancer.
Agents that may determine the outcome of disease	Malnutrition.	Medical treatment and medical nutrition therapy.

Source: This information was published in Coulston A, Rock C, Monsen E. *Nutrition in the Prevention and Treatment of Disease.* Copyright Academic Press (2001). Reprinted with permission.

Types of Public Health Nutritional Epidemiology Research

Public health nutritional epidemiology research and research design can be divided into observational and experimental/clinical categories. The difference between an experimental and an observational study is the control the researcher may have over participants, the methods and procedures, and the exposures (see **Table 3.2**). In an experimental/clinical study, the researchers can control some of the clients' entire dietary intake. In an observational study, the researcher does not intervene in or manipulate the clients' dietary intake.[70] We will first discuss observational studies. The types of observational studies for individuals include *cross-sectional, case-control, and cohort/prospective studies*; studies of groups are referred to as *ecologic studies*. After that, we will discuss experimental studies.

TABLE 3.2 **Types of Epidemiological Research Design**

Observational Studies of Individuals

In a *cross-sectional study*, sometimes described as prevalence or descriptive surveys, nutrient intake and outcome are both measured at the same point in time. The aim of the study is to describe the relationship between diseases and dietary intake in a specified community at a particular time. It can provide a "snapshot" of the frequency and characteristics of a disease in a population at a particular point in time.[71] An example of a cross-sectional study question would be: What is the association between nutrient intake and disease outcome? For example, the National Health and Nutrition Examination Survey (NHANES) and the International Study on Macronutrients and Blood Pressure (INTERMAP) are cross-sectional studies. INTERMAP is a cross-sectional study of associations between macronutrients and blood pressure. In this study, participants had their blood pressure measured twice on each of four occasions and completed a 24-hour recall on each day that their blood pressure was measured.[70,72] Similarly, the National Center for Health Statistics conducts the NHANES survey biannually to measure the health and nutritional condition of adults and children living in the United States. The survey utilizes both questionnaire and examination techniques. In this study, a sample of 1,890 12- to 16-year-olds with measured height and weight were obtained from the NHANES III survey to identify factors to potentially combat obesity in 12- to 16-year-olds with one or two obese parents and those with no obese parents. NHANES III surveys were conducted in two stages: 1) an initial interview was conducted in the respondents' homes where health histories and sociodemographic characteristics were obtained and 2) 3 weeks later, dietary intake assessments and physical examinations were conducted on the participants in a mobile examination center.

Results show that eating breakfast every day or some days was significantly protective against obesity in adolescents with obese parent(s), and this proved to be the strongest protective factor in this group of children. Findings from the NHANES studies have been used to create public health education and intervention programs.[73,74]

In nutritional *case-control studies*, also referred to as retrospective and case-referent studies, persons recently diagnosed with a diet-related disease and a group of persons without the disease (the control) from the same population are interviewed concerning their dietary habits. The differences between both groups' findings are compared. Case-control studies are a commonly used method of observational epidemiologic studies. The aim of this type of study is to identify the cause of a disease among a group of people, or the cause-and-effect relationships of the health condition.[75] A typical study question could be: Do people with the disease or health condition have a different lifestyle than persons who have not been diagnosed with the health condition? Or, do people diagnosed with hypertension smoke cigarettes and consume foods higher in sodium than persons without hypertension?[70] For example, in 2004 Lubin et al. conducted a case-control study in Israel.[76] The aim of the study was to determine the association between body size and the risk of breast cancer. The study used a population of 1,065 breast cancer patients, 964 surgical controls, and 981 neighborhood controls. Heights and weights at three periods throughout the participants' lives (at age 18, for "most of adult life," and most recent) were ascertained. The authors analyzed these parameters and the body mass index for each period, as well as BMI changes throughout life, controlling for age, menstrual status, and ethnic origin. Result show an increase in risk for breast cancer with greater recent BMI among postmenopausal women aged 60+ for breast cancer.[76]

In *cohort studies*, sometimes called prospective, follow-up, and longitudinal studies, baseline risk factors are evaluated and participants are followed over time to monitor disease occurrence. It is the analytic method of epidemiological studies. Participants are typically free of disease. A typical study question would be: Do people with a higher intake of a nutrient develop or die from a particular disease more frequently or sooner than persons with a lower intake? Cohort studies are usually very large, exceeding 50,000 participants; may take many years to be conducted; and are expensive.[77] An example of a cohort study is the Women's Health Initiative (WHI), a 15-year study investigating the degree to which diet, hormone replacement therapy (HRT), calcium, and vitamin D might prevent heart disease, breast and colorectal cancer, and osteoporosis in postmenopausal women. The main advantage of cohort studies is that exposure to potential risk factors is assessed before the development of the disease. **Tables 3.3** and **3.4** present examples of cohort studies that utilized some form of nutritional assessment.

Observational Studies of Groups

Ecologic studies compare collective data that represent entire populations. An ecologic study focuses on the comparison of groups, not individuals. The purpose of an ecologic analysis may be to make biologic implications about the association between exposure (water contaminant) and disease outcome in various communities within a population or to make ecologic inferences about effects on group rates.[78] Ecologic studies may be very useful for monitoring national trends in health, social, cultural, economic, and environmental factors that influence health that cannot be measured at an individual level. For example, migration studies, a type of ecologic study, show a significant increase in the risk of several chronic diseases, such as breast cancer, when people move from an Eastern to a Western country.[79,80]

<table>
<tr><td colspan="2">

TABLE 3.3   **Dietary Assessment in Different Study Situations**

</td></tr>
</table>

Study Situation	Methods Commonly Used
Cross-sectional	24-hour recall; food-frequency questionnaire (FFQ); brief methods
Case-control (retrospective)	FFQ; diet history
Cohort	FFQ; diet history; 24-hour recall
Intervention	FFQ; brief methods; 24-hour recall
Clinical screening	24-hour recall; brief methods; diet history
Surveillance	24-hour recall; brief methods

Modified from: Coulston A, Rock C, Monsen E. *Nutrition in the Prevention and Treatment of Disease*. Copyright Academic Press (2001). Reprinted with permission.

utilization and storage in relation to obesity and diabetes), metabolic processes (e.g., absorption, transport, and utilization of minerals, vitamins, and protein), and specific enzyme systems in experimental animals and humans.[81] An example of an experimental study is a metabolic ward study that reported changes in total cholesterol from changes in intakes of saturated and polyunsaturated fatty acids and dietary cholesterol.[70,82–84] Crossover research design is common in metabolic/feeding studies. In this design, each volunteer participant serves as his or her own control.

Another type of experimental study is the randomized clinical trial, which is a prospective study in which participants are randomly assigned to intervention and control groups. The participants are followed over time to assess the effectiveness and safety of the intervention after randomization.[79] An example of a randomized study is the Fracture Intervention Trial, which was designed to test the hypothesis that hormone replacement therapy will reduce the rate of fracture in postmenopausal women.[85]

Genetic Epidemiologic Studies

Genetic epidemiologic studies use genetic epidemiology and molecular epidemiology. The investigation could be a cross-sectional and/or an intervention study. In genetic epidemiology, a question could be: Do genes determine eating behaviors, such as how much one eats, preferences for certain types of foods, and frequency or patterns of eating?[70,81] Research implies that there is a resemblance among family members for these behaviors, but it is not clear whether genes, shared environments, or both are the cause.[86] In molecular epidemiology, questions relate to the physical and hormonal mechanisms leading to taste preferences, hunger, and satiety. For example, taste receptors

Experimental Studies

Experimental studies involve intentional alteration or intervention in the course of a disease. Nutritional intervention studies include metabolic studies and randomized clinical trials.[70] In metabolic or feeding studies, the researcher develops nutritionally adequate diets that vary on one or more components, to investigate the effect of this diet on internal physiological reactions (e.g., carbohydrate, lipid, and energy

<table>
<tr><td colspan="5">

TABLE 3.4   **Examples of Cohort Studies Utilizing Nutrition Assessments**

</td></tr>
</table>

Cohort Study	Years Conducted	Sample Studied	Outcome	Nutritional Intake Measurement
Coronary Artery Risk Development in Young Adults (CARDIA)	Baseline: 1985–1986 Year 2: 1987–1988	5,116 sampled men and women, blacks and whites, 18–30 years old	Coronary heart disease risk factors	Baseline: Diet history questionnaire (interview-administered) Year 2: NCI (Block) food frequency questionnaire
Framingham Study: Heart and Vascular Disease Program	1949–1989	5,209 sampled men and women, primarily whites, 30–62 years old	Cardiovascular risk factors	Semi-Quantitative Food Frequency Questionnaire (Willet)
Framingham Offspring and Spouse Study	1971–1988	5,135 sampled men and women, primarily whites, 12–60 years old	Cardiovascular risk factors	24-hour dietary recall
RENO (Relationship of Energy and Nutrition to Obesity) Diet-Heart Study	1985–1993	508 sampled men and women, primarily whites, 20–69 years old, normal/overweight	Cardiovascular risk factors	24-hour dietary recall, 7-day food record NCI (Block) food frequency questionnaire
Nurses' Study	1976–1996	121,700 sampled female registered nurses, primarily whites, 30–55 years old	Cancer risk factors	Semi-Quantitative Food Frequency Questionnaire (Willet)
Health Professionals Follow-Up Study	1986–1994	51,529 sampled male health professionals, primarily whites, 40–75 years old	Heart disease and cancer risk factors	Semi-Quantitative Food Frequency Questionnaire (Willet)

Modified from: Berdanier CD, Feldman E, Flatt W, Sachiko J. *Handbook of Nutrition and Food*. New York: CRC Press; 2002. Reprinted with permission.

are clearly genetically determined, although the gene(s) may not all be identified yet.[87] For example, genes encoding hormones and proteins that regulate hunger and satiety have just been identified recently.[88–89] It has been known for some time that certain enzyme deficiencies, which have a genetic cause, give rise to specific nutritional problems; examples of these are phenylketonuria and galactosemia.[88]

Interpretation of Cause and Effect in Nutritional Epidemiology

Epidemiology is the study of associations, and statistical methods are used to test the strength of these associations. However, it is important to note that the existence of a statistically significant association does not indicate that the observed relationship is one of cause and effect. For any observed association, the following should be considered:[56]

- The observed association may be due to chance.
- The association may be due to improper study design or implementation or inappropriate analysis of data.

- The association may be weak or strong.
- A credible biologic mechanism may exist.
- There could be an association between exposure and the outcome.
- The significance of the results depends on the context of all the available evidence. Causality is supported when studies that are conducted at different times, using different methods, and performed among different populations show similar results.
- The result correlates with other criteria of causality (given in **Table 3.5**).

It is not uncommon in the field of nutritional epidemiology for a cause-and-effect relationship to be beyond doubt. However, research information should not be ignored or discarded.[90] One must exercise caution and use thoughtful consideration before acting on epidemiologic evidence. This chapter's Successful Community Strategies feature presents a successful cohort research study that verified the association between plant-based diets and the rate of mortality.

TABLE 3.5	Guidelines for Assessing Evidence of Causation
Criteria	**Association**
Strength	The cause and effect should not be dismissed easily because the observed association seems minor. This means that a small association does not imply that a causal effect does not exist.
Consistency	Consistent findings observed by different individuals in different places with different samples strengthen the likelihood of cause and effect. For example, several research studies established that there is an association between cigarette smoking and lung cancer.
Specificity	Causation is likely if a very specific population at a specific site has a disease with no other likely explanation. This means that the health condition is limited to specific individuals at a particular location.
Temporality	The effect has to occur after the cause (and if there is an expected delay between the cause and expected effect, then the effect must occur after that delay). The investigator may consider this question: Does a high-fat diet lead to heart disease or do the early stages of heart disease lead to poor dietary habits?
Biological gradient	Greater exposure should lead to greater incidence of the effect. For example, the evidence that the death rate from lung cancer increases linearly with the number of cigarettes smoked every day adds significantly to the simpler evidence that cigarette smokers have a higher lung cancer death rate than nonsmokers.
Plausibility	A credible mechanism between cause and effect is helpful. However, an association that is not biologically credible at one time may eventually prove to be so in the future. Implausible associations may be the beginning of the advancement of knowledge.
Coherence	Coherence between epidemiologic and laboratory findings increases the likelihood of an effect. However, lack of such laboratory evidence cannot nullify the epidemiologic findings.
Experiment	Sometimes it is possible to request experimental evidence. The investigator may ask this question: Does increased consumption of diets high in calcium prevent colon cancer or osteoporosis?
Analogy	The effects of similar substances may be considered supportive of causality. The investigator may ask this question: Can parallels be drawn with examples of other well-established cause-and-effect relationships (e.g., the relationship between obesity and heart disease)?

Sources: Hennekens CH, Buring JE. *Epidemiology in Medicine.* Mayren SL, ed. Boston: Little, Brown; 1965; and Hill AB. The environment and disease: association or causation? *Proc Royal Soc Med.* 1965; 58:295–300. Reprinted with permission.

Successful Community Strategies 🏠🏠🏠

EPIC Elderly Cohort Research Study[5,91–109]

The Mediterranean diet has been reviewed in many studies because several of its components have been related to decreases in common chronic diseases. Ecological evidence suggests that such a diet may be beneficial to health, and variants of this diet have improved the prognosis of patients with coronary heart disease. The Mediterranean diet is characterized by a high intake of vegetables, legumes, fruits, and cereals; a moderate to high intake of fish; a low intake of saturated lipids but a high intake of unsaturated lipids, particularly olive oil; a low to moderate intake of dairy products, mostly cheese and yogurt; a low intake of meat; and a modest intake of ethanol, mostly as wine. Several studies have reported that a diet that adheres to the principles of the traditional Mediterranean one is associated with longer survival. Trichopoulou and Vasilopoulou used a 10-unit dietary score to determine whether adherence to a Mediterranean diet was associated with a longer life expectancy among elderly Europeans.[90] However, several studies have used variations of this score and reported opposite associations with overall mortality. These studies, however, relied on small samples of mostly elderly participants or only on the Greek population.

The European Prospective Investigation into Cancer and Nutrition (EPIC) study used a multi-center, prospective cohort study to investigate the role of biological, dietary, lifestyle, and environmental factors in cancer and other chronic diseases and to examine whether adherence to the modified Mediterranean diet, in which unsaturated fats were substituted for monounsaturated fats, is associated with longer life expectancy among elderly persons.

Between 1992 and 2000, 519,978 healthy volunteers were recruited in 23 centers from 10 European countries (Denmark, France, Germany, Greece, Italy, the Netherlands, Norway, Spain, Sweden, and the United Kingdom). After initial screening, only 74,607 individuals were included in the study. Data were collected from participants ages 60 or over. Information on the vital status of participants was obtained from mortality registries and by active follow-up. The earliest and latest years of follow-up were 1999 (some participants in the Netherlands) and December 2003 (most of the centers). Participants were classified as alive at last follow-up, dead, emigrated, refused to participate further, or unknown.

Dietary intakes were assessed through compatible instruments (food frequency questionnaires and, in some centers, records of intake over 7 or 14 days) that had been developed and validated within each center. In addition, a computerized instrument for recall of dietary intake over 24 hours was developed to collect information from a standardized random sample of the aggregate cohort. The aim was to calibrate the measurements across countries.

Nutrient intakes were calculated using food composition tables specific to the country. Fourteen food groups and nutrients were considered: potatoes, vegetables, legumes, fruits, dairy products, cereals, meat and meat products, fish and seafood, eggs, monounsaturated lipids, polyunsaturated lipids, saturated lipids, sugar and confectionery (candy, pastry, etc.), and nonalcoholic beverages.

Results showed that an increase in the modified Mediterranean diet score was associated with lower overall mortality. When dietary exposures were calibrated across countries, the reduction in mortality was 7 percent (ranging from 1 to 12 percent). The study concluded that the Mediterranean diet, modified so as to apply across Europe, was associated with increased survival among older people.

Chapter Summary

- The research process involves assessment, planning, implementation, evaluation, and action.
- Research questions and methodologies guide the plan for data analysis. It is important to consult a statistician before carrying out a research study.
- It is important to submit the research proposal to the institutional review board for approval. This is done to protect human research participants from physical or mental harm as well as to protect the researcher from unnecessary complaints.
- Pilot studies can be used to test data-gathering methods and to apply the data analysis plan. It is important to test these when the data-gathering methods and procedures are new to the investigator.
- A community nutritionist is a member of a multidisciplinary team and can conduct research studies that can benefit the public.
- Successful collaboration requires that the multidisciplinary team develop a common purpose, communicate to coordinate efforts, and recognize the unique and complementary skills possessed by each team member.
- The three components of the epidemiologic triangle model are agent, host, and environment, and they are used to explore health and disease.
- In experimental studies, the investigator has control over participants, procedures, and exposures.
- Epidemiology is the study of associations, and statistical methods are used to test the associations. The existence of a statistically significant association does not indicate that the observed relationship is one of cause and effect. Causality is supported when a number of studies that are conducted at different times, using different methods, and performed among different populations show similar results.

Critical Thinking Activities

- Identify a research study in the literature relevant to community and public health nutrition. Then identify the strengths and limitations of the research.
- Communicate/present the research findings in class.
- Meet with the librarian as a class/group and learn how to use the Medline database; ERIC database; CINAHL database; and Ingenta: The Global Research Gateway (http://www.ingenta.com), a portal to online information around the world; and other search engines for finding grant sources.

Case Study 3-1

Damian and Monica, two senior baccalaureate nutrition students in a community nutrition course, had their community outreach experience at a rural community clinic. They were involved with the owner of a local candy factory in planning for disease prevention and health promotion activities for the employees. After consulting with the faculty member responsible for the course and the director of the community clinic, they designed a survey to distribute to employees to assess their needs for health education programming. The students submitted the survey to the university's institutional review board for approval before distributing it to the employees.

One of the employee priorities identified from the survey data was to establish a smoking cessation and weight loss program for factory employees. The students met with the factory owner, the faculty member, and a representative of the local chapter of the American Lung Association to plan for implementation of this initiative. A time line was established to notify employees of an opportunity to participate in the weight loss and smoking cessation program. This included notices distributed in employee paychecks and signs posted in prominent locations throughout the factory. The students discussed plans for conducting a research study related to implementation and evaluation of the weight loss and smoking cessation program with the faculty member.

Activities

- Generate a research problem.
- Develop hypotheses/objectives to investigate the problem.
- Identify and present the type of epidemiologic method that can be used to investigate the problem.
- Use the most current literature to identify eight smoking cessation and five weight loss strategies and present the information gathered.
- Determine how to disseminate the information gathered and other different methods of dissemination of research findings.

References

1. Israel BA, Schulz AJ, Parker EA, Becker AB. Review of community-based research: assessing partnership approaches to improve public health. *Ann Rev Public Health.* 1998; 19:173–202.

2. Frank-Spohrer G. *Community Nutrition: Applying Epidemiology to Contemporary Practice.* Rockville, MD: Aspen; 2007.

3. Brachman PS. *Epidemiology General Concepts.* 4th ed. Galveston: The University of Texas Medical Branch at Galveston; 1996.

4. Morgan R, Jain M, Miller A, Choi N, Matthews V, Munan L, Burch J, Feather G, Kelly A. A comparison of dietary methods in epidemiologic studies. *Amer J Epidemiol.* 2006; 107(6):488–498.

5. Stanhope M, Lancaster J. *Community and Public Health Nursing.* 5th ed. New York: Mosby; 2000.

6. Trochim WMK. Research Methods Knowledge Base. Available at: http://www. socialresearchmethods.net/kb/strucres.htm. Accessed November 28, 2006.

7. Roberts WC. High salt intake, its origins, its economic impact, and its effect on blood pressure. *Am J Cardiol.* 2001; 88(11):1338–1346.

8. Huff R, Kline M. *Promoting Health in Multicultural Populations. A Handbook for Practitioners.* Thousand Oaks, CA: Sage; 1999.

9. Abramson JJ, Abramson ZH. *Survey Methods in Community Medicine: Epidemiological Research, Programme Evaluation, Clinical Trials.* 5th ed. London: Churchill Livingstone; 1999.

10. Monsen ER. *Research: Successful Approaches.* 2nd ed. Chicago: American Dietetic Association; 2003.

11. Grant M. Women's health beliefs regarding hypertension. *West Indian Med J.* 1993; 42(4):158–160.

12. Tussing L, Chapman-Novakofski K. Osteoporosis prevention education: behavior theories and calcium intake. *J Am Diet Assoc.* 2005; 105(1):92–97.

13. Abood DA, Black DR, Feral D. Nutrition education worksite intervention for university staff: application of the health belief model. *J Nutr Educ Behav.* 2003; 35(5):260–267.

14. Ueland A, Hornung PA, Greenwald B. Colorectal cancer prevention and screening: a Health Belief Model-based research study to increase disease awareness. *Gastroenterol Nurs.* 2006; 29(5):357–363.

15. Anderson E, McFarlane J. *Community as Partner: Theory and Practice in Nursing.* 3rd ed. Philadelphia: Lippincott; 2000.

16. Varkevisser CM, Brownlee B. *Designing and Conducting Health Systems Research.* International Development Research Centre. Ottawa, Canada: World Health Organization; 2003.

17. Frank K. The impact of a confounding variable on the inference of a regression coefficient. *Sociol Methods Res.* 2002; 29(2):147–194.

18. Pelto GH, Freake HD. Social research in an integrated science of nutrition: future directions. *J Nutr.* 2003; 133:1231–1234.

19. Munhall PL, Boyd CO. *Nursing Research: A Qualitative Perspective.* New York: National League for Nursing; 1993.

20. Murtagh MJ, Thomson RG, May CR, Rapley T, Heaven B, Graham R, Kaner E, Stobbart L, Eccles M. Qualitative methods in a randomized controlled trial: the role of an integrated qualitative process evaluation in providing evidence to discontinue the intervention in one arm of a trial of a decision support tool. *Qual Saf Health Care.* 2007; 16:224–229.

21. McGee R. Analysis of poverty assessment (PPA) and household survey findings on poverty trends in Uganda. Institute of Development Studies. Available at: http://www.finance.go.ug/docs/Kigusa%20Muterere.pdf. Accessed April 6, 2008.

22. DeLeeuw E. Reducing missing data in surveys: an overview of methods. *Qual Quant.* 2001; 35(2):147–160.

23. Gibson RS. *Principles of Nutritional Assessment.* 2nd ed. Dunedin, New Zealand: Oxford University Press; 2005.

24. RD Direct. Your research project: how and where to start? Available at: http://www.rdinfo.org.uk/flowchart/Flowchart.html. Accessed April 6, 2008.

25. Hinke M, Maurits W, Seidell C, Thijs A, Ader H. Effectiveness and cost-effectiveness of early screening and treatment of malnourished patients. *Am J Clin Nutr.* 2005; 82:1082–1089.

26. Vazirani S, Hays RD, Shapiro, MF, Cowan M. Effect of a multidisciplinary intervention on communication and collaboration among physicians and nurses. *Am J Crit Care.* 2005; 14(1):71–77.

27. Sullivan MB, Camer L, et al. Benefits, barriers and enablers of university-community research: input from health and social service agencies. *Soc Mark Q.* 2000; 4:9–25.

28. Institute of Medicine. *The Future of Public Health.* Washington, DC: National Academy Press; 1998.

29. Vega WA. Theoretical and pragmatic implications of cultural diversity for community research. *Am J Community Psychol.* 1992; 20:375–391.

30. Clark MJ. *Nursing in the Community.* 3rd ed. Stamford, CT: Appleton & Lange; 1999.

31. Malone TW, Crowston K. *Toward an Interdisciplinary Study of Coordination.* Cambridge, MA: Center for Coordination Science, MIT; 1991.

32. Amuwo S, Jenkins E. True partnership evolves over time. In: Sullivan AK, ed. *Collaborative Research: University and Community Partnership.* Washington, DC: American Public Health Association; 2001:25–43.

33. Hitchcock J, Schubert PE, Thomas SA. *Community Health Nursing.* 2nd ed. Clifton Park, NY: Thomson Delmar Learning; 2003.

34. Schneider MJ. *Introduction to Public Health.* Sudbury, MA: Jones and Bartlett; 2006.

35. Franco OH, Peeters A, Bonneux L, de Laet C. Blood pressure in adulthood and life expectancy with cardiovascular disease in men and women: life course analysis. *Hypertension.* 2005; 46(2):280–286.

36. Sheats N, Lin Y, Zhao W, Cheek DE, Lackland DT, Egan BM. Prevalence, treatment, and control of hypertension among African Americans and Caucasians at primary care sites for medically under-served patients. *Ethnicity Dis.* 2005; 15(1):25–32.

37. Arnold AM, Psaty BM, Kuller LH, et al. Incidence of cardiovascular disease in older Americans: the cardiovascular health study. *J Am Geriatr Soc.* 2005; 53(2):211–218.

38. National Center for Health Statistics. *National Vital Statistics Reports.* Available at: http://www.cdc.gov/nchs/products/pubd/nvsr/nvsr.htm. Accessed February 15, 2008.

39. Freeman J, Hutchison G. Prevalence, incidence and duration. *Amer J Epidemiol.* 2005; 112(5):707–723.

40. Flanders WD, O'Brien TR. Inappropriate comparisons of incidence and prevalence in epidemiologic research. *Am J Public Health.* 1989; 79(9):1301–1303.

41. Robinson JR, Young TK, Roos LL, Gelskey DE. Estimating the burden of disease. *Med Care.* 1997; 35:932–947.

42. Higginson I. Epidemiological methods in studies of symptoms in advanced disease. *Interactive Textbook on Clinical Symptom Research*; 2006. Available at: http://symptomresearch.nih.gov/chapter_19/cihauthbio.htm. Accessed April 5, 2008.

43. Paulette GB. Populations at risk across the lifespan reducing infant mortality rates using the perinatal periods of risk model. *Public Health Nurs.* 2005; 22(1):2–7.

44. Kramer MS, Platt RW, Yang H, Haglund B, Cnattingius S, Bergsjo P. Registration artifacts in international comparisons of infant mortality. *Paediatr Perinat Epidemiol.* 2002; 16(1):16–22.

45. Silva AA, Barbieri MA, Gomes UA, Bettiol H. Trends in low birth weight: a comparison of two birth cohorts separated by a 15-year interval in Ribeirao Preto, Brazil. *Bull World Health Organ.* 1998; 76(1):73–84.

46. Wakeford R, McElvenny D. From epidemiological association to causation. *Occup Med.* 2007; 57(7):464–465.

47. McDonald JC, McDonald AD, Hughes JM, Rando RJ, Weill H. Mortality from lung and kidney disease in a cohort of North American industrial sand workers: an update. *Ann Occup Hyg.* 2005; 49(5):367–373.

48. Alexander GL. Dietary sodium intake and its relation to human health: a summary of the evidence. *J Am Coll Nutr.* 2006; 25(3):165–169.

49. Barry MP. Urbanization, lifestyle changes and the nutrition transition. *World Dev.* 1999; 27:1905–1916.

50. Pryer J, Cappuccio F, Elliott P. Dietary calcium and blood pressure: a review of the observational studies. *J Hum Hypertens.* 1995; 9(8):597–604.

51. Crawford MD, Gardner MJ, Morris JN. Mortality and hardness of local water supplies. *Lancet I.* 1968; 1(7547):827–831.

52. Sacks FM, Svetkey LP, Vollmer WM, et al. Effects on blood pressure of reduced dietary sodium and the Dietary Approaches to Stop Hypertension (DASH) diet. DASH-Sodium Collaborative Research Group. *N Engl J Med.* 2001; 344(1):3–10.

53. Sacks FM, Appel LJ, Moore TJ. A dietary approach to prevent hypertension: a review of the Dietary Approaches to Stop Hypertension (DASH) study. *Clin Cardiol.* 1999; 22(7 Suppl):1116–1110.

54. Trichopoulou A, Orfanos P, Norat T, Bueno-de-Mesquita B. Modified Mediterranean diet and survival: EPIC elderly prospective cohort study. *BMJ.* 2005; 330:7498.

55. INTERSALT Cooperative Research Group. INTERSALT: an international study of electrolyte excretion and blood pressure. results for 24 hour urinary sodium and potassium excretion. *BMJ.* 1988; 297(6644):319–328.

56. Coulston A, Rock C, Monsen E. *Nutrition in the Prevention and Treatment of Disease.* New York: Academic Press; 2001.

57. INTERSALT Cooperative Research Group. Sodium, potassium, body mass, alcohol and blood pressure: the INTERSALT study. *J Hypertens.* 1988; 6(4 Suppl):S584–S586.

58. Beevers DG. The epidemiology of salt and hypertension. *Clin Autonom Res.* 2002; 12(5):353–357.

59. Law MR, Frost CD, Wald NJ. Analysis of data from trials of salt reduction. *BMJ.* 1991; 302:819–824.

60. Haddy FJ, Vanhoutte PM, Feletou M. Role of potassium in regulating blood flow and blood pressure. *Am J Physiol Regul Integr Comp Physiol.* 2006; 290:R548–R552.

61. Lawrence J. Lifestyle modification as a means to prevent and treat high blood pressure. *J Am Soc Nephrol.* 2003; 14:S99–S102.

62. Frank M, Sacks WC, Willett A, Smith LE, Brown BR, Thomas JM. Effect on blood pressure of potassium, calcium, and magnesium in women with low habitual intake. *Hypertens.* 1998; 31:131.

63. Persky V, McDonald A, Molteni A, Liu K. The effect of dietary sucrose of blood pressure in spontaneously hypertensive rats. *Nutr Res.* 1986; 6(9):1111–1115.

64. Karanja NM, Obarzanek E, Lin PH, et al. Descriptive characteristics of the dietary patterns used in the Dietary Approaches to Stop Hypertension trial. DASH Collaborative Research Group. *J Am Diet Assoc.* 1999; 99(8):S19–S27.

65. Mellora JM, Milyo J. Exploring the relationships between income inequality, socioeconomic status and health: a self-guided tour? *Int J Epidemiol.* 2002; 31:685–687.

66. Maletnlema TN. A Tanzanian perspective on the nutrition transition and its implications for health. *Public Health Nutr.* 2002; 5(1A):163–168.

67. Armstrong BK, White E, Saracci R. Monographs in epidemiology and biostatistics. *Principles of Exposure Measurement in Epidemiology.* Vol. 21. Oxford: Oxford University Press; 1994.

68. Zimlichman E, Kochba I, Mimouni FB, et al. Smoking habits and obesity in young adults. *Addiction.* 2005; 100(7):1021–1025.

69. Ness AR, Powles JW. Fruit and vegetables, and cardiovascular disease: a review. *Int J Epidemiol.* 1997; 26:1–13.

70. Berdanier C, Feldman E, Flatt W, Sachiko J. *Handbook of Nutrition and Food.* New York: CRC Press; 2002.

71. Abramson JH, Abramson ZH. *Survey Methods in Community Medicine.* 5th ed. London: Livingstone; 2000.

72. Stamler J, Elliott P, Dennis B, Dyer AR, Kesteloot H, Liu K, Ueshima H, Zhou B. INTERMAP: background, aims, design, methods, and descriptive statistics (nondietary). *J Hum Hypertens.* 2003; 17:591–608.

73. Tande DL, Hotchkiss L, Cotugna N. The associations between blood lipids and the Food Guide Pyramid: findings from the Third National Health and Nutrition Examination Survey. *Prev Med.* 2004; 38(4):452–457.

74. Fiore H, Travis S, Whalen A, Auinger P, Ryan S. Potentially protective factors associated with healthful body mass index in adolescents with obese and nonobese parents: a secondary data analysis of the Third National Health and Nutrition Examination Survey, 1988–1994. *J Am Diet Assoc.* 2006; 106(1):55–64.

75. Eugene W, Kaplan H, James S, Wagner E, Schoenbach V, Grimson R, Siegfried H, Gosta T, Gehlbach S. The epidemiologic evidence for a relationship between social support and health. *Amer J Epidemiol.* 2005; 117(5):521–537.

76. Lubin F, Ruder M, Wax Y, Modan B. Overweight and changes in weight throughout adult life in breast cancer etiology. *Amer J Epidemiol.* 2004; 122(4):579–588.

77. Cade JE, Burley VJ, Greenwood DC; UK Women's Cohort Study Steering Group. The UK Women's Cohort Study: comparison of vegetarians, fish-eaters and meat-eaters. *Public Health Nutr.* 2004; 7(7):871–878.

78. Morgenstern H. Ecologic studies in epidemiology: concepts, principles, and methods. *An Rev Public Health.* 1995; 16:61–81.

79. Kant A, Block G, Schatzkin A, Ziegler RG, Nestle M. Dietary diversity in the U.S. population. NHANES II 1976–1980. *J Am Diet Assoc.* 1991; 91:34–38.

80. Grant WB. A multicountry ecologic study of risk and risk reduction factors for prostate cancer mortality. *Eur Urol.* 2004; 45(3):271–279.

81. Winitz M, Seedman DA, Graff J. Studies in metabolic nutrition employing chemically defined diets. I. Extended feeding of normal human adult males. *Am J Clin Nutr.* 1970; 23(5):525–545.

82. Dreon DM, Fernstrom HA, Campos H, et al. Change in dietary saturated fat intake is correlated with change in mass of large low-density-lipoprotein particles in men. *Am J Clin Nutr.* 1998; 67:828–836.

83. Sukhinder KC, Luis BA. Metabolism of cholesterol is altered in the liver of C3H mice fed fats enriched with different C-18 fatty acids. *J Nutr.* 1999; 129:1718–1724.

84. Greenspan SL, Resnick NM, Parker RA. Combination therapy with hormone replacement and alendronate for prevention of bone loss in elderly women: a randomized controlled trial. *JAMA.* 2003; 289:2525–2533.

85. Perusse LB, Bouchard CE. The genetics of obesity. In: Bouchard CE, ed. *Family studies.* Boca Raton, FL: CRC Press; 1994:125.

86. Prutkin J, Fisher EM, Etter L, et al. Genetic variation and inferences about perceived taste intensity in mice and men. *Physiol Behav.* 2000; 69:161–173.

87. Cummings DE, Schwartz MW. Genetics and pathophysiology of human obesity. *Annual Review of Medicine.* 2003; 54:453–471.

88. Behrens MM. The human taste receptor hTAS2R14 responds to a variety of different bitter compounds. *Biochem Biophys Res Comm.* 2004; 319(2):479–485.

89. Smith J, Lensing S, Horton JA, et al. Prevalence of self-reported nutrition-related health problems in the Lower Mississippi Delta. *Am J Public Health.* 1999; 89:1418–1421.

90. Hill AB. The environment and disease: association or causation? *Proc Roy Soc Med.* 1965; 65:58–295.

91. Trichopoulou A, Vasilopoulou E. Mediterranean diet and longevity. *Br J Nutr.* 2000; 84(2):S205–S209.

92. De Groot LC, van Staveren WA, Burema J. Survival beyond age 70 in relation to diet. *Nutr Rev.* 1996; 54:211–212.

93. World Cancer Research Fund and American Institute for Cancer Research. *Food, Nutrition and the Prevention of Cancer: A Global Perspective.* Washington, DC: World Cancer Research Fund International; 1997.

94. Willett WC. *Diet and Coronary Heart Disease: Nutritional Epidemiology.* 2nd ed. New York: Oxford University Press; 1998.

95. Keys A. *Seven Countries: A Multivariate Analysis of Death and Coronary Heart Disease.* Cambridge, MA: Harvard University Press; 1980.

96. De Lorgeril M, Renaud S, Mamelle N, et al. Mediterranean alpha-linolenic acid-rich diet in secondary prevention of coronary heart disease. *Lancet.* 1994; 343:1454–1459.

97. Singh RB, Dubnov G, Niaz MA, et al. Effect of an Indo-Mediterranean diet on progression of coronary artery disease in high risk patients (Indo Mediterranean diet heart study): a randomised single-blind trial. *Lancet.* 2002; 360:1455–1461.

98. Trichopoulou A, Costacou T, Bamia C, Trichopoulos D. Adherence to Mediterranean diet and survival in a Greek population. *N Engl J Med.* 2003; 348:2599–2608.

99. Trichopoulou A, Kouris-Blazos A, Wahlqvist ML, et al. Diet and overall survival in elderly people. *BMJ.* 1995; 311:1457–1460.

100. Osler M, Schroll M. Diet and mortality in a cohort of elderly people in a north European community. *Int J Epidemiol.* 1997; 26:155–159.

101. Lasheras C, Fernandez S, Patterson AM. Mediterranean diet and age with respect to overall survival in institutionalized, nonsmoking elderly people. *Am J Clin Nutr.* 2000; 71(4):987–992.

102. Knoops KT, de Groot LC, Kromhout D, et al. Mediterranean diet, lifestyle factors, and 10-year mortality in elderly European men and women: the HALE project. *JAMA.* 2004; 292:1433–1439.

103. Willett WC, Sacks F, Trichopoulou A, et al. Mediterranean diet pyramid: a cultural model for healthy eating. *Am J Clin Nutr.* 1995; 61(Suppl 6):S1402–S1406.

104. Slimani N, Kaaks R, Ferrari P, et al. European Prospective Investigation into Cancer and Nutrition (EPIC) calibration study: rationale, design and population characteristics. *Public Health Nutr.* 2002; 5:1125–1145.

105. Riboli E, Hunt KJ, Slimani N, et al. European Prospective Investigation into Cancer and Nutrition (EPIC): study populations and data collection. *Public Health Nutr.* 2002; 5:1113–1124.

106. U.K. Department of Health. *Dietary Reference Values for Food Energy and Nutrients for the UK Department of Health Report on Health and Social Subjects.* No. 41. London: United Kingdom Stationery Office; 1991.

107. Margetts BM, Pietinen P. European Prospective Investigation into Cancer and Nutrition: validity studies on dietary assessment methods. *Int J Epidemiol.* 1997; 26(Suppl 1):S1–S5.

108. Kaaks R, Riboli E. Validation and calibration of dietary intake measurements in the EPIC project: methodological considerations. European Prospective Investigation into Cancer and Nutrition. *Int J Epidemiol.* 1997; 26(Suppl 1):S15–S25.

109. Deharveng G, Charrondiere UR, Slimani N, Southgate DA, Riboli E. Comparison of nutrients in the food composition tables available in the nine European countries participating in EPIC. European Prospective Investigation into Cancer and Nutrition. *Eur J Clin Nutr.* 1999; 53:60–79.

U.S. Nutrition Monitoring and Food Assistance Programs

LEARNING OBJECTIVES

- Describe the purpose of U.S. food assistance programs.
- Identify entitlement and non-entitlement programs.
- Define *nutrition monitoring* in the United States.
- Outline and describe the adult and child nutrition programs in the United States.
- Discuss the status of food insecurity in the United States.
- Discuss the impact of welfare reform.
- Identify the federal domestic nutrition assistance programs.

Introduction

Providing guidelines or food selection information to someone does not guarantee optimal nutrition if that person doesn't have access to adequate food or the money to buy it. A variety of food and nutrition programs have become available to assist low-income families in obtaining a safe and wholesome food supply in adequate amounts. Among some of the U.S. landmark programs are the **National School Lunch Program**, the **WIC program** (Special Supplemental Nutrition Program for Women, Infants, and Children), the **Food Stamp Program**, food distribution programs, and senior adult meals.

The nutrition assistance programs are a uniquely American invention, with nearly all the resources provided by the federal government but with most of the operational responsibility located as close as possible to the communities they serve. The success of U.S. nutrition assistance programs means that extreme forms of hunger and malnutrition, common in developing countries, have been practically eliminated.

However, less severe forms of food insecurity and hunger are still found within the United States and remain a reason for concern.[1] This chapter discusses nutrition monitoring in the United States, food insecurity, and food assistance programs.

The History of Food Assistance Programs in the United States

W.O. Atwater discovered the link among food composition, dietary intake, and health in 1890. The predominant nutritional problems then were low caloric and inadequate intakes of certain vitamins and minerals.[2,3] Because of food restrictions and shortages during World War I, scientific discoveries in nutrition were translated quickly into public health policy. In 1917, the U.S. Department of Agriculture (USDA) issued the first dietary recommendations based on five food groups.[4]

In 1921, the Maternal and Infancy Act, formerly known as the Sheppard-Towner Act, was adopted by Congress and remained in effect until 1929. The passage of the act resulted in federal grant-in-aid to states for child and adult health programs. Another major result of the act was the development of full-time units of maternal and child health services in state health departments. The act also enabled state health departments to employ nutritionists. During the 1930s, the federal government developed food relief and food commodity distribution programs, including school feeding, nutrition education programs, and national food consumption surveys.[5,6]

The growth of publicly funded nutrition programs accelerated during the early 1940s because of reports that 25 percent of military draftees showed evidence of past or present malnutrition. A frequent cause of rejection from military service was tooth decay or loss caused by conditions that might have been prevented or corrected by adequate nutrition in early childhood.[6,7]

U.S. Department of Agriculture Food Plans

In the 1930s, the USDA began developing family food plans at four separate cost levels: Economical, Low-Cost, Moderate-Cost, and Liberal. In 1974, the USDA replaced the Economical Plan with the Thrifty Plan. These plans are still the official food plans maintained by the USDA Center for Nutrition Policy and Promotion (CNPP).[8]

Each plan represents a set of market baskets applicable to one of 12 age/gender groups. Each market basket contains a selection of foods in quantities that reflect dietary recommendations, food consumption patterns, food composition data, and food prices. The four plans have various policy uses, including:[8,9]

- Bankruptcy courts often use the value of the Low-Cost Plan to determine the portion of a bankruptee's income to allocate for necessary food expenses.
- The Department of Defense uses the values of the Moderate-Cost and Liberal Food Plans to set the Basic Allowance for Subsistence rate for all enlistees.
- Many divorce courts use the value of the food plans to set alimony payments, and all three plans are used in the USDA's Expenditures on Children by Families Report, which is used to set state child support guidelines and foster care payments.
- Policymakers and others use the food plans as national standards in educational programs and as references for policies that are designed to help families budget their food dollars effectively and improve their diets.

In 1955, the USDA National Food Consumption Study found that the average U.S. family spent about one-third of its net income on food.[10] Therefore, the poverty line was established at three times the cost of the USDA's Low-Cost Food Plan for a family of four. After the USDA established the Thrifty Plan in 1974—using more frugal food choices than the Low-Cost Food Plan—they switched to that plan. The Thrifty Plan is now multiplied by three and adjusted for the size of the family and the current consumer price index to determine the official poverty income guidelines each year. The Thrifty Plan is also used to calculate food stamp allowances. These guidelines are used by federal agencies as criteria for eligibility for different federal assistance programs and as a basis for compiling data on poverty. **Table 4.1** lists an example of estimated weekly costs of the four USDA food plans for the month of May 2006.[11]

Monitoring Nutrition in the United States

Nutrition monitoring provides an ongoing description of nutrition conditions in the population, paying particular attention to subgroups defined in socioeconomic terms. It is used to plan, analyze the effects of policies and programs on nutrition problems, and predict future trends.[12]

Nutrition programs rely on data from nutrition monitoring surveys to identify the needs of those they serve. Data from national surveys are used to monitor the dietary status of the population, assess the nutritional adequacy of the food supply, measure the economics of food consumption, make public policies related to nutrition education programs, evaluate the effects of food assistance and regulatory programs, and provide the public with guidelines for food selection.[13,14] The data are also used to direct program development and to determine national, state, and local funding.

The United States is recognized as having one of the most comprehensive nutrition monitoring programs in the world. The United States and some other developed countries, such as the United Kingdom, France, Japan, Norway, and Canada, have integrated a data collection and reporting system into a national nutrition monitoring program to provide comprehensive nutrition and diet and health information. Programs in the United States such as the Food Stamp Program, National School Lunch Program, and WIC support a myriad of nutrition and health policy needs, regulatory reviews, and research studies.

The food and nutrient intakes reported from national food consumption surveys reflect either daily or usual consumption patterns; information is obtained on the types of foods consumed, commercially

---

National School Lunch Program Child nutrition program started in 1946 that provides cash reimbursement to schools so they can provide a free or reduced price lunch that meets specified nutritional requirements.

WIC The Special Supplemental Nutrition Program for Women, Infants, and Children was established in 1972 to improve the nutritional status of medically high-risk pregnant and lactating women as well as children up to 5 years of age from low-income families. WIC is funded through the USDA.

Food Stamp Program A federal entitlement program established in 1964 and administered by the U.S. Department of Agriculture (USDA) to give more food-buying power to low-income persons or families through monthly allotments of stamps.

nutrition monitoring An ongoing description of nutrition conditions in the population with particular attention to subgroups defined in socioeconomic terms, for purposes of planning, analyzing the effects of policies and programs on nutrition problems, and predicting future trends.

TABLE 4.1 **Official USDA Food Plans: Cost of Food at Home at Four Levels**

AGE-GENDER GROUPS	U.S. Average, May 2006[a] WEEKLY COST[b] (in dollars)			
	Thrifty Plan	Low-Cost Plan	Moderate-Cost Plan	Liberal Plan
Individuals:[c]				
CHILD:				
1 year	17.90	22.60	26.40	31.60
2 years	17.90	22.40	26.60	32.10
3–5 years	19.90	24.60	30.40	36.60
6–8 years	25.50	33.30	40.10	48.00
9–11 years	29.50	37.50	48.00	55.90
MALE:				
12–14 years	30.60	42.50	52.40	62.00
15–19 years	30.80	44.00	54.60	63.50
20–50 years	33.90	43.70	54.30	66.40
51 years and over	30.80	41.40	51.10	61.60
FEMALE:				
12–19 years	30.50	36.70	44.30	53.70
20–50 years	30.60	38.00	46.40	59.70
51 years and over	30.00	36.80	45.80	55.10
Families:				
FAMILY OF 2:[d]				
20–50 years	71.00	89.80	110.80	138.80
51 years and over	66.90	86.10	106.60	128.30
FAMILY OF 4:				
Couple, 20–50 years and children				
2 and 3–5 years	102.40	128.60	157.70	194.90
6–8 and 9–11 years	119.10	152.50	189.90	230.10

[a]Based on all meals and snacks purchased at stores and prepared at home. For specific foods and quantities of foods in the Thrifty Food Plan, see *Family Economics and Nutrition Review*, Vol. 13, No. 1 (2001), pp. 50–64; for specific foods and quantities of foods in the Low-Cost, Moderate-Cost, and Liberal Plans, see *The Low-Cost, Moderate-Cost, and Liberal Food Plans, 2003 Administrative Report* (2003). All four Food Plans are based on 1989–91 data and are updated to current dollars using the Consumer Price Index for specific food items.

[b]All costs are rounded to the nearest 10 cents.

[c]The costs are given for individuals in four-person families. For individuals in other size families, the following adjustments are suggested: one person: add 20 percent; two people: add 10 percent; three people: add 5 percent; four people: no adjustment; five or six people: subtract 5 percent; seven or more people: subtract 10 percent. To calculate overall household food costs, 1) adjust food costs for each person in the household, and then 2) add these adjusted food costs.

[d]Ten percent added for family size adjustment.

Source: U.S. Department of Agriculture. Income Eligibility Guidelines. Available at: http://www.fns.usda.gov/cnd/Governance/notices/iegs/IEGs.htm. Accessed April 14, 2005.

prepared or home-prepared foods, quantities of food consumed per meal or per day, and food preparation methods and recipe ingredients. Nutrition monitoring programs provide broad management capability to ensure that surveillance surveys exist to detect and report changes so that appropriate actions can be taken.[15,16]

In 1990 the National Nutrition Monitoring System (NNMS) was renamed the National Nutrition Monitoring and Related Research Program (NNMRRP).[17-19] The aim of this nutrition monitoring program is to strengthen nutrition monitoring efforts in the United States, and have a coordinated, comprehensive system that provides information about the dietary and nutritional status of the U.S. population, the conditions that affect the dietary and nutritional status of individuals, and the relationships between diet and health.[20,21]

National Center for Health Statistics (NCHS)/ Centers for Disease Control and Prevention (CDC) Growth Charts

The NCHS/CDC growth charts are one example of how nutrition monitoring data have been used for the development of population reference standards.[22] In 2000, data from the third National Health and Nutrition Examination Survey (NHANES III) were used to develop the revised NCHS/CDC growth charts.[23] The revised charts represent racial and ethnic diversity in the United States and contain a mixture of growth data from infants who were breast- and formula-fed that is more accurate than the 1977 NCHS reference growth charts.[24,25] They also include information for children from infancy up through 20 years of age as well as a new chart for body mass index (BMI) by age.[23,26] Visit the CDC website at http://www.cdc.gov/growthcharts to view or download the charts.

Programmatic Uses

National nutrition monitoring programs provide information for developing and promoting nutrition education activities and programs such as the *Dietary Guidelines for Americans*[27] and Fruits and Veggies More Matters program,[28] public health programs such as the National Cholesterol Education Program[29] and the National High Blood Pressure Education Program,[30] and federally supported food assistance programs such as the Food Stamp Program and WIC.[31,32]

Regulatory Uses

Nutrition monitoring data have been used by regulatory agencies to develop and examine U.S. food fortification,[33,34] food safety, and food labeling policies to enlighten and educate consumers.[35] The data have been used to provide dietary estimates for nutrient and non-nutrient food components. For instance, national nutrition monitoring data collected in NHANES III were used to evaluate folate status and the relationship among serum determinations, diet, and other nutrition and health variables before the Food and Drug Administration (FDA) ruled on the need for folate food fortification.[34,36]

Scientific Uses

Nutrition monitoring data are used by scientists to revise the standards of human nutrient requirements and to study the relationship among diet, nutrition, and health.[37,38] National data on the population's dietary intake and serum nutrient levels have been used to investigate nutrient requirements throughout the lifecycle, to identify areas of nutrition research that are needed to increase the knowledge base, and for the development of the Dietary Reference Intakes by the National Academy of Sciences (NAS).[37-39] Current research, such as the Human Genome Project, are being used to develop nutrition status indicators, which will be important for future monitoring efforts.

Nutrition monitoring data also are used to evaluate progress toward the 2010 Healthy People Objectives and to determine and prioritize the food and nutrition research needs of the community and public.[39-43] For example, national nutrition monitoring data have been used in the Surgeon General's *Report on Nutrition and Health* to provide important information about the link between diet and chronic health conditions[44] and the NAS report *Diet and Health: Implications for Reducing Chronic Disease Risk*.[39] **Table 4.2** presents a summary of federal nutrition monitoring surveys and surveillance activities since 1990.

TABLE 4.2	Federal Nutrition Monitoring Surveys and Surveillance Activities Since 1990		
Date (initiated)	**Dept.**	**Survey**	**Sample Size and Target U.S. Population**
Nutrition and Related Health Measurements			
Continuous (1915)	HHS	National Vital Registration System	All births and deaths in the total U.S. population
Annual (1957)	HHS	National Health Interview Survey (NHIS)	Civilian, non-institutionalized household population (N = 103,477 individuals and N = 39,832 households in 1997)
1985, 1990, 1998	HHS	National Health Interview Survey on Health Promotion and Disease Prevention	Civilian, non-institutionalized household population in the U.S., ages 18+ years (N = 41,104 households in 1990)
1987, 1992	HHS	National Health Interview Survey on Cancer Epidemiology and Cancer Control	Civilian, non-institutionalized household population ages 18+ years in the United States (N = 12,000 households in 1992)
1991	HHS	1991 National Health Interview Survey on Health Promotion and Disease Prevention	Civilian, non-institutionalized, household population in the United States, ages 18+ years (N = 43,732 households)
1992–1993	HHS	National Health Interview Survey on Youth Behavior Supplement	Youth ages 12–21 years (N = 10,645 households)

TABLE 4.2	(Continued)		

Date (initiated)	Dept.	Survey	Sample Size and Target U.S. Population
Nutrition and Related Health Measurements (Cont.)			
1994	HHS	National Health Interview Survey on Disability	Civilian, non-institutionalized household population (*N* = 107,469 households)
1993, 1995	HHS	National Health Interview Survey Year 2000 Objectives Supplement	Civilian, non-institutionalized household population in the U.S., ages 18+ years (*N* = 17,317 households in 1995)
1990, 1995 (1973)	HHS	National Survey of Family Growth	Women, 15–44 years (*N* = 10,847 households in 1995)
Continuous (1973)	HHS	Pregnancy Nutrition Surveillance System (PNSS)	Low-income, high-risk pregnant women participating in programs in 18 states, the Navajo Nation, and the Intertribal Council of Arizona (*N* = 599,000 records in 1995)
Continuous (1973)	HHS	Pediatric Nutrition Surveillance System (PedNSS)	Low-income, high-risk children, birth–17 years in participating programs in 43 states and Washington, DC, Puerto Rico, and 6 Indian reservations (*N* = 8,800,000 records in 1995)
1988–1990	HHS	National Maternal and Infant Health Survey	Women, hospitals, and prenatal care providers associated with live births (*N* = 9,953), still births (*N* = 3,309), and infant deaths (*N* = 5,332)
1988–1994	HHS	Third National Health and Nutrition Examination Survey (NHANES III); a follow-up study is under consideration	U.S. non-institutionalized, civilian population, 2+ months; oversampling of African Americans and Mexican Americans, children 0–5 years, and individuals 60+ years (*N* = 33,994 individuals interviewed; *N* = 31,311 individuals examined)
1989–1993	HHS	National Health and Nutrition Examination III Supplemental Nutrition Survey (SNS) of Older Americans	NHANES III (1988–91) examinees 50+ years (*N* = 2,602 completed NHANES III dietary recall (DR) and first SNS interview; *N* = 2,519 completed NHANES III DR and second SNS interview; *N* = 2,261 completed NHANES III DR and two SNS interviews)
1990–1991	HHS	Survey of Heights and Weights of American Indian School Children	American Indian school children, ages 5–18 years (*N* = 9,464 children in 1990–91 school year)
1991–1992	HHS	Navajo Health and Nutrition Survey	Persons ages 12+ years residing on or near the Navajo reservation in Arizona, New Mexico, and Colorado (*N* = 985 examined)
1991–1992	HHS	Longitudinal Follow-up to the National Maternal and Infant Health Survey (NMIHS)	Participants in the 1988 NMIHS (*N* = 9,400 mothers of 3-year-olds; *N* = 1,000 women who had infant deaths; *N* = 1,000 women who had late fetal deaths in 1988)
1992	HHS	NHANES I Epidemiologic Follow-up Study	Individuals examined in NHANES I, 25–74 years at baseline, 1971–74 (*N* = 9,281, 1992 cohort)
Continuous (1992)	HHS	NHANES II Mortality Follow-up Survey	Individuals examined in NHANES II, 30–74 years at baseline, 1976–80 (*N* = 9,252)
Continuous (1992)	HHS	Hispanic HANES (HHANES) Mortality Follow-up Survey	Individuals interviewed in HHANES, 20–74 years at baseline, 1982–84
Annual (1992)	HHS	National Health Care Survey (integrates National Home and Hospice Care Survey (1992–94; 1996), National Nursing Home Survey (since 1973–74) and follow-up (1995, 1997), National Hospital Discharge Survey (since 1965), National Ambulatory Medical Care Survey (since 1973), National Hospital Ambulatory Medical Care Survey (1992), and National Survey of Ambulatory Surgery (1994–96)	Record-based healthcare provider surveys including: visits to hospital emergency and outpatient departments of nonfederal, short-stay, general, and specialty hospitals and ambulatory surgical centers; office visits to nonfederal, office-based physicians; and home health agencies and nursing homes (*N* = 11,396 for 1996 NHHCS; *N* = 9,556 for 1995 NNHS; *N* = 282,525 for 1995 NHDS; *N* = 32,978 for 1996 NAMCS; *N* = 52,194 for 1996 NHAMCS; *N* = 125,751 for 1996 NSAS)

(continues)

TABLE 4.2	(Continued)		

Date (initiated)	Dept.	Survey	Sample Size and Target U.S. Population
Nutrition and Related Health Measurements (Cont.)			
Continuous (1992)	HHS	NHANES III Mortality Follow-up Survey	Individuals interviewed and examined in NHANES III, 20+ years at baseline, 1988–94
1996–1999	HHS	Demonstration sites for PedNSS and PNSS	Low-income, high-risk women, infants, and children who participate in government food assistance programs and participate in PedNSS and PNSS (N = minimum of 1,000 children in WIC for PedNSS; N = minimum of 300 women in WIC for PNSS)
1999+	HHS	National Health and Nutrition Examination Survey	Civilian, non-institutionalized individuals; oversampling of African Americans, Mexican Americans, adolescents, older persons, and pregnant women in the first 3 years
Food and Nutrient Consumption			
Continuous (1917)	DOD	Nutritional Evaluation of Military Feeding Systems and Military Populations	Enlisted personnel of the Army, Navy, Marine Corps, and Air Force (N = 20–240 depending on study focus)
Annual supplement (1995)	BLS; CB; USDA	Current Population Survey, Supplement of Food Security	Civilian, non-institutionalized U.S. population (N = approx. 59,500 for CPS)
Continuous (1980)	DOL	Consumer Expenditure Survey	Civilian, non-institutionalized, population and a portion of the institutionalized population (N = 5,000 in quarterly interview survey of consumer units; N = 6,000 diary surveys of consumer units kept for two consecutive 1-week periods)
Continuous (1983)	DOC	Survey of Income and Program Participation (SIPP)	Civilian, non-institutionalized population of the U.S. (N = 11,600–36,800 households in a continuous series of panels)
1994, 1996 (1984)	USDA	Study of WIC Participants and Program Characteristics	WIC participants, using mail surveys of state and local WIC agencies, record abstractions at local WIC service sites and, in 1988, interviews with participants (N = 7 million+ individuals in 1996)
1988–1994	HHS	NHANES III and Supplemental Nutrition Survey of Older Americans	See NHANES III listing above. Individuals ages 50+ years examined in NHANES III by telephone (see listing above for number of participants)
1989–1991, annual 1994–1996, annual (1985–1986)	USDA	Continuing Survey of Food Intakes by Individuals (CSFII) (Intake of Pyramid Servings and Servings database, 1994–1996)	Females 19–50 years and their children 1–5 years, and males 19–50 years residing in households in the 48 contiguous states in 1985–86, individuals of all ages residing in households in 48 conterminous states in 1989–91, and nationwide in 1994–96; oversampling of individuals in low-income households; individuals 2+ years from CSFII 1994–96 (N = 15,303 in 1994–96)
1989–1991	HHS	Strong Heart Dietary Survey	American Indian adults ages 45–74 years in South Dakota, Oklahoma, and Arizona (N = 888)
1991–1992	DOC	Development of a National Seafood Consumption Survey Model	Individuals residing in eligible households and recreational/subsistence fishermen
1992	USDA	School Nutrition Dietary Assessment Study	School-age children in grades 1–12 in 48 contiguous states and Washington, DC (N = 380 school districts; N = 607 schools; N = 4,489 students)
1992	USDA	Adult Day Care Program Study	Adult daycare centers and adults participating in the Child and Adult Care Food Program (N = 282 CACFP centers; N = 282 non-CACFP centers; N = 942 participating adults)
1994–1995	USDA	WIC Infant Feeding Practices Study	Nationally representative sample of WIC mothers and infants living in the 48 contiguous states, Washington, DC, and the 33 WIC agencies on Indian reservations (N = 971)

TABLE 4.2	(Continued)		

Date (initiated)	Dept.	Survey	Sample Size and Target U.S. Population
Food and Nutrient Consumption (cont.)			
1995	USDA	Early Childhood and Child Care Study	Childcare sponsors, providers, and children participating in the CACFP (*N* = 566 sponsors; *N* = 1,962 providers; *N* = 1,951 households; *N* = 2,174 child-day observations)
1997–1998	USDA	Supplemental Children's Survey	Non-institutionalized children 0–9 years in households in the U.S.; oversampling of low-income households (*N* = approx. 5,000)
1998	USDA	School Nutrition Dietary Assessment Study II	School-age children in grades 1–12 in 48 contiguous states and Washington, DC (*N* = approx. 1,152 schools)
1999+	HHS	National Health and Nutrition Examination Survey	Civilian, non-institutionalized individuals; oversampling of African Americans, Mexican Americans, adolescents, older persons, and pregnant women in the first 3 years (*N* = approx. 3,200)
Knowledge, Attitudes, and Behavior Assessments			
Continuous (1984)	HHS	Behavioral Risk Factor Surveillance System	Individuals 18+ years residing in households with telephones in participating states (*N* = approx. 2,039 per state in all 50 states for 1995)
1990, 1994 (1982)	HHS	Health and Diet Survey	Civilian, non-institutionalized individuals in households with telephones, 18+ years (*N* = 5,005 in 1995)
1989–1991, 1994–1996	USDA	Diet and Health Knowledge Survey	Main meal-planner/preparer in households participating in 1989–91 and 1994–96 CSFII (*N* = 5,765 for 1994–96)
Annual (1990)	HHS	Youth Risk Behavior Survey (YRBS)	Youths attending school in grades 9–12 and 12–21 years of age in households in 50 states, Washington, DC, Puerto Rico, and Virgin Islands (*N* = approx. 12,000 for the national surveys and *N* = approx. 2,000 for the state and local surveys)
1990	HHS	Cholesterol Awareness Survey—Physicians' Survey	Physicians practicing in the conterminous U.S. (*N* = 1,604)
1990–1991	HHS	Nationwide Survey of Nurses' and Dietitians' Knowledge, Attitudes, and Behavior Regarding Cardiovascular Risk Factors	Registered nurses and registered dietitians currently active in their professions (*N* = 7,200 registered nurses; *N* = 1,621 occupational health nurses oversample; *N* = 1,782 registered dietitians)
1990–1991	HHS	Nutrition Label Format Studies	Primary food shoppers, ages 18+ years (*N* =2,676)
1991	HHS	Weight Loss Practices Survey	Individuals currently trying to lose weight, ages 18+ years, in households with telephones (*N* = 1,232 current dieters; *N* = 205 African American oversample; *N* = 218 nondieting controls)
1991	HHS	5 A Day for Better Health Baseline Survey	Individuals ages 18+ years with telephones (*N* = approx. 2,059)
1992–1993; 1998	HHS	Consumer Food Handling Practices and Awareness of Microbiological Hazards Screener	Individuals in households with telephones, 18+ years (*N* = 1,620)
1993–1994	HHS	Infant Feeding Practices Survey	New mothers and healthy, full-term infants 0–1 year (*N* = 1,200)
1994–1995	USDA	WIC Infant Feeding Practices Survey	Prenatal and postnatal women and their infants participating in the WIC program (*N* = 971)
Food Composition and Nutrient Databases			
Continuous (1892)	USDA	National Nutrient Data Bank Food Composition Laboratory	Not available
Annual (1961)	HHS	Total Diet Study	Representative diets of specific age/sex groups
1991–1993, 1993–1994, 1995–1996 (1977)	HHS	Food Label and Package Survey	*N* = 1,250 food brands

(continues)

| TABLE 4.2 | | (Continued) | | |

Date (initiated)	Dept.	Survey	Sample Size and Target U.S. Population
Food Composition and Nutrient Databases (cont.)			
Continuous (1977)	USDA	Survey Nutrient Data Base for CSFH 1989–91, 1994–96; NHANES III 1988–94	Not available
1988–1994	HHS	Technical Support Information for the NHANES III, 1988–94 Dietary Interview Data Files	Not available
1994–1996	USDA	CSFII 1994–96 Technical Support Files Food Coding Database, Recipe Database, Survey Nutrient Database, and Related Files	Not available
Food Supply Determinations			
Annual (1909)	DOC	Fisheries of the United States	Not available
	USDA	U.S. Food and Nutrition Supply Series	
	USDA	Estimates of Food Available	
		Estimates of Nutrients	
Continuous (1985)	USDA	A.C. Nielsen SCANTRACK	N = 3,000 supermarkets since 1988

Abbreviations: ARS, Agricultural Research Service; BLS, Bureau of Labor Statistics; CACFP, Child and Adult Care Food Program; CB, Census Bureau; CDC, Centers for Disease Control and Prevention; DOC, Department of Commerce; DOD, Department of Defense; DOL, Department of Labor; FDA, Food and Drug Administration; FNS, Food and Nutrition Service; HHS, Department of Health and Human Services; IHS, Indian Health Service; NCHS, National Center for Health Statistics; USDA, U.S. Department of Agriculture.

Modified from: Berdanier CD, Feldman E, Flatt, St. Jeor ST. *Handbook of Nutrition and Food*. New York: CRC Press; 2002. Reprinted with permission.

Food Insecurity

Nutrition monitoring data are also used to estimate food insecurity. In the United States, food security is defined as access to enough food for an active, healthy life and includes at a minimum: 1) the ready availability of nutritionally adequate and safe foods and 2) the assured ability to acquire acceptable foods in socially acceptable ways (e.g., without resorting to emergency food supplies or other coping strategies).[45]

> **food insecurity** The inability to obtain sufficient food for any reason.

Food insecurity exists whenever the availability of nutritionally adequate and safe foods or the ability to acquire acceptable foods in socially acceptable ways is limited or uncertain.[46,47] Four main conceptual elements define this phenomenon:[48]

- Food insecurity is experienced at the household and individual levels in different ways. Individual-level experience relates to issues of food consumption and allocation and includes the physiological sensation of hunger. Food supply management and acquisition issues define the household situation.[49]
- The experience of food insecurity is not static but dynamic in nature, defined by a sequence of events and experiences that can be considered in terms of frequency, duration, and periodicity.
- The sequence of stages that define the experience reflects graded levels of severity, ranging from qualitative compromises in food selection and consumption to quantitative compromises in intake and the physical sensation of hunger, as resources become depleted. At its most severe stage, food insecurity is experienced as absolute food deprivation (i.e., individuals not eating at all).
- Within households, individuals' experiences of food insecurity differ. Mainly, adults seem to compromise their own intakes first in an effort to minimize the extent and nature of compromise experienced by children in the household. This suggests that food insecurity is a managed process in which the sequence of events and severity of experience for different household members is, to some extent, controlled and predictable.[50-52]

The four aspects of this conceptual framework are summarized in **Table 4.3**.

Assessing Food Insecurity

Since 1995, the U.S. Census Bureau has conducted an annual survey of food security among a nationally representative sample of people living in the United States using the food security module in the Current Population Survey (CPS). The questions asked were about the following:[53]

- Anxiety or the perception that the household budget is inadequate to buy enough food
- A perception of inadequacy in the quantity or quality of food eaten by adults and children in the household
- Instances of reduced food intake or consequences of reduced food intake for adults and children
- Periods of a decrease in food intake, hunger, and/or weight loss by household members

TABLE 4.3	Dimensions of Food Insecurity Elucidated from Qualitative Research by Radimer 1990

	Individual Level	Household Level
Quantitative	Insufficient intake	Food depletion
Qualitative	Nutritional inadequacy	Unsuitable food
Psychological	Lack of choice, feelings of deprivation	Food anxiety
Social	Disrupted eating patterns	Food acquisition in socially unacceptable ways

From: Kendall A, Olson CM, Frongillo EA. Validation of the Radimer/Cornell measures of hunger and food insecurity. *J Nutr.* 1995; 125:2793–2801. Reprinted with permission.

The CPS questionnaire contains 18 items. Households without children were asked to respond to 10 questions and households with children were asked to respond to all 18 questions. Questions 1, 1a, and 1b are not used to calculate the food security/hunger scale and may be used, in conjunction with income, as a preliminary screener to reduce respondent burden for high-income households. Therefore, question 1 was not included in **Table 4.4**. The CPS can be administered in about 2 minutes.[53] The questions reflect the different classifications of households' food insecurity levels. For example, the least severe item is an adult-referenced item, which asks whether the household members worried that food would run out before they got money to buy more. See **Box 4-1** for measure of severity of household food insecurity and hunger. Households are classified into one of four categories of food security:[53]

- *Food Secure:* Households with no or minimal evidence of food insecurity.
- *Food Insecure without Hunger:* Food insecurity is evident in the household's concerns and in adjustments to household food

TABLE 4.4	Questions Included in the Core Food Security Scale[53,55]

	Stage 1 (Screen 1 asked of all households)
	Now I'm going to read you several statements that people have made about their food situation. Please tell me whether the statement was *often*, *sometimes*, or *never true* in the last 12 months:
Q2	"I worried whether our food would run out before we got money to buy more." Was that often, sometimes, or never true for you in the last 12 months?
Q3	"The food that we bought just didn't last, and we didn't have money to get more." Was that often, sometimes, or never true for you in the last 12 months?
Q4	"We couldn't afford to eat balanced meals." Was that often, sometimes, or never true for you in the last 12 months?
Q5	"We relied on only a few kinds of low-cost food to feed the children because we were running out of money to buy food." Was that often, sometimes, or never true for you in the last 12 months?
Q6	"We couldn't feed the children a balanced meal because we couldn't afford that." Was that often, sometimes, or never true for you in the last 12 months?
	Stage 2 (Asked of households after passing of the first screen)
Q7	"The children were not eating enough because we just couldn't afford enough food." Was that often, sometimes, or never true for you in the last 12 months?
Q8	In the last 12 months, did you or other adults in your household ever cut the size of your meals or skip meals because there wasn't enough money for food?
Q9	In the last 12 months, did you ever eat less than you felt you should because there wasn't enough money to buy food?
Q10	In the last 12 months, were you ever hungry, but didn't eat because you couldn't afford enough food?
Q11	Sometimes people lose weight because they don't have enough to eat. In the last 12 months, did you lose weight because there wasn't enough food?
	Stage 3 (Asked of households after passing the second level screen)
Q12	In the last 12 months, did you or other adults in your household ever not eat for a whole day because there wasn't enough money for food? How often did this happen—almost every month, some months but not every month, or in only one or two months?
Q13	In the last 12 months, did you ever cut the size of any of the children's meals because there wasn't enough money for food?
Q14	In the last 12 months, did any of the children ever skip meals because there wasn't enough money for food? How often did this happen—almost every month, some months but not every month, or in only one or two months?
Q15	In the last 12 months, were the children ever hungry, but you just couldn't afford more food?
Q16	In the last 12 months, did any of the children ever not eat for a whole day because there wasn't enough money for food?

Box 4-1 Measure of Severity of Household Food Insecurity and Hunger[53,55]

Conditions/Experiences/Behaviors Indicative of Food Insecurity and Hunger:
(sequential set of increasingly severe indicators)

No such indications: **Presumed food secure**	One or two indications: **At-risk**	Multiple indications: **Few or no hunger indicators**	More, and more severe, indications: **Multiple indicators of adult hunger**	Many indications, including: **Child hunger indicators and more severe adult hunger indicators**

0   1.0   2.0   3.0   4.0   5.0   6.0   7.0   8.0   9.0   10

Household Food Security Scale—continuous measure

management, including reduced quality of diets. Little or no reduction in household members' food intake is reported.

- *Food Insecure with Moderate Hunger:* Food intake for adults in
the household has been reduced to an extent that it implies the
adults have repeatedly experienced the physical sensation of
hunger. Such reductions are not observed at this stage for children in the household.

- *Food Insecure with Severe Hunger:* Households with children
that have reduced the children's food intake to an extent that
it implies the children have experienced the physical sensation
of hunger. Adults in households with and without children have
repeatedly experienced more extensive reductions in food intake
at this stage.

The food security scale measures the respondents' levels of food security or insecurity in terms of a numeric value that ranges between 0 and
18. A respondent who has not experienced any of the food insecurity
situations would have a scale value of zero. A respondent who has
experienced all of the situations covered in the questions would have
a scale value of 10 or 18, depending on which version of the survey
they took. For categorizing or assigning respondents to levels of food
insecurity, the maximum raw score for being classified as food insecure
based on the standard value is level 3 in households with or without
children. Respondents with a score of zero are classified as food secure.
At the other extreme, respondents who reported experiencing all or
nearly all of the conditions receive high scale values of level 3 and are
classified as food insecure with severe hunger. See **Table 4.4** for measures of severity of household food insecurity and hunger.[54] The CPS
questionnaire and instructions can be downloaded in PDF format from
http://www.ers.usda.gov. The Spanish version has been validated and
is also available.

The Current Status of Food Insecurity in the United States

In 2005, 35 million people in the United States lived in households
experiencing food insecurity, down from 38.2 million in 2004 and 36.3

million in 2003.[56,57] In 2005, 89 percent of U.S. households were food
secure throughout the entire year, implying that they had access, at all
times, to enough food for an active, healthy life for all household members.[57-59] The remaining 11 percent of households were food insecure
at least some time during that year. (See **Figure 4-1**.) The prevalence of
food insecurity increased from 10.7 percent in 2001 to 11.9 percent in
2004, but decreased slightly to 11 percent in 2005. The prevalence of
low food security increased from 3.7 percent in 2004 to 7.1 in 2005. In
2005, 3.9 percent of households experienced very low food security
(food security with hunger). See **Table 4.5** for the revised description of
ranges of food security.[53,57,60] **Table 4.6** shows a summary of the trends
in U.S. food insecurity and hunger from 1995 to 2005. The rates of the
prevalence of food insecurity and food insecurity with hunger were not
statistically significant from 2002 to 2003, and stayed below the levels
of the 1995 prevalence rate, when it was first measured.

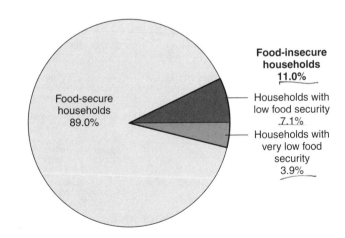

FIGURE 4-1 U.S. Households by Food Security Status, 2005

Source: Economic Research Service/USDA. Household Food Security in the
United States, 2005.

TABLE 4.5	USDA's New Labels Describing the Ranges of Food Security

		Detailed Categories	
General Categories	**Old Label**	**New Label**	**Description of Conditions in the Household**
Food security	Food security	High food security	No reported indications of food-access problems or limitations
		Marginal food security	One or two reported indications—typically of anxiety over food sufficiency or shortage of food in the house
			Little or no indication of changes in diets or food intake
Food insecurity	Food insecurity without hunger	Low food security	Reports of reduced quality, variety, or desirability of diet
			Little or no indication of reduced food intake
	Food insecurity with hunger	Very low food security	Reports of multiple indications of disrupted eating patterns and reduced food intake

Source: USDA/ERS. Recommendation by the Committee on National Statistics (CNSTAT) of the National Academies. Available at: http://www.ers.usda.gov/Briefing/FoodSecurity/labels.htm. Accessed January 2, 2007.

TABLE 4.6	Trends in Prevalence of Food Insecurity and Food Insecurity with Hunger in U.S. Households, 1995–2005[62]

Years	All Households Percentage	Food Secure Percentage	Low Food Security Percentage	Very Low Food Security Percentage
1995	10.3	89.6	6.4	3.9
1996	10.4	89.6	6.3	4.4
1997	8.7	91.3	5.6	3.1
1998	10.2	88.2	6.6	3.6
1999	10.1	89.9	7.1	3.1
2000	10.5	89.5	7.3	3.1
2001	10.7	89.3	7.4	3.3
2002	11.1	88.9	7.6	3.5
2003	11.2	88.8	7.7	3.5
2004	11.9	88.1	8.0	3.9
2005	11.0	89.0	7.1	3.9

Adapted from: Nord M, Andrews M, Carlson S. *Household Food Security in the United States, 2003*. Washington, DC: USDA; 2004. Available at: http://www.ers.usda.gov/publication/fanrr42/fanrr42.pdf. Accessed March 3, 2008.

Figures 4-2 and **4-3** show the prevalence of food insecurity and hunger among various socioeconomic, geographic, and demographic groups. The difference in the rates of food insecurity and hunger was not statistically significant. However, they show that poverty and hunger continued in households with children headed by single women, African Americans, Hispanics, and those with income below the poverty threshold.[57,61] The data also indicated that households were more likely to be hungry or food insecure if they lived in states in the Southern region of the country.[61,62] Overall, households with children reported food insecurity more than households without children. The following sections describe the groups that are experiencing the most food insecurity and hunger in the United States today.

Low-Income People

Poverty is one of the contributing factors to food insecurity and hunger. For example, in 2005, food insecurity was more than five times as prevalent in households with annual incomes below 185 percent of the poverty line as in households with incomes above that range. However, many factors that might affect a household's food security (such as job loss, divorce, or other unexpected events) are not recognized by any annual income measure.[63,64] One in three low-income households with annual incomes below 130 percent of the poverty line was food insecure in 2005. Reports show that low-income households with children were more affected by food insecurity than low-income households without children (40.6 percent vs. 27.7 percent). Low-income single mothers with children were more vulnerable to both food insecurity and hunger; 45 percent of these households were food insecure.[65,59] Households with income below 130 percent of the poverty line can receive food stamps, and children in these households are eligible for free meals in the National School Lunch and School Breakfast Programs.

The Working Poor

In 2005, 37 million people (12.6 percent of the population) lived at or below the official poverty threshold; this is not statistically different from 2004, when 37 million (12.7 percent) were at or below the threshold. Although the nation's poor were mainly children and adults who were not in the labor force, one in every five (7.8 million individuals) was classified as *working poor*. The working poor are those who spent at least 27 weeks of the year in the labor force (working

working poor Those who spent at least 27 weeks in the labor force (working or looking for work), but whose income is below the official poverty threshold.

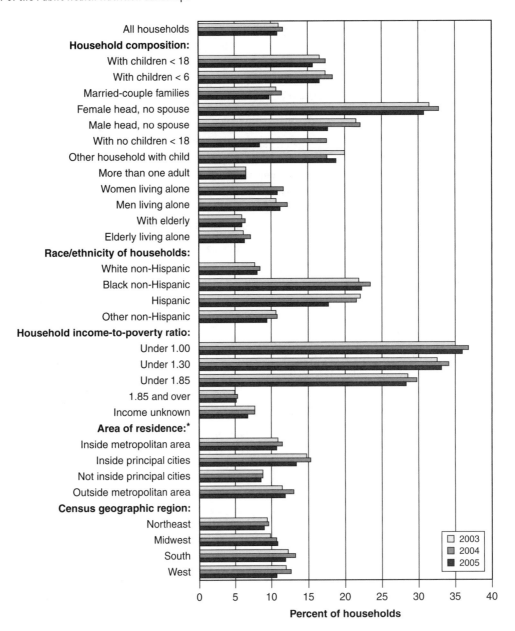

*Prevalence rates by area of residence in 2004 are not comparable with those for 2003 and earlier years because they represent somewhat different geographic areas. The 2004 survey classified metropolitan area residence based on revised metropolitan statistical areas delineated by the Office of Management and Budget in 2003.

FIGURE 4-2 Prevalence of Food Insecurity by Selected Household Characteristics, 2003, 2004, and 2005

Source: Calculated by Economic Research Service/USDA based on Current Population Survey Food Security Supplement data, December 2003, December 2004, and December 2005.

or looking for work), but whose incomes are below the official poverty threshold. (See **Table 4.7.**) Additional highlights from the 2005 data include:[65–69]

- 2.8 percent of those employed full time were classified as working poor, compared with 12.8 percent of part-time workers.
- The likelihood of being classified as working poor greatly diminishes as workers achieve higher levels of education. Only 1.7

percent of college graduates were counted among the working poor, compared with 15.2 percent of people with less than a high school diploma.
- Women who maintain families are twice as likely as their male counterparts to be among the working poor.

Of all individuals in the labor force for at least half of the year, more women than men head of households were poor (28.7 vs. 13.0 per-

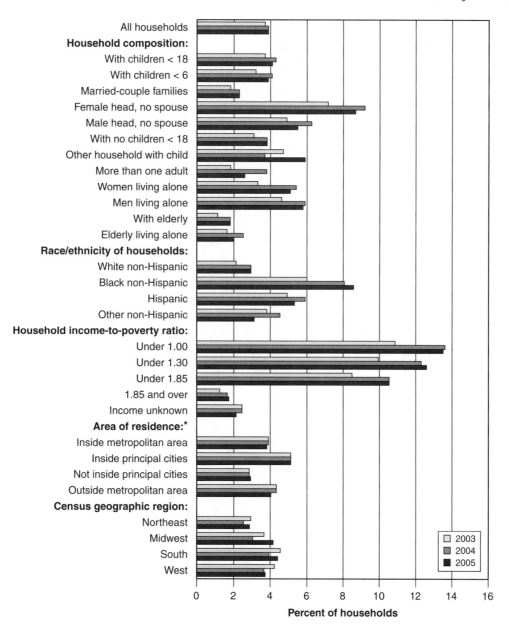

*Prevalence rates by area of residence in 2004 are not comparable with those for 2003 and earlier years because they represent somewhat different geographic areas. The 2004 survey classified metropolitan area residence based on revised metropolitan statistical areas delineated by the Office of Management and Budget in 2003.

FIGURE 4-3 Prevalence of Food Insecurity with Hunger, 2003, 2004, 2005

Source: Calculated by Economic Research Service/USDA based on Current Population Survey Food Security Supplement data, December 2003, 2004, and December 2005.

cent). Although about 7 in every 10 of the working poor were European American workers, African American and Hispanic workers were more than twice as likely as their European American counterparts to be among the working poor. The poverty rate for African Americans was 24.9 percent, for Hispanics 21.8 percent, for European Americans 8.3 percent, and for Asians 11.1 percent.[67,68]

Reports show that younger workers were more vulnerable to being poor than older workers. The poverty rate for children under age 18 was 17.6 percent. A recent, government-sponsored survey of clients at food pantries estimated that more people will use food pantries this year than compared to last year.[70] The survey showed that the majority of families that go to food pantries for emergency help work or have children. The use of food pantries varied considerably by household structure and by race and ethnicity.[68] Households with children were nearly twice as likely as those without children to use food pantries (5.5 vs. 3.2 percent). Food pantry use was high among

TABLE 4.7	Poverty Status of Persons and Primary Families in the Labor Force for 27 Weeks or More, 2001–2005 (Numbers in Thousands)				
Characteristics	**2001**	**2002**[a]	**2003**[b]	**2004**	**2005**
Total Persons[c]	138,143	139,728	140,007	140,876	142,824
In poverty	6,802	7,359	7,429	7,837	7,744
Poverty rate	4.9	5.3	5.3	5.6	5.4
Unrelated individuals	29,387	29,847	29,898	30,373	31,422
In poverty	2,388	2,584	2,472	2,720	2,846
Poverty rate	8.1	8.7	8.3	9.0	9.1
Primary families[d]	62,251	63,352	63,567	64,063	64,360
In poverty	3,697	3,973	4,167	4,279	4,094
Poverty rate	5.9	6.3	6.6	6.7	6.4

[a]Data, beginning in 2002 with the collection of the 2003 Annual Social and Economics Supplement to the Current Population Survey, are not strictly comparable with data for earlier years because of the introduction in the January 2003 survey of revised population controls.

[b]Data, beginning in 2003 with the collection of the 2004 Annual Social and Economic Supplement to the Current Population Survey, are not strictly comparable with data for earlier years because of the introduction in the January 2004 survey of revised population controls.

[c]Includes persons in families, not shown separately.

[d]Refers to primary families with at least one member in the labor force for more than half the year. A primary family includes the reference person (householder) and all people living in the household who are related to the reference person.

Source: U.S. Department of Labor, U.S. Bureau of Labor Statistics. A profile of working poor, September 2007. Available at: http://www.bls.gov/cps/cpswp2005.pdf. Accessed February 20, 2008.

female-headed households with children (10.5 percent), whereas use by married couples with children was lower than the national average (2.9 percent). Few households with elderly members used food pantries (2.3 percent).

The use of food pantries was higher among African Americans (7.8 percent) and Hispanics (3.9 percent) than among European Americans (2.7 percent). In spite of their lower use rate, European Americans comprised a majority (55 percent) of food pantry users because of their larger share in the general population. About 16 percent of households with incomes below the poverty line received food from food pantries, compared with 0.9 percent of households with incomes above 185 percent of the poverty line.[71]

The use of food pantries was higher in principal metropolitan cities (households within incorporated areas of the largest cities in each metropolitan area) (4.3 percent) and in non-metropolitan areas (4.3 percent) than in metropolitan areas (2.4 percent). There was no significant regional variation in the use of food pantries; however, the use of food pantries was more common in the Midwest (3.8 percent) and

the West (3.9 percent).[72] In addition, the prevalence rate of food insecurity for households located in principal metropolitan cities was 2.9 percent compared to 4.0 percent in non-metropolitan areas. Regionally, the prevalence of food insecurity was higher in the South (4.4 percent), Midwest (4.1 percent), and West (3.7 percent) than in the Northeast (2.8 percent).[71]

Ethnic Groups

Low-income and minority persons are more likely to suffer from food insecurity than those in the majority group. The prevalence of food insecurity with hunger for African American households was 8.6 percent, and for Hispanic households was 5.3 percent. Food insecurity represents lack of enough food and lack of nutritious food. Both socioeconomic status and race have been shown to affect household diets.[73]

The Elderly

In 2005, the poverty rate for the elderly increased to 3.6 million (10.1 percent) after it reached a historic low of 3.5 million in 2004.[74] Additionally, in 2005, 2.6 percent of the elderly population lived in severe poverty (below 50 percent of the poverty threshold), and 16.7 percent were classified as near poor (incomes between 100 percent and 125 percent of poverty).[68] A significant number of elderly encounter poverty at some time during their lifetimes. After age 65, the probability of a person experiencing a year below the poverty line at some point was 40 percent.[68]

Rates of food insecurity and hunger among elderly households depended on household composition, household income, race and ethnicity, and area of residence. The rates of food insecurity were higher among those living alone (6.4 percent). The rates of food insecurity among elderly households with incomes below the federal poverty line were higher compared to those of elderly households with incomes above 185 percent of the poverty line. Food insecurity and hunger were more common among African American (22.4 percent) and Hispanic (17.9 percent) elderly persons than among European Americans (8.2 percent).[68]

State-by-State Variations

The rates of food insecurity and food insecurity with hunger vary from state to state. Data compiled from 2003 to 2005 showed a food insecurity range from 6.4 percent in North Dakota to 16.8 percent in New Mexico; measured prevalence rates of food insecurity with hunger ranged from 1.9 percent in Delaware to 6.3 percent in South Carolina. Taking the margin of error of the state and U.S. estimates into consideration, the prevalence of food insecurity was higher than the national average in 11 states, lower than the national average in 20 states, and not statistically different in 19 states and the District of Columbia.[75]

The Homeless

Homeless people are individuals who do not have a fixed, regular, and adequate nighttime residence. They may be sleeping on the streets, with friends or family, in cars, in abandoned buildings, or in shelters.[76] In 2006, the demand for emergency shelter for homeless people increased by about 68 percent and for homeless families by 59 percent.

Homelessness affects the health and well-being of individuals throughout the life span. Consider the effect of homelessness on children, pregnant women, adolescents, or older persons. Each group has different nutritional needs, and dietitians need to be aware of their unique needs. For example, homeless pregnant women have less access to prenatal care, poorer nutritional status, and a higher incidence of poor birth outcomes (lower-birth-weight infants).[77] Homeless children are at greater risk for inadequate nutrient intake that can contribute to failure to thrive, obesity, and poor growth.[78] In addition, homeless older persons suffer from untreated nutrition-related conditions such as obesity, heart disease, hypertension, and malnutrition.[79] Similar to other homeless people, older persons must focus their energy on survival.

It is not easy to know the number of homeless people and who they are. The high cost of housing, mental illness, low-paying jobs, substance abuse, domestic violence, and unemployment limits the food budget and creates the problems of hunger and homelessness.

Becoming homeless is a gradual process. Once the individual or family loses their home, they may live with family or friends and only go to the shelter or seek refuge on the streets when all other options are depleted.[80] Several factors can contribute to homelessness and hunger, including poverty, unemployment, and emergency demands on income. However, the two factors that contribute most to homelessness and hunger are unaffordable housing units and income. The national *housing wage* (the amount a person working full time must earn to pay for a two-bedroom rental unit at fair market rent [80]) for 2006 was $16.31 an hour, or $33,925 a year. This is almost three times the federal minimum wage of $6.55 an hour. The Housing Wage has increased 37 percent since 1999, when a person had to earn $11.08 an hour to pay for fair market rent.[80] Additional contributing factors to homelessness are presented in **Box 4-2**.

Homeless people are at high risk of food insecurity because they lack both money and cooking facilities.[57] They regularly depend on soup kitchens and shelters to obtain adequate food. The consequences of inadequate food intake are poor nutritional status (due to lack of folate, vitamin A, vitamin C, magnesium, zinc, vitamin B$_{12}$, iron, etc.),

and nutrition-related health conditions such as anemia, dental caries, stunted growth, failure to thrive, low-birth-weight infants, infant mortality, and obesity.[81–83] Homeless individuals, however, are not required to provide an identification card or home address in order to participate in WIC or Food Stamp programs.

Homeless individuals have minimal (on an emergency basis only) or no access to healthcare and have problems following a prescribed diet. For example, it is impossible for a homeless diabetic woman who lives on the street or in a shelter to eat regular meals, get adequate rest and exercise, and administer insulin on schedule. Also, crowded living conditions put homeless people at risk for exposure to viruses and bacteria that cause pneumonia, food poisoning (e.g., *E. coli*), and tuberculosis.[84] The number of homeless individuals with AIDS has increased because of high housing and medical costs. HIV infection in the homeless is estimated to be at least double that found in the general population.[85,86]

Community nutritionists have an important role to play in providing nutrition services to the poor or homeless. They can advocate for accessible nutrition services, and coordinate a network of services and providers to help prevent malnutrition. Some homeless individuals are eligible for programs such as WIC and food stamps (see examples of food programs later in the chapter in Table 4.10). Even with federal assistance programs, many poor people depend on churches and charitable emergency food services to provide for their nutritional needs. For example, Second Harvest, the nation's largest charitable hunger relief organization, provides foods to about 23 million people each year.[87] See the Successful Community Strategies feature for exemplary programs for responding to hunger.

Welfare Reform

On August 22, 1996, the Personal Responsibility and Work Opportunity Reconciliation Act of 1996, P.L. 104-193 (PRWORA) became law. This comprehensive, bipartisan legislation changed the U.S. welfare system to one that requires work in exchange for time-limited cash assistance. It created the *Temporary Assistance for Needy Families* (TANF) program, which replaced the Aid to Families with Dependent Children (AFDC), Emergency Assistance (EA), and Job Opportunities and Basic Skills Training (JOBS) programs under Title IV of the Social Security Act. The law marked the end of federal entitlement to assistance that began in 1935 when the AFDC was established to provide monetary public assistance to poor single mothers and their children.[88] TANF was reauthorized in February 2006 under the Deficit Reduction Act of 2005. States and territories operate programs, and Native American tribes have the option to carry out their own programs in TANF. States, territories, and tribes each receive a block grant allocation, and states, territories, and tribes must maintain a historical level of state spending known as maintenance of effort. The basic block grant includes cash benefits, administrative expenses, and services targeted to needy families. PRWORA significantly changed the structure

---

Box **4-2 Contributing Factors to Homelessness and Hunger[86]**

- Low-paying job
- High housing costs
- Medical or health costs
- Substance abuse
- Mental illness
- Reduced public benefits
- Childcare costs
- Limited life skills (lack of education)
- Weakening of the economy
- Transportation expenses or lack of transportation
- Lack of information about food stamps
- Lack of nutrition education and income in older population
- Divorce
- Jail or prison (prison release)
- Domestic violence
- Reluctance to participate in food assistance programs, especially among older persons, due to the stigma associated with being on welfare

---

homeless people Individuals who do not have a fixed, regular, and adequate nighttime residence.

housing wage The amount a person working full time must earn to pay for a two-bedroom rental unit at fair market rent.

Temporary Assistance for Needy Families A program created by 1996 welfare reform to replace AFDC. It is the major source of funding for cash welfare for needy families with children. There are federal requirements about work and time limits for families receiving assistance.

Head Start program A comprehensive child development program for low-income preschool children and their families.

non-entitlement programs Programs that compete for funds through the congressional appropriation process and establish eligibility requirements for recipients.

Emergency Food Assistance Program (TEFAP) Distributes commodities to state agencies (food banks), which distribute the foods to the public including homeless people via soup kitchens and food pantries.

electronic benefit transfer (EBT) system An electronic system that allows a recipient to authorize transfer of their government benefits from a federal account to a retailer.

of income support for poor single parent families in the United States by:[88]

- Eliminating the entitlement to cash assistance
- Imposing a time limit on federal aid
- Granting broad discretion to states in designing a "work-based safety net" for poor families with children

The provisions in federal law often identified as the key elements of TANF's "work-based safety net" include the elimination of the entitlement to cash assistance, block grant funding, mandatory work requirements, sanctions, and a 5-year time limit on cash assistance (see **Table 4.8**).

The Impacts of Welfare Reform

The impacts of welfare reform on families may be positive due to greater self-esteem associated with joining the workforce. However, this advantage may not result in increased financial security. Studies show that welfare reform causes a higher incidence of depression, poorer child health status, household food insecurity, and loss of federal financial support and food stamps.[89] Symptoms of depression were also observed in inner-city pediatric

clinical populations [90–91] and children participating in a **Head Start program**.[92] The incidence of depression was associated with changes in federal financial assistance and food stamp support. In addition, families were more likely to face a decrease in income from direct loss of benefits and also from related barriers to employment such as poor physical and mental health, inadequate past employment experience, discrimination, and low education.[91] Mothers' emotional state has been shown to be associated with material circumstances. Worry about debt was the strongest independent socioeconomic predictor of maternal depression.

The most quoted impact of welfare reform is the decrease in the number of families receiving cash public assistance. The national welfare caseload reached its peak in 1994, with 5 million families receiving cash public assistance. Before the passage of welfare reform in 1996, the caseload had decreased to 4.4 million families. After welfare reform it decreased further to 2.5 million in 1999.[92,93]

Another often-quoted impact of welfare reform is the increase in the employment rates of various groups of single mothers. National labor force data show that the number of all mothers participating in paid work was 70.9 percent in 2006, the same as the previous year. The participation rate for single mothers (widowed, divorced, separated, or never married) was 76.1 percent in 2006.[86,94,95] State and national studies consistently show that about 60 percent of those who have left the TANF program were employed shortly after leaving the program.[86,96,97]

Studies have also shown that although the rate of employment has increased, these mothers' earnings, income, and poverty did not improve. For example, those leaving welfare for employment usually take jobs that pay below poverty-level wages and have no employer-provided benefits, such as health insurance and paid sick or vacation leave. In addition, many of these families do not receive important public income supports including Medicaid, childcare assistance, and food stamps, although their incomes are low enough to meet eligibility requirements.[94,98,99]

Successful Community Strategies

Responding to Problems of Hunger[87]

Chicago

The Greater Chicago Food Depository (GCFD) reduced the problems of hunger by developing a food program that picked up foods from supermarket delis, restaurants, hotels, and other institutional kitchens in refrigerated trucks and delivered the foods to Chicago Community Kitchens. Chicago Community Kitchens trains underemployed and unemployed individuals for careers in food service. The students were challenged by the variety of foods GCFD delivered to the kitchen to create nutritious and appealing meals for children. The food was then frozen and delivered again in Food Depository refrigerated

vehicles to Kids Cafés across the city. The meals released the Kids Café volunteers and staff from preparing the meals, which made them more available to spend time with the children, often latch key kids living in dangerous neighborhoods.

San Antonio[87]

Another exemplary program can be found in the city of San Antonio. The San Antonio Food Bank started a program called Project HOPE. This program served hungry senior citizens by acting as a direct partner with the city's Senior Nutrition Centers. These centers are safe nurturing places where neighborhood seniors go to receive a hot

lunch. In addition, the San Antonio Food Bank provided the seniors with two bags of groceries each month. Most of the Project HOPE participants were single and low-income individuals. Some of the achievements of the joint project were that it strengthened the communities and families and created the opportunity to form friendships. Also, participants shared meals together and restocked their pantries. In October 2003, the city invested an additional $270,000 in the program. The San Antonio Food Bank plans to expand the program by including a food stamp education program and nutrition classes.

In addition, "dire" or "deep" poverty (i.e., family income below 50 percent of the poverty level) has increased among some families headed by single mothers. This means that some groups of poor single mothers and children remained poor after welfare reform.[99–104]

The Importance of Food Assistance Programs

The goal of food assistance programs is to achieve food security for all Americans.[105,106] The USDA and DHHS conduct a variety of health-related programs that significantly affect the nutritional status of the population, from newborn infants to the elderly. Some of these programs are known as non-entitlement programs. *Non-entitlement programs* compete for funds through the congressional appropriation process and establish eligibility requirements for recipients. The National School Lunch Program and WIC program are examples of non-entitlement program. The Food Stamp Program, in contrast, is an entitlement program.[10,107]

U.S. food assistance programs are designed to improve the nutrition and health status of target recipients/beneficiaries by improving their access to food. The other aims of these programs are to support agriculture and ultimately to reduce food insecurity in many U.S. households.[107,108] All the assistance programs, including those administered by the Department of Health and Human Services and Department of Homeland Security (DHS), are often referred to as a food or nutrition "safety net."[104]

Federal Domestic Nutrition Assistance Programs

In the United States, the major food assistance programs designed to make sure that all people have access to an adequate diet are the Food Stamp Program (FSP); Special Supplemental Nutrition Program for Women, Infants, and Children (WIC); Child Nutrition Program; and *Emergency Food Assistance Program (TEFAP)*. Under TEFAP, the USDA distributes commodities to states, which then provide the food to local agencies that they have selected, usually food banks, which in turn distribute the food to soup kitchens and food pantries that serve the public. The commodities vary depending on market conditions. Products that are typically available include canned and dried fruits, canned vegetables, canned meats, cheese, peanut butter, butter, and pasta products.

It was estimated that 1 in 5 Americans participated in at least 1 of the 15 USDA domestic food assistance programs during 2005. In fiscal year 2005, the USDA's expenditures for the 15 food assistance programs were $51 billion, compared to $46.0 billion and $41.6 billion that was spent on food assistance in fiscal 2004 and 2003, respectively.[109] Programs that target specifically women, infants, children, and the elderly will be discussed in detail in Chapters 8, 9, and 11. A brief description of some of the food assistance programs is presented in this section.

Food Stamp and Related Programs

The Food Stamp Program (FSP) provides a basic safety net to millions of people. The program provides monthly coupons to eligible low-income families, which can be used to purchase food. However, *electronic benefit transfer (EBT) systems* are quickly replacing the use of coupons. The EBT system replaces paper coupons with a benefits card, similar to a bankcard. The USDA reports that all 50 states; Washington, DC; and Puerto Rico are now using EBT systems.

The Food Stamp Program is designed to supplement the food-buying power of eligible low-income people. About 38.4 percent of food stamp households have gross incomes at or below half of the poverty line. In fiscal year 2005, the average monthly number of participants was 25.7 million individuals.

TABLE 4.8	**Key Provisions: The Personal Responsibility and Work Opportunity Reconciliation Act**

Establishes Temporary Assistance for Needy Families (TANF)
- Replaces former entitlement programs with federal block grants
- Transfers authority and responsibility for welfare programs from federal to state government
- Emphasizes moving from welfare to work through time limits and work requirement

Changes eligibility standards for Supplemental Security Income (SSI) child disability benefits
- Restricts certain formerly eligible children from receiving benefits
- Changes eligibility rules for new applicants and eligibility predetermination

Requires states to enforce a strong child support program for collection of child support payments

Restricts aliens' eligibility for welfare and other public benefits
- Denies illegal aliens most public benefits, except emergency medical services
- Restricts most legal aliens from receiving food stamps and SSI benefits until they become citizens or work for at least 10 years
- Allows states the option of providing federal cash assistance to legal aliens already in the country
- Restricts most new legal aliens from receiving federal cash assistance for 5 years
- Allows states the option of using state funds to provide cash assistance to nonqualifying aliens

Provides resources for foster care data systems and a national child welfare study

Establishes a block grant to states to provide childcare for working parents

Alters eligibility criteria and benefits for child nutrition programs
- Modifies reimbursement rates
- Makes families (including aliens) that are eligible for free public education also eligible for school meal benefits

Tightens national standards for food stamps and commodity distribution
- Institutes an across-the-board reduction in benefits
- Caps standard deduction at fiscal year 1995 level
- Limits receipt of benefits to 3 months in every 3 years by childless able-bodied adults ages 18–50 unless working or in training

Source: Economic Research Service. United States Department of Agriculture. Food and Nutrition Assistance Programs: Welfare Reform and Food Assistance Briefing Room. Available at: http://www.ers.usda.gov/briefing/foodnutritionassistance/gallery/keyprovisions.htm. Accessed February 20, 2008.

In April 2003, all legal immigrants who had worked in the United States continuously for 5 years became eligible to apply for food stamps. In October 2003, all legal immigrants' children, regardless of date of entry to the United States, became eligible to apply. In 2005, the USDA spent about $31 billion on food stamps. The Food Stamp Program is the largest of the food assistance programs. From November 2004 to August 2005, participation was between 25.2 million and 25.8 million people per month, and over half of the participants are children. Participation increased to 27.5 million in September 2005, mainly due to the Disaster Food Stamp Program for victims of Hurricane Katrina. One of the strengths of the Food Stamp Program is its ability to respond to local, state, and national economic changes and emergencies.[110]

Changes from PRWORA affected the Food Stamp Program. FSP expenditures declined by 33 percent from 1996 to 2000, and average monthly participation rates also decreased from 25.5 million to 17.2 million recipients.[111] It is estimated that 65 percent of the decrease in FSP participation was due to welfare reform, and 35 percent was due to an improved economy.[112]

Data from the Census Bureau's Current Population Survey indicated that from 1995 to 1997, disposable income increased for many families, but total monetary resources decreased among families with the lowest income.[113] In addition, some states have not increased their welfare benefit levels since the passage of PRWORA in 1996, causing a decrease in benefits over time.[114] Consequently, the poorest families have less money to spend on food and are in greater need of food and nutrition assistance programs.[104]

In fiscal year 2005, 62 percent of all food stamp benefits went to households with children, 17 percent of food stamp households had an elderly person, and 23 percent had a disabled person. About 88 percent of food stamp households had gross incomes below the poverty line. The following provides the USDA's Office of Analysis, Nutrition and Evaluation 2005 characteristics of food stamp households:[115]

- Over half (54 percent) of all food stamp participants are children.
- 42 percent are non-elderly adults (60 years and older).
- 8 percent are elderly.
- 62 percent of all food stamp benefits go to households with children.

Food Stamp Nutrition Education (FSNE) Provides educational programs that help all food stamp recipients make healthy food choices consistent with the most recent dietary advice as reflected in the *Dietary Guidelines for Americans* and MyPyramid.

Commodity Supplemental Food Program (CSFP) Provides food and administrative funds to states to supplement the diets of low-income pregnant and breastfeeding women, infants, and children up to age 6, and elderly people at least 60 years of age.

Food Distribution Program on Indian Reservations (EDPIR) The USDA purchases commodities and ships them to Indian Tribal Organizations (ITOs) to help low-income American Indian and non-Indian households living on a reservation to maintain a nutritionally balanced diet.

Nutrition Services Incentive Program (NSIP) Provides incentives to states and tribes for the effective delivery of nutritious meals to older adults. The USDA provides cash and/or commodities to supplement meals provided under the authority of the Older Americans Act (OAA).

- 33.3 percent of all children receiving food stamps are age 4 or younger.
- 66 percent of children receiving food stamps are school-age.
- Among adult participants, 68 percent are non-elderly women.

As part of an effort to more fully understand the factors that influence Food Stamp Program participation, Economic Research Service (ERS) funded the Food Stamp Program Access Study, which examined the extent to which policies implemented at the local level, as well as local office practices, affect households' decision to apply for food stamps and their decision to continue participating once they are approved for food stamp benefits. Although most non-participant households (69 percent) said that they would apply for food stamp benefits if they were sure they were eligible, 27 percent would not apply even in those circumstances. Other factors that would prevent some households from participating in the Food Stamp Program include:[116]

- Stigma (41 percent)
- Previous bad experience (24 percent)
- Costs of application or participation (61 percent)
- Personal independence (91 percent)
- Did not know how to apply (12 percent)

The Food Stamp Program Map Machine is a very important interactive web-based mapping utility that shows program participation and benefit levels up to the county level. The Map Machine can show per capita participation, per capita benefits, changes from year to year, and more. For example, an individual can select any state or region of the United States and display a map showing how program participation changed in each county between 1994 and 2000. To access the Map Machine, visit http://maps.ers.usda.gov/fsp.

Food Stamp Nutrition Education (FSNE)

In the 1990s, the USDA's Food and Nutrition Service (FNS) began to provide funds for **Food Stamp Nutrition Education (FSNE)** by matching the dollars a state spends on FSNE activities. This provided links to state-level maps and data, and posted tools to assist in assessing the impact of FSNE. The goal of the FSNE program is to provide educational programs that increase, within a limited budget, the possibility that all food stamp recipients will make healthy food and lifestyle choices consistent with the most recent dietary advice (the *Dietary Guidelines for Americans* and MyPyramid).[117] The goals of FSNE include:[118]

- Assisting food stamp households to implement healthy eating and active lifestyles that are consistent with the *Dietary Guidelines for Americans* and MyPyramid
- Increasing practices related to economical shopping and preparation of nutritious foods
- Increasing food security of food stamp households and making certain that people eligible for FSP but not participating are aware of its benefits and how to apply for them as part of nutrition education activities
- Increasing food stamp households' safe handling, preparation, and storage of food

Studies show that FSP and WIC clients enrolled in FSNE increased their vegetable, fruit, dairy product, and grain intake to an amount consistent with the *Dietary Guidelines for Americans* and MyPyramid. In addition, the participants engaged in behaviors that reflected improvements in safe food handling practices.[119–121]

Food Distribution Programs

Several commodity distribution programs assist in preventing food insecurity and hunger. The purpose of food distribution programs is to strengthen the food and nutrition safety net through commodity distribution and other nutrition assistance to low-income individuals and families.[122] Some of the food distribution programs include the Commodity Supplemental Food Program (CSFP), Food Distribution Program on Indian Reservations (FDPIR), the Emergency Food Assistance Program (TEFAP), Nutrition Services Incentive Programs, and School/Child Nutrition Commodity Programs.

Commodity Supplemental Food Program (CSFP)

The aim of the **Commodity Supplemental Food Program (CSFP)** is to improve the health of low-income pregnant and breastfeeding women, infants, and children up to age 6, and elderly people at least 60 years of age by supplementing their diets with nutritious USDA commodity foods. CSFP provides food and administrative funds to states to supplement the diets of these groups. The CSFP state agencies are responsible for determining the income eligibility for participants. Some states may need the participants to be at nutritional risk before they can participate. The assessments that can be used to determine whether individuals are at nutritional risk include blood tests and height and weight measurements. Examples of nutritional risk conditions are anemia and underweight.[123]

The commodities available each year vary depending on the market conditions. Food packages include a variety of foods, such as infant formula and cereal; non-fat dry and evaporated milk; juice; farina; oats; ready-to eat cereal; rice; pasta; egg mix; peanut butter; dry beans or peas; canned meat, poultry, or tuna; and canned fruits and vegetables. The packages are designed to address the nutritional needs of the clients. In fiscal year 2004, about 521,000 people participated in the program each month, including more than 458,000 elderly people and more than 62,000 women, infants, and children. (Clients may not participate in WIC and CSFP at the same time.)

Food Distribution Program on Indian Reservations

The purpose of the **Food Distribution Program on Indian Reservations (FDPIR)** is to help low-income American Indian and non-Indian households living on a reservation to maintain a nutritionally balanced diet. Those who do not have access to food stamp offices or authorized food stores can participate in the FDPIR. The Indian Tribal Organizations (ITOs) or an agency of the state government administers FDPIR locally. About 243 tribes receive benefits under the FDPIR through 98 ITOs and 5 state agencies. The USDA purchases the commodities, based on a list of available foods, and ships them to the ITOs and state agencies. However, some commodities offered through FDPIR may be donated to the program from agricultural surpluses. These administering agencies store and distribute the food, determine applicant eligibility, and provide nutrition education to recipients. The USDA also provides the administering agencies with funds for program administrative costs.[124] Participants may select from over 70 products (see **Box 4-3**).

In fiscal year 2005, the average monthly participation was 99,011 individuals. In fiscal year 2006, the federal government appropriated $25.1 million for a special purchase of bison meat, which made the food selection more culturally appropriate.[124]

Participants on most reservations can choose fresh produce instead of canned fruits and vegetables and may decide from month to month whether to participate in the Food Stamp Program or the Food Distri-

---

$\mathcal{B}ox$ 4-3 Examples of Commodity Foods[124]

Frozen ground beef	Chicken
Canned meats	Reduced sodium crackers
Poultry and fish	Dried beans
Canned fruits and vegetables	Low-fat refried beans
Canned soups	Dehydrated potatoes
Spaghetti sauce	Vegetable oil
Macaroni and cheese	Juices
Pastas	Dried fruit
Cereals	Peanuts
Rice	Peanut butter
Grains	Corn syrup
Cheese	Shortening
Egg mix	Canned juices
Non-fat dry evaporated milk	Bakery mix
Flour	Cornmeal

---

bution Program. Administering agencies are responsible for providing nutrition education to participants, which can include individual nutrition counseling, cooking demonstrations, proper storage of commodities, nutrition classes, and information on how to use commodities to make a nutritious diet. A collection of test recipes submitted by program participants can be found at http://www.fns.usda.gov.

Emergency Food Assistance Program

The purpose of the Emergency Food Assistance Program (TEFAP), formerly known as the Temporary Emergency Food Assistance Program, (TEFAP) is to reduce federal food inventories and storage costs and help poor people, including the elderly, at the same time. The amount that each state receives from the USDA depends on its low-income and unemployed population. TEFAP distributes the commodities to state agencies (food banks), which distribute the foods to the public including homeless people via soup kitchens and food pantries. The state is responsible for setting the eligibility criteria. The foods TEFAP distributes vary depending on the preferences of states and agricultural market conditions. More than 60 products were made available for fiscal year 2006, including canned and dried fruits, canned vegetables, fruit juice, dried egg mix, meat, poultry, fish, non-fat dry milk, pasta, peanut butter, rice, grits, cereal, and soups.

In fiscal year 2006, Congress appropriated $189.5 million for TEFAP, $140 million to purchase food, and another $49.5 million for administrative support for state and local agencies.[125]

Nutrition Services Incentive Program

The purpose of the **Nutrition Services Incentive Program (NSIP)** is to provide incentives to states and tribes for the effective delivery of nutritious meals to older adults. The program originally was administered by the USDA, which provided cash and/or commodities to supplement meals provided under the authority of the Older Americans Act (OAA). The OAA was amended in 2003 to transfer the NSIP from the USDA to the Administration on Aging (AOA) within the Department of Health and Human Services.[126] The only eligibility criterion is age. People 60 years of age or older and their spouses, regardless of age, are eligible for NSIP benefits. ITOs may choose an age below 60 for defining an older person for their tribes. Additionally, the following individuals may also receive meals through NSIP:[126]

- Disabled people under age 60 who live in elderly housing facilities where congregate meals are served
- Disabled persons who reside at home and accompany elderly participants to meals
- Volunteers who assist in the meal service

Food Distribution Disaster Assistance

Food distribution disaster assistance programs distribute commodity foods directly to households that are in need as a result of an emergency. Such direct distribution takes place when normal commercial food supply channels such as grocery stores have been disrupted, damaged, or destroyed, or can't function (e.g., lack of electricity). The Food and Nutrition Service (FNS) of the USDA is the agency in charge of food during a period of disaster. The Federal Emergency Management Agency (FEMA) in the Department of Homeland Security coordinates overall disaster relief efforts.[127] In an emergency situation, the USDA can authorize states to release food stocks to disaster relief agencies (e.g., Salvation Army, Red Cross) to feed people at shelters and mass feeding sites. If the President declares a disaster, states, with USDA approval, can also distribute commodity foods directly to households that are in need as a result of an emergency.[127]

FNS uses the term *situation of distress* when a natural catastrophe or other event has not been declared by the president to be a disaster, but in the judgment of the state distributing agency or FNS warrants the use of USDA-donated foods for congregate feeding or household distribution or the issuance of emergency food stamps. A situation of distress could be caused by a hurricane, tornado, storm, flood, tidal wave, tsunami, earthquake, volcanic eruption, landslide, mudslide, snowstorm, drought, fire, explosion, or other natural catastrophe. There are also situations other than natural catastrophes, such as strikes or explosions, that in the judgment of FNS may warrant the use of donated foods. It is recommended that state distributing agencies use commodities provided through the National School Lunch Program whenever possible. These commodities are easy for disaster feeding organizations to use in preparing congregate meals, and they are easy for FNS to replace or reimburse.

Child Nutrition and Related Programs

There are several nutrition programs that target children. This section discusses some of these programs. Chapter 10 and **Table 4.10** (later in this chapter) provide more information on child nutrition programs, including the Head Start Program.

The National School Lunch Program and School Breakfast Program

Both the National School Lunch Program and the School Breakfast Program were designed to improve children's diet, nutrient intake, and well-being. These meals make a very important contribution to children's mental and physical development. Both meals must meet the nutritional requirements outlined in the *Dietary Guidelines for Ameri-*

cans, published jointly by the USDA and the U.S. Department of Health and Human Services, which recommends that no more than 30 percent of an individual's calories come from fat, and less than 10 percent from saturated fat. In addition, breakfasts must provide one-fourth of the Recommended Dietary Allowance for protein, calcium, iron, Vitamin A, Vitamin C, and calories. The **School Breakfast Program (SBP)** provides children with nutritious foods before their school day begins; this helps improve their diets and encourages the learning process. An example of a good breakfast consists of a serving of orange juice, toast with jelly, and oatmeal with milk and raisins. This breakfast provides about 450 calories plus protein; B vitamins; vitamins C, A, and D; and the minerals calcium and iron.[128] The School Lunch Program must provide one-third of the children's nutritional requirements for the day.

Most of the support the USDA provides to schools in the School Breakfast and Lunch Programs comes in the form of a cash reimbursement for each meal served. In addition to cash reimbursements, schools are entitled by law to receive commodity foods, called **entitlement programs** foods, at a value of 17.25 cents for each meal served. Schools can also receive "bonus" commodities, as they are available from surplus agricultural stocks.

These school programs help children from families with income at or below 130 percent of the federal poverty level obtain free meals. Those with income between 130 percent and 185 percent of the poverty level are eligible for reduced-price meals. (For the period July 1, 2006, through June 30, 2007, 130 percent of the poverty level was $25,155 for a family of four; 185 percent was $35,798.) (See **Table 4.9.**) Children from families over 185 percent of poverty level pay full price. Children from families that qualify for the Food Stamp Program automatically qualify for free school breakfasts and lunches. In fiscal year 2005, more than 29.6 million children participated in the School Lunch Program each day at a cost of $7.9 billion, and 9.3 million children participated in the School Breakfast Program.[129]

TABLE 4.9	**2006 HHS Poverty Guidelines**		
Size of Family Unit	48 Contiguous States and Washington, DC	Alaska	Hawaii
1	$9,800	$12,250	$11,270
2	13,200	16,500	15,180
3	16,600	20,750	19,090
4	20,000	25,000	23,000
5	23,400	29,250	26,910
6	26,800	33,500	30,820
7	30,200	37,750	34,730
8	33,600	42,000	38,640
For each additional person, add:	3,400	4,250	3,910

Tables containing various percentage multiples (i.e., 100 percent, 120 percent, 133 percent, etc.) of the 2006 poverty guidelines commonly used in federal and state programs are available online.

Source: *Federal Register*, Vol. 71, No. 15, January 24, 2006, pp. 3848–3849.

After-School Snack Program

An after-school snack gives children a nutritional enhancement and encourages them to participate in supervised activities that are safe and filled with learning opportunities. The National School Lunch Program offers cash reimbursement to help schools that serve snacks to children. *After-school snack programs* are designed to promote the health and well-being of children and youth through the age of 18. In order for schools to qualify for the program they must provide children with regularly scheduled activities in an organized, structured, and supervised environment. The activities must be educational or enrichment-based (e.g., mentoring or tutoring programs). Competitive interscholastic sports teams are not eligible for the after-school program. The programs must meet state or local licensing requirements, if available, or state or local health and safety standards.[130] The USDA reimburses the schools for the snacks. From July 1, 2006, through June 30, 2007, reimbursement was $0.65 for free snacks, $0.32 for reduced-price snacks, and $0.06 for paid snacks. These rates are adjusted annually.[130]

Special Milk Program

The Food and Nutrition Service of the USDA administers the *Special Milk Program* at the federal level. The Special Milk Program provides milk to children in schools, childcare institutions, and eligible camps that do not participate in other federal child nutrition meal service programs. The program reimburses schools and institutions for the milk they serve to the children. In 2005, about 5,375 schools and residential childcare institutions, 1,011 summer camps, and 642 non-residential childcare institutions participated in the Special Milk Program. That year, more than 100 million half-pints of milk were served through the program. The federal reimbursement for each half-pint of milk given for free to children in school year 2006–2007 was 0.145 cents.[129]

Summer Food Service Program for Children

Millions of low-income children lose access to the school breakfasts, lunches, and after-school snacks when school is no longer in session. The *Summer Food Service Program* (SFSP) fills this gap. Many of the children served may be at nutritional risk if they do not have access to school meals. SFSP provides free meals to all eligible participants and children up to the age of 18 years from households with incomes at or below 185 percent of the poverty guidelines. Most SFSP sites can provide up to two meals (breakfast and lunch or breakfast and dinner) or one meal and a snack a day.

Sites that serve migrant children and certain types of summer camps are "open sites," which means that they are open to all children who go to the site during meal service times. These sites are especially important for migrant workers' children, who may not have the opportunity to officially enroll in the program. An open site is eligible for federal SFSP funds for all the children if it is located in a geographic area in which at least 50 percent of the children are from low-income families. Some sites are called "enrolled sites;" these sites serve only children who are officially enrolled in the program. An enrolled site is eligible for federal funds to serve all the children enrolled in the program if at least 50 percent of the children enrolled can qualify for free or reduced price school meals (documented). In fiscal year 2005, the total federal funding for the SFSP was $266.0 million, and Congress appropriated $293.7 million in 2007.

Many SFSP sites provide not just meals, but educational enrichment and recreational activities that help children continue to learn and stay safe when school is not in session. Accordingly, the National Youth Sports Program (NYSP) provides youth from low-income communities the opportunity to receive benefits from structured sports and education programs and at least one USDA-approved meal daily. Local universities, colleges, schools, parks and recreation departments, summer camps, community action agencies, and other nonprofit organizations manage NYSP.[131] About 76,000 disadvantaged children ages 10 to 16 were served in 2005.

Child and Adult Care Food Program

The purpose of the *Child and Adult Care Food Program (CACFP)* is to serve nutritious meals and snacks to eligible children and adults who are enrolled for care at participating childcare centers, daycare homes, and adult daycare centers. CACFP also provides meals to children residing in homeless shelters, and snacks to youths participating in after-school care programs. The USDA's FNS administers CACFP through grants to states. The program is administered within most states by the state educational agency.

Childcare centers and daycare homes may be approved to claim up to two reimbursable meals (breakfast, lunch, or dinner) and one snack, or two snacks and one meal, to each eligible participant, each day. Shelters may serve each child up to three reimbursable meals (breakfast, lunch, and dinner) each day. After-school care programs may claim reimbursement for serving each child one snack each day. In childcare centers, participants from households with incomes at or below 130 percent of poverty level are eligible for free meals. Participants with household incomes between 130 percent and 185 percent of poverty level are eligible for meals at a reduced price. Institutions must determine each enrolled participant's eligibility for free and reduced-price meals served in centers. Children whose families receive benefits from the Food Stamp Program, Food Distribution Program on Indian Reservations (FDPIR), or state programs funded through Temporary Assistance for Needy Families (TANF) are categorically eligible for free meals. Children who were eligible to participate in the Head Start program are automatically eligible for free meals. In fiscal year 2007, the USDA reimbursed $2.23 billion to institutions participating in CACFP.[132,133]

---

food distribution disaster assistance programs Distribute commodity foods directly to households that are in need as a result of an emergency. Such direct distribution takes place when normal commercial food supply channels, such as grocery stores, have been disrupted, damaged, or destroyed, or can't function (e.g., lack of electricity).

School Breakfast Program Provides a nutritious breakfast to children in participating schools or institutions.

entitlement programs Programs funded by Congress for persons who qualify due to level of income or other eligibility requirements; food stamps and the majority of other food assistance programs are included in this category.

after-school snack program Gives children a nutritional enhancement and encourages them to participate in supervised activities that are safe and filled with learning opportunities.

Special Milk Program Provides milk to school-age children in childcare centers and in schools or institutions where there is no School Lunch Program.

Summer Food Service Program Provides nutritious meals to children during summer as a substitute for the National School Lunch and School Breakfast Programs.

Child and Adult Care Food Program Serves nutritious meals and snacks to eligible children and adults who are enrolled for care at participating childcare centers, daycare homes, and adult daycare centers.

Programs for Women and Young Children

Among many nutrition programs designed to serve vulnerable people are programs to assist low-income women and their children obtain nutritious foods. (See Chapters 8 and 9 and later in the chapter for more information.) This section provides a brief discussion of women and young children's programs.

Special Supplemental Nutrition Program for Women, Infants, and Children (WIC)

WIC is a federally funded program that provides healthy supplemental foods and nutrition counseling for pregnant women, new mothers, infants, and children up to age 5. The program has an extraordinary record of over 25 years of preventing children's health problems and improving their long-term health, growth, and development. WIC is not an entitlement program; that is, Congress does not set aside funds to allow every eligible individual to participate in the program. Instead, WIC is a federal grant program for which Congress authorizes a specific amount of funding each year for program operations. The Food and Nutrition Service, which administers the program at the federal level, provides these funds to WIC state agencies (state health departments or comparable agencies) to pay for WIC foods, nutrition counseling and education, and administrative costs. A few WIC state agencies distribute the WIC foods through warehouses or deliver the foods to participants' homes. The foods provided are high in one or more of the following nutrients: protein, calcium, iron, and vitamins A and C.

In most WIC state agencies, WIC participants receive the following:[134]

- Checks or vouchers to purchase specific foods each month that are designed to supplement their diets. Different food packages are provided for different categories of participants.
- Special therapeutic infant formulas and medical foods are provided when prescribed by a physician for a specified medical condition.
- Nutrition education and counseling.
- Referrals to other healthcare services.

An individual whose income is at or below 185 percent of the U.S. Poverty Income Guidelines is eligible to participate. A person who participates or has family members who participate in certain other benefit programs, such as the Food Stamp Program, Medicaid, or Temporary Assistance for Needy Families, automatically satisfies the income eligibility requirement. In fiscal year 2004, the average monthly participation was about 7.9 million. Children were the largest population served—of the 7.9 million, about 4.0 million were children, 2.0 million were infants, and 1.9 million were women. Congress appropriated $5.204 billion for WIC in fiscal year 2006. By comparison, the WIC program appropriation was $20.6 million in 1974, $750 million in 1980, $1.5 billion in 1985, and $2.1 billion in 1990.[134]

WIC Farmers' Market Nutrition Program Provides fresh, unprepared, locally grown fruits and vegetables to WIC participants; also expands the awareness, sales, and use of farmers' markets.

WIC Farmers' Market Nutrition Program

The *WIC Farmers' Market Nutrition Program (FMNP)* was established in 1992 to provide fresh, unprepared, locally grown fruits and vegetables to WIC participants and to expand the awareness, sales, and use of farmers' markets. FMNP participants receive vouchers in addition to their regular WIC food provisions. The vouchers issued to the participants may not be less than $10 and not more than $30 per year.[135] However, state agencies may supplement the benefit level. These are used to buy fresh, unprepared locally grown fruits, vegetables, and herbs from farmers' markets or roadside stands that have been approved by the state agency to accept FMNP coupons. Participants also receive nutrition education through an arrangement with the local WIC agency. The nutrition education is designed to encourage FMNP participants to improve and expand their diets by adding fresh fruits and vegetables, as well as to educate them on how to select, store, and prepare the fresh fruits and vegetables.

During fiscal year 2005, more than 2.5 million WIC clients participated in FMNP. This program is currently authorized in 45 states. About $19.8 million was appropriated for FMNP for fiscal year 2006.[135]

Expanded Food and Nutrition Education Program (EFNEP)

The Expanded Food and Nutrition Education Program (EFNEP) is a unique program that currently operates in all 50 states and in American Samoa, Guam, Micronesia, Northern Marianas, Puerto Rico, and the Virgin Islands. It provides community-based nutrition education programs designed to help individuals, families, and communities acquire knowledge, skills, attitudes, and changed behavior needed to support health, economic, and social well-being. EFNEP is offered to families who are eligible for WIC and the Food Stamp Program.

County extension professionals provide on-the-job training and supervise paraprofessionals and volunteers who teach EFNEP. The paraprofessionals usually live in the communities where they work. They recruit families and receive referrals from neighborhood contacts and community agencies (e.g., Food Stamps and WIC). EFNEP activities may include:[136]

- Direct teaching in group or one-to-one situations
- Mailings and telephone teaching
- Mass media efforts to promote the educational program
- Development and training of volunteers to assist with direct teaching of adults and youth
- Assisting limited-resources individuals and families improve their physical activity

The Cooperative State Research Education Extension Service (CSREES) provides funds for the EFNEP programs. CSREES's goal is to advance knowledge for agriculture, the environment, human health and well-being, and communities by supporting research, education, and extension programs in the land-grant university system and other partner organizations (e.g., Economics and Commerce; Families, Youth, and Communities; Food, Nutrition, and Health; and Natural Resources and Environment).[137,138]

Research shows that EFNEP has made a significant impact in improving low-income families' nutrient intake. For example, dietary intake of six important nutrients that are frequently limited in the diets of low-income people (protein, iron, calcium, vitamin A, vitamin C, and vitamin B_6) increased considerably due to participation in EFNEP.[139]

Programs for Older Adults

There are many federal, local, and private programs designed to promote the nutritional health of older persons in the United States. Chapter 11 and **Table 4.10** provide more information about the programs. This section provides a brief discussion of some of the programs.

TABLE 4.10	Federally Funded Food and Nutrition Programs				
Food Assistance and Nutrition Programs	**Service Provider**	**Who Qualifies**	**Service/Benefits**	**Funding**	**Administrative Agency**
National School Lunch Program					
Provides nutritious low-cost lunches to children enrolled in school	All public schools; voluntary in private schools	All children attending school may participate; reduced-price meals to children from families with incomes between 130% and 185% of poverty level; free meals to children from families with income at or below 130% of poverty level	Nutritious low-cost lunch at full or reduced prices or free	USDA	State departments of education; local school districts
School Breakfast Program					
Provides nutritious breakfast to children in participating schools or institutions	Voluntarily by public and private schools	All children attending schools where the breakfast program operates may participate; reduced-price breakfast available to children from families with income between 130% and 185% of poverty level; free breakfast to children from families with incomes at or below 130% of poverty level	Nutritious low-cost breakfast at full or reduced prices or free	USDA	State departments of education; local school districts
Special Milk Program					
Provides milk to school-age children in childcare centers and in schools or institutions where there is no school lunch program	Schools, camps, and childcare institutions not participating in other school nutrition programs	All children attending schools or institutions with this program	Milk at reasonable price or free	USDA	State departments of education; local school districts
Summer Food Service Program for Children					
Provides one nutritious meal to children as a substitute for the National School Lunch and School Breakfast programs during summer vacation	Public and nonprofit private schools; public or nonprofit private residential facilities of local, municipal, or county government	Children under 18 years and persons over 18 years who are handicapped and participate in a sponsored program of county government; no income requirements; eligibility is determined by location and sponsor	Nutritious meals (breakfast, lunch, and/or snacks)	USDA	State departments of education; local sponsors
Child Care Food Program					
Provides financial assistance for nutritious food in childcare settings	Licensed childcare centers or family daycare homes; Head Start programs	Children 12 years and under; children of migrant workers 15 years and younger; physically/ mentally handicapped individuals provided care in a center where majority are age 18 or younger	Free or reduced-price meals to eligible children in centers and free meals to all children in family daycare homes; reimbursements for up to two meals and one snack daily	USDA	State departments of education; local providers

(continues)

TABLE 4.10 (Continued)

Food Assistance and Nutrition Programs	Service Provider	Who Qualifies	Service/Benefits	Funding	Administrative Agency
Head Start					
Provides comprehensive health, educational, nutrition, social, other services to low-income preschool children and their families	Local Head Start program	Children ages 3–5 years from low-income families receiving public assistance or total annual income not more than 100% of poverty level; at least 10% total enrollment available for handicapped children	Education, comprehensive medical, dental, nutrition, and social services through assessment, early intervention, and prevention; nutritious meals and snacks (through Child Care Food Program); nutrition education; family counseling and referrals for social services	DHHS	DHHS regional offices; local providers
Special Supplemental Food Program for Women, Infants, and Children (WIC)					
Provides supplemental food and nutrition education as an adjunct to healthcare to low-income pregnant, postpartum, and breast-feeding women, infants, and children at nutritional risk	Health agencies, social services, community action agencies	Pregnant women, postpartum women (6 months), breast-feeding women (up to 1 year); infants and children (up to 5 years); must be certified to be at nutritional risk; household income determined to be at or below 185% of poverty levels	Monthly foods or coupons for milk, cheese, eggs, fruit juice, cereal, peanut butter or legumes, infant formula, and infant cereal, nutrition education	USDA	State health agencies; local agencies
Commodity Supplemental Food Program (CSFP)					
Provides commodity foods to low-income women (pregnant, breastfeeding, or postpartum), infants, and children to 6 years of age, and the elderly in certain cases	Public and private nonprofit agencies (community health or social service agencies)	Pregnant women, postpartum women, breastfeeding women, infants, and children (up to 6 years); household income determined to be at or below 185% of poverty level; low-income elderly may be served if it does not reduce the benefits to eligible women, infants, and children	Monthly commodity canned or packaged food including fruits, vegetables, meats, infant formula, farina, beans, and others as available	USDA	State health agencies
Food Stamps					
Provides low-income households with coupons to increase food purchasing power	Local public assistance or social services offices	U.S. citizen; recognized refugee with visa status or legal alien; households with low income and with resources (aside from income) of $2,000 or less/$3,000 or less with at least one elderly person (age 60 or older); eligibility determined after formal application to local public assistance or social services	Food coupons to purchase foods at participating food markets	USDA	State welfare, social service, or human service agencies

TABLE 4.10 (Continued)					
Food Assistance and Nutrition Programs	**Service Provider**	**Who Qualifies**	**Service/Benefits**	**Funding**	**Administrative Agency**
Temporary Emergency Food Assistance Program (TEFAP)					
Provides commodity foods to low-income households through local public or private nonprofit agencies; quarterly distributions by emergency providers	Public and private nonprofit agencies (community action agencies, councils on aging, or local health/local school districts)	Households with incomes at or below 150% of poverty level	Quarterly distribution of cheese, butter, rice, and occasionally flour, cornmeal, and dry milk; emergency food available once per month; dairy products, rice, flour, cornmeal	USDA	State and local agencies
Nutrition Assistance Program (NAP) for Puerto Rico					
Block grant program in which Puerto Rico receives the cost of food assistance benefits (provided to recipients and half of the Commonwealth) and administrative costs, up to a legislatively set total	Commonwealth of Puerto Rico	Program operates under eligibility rules similar to the Food Stamp Program	Cash to be used by recipients to supplement their food budget	USDA	Puerto Rico Commonwealth government
Food Distribution Program on Indian Reservations (FDPIR)					
Operates as a substitute for food stamps for eligible needy families living on or near Indian reservations	Local agency	Indian families living on or near reservations	Offers USDA commodities monthly	USDA	Indian tribal councils
Meal Program for the Elderly ENP					
Provides older Americans with meals and nutrition education in congregate setting or delivered to their homes	Area agency on aging or other aging services provider	People age 60 or older with social or economic needs; spouses of eligible people; handicapped or disabled people under 60 who reside in housing occupied primarily by the elderly	Nutritious meals; nutrition education; access to social and rehabilitative services; transportation	DHHS; Administration on Aging; state; individual donations	State agencies on aging; area agencies on aging
Cooperative Extension—Expanded Food and Nutrition Education Program (EFNEP)					
Provides nutrition education to low-income families and individuals	Local cooperative extension office where program is available	Families with children under 19 years; income at or below 125% of federal poverty level; at nutritional risk	Education and training on food and nutrition for homemakers and youth	USDA	State land grant universities; cooperative extension

Adapted from: Kaufman M. *Nutrition in Public Health: A Handbook for Developing Programs and Services.* Rockville, MD: Aspen; 1990.

Elderly Nutrition Program

The U.S. Department of Health and Human Services Administration on Aging provides funding for the ***Elderly Nutrition Program (ENP)***. All seniors 60 years of age and older and their spouse of any age, regardless of income, are eligible to participate in the ENP. (Some tribal organizations set the age eligibility limit lower than 60.) Although the programs do not set particular income limits to participate, outreach efforts are focused on low-income older persons and low-income minority older persons.

The purpose of the ENP is to:[140]

- Improve the dietary intakes of older persons
- Create informal support networks
- Provide positive social contacts with other seniors at the group meal sites
- Make community-based services available to older adults who may be at risk of losing their independence

Elderly Nutrition Program
A federal program established in 1965 to provide congregate and home-delivered meals and related nutrition services to older adults.

- Educate them on how to shop, plan, and prepare nutritious meals that are economical
- Enhance their health and well-being

The Elderly Nutrition Program provides a Congregate Meal Program at locations such as churches and senior community centers. Sometimes called "Meals on Wheels," home-delivered meals are delivered to homebound seniors who are unable to travel to a congregate meal site. The program must provide at least one-third of the recommended dietary allowances established by the Food and Nutrition Board of the Institute of Medicine of the National Academy of Sciences, as well as the *Dietary Guidelines for Americans*. In practice, the Elderly Nutrition Program's 3.1 million elderly participants are receiving an estimated 40 to 50 percent of most required nutrients.[141]

Senior Farmers' Market Nutrition Program Provides low-income older persons coupons that can be used to purchase locally grown fresh, unprepared fruits, vegetables, and herbs at farmers' markets, roadside stands, and community-supported agriculture programs.

Senior Farmers' Market Nutrition Program (SFMNP)

In fiscal year 2001, the *Senior Farmers' Market Nutrition Program* (SFMNP) was established. The purpose of the program is to provide low-income older persons coupons that can be used to purchase locally grown fresh, unprepared fruits, vegetables, and herbs at farmers' markets, roadside stands, and community-supported agriculture programs. The eligibility criteria are set on income not more than 185 percent of poverty level, age 60 years or older (with some exceptions). In fiscal year 2007, $15 million was used to operate SFMNP in 46 states, and federally recognized Indian tribal governments are supposed to operate the SFMNP.[142] **Table 4.9** presents the poverty guidelines and **Table 4.10** presents federally funded food and nutrition programs.

Chapter Summary

- In the 1930s, the USDA began developing family food plans at four separate cost levels. The Thrifty Food Plan continues to be used as the nutritional basis for the benefits of the Food Stamp Program.
- National nutrition monitoring programs provide data to assess food and nutrient inadequacies as well as malnutrition and chronic diseases related to overconsumption. Scientific research utilizes nutrition monitoring data to revise the standards of human nutrient requirements and to study the relationship among diet, nutrition, and health.
- The prevalence of food insecurity decreased to 11.0 percent in 2005 from 11.9 percent in 2004; however, the prevalence of food insecurity with hunger increased from 3.5 percent to 3.7 percent. Households with children experience food insecurity more than households without children.
- During the 1930s, the federal government developed food relief and food commodity distribution programs, including school food programs, nutrition education programs, and the national food consumption survey.
- The Department of Health and Human Services (DHHS) administers the majority of public health and nutrition programs. It is the second largest federal agency in terms of dollars received from the federal budget for its programs.
- The National School Lunch Program, established in 1946, provides nutritious lunches and the opportunity to practice skills learned in nutrition education classrooms.
- Federal cash reimbursements and donated foods from the Commodity Food Program are provided to schools that serve a lunch meeting the specified nutritional requirements under the School Lunch Program.
- The Special Milk Program, established in 1955 by the USDA, provides reimbursement for milk served to children.
- The Special Supplemental Nutrition Program for Women, Infants, and Children (WIC) and the National School Lunch Program (NSLP) are non-entitlement programs.
- WIC was established as a pilot program in 1972 and was made permanent in 1974. The Food and Nutrition Service administers WIC at the federal level.
- The Food Stamp Program is an entitlement program; eligible individuals are entitled to receive benefits. To qualify for the FSP, households must have gross incomes below 130 percent of the official poverty level.
- The National Youth Sports Program is a federal program designed to assist low-income children ages 10 to 16 in a summer program. It provides a comprehensive developmental and instructional sports program to low-income children as well as one USDA-approved meal per day.
- School nutrition services integrate nutritious, affordable, and appealing meals; nutrition education; and an environment that promotes healthful eating behaviors.
- The Emergency Food Assistance Program (TEFAP) provides commodity foods to emergency kitchens (often referred to as soup kitchens), homeless shelters, and similar organizations that serve meals to low-income individuals. An eligibility criterion is set between 130 and 150 percent of the poverty line for some states.
- Federally funded food and nutrition programs are the safety net through which families are provided a reasonable supply of nutritious food, knowledge, and the skills required to make healthy food choices.

Critical Thinking Activities

- Assist a community nutritionist to provide nutrition education on how to plan and prepare low-cost meals using MyPyramid and other educational tools.
- Observe a community nutritionist for 2 days and write a reflective journal/log about the experiences/observations.
- Obtain and critique a research article about working poor issues that are related to nutrition.
- Collect data on population groups that are new to the community, such as migrant workers, Asian groups, or refugees, to determine the availability of food and their eligibility for any of the federal programs.

Case Study 4-1

Population characteristics impact the health of individuals, families, and aggregates. However, community nutritionists can address nutritional needs and minimize health risks by creating interventions for those populations at risk, such as those who are homeless, elderly, or hungry. A city with a population of 200,000 was experiencing an increase in homeless people, high infant mortality, and an increase in the elderly population. Students enrolled in a community nutrition course in that city were assigned to help reduce the incidence of hunger and malnutrition in this community by providing services as needed at various community sites. They served meals to the homeless and the elderly, and provided nutrition education to pregnant and lactating women, and low-income families receiving help at food pantries. At the end of the school year, the students decided to establish a community-based emergency food delivery network by involving different student organizations and local businesses in the community.

Activities

- Create a list for individuals participating in a food pantry, showing where and how to shop for the most economical nutritious foods in the community.
- Survey two participants in food pantries, a homeless shelter, the WIC program, or the like about the effectiveness of food assistance programs.
- Interview a community nutritionist to determine the impact of welfare reform on food security in the community.
- Contact different businesses (such as restaurants, grocery stores, churches, and senior citizen clubs) to donate time, food items, and other products to organizations such as homeless shelters, the Salvation Army, Catholic Charity sites, and so on.
- Divide students into groups of two for service-learning activities. Each group should observe and participate/work in a community-based food assistance program for 1 to 3 days. It is more rewarding to vary the experiences by working at two different sites. Examples of assistance programs include homeless shelters, WIC, Peace Meal/Congregate Meal Programs, food banks/

pantries, and Catholic meal programs in the community. You can help serve meals and/or engage in conversation with the clients. (Older clients in the Congregate Meal Program are especially very receptive to students.)

- Keep a reflective journal/log about how you felt after accomplishing these activities. Describe the quality of your interactions with the clients at the site and what you learned during these interactions. How will these experiences be useful to you as a community nutritionist in the future?
- Ask the supervisor/coordinator of the sites some of the following questions:
  - Who does the program serve?
  - What are the eligibility requirements?
  - Who helps carry out the duties of the program?
  - How many people (staff) work for the program and what are the skills required?
  - What is the purpose of the program?
  - Who funds the program and what are the eligibility criteria for funding?
  - What are the challenges/difficulties the program encounters?

Use this information for in-class discussion.

References

1. Jung SL, Frongillo EA. Understanding needs is important for assessing the impact of food assistance program participation on nutritional and health status in U.S. elderly persons. *J Nutr.* 2001; 131:765–773.
2. Hess AF. Newer aspects of some nutritional disorders. *JAMA.* 1921; 76:693–700.
3. Atwater WO. Food: nutritive value and cost. *USDA Farmer's Bulletin.* 1894; 23:1–32.
4. Langer PL. *History of goitre: in endemic goitre.* Geneva, Switzerland: World Health Organization; 1960.
5. Centers for Disease Control and Prevention. Achievements in public health, 1900–1999: safer and healthier foods. *MMWR.* 1999; 48(40):905–913.
6. Centers for Disease Control and Prevention. Achievements in public health, 1900–1999: safer and healthier foods. Available at: http://www.cdc.gov/epo/mmwr/preview/mmwrhtml/mm4840a1.htm. Accessed April 15, 2005.
7. Kaufman M. *Nutrition in promoting the public's health: Strategies, principles, and practice.* Sudbury, MA: Jones and Bartlett; 2007.
8. Economic Research Service, U.S. Department of Agriculture. Household Food Security in United States. Appendix C: USDA's Thrifty Food Plan. Available at: http://www.ers.usda.gov/publications/fanrr35/fanrr35appc.pdf. Accessed April 15, 2005.
9. Andrews M, Kantor SL, Lino M, Ripplinger D. Using USDA's Thrifty Food Plan to Assess Food Availability and Affordability: U.S. Department of Agriculture. Available at: http://www.findarticles.com/p/articles/mi_m3765/is_2_24/ai_80517266. Accessed April 19, 2005.
10. Kaufman M. *Nutrition in Public Health: A Handbook for Developing Programs and Services.* Rockville, MD: Aspen; 1990.
11. U.S. Department of Agriculture. Income Eligibility Guidelines. Available at: http://www.fns.usda.gov/cnd/Governance/notices/iegs/IEGs.htm. Accessed April 14, 2005.
12. Mason JB, Habicht JP, Tabatabai H, Valverde V. *Nutritional Surveillance.* Geneva, Switzerland: World Health Organization; 1984.
13. U.S. Department of Agriculture. *Dietary Guidelines for Americans.* Available at: http://www.healthierus.gov/dietaryguidelines. Accessed June 20, 2005.
14. Sims LS. Research aspects of public policy in nutrition generating research questions to determine the impact of nutritional, agricultural, and healthcare policy and regulations on the health and nutritional status of the public. The research agenda for Dietetics Conference. In: American Dietetic Association, ed. *Proceedings.* Chicago, IL: 1993:25–38.
15. Caballero B, Allen L. *Encyclopedia of Human Nutrition.* 1st ed. St. Louis, MO: Elsevier Academic Press; 1999.
16. St-Onge MP, Keller KL, Heymsfield SB. Changes in childhood food consumption patterns: a cause for concern in light of increasing body weights. *Am J Clin Nutr.* 2003; 78(6):1068–1073.
17. Mitchell CO. *Geriatric Nutrition: The Health Professional's Handbook.* 2nd ed. Gaithersburg, MD: Aspen; 1999.
18. U.S. Congress. *P.L. 101-445. National Nutrition Monitoring and Related Research Act of 1990.* Washington, DC: 101st Congress; October 22, 1990.
19. U.S. Department of Health and Human Services, U.S. Department of Agriculture. Ten-year comprehensive plan for the national nutrition monitoring and related research program. *Fed Reg.* 1993; 58:32752–32806.
20. Briefel RR. Assessment of the U.S. diet in national nutrition surveys: national collaborative efforts and NHANES. *Am J Clin Nutr.* 1994; 59:164S–167S.
21. Berdanier CD, Feldman E, Flatt W. *Handbook of Nutrition and Food.* New York: CRC Press; 2002.
22. Centers for Disease Control and Prevention, National Center for Health Statistics. *National Center for Health Statistics-at-a-Glance.* Available at: http://www.cdc.gov/nchs/data/misc/proact02.pdf. Accessed February 20, 2008.
23. Kuczmarski RJ, Ogden CL, Grummer-Strawn LM, et al. CDC growth charts: United States. *Adv Data.* 2000; 8(314):1–27.
24. Cole TJ, Bellizzi MC, Flegal KM, Dietz WH. Establishing a standard definition for child overweight and obesity worldwide: international survey. *BMJ.* 2000; 320:1240–1243.
25. Beker L. Principles of Growth Assessment. *Pediatrics in Review.* 2006; 27:196–198.
26. Ogden CL, Kuczmarski RJ, Flegal KM, et al. Centers for Disease Control and Prevention 2000 growth charts for the United States: improvements to the 1977 National Center for Health Statistics version. *Pediatrics.* 2002; 109(1):45–60.
27. U.S. Department of Agriculture, U.S. Department of Health and Human Services. *Nutrition and Your Health: Dietary Guidelines for Americans.* 5th ed. Washington, DC: U.S. Government Printing Office; 2000. Available at: http://www.health.gov/dietaryguidelines/dga2005/document/default.htm. Accessed February 20, 2008.
28. Centers for Disease Control and Prevention. How many fruits and vegetables do you need? Fruits and Veggies More Matters. Available at: http://www.fruitsandveggiesmatter.gov. Accessed February 20, 2008.
29. National Cholesterol Education Program (NCEP). Summary of the second expert panel of the National Cholesterol Education Program (NCEP) Expert Panel on Detection, Evaluation, and Treatment of High Blood Cholesterol in Adults (Adult Treatment Panel II). *JAMA.* 1993; 269:3015–3023.
30. National Heart Lung and Blood Institute. *Sixth Report of the Joint National Committee on Detection, Evaluation, and Treatment of High Blood Pressure.* Washington, DC: U.S. Department of Health and Human Services; November 1997.
31. Koplan J, Liverman CT, Kraak VI. *Preventing Childhood Obesity: Health in the Balance.* Washington, DC: National Academies Press; 2005.
32. Centers for Disease Control and Prevention. Nutritional status of children participating in the Special Supplemental Nutrition Program for Women, Infants, and Children—United States, 1988-91. *MMWR.* 1995; 45(3):65–69.
33. Crane NT, Wilson DB, Lewis CJ, Cook DA, Rader JI, Yetley EA. Evaluating Food Fortification Options: General Principles Revisited with Folic Acid. *Am J Public Health.* 1995; 85:660–666.
34. Lewis C, Crane NT, Wilson DB, Yetley EA. Estimated folate intakes: data updated to reflect food fortification, increased bioavailability, and dietary supplement use. *Am J Clinical Nutr.* 1999; 70:198–207.
35. U.S. Department of Health and Human Services, Food and Drug Administration. Notice of final rule: food labeling: health claims and label statements; dietary

fiber and cardiovascular disease; dietary fiber and cancer. *Fed Reg*. January 5, 1993: 2537–2605.

36. Wright J, Bialostosky K, Gunter EW, Najjar MF, Bowman BA, Johnson CL. Blood folate and vitamin B12: United States, 1988–1994.*Vital Health Stat*. 1998; 11(243):1–13.

37. Institute of Medicine, Food and Nutrition Board. *Dietary Reference Intakes for Calcium, Phosphorus, Magnesium, Vitamin D, and Fluoride. A Report of the Standing Committee on the Scientific Evaluation of Dietary Reference Intakes*. Washington, DC: National Academy Press; 1997.

38. Institute of Medicine, Food and Nutrition Board. *A Report of the Standing Committee on the Scientific. Evaluation of Dietary Reference Intakes and Its Panel on Folate, Other B Vitamins, and Choline and Dietary Reference Intakes for Thiamin, Riboflavin, Niacin, Vitamin B6, Folate, Vitamin B12, Pantothenic Acid, Biotin, and Choline*. Washington, DC: Subcommittee on Upper Reference Levels of Nutrients: National Academy Press; 1998.

39. National Research Council. *Diet and Health. Implications for Reducing Chronic Disease Risk*. Washington, DC: National Academy Press; 1989.

40. U.S. Department of Health and Human Services. *Healthy People 2000, National Health Promotion and Disease Objectives*. PHS Publication No. 91-50212. Washington, DC: Author; 1991.

41. U.S. Department of Health and Human Services. *Healthy People 2010. Conference Edition in Two Volumes*. Washington, DC: Author; 2000.

42. Sims LS. Public policy in nutrition: a framework for action. *Nutr Today*. 1993; 28(2):10–20.

43. Office of Science and Technology Policy (OSTP). *Meeting the Challenge. A Research Agenda for America's Health, Safety, and Food*. Washington, DC: Government Printing Office; February 1996.

44. U.S. Department of Health and Human Services. *The Surgeon General's Report on Nutrition and Health*. PHS Publication No. 88-50210. Washington, DC: Author; 1988.

45. Anderson SA. The 1990 Life Sciences Research Office (LSRO) Report on Nutritional Assessment defined terms associated with food access. Core indicators of nutritional state for difficult to sample populations. *J Nutr*. 1990; 102:1559–1660.

46. Radimer K. Measurement of household food security in the USA and other industrialized countries. *Pub Health Nutrit*. 2002; 5:859–864.

47. Life Sciences Research Office, Federation of American Societies for Experimental Biology. Core indicators of nutritional state for difficulty-sample populations. *J Nutr*. 1990; 120(Suppl):1559–1600.

48. Health Canada. What Is Food Insecurity? Available at: http://www.hc-sc.gc.ca/fn-an/nutrition/pol/food_sec_entire-sec_aliments_entier-02_e.html. Accessed July 23, 2006.

49. Campbell C, Desjardins E. A model and research approach for studying the management of limited food resources by low income families. *J Nutr Educ*. 1989; 21(4):162–171.

50. Radimer KL, Olson CM, Greene JC, Campbell CC, Habicht JP. Understanding hunger and developing indicators to assess it in women and children. *J Nutr Educ*. 1992; 24(1):36S–45S.

51. Radimer KL, Olson CM, Campbell CC. Development of indicators to assess hunger. *J Nutr*. 1990; 120:1544–1548.

52. Campbell CC, Desjardins E. A model and research approach for studying the management of limited food resources by low income families *J Nutr Educ*. 1989; 21(4):162–171.

53. U.S. Department of Agriculture. Food Security. Available at: http://www.ers.usda.gov/Briefing/FoodSecurity/surveytools.htm. Accessed April 20, 2005.

54. Hamilton WL, Cook JT, Thompson WW, et al. *Household Food Security in the United States in 1995—Summary Report of the Food Security Measurement Project*. Washington, DC: Office of Analysis and Evaluation, Food and Consumer Service; 1997.

55. Furness BW, Simon PA, Wold CM, Asarian-Anderson J. Prevalence and predictors of food insecurity among low-income households in Los Angeles County. *Public Health Nutr*. 2004; 7(6):791–794.

56. Nord M, Andrews M, Winicki J. Frequency and duration of food insecurity and hunger in US households. *J Nutr Educ Behav*. 2002; 34(4):194–200.

57. Nord M, Andrews M, Carlson S. *Household Food Security in the United States, 2005*. Economic Research Report No. ERR-29. November 2005. Available at: http://www.ers.usda.gov/Publications/ERR29/ERR29.pdf. Accessed February 20, 2008.

58. Olson CM, Anderson K, Kiss E, et al. Factors protecting against and contributing to food insecurity among rural families. *Fam Econ Nutr Rev*. 2004; 16(1):12–20.

59. Nord M, Andrews M, Carlson S. *Household Food Security in the United States, 2004*. Economic Research Report No. ERR-11. October 2005. Available at: http://www.ers.usda.gov/publications/err11. Accessed February 20, 2008.

60. Nord M, Tiehen L, Andrews M, Bickel G, Carlson S. *Household Food Security in the United States, 2000*. FANRR-21. Alexandria, VA: U.S. Department of Agriculture; 2002.

61. Economic Research Service, U.S. Department of Agriculture. Food Security in the United States: Conditions and Trends. Available at: http://www.ers.usda.gov/Briefing/FoodSecurity/trends.htm. Accessed April 27, 2005.

62. Bogle M. Nutrition Intervention Research in the Mississippi Delta of Arkansas, Louisiana, and Mississippi. Washington, DC. U.S. Department of Agriculture. Available at: http://www.ars.usda.gov/research/projects/projects.htm?ACCN_NO=408537. Accessed April 6, 2008.

63. Nord M, Brent CP. Food Insecurity in Higher Income Households. Available at: http://www.ers.usda.gov/publications/efan02016. Accessed February 20, 2008.

64. Gundersen C, Gruber J. The dynamic determinants of food insecurity. In: Andrews M, Prell M, eds. *Second Food Security Measurement and Research Conference*. Vol. II. USDA, Economic Research Service No. 91-109. 2001. Available at: http://www.ers.usda.gov/publications/efanrr/11-2. Accessed February 20, 2008.

65. Nord M, Andrews M, Carlson S. Measuring Food Security in the United States: Household Food Security in the United States, 2003. Available at: http://www.ers.usda.gov/publications/fanrr42/fanrr42.pdf. Accessed February 20, 2008.

66. DeNavas-Walt C, Bernadette DP, Hill L. *Current Population Reports, P60-231, Income, Poverty, and Health Insurance Coverage in the United States: 2005*. Washington, DC: U.S. Census Bureau; 2006.

67. U.S. Bureau of Labor Statistics. Adjustments to Household Survey Population Estimates in January 2005. Available at: http://www.bls.gov/cps/cps05adj.pdf. Accessed July 28, 2006.

68. America's Second Harvest. Hunger Study 2006. Available at: http://www.hungerinamerica.org/key_findings. Accessed January 1, 2007.

69. Economic Research Service, U.S. Department of Agriculture. Food Security in the United States: Conditions and Trends. Available at: http://www.ers.usda.gov/Briefing/FoodSecurity/trends.htm. Accessed January 1, 2007.

70. Nord M. Food Security in the United States. August 2005. Available at: http://www.ers.usda.gov/Briefing/FoodSecurity. Accessed July 2005.

71. U.S. Department of Labor. A Profile of the Working Poor, 2003. Available at: http://www.bls.gov/cps/cpswp2003.pdf. Accessed August 5, 2005.

72. Proctor BD, Delaker J. Poverty in the United States: 2001. *Current Population Reports*. 2002; P60-214. Available at: http://www.census.gov/prod/2002pubs/p60-219.pdf. Accessed February 22, 2008.

73. Nord M, Andrews M, Carlson S. Use of Federal and Community Food Assistance Programs. In: *Household Food Security in the United States, 2005*. Available at: http://www.ers.usda.gov/publications/err29/. Accessed January 1, 2007.

74. Project H.O.M.E. Facts on Homelessness. Available at: http://www.projecthome.org. Accessed February 22, 2008.

75. Beal AC, Redlener I. Enhancing perinatal outcome in homeless women: the challenge of providing comprehensive health care. *Semin Perinatol*. 1995; 19(4):307–313.

76. Kelly E. Assessment of dietary intake of preschool children living in a homeless shelter. *Appl Nurs Res*. 2001; 14(3):146–154.

77. Johnson LJ, McCool AC. Dietary intake and nutritional status of older adult homeless women: a pilot study. *J Nutr Elderly*. 2003; 23(1):1–21.

78. National Low Income Housing Coalition. Housing Remains "Out of Reach" for Millions of Americans. Available at: http://www.nlihc.org. Accessed February 22, 2008.

79. Tarasuk V, Dachner N, Li J. Homeless youth in Toronto are nutritionally vulnerable. *J Nutr*. 2005; 135(8):1926–1933.

80. Luder E, Ceysens-Okada E, Koren-Roth A, Martinez-Weber C. Health and nutrition survey in a group of urban homeless adults. *J Am Diet Assoc*. 1990; 90(10):1387–1392.

81. Drake MA. The nutritional status and dietary adequacy of single homeless women and their children in shelters. *Pub Health Rep*. 1992; 107(3):312–319.

82. Whit MC, Tulsky JP, Dawson C, Zolopa AR, Moss AR. Association between time homeless and perceived health status among the homeless in San Francisco. *J Comm Health*. 1997; 22(4):271–282.

83. Busen NH, Beech, BL. A collaborative model for community-based healthcare screening of homeless adolescents. *J Prof Nurs*. 1997; 13(5):316.

84. Miller CL, Spittal PM, Frankish JC, Li K, Schechter MT, Wood E. HIV and hepatitis C outbreaks among high-risk youth in Vancouver demands a public health response. *Can J Public Health*. 2005; 96(2):107–108.

85. America's Second Harvest. Creating a Hunger-Free America. Available at: http://www.secondharvest.org. Accessed February 22, 2008.

86. U.S. Conference of Mayors. Hunger and Homelessness Continues to Rise in U.S. Cities. Available at: http://www.citymayors.com/features/uscity_poverty.html#Anchor-Homelessness-35882. Accessed February 22, 2008.

87. U.S. Conference of Mayors, Sodexho USA. Hunger and Homelessness Survey. Available at: http://www.usmayors.org/uscm/hungersurvey/2004/onlinereport/HungerAndHomelessnessReport2004.pdf. Accessed February 22, 2008.

88. Jones-DeWeever A, Peterson J, Song X. Before and After Welfare Reform: The Work and Well-Being of Low-Income Single Parent Families. Available at: http://www.iwpr.org/pdf/D454.pdf. Accessed August 12, 2005.

89. Casey P, Goolsby S, Berkowitz C, et al. Maternal depression, changing public assistance, food security, and child health status. *Pediatr*. 2004; 113(2):298–304.

90. Bartlett SJ, Kolodner K, Butz AM, et al. Maternal depressive symptoms and emergency department use among inner-city children with asthma. *Arch Pediatr Adolesc Med*. 2001; 155:347–353.

91. Heneghan AM, Silver EJ, Bauman LJ, Stein RE. Do pediatricians recognize mothers with depressive symptoms? *Pediatr*. 2000; 106:1367–1373.

92. Lanzi RG, Pascoe JM, Keltner B, Ramey SL. Correlates of maternal depressive symptoms in a national Head Start Program sample. *Arch Pediatr Adolesc Med*. 1999; 153:801–807.

93. Smith LA, Wise PH, Chavkin W, Romero D, Zuckerman B. Implications of welfare reform for child health: emerging challenges for clinical practice and policy. *Pediatr*. 2000; 106:1117–1125.

94. Kaestner R, Tarlov E. Changes in the welfare caseload and the health of low-educated mothers. *JPAM*. 2006; 25(3):623–643.

95. Greenberg M, Laracy M. *Welfare Reform: Next Steps Offer New Opportunities*. Neighborhood Funders Group Policy Paper No. 4. Washington, DC: Center for Law and Social Policy; 2000.

96. U.S. Department of Labor Statistics. Employment Characteristics of Families Summary. Available at: http://www.bls.gov/news.release/famee.nr0.htm. Accessed January 2, 2007.

97. Haskins R, Sawhill I, Weaver K. Welfare Reform: An Overview of Effects to Date. Welfare Reform & Beyond. Policy Brief no. 1. Washington, DC: Brookings Institution; 2001.

98. Soss J, Sanford FA. Public Transformed? Welfare reform as policy feedback. *American Political Science Review*. 2007;101:111–127.

99. Nnakwe N. Dietary patterns and prevalence of food insecurity among low-income families participating in community assistance programs in a Midwest town. *Family & Consumer Sciences Research Journal*. 2008; 36(3):229–242.

100. Pati S, Romero D, Chavkin W. Changes in use of health insurance and food assistance programs in medically underserved communities in the era of welfare reform: an urban study. *Amer J Public Health*. 2002; 92(9):1441–1445.

101. Porter K, Dupree A. *Poverty Trends for Families Headed by Working Single Mothers, 1993–1999*. Washington, DC: Center on Budget and Policy Priorities; 2001.

102. Pavetti L. Welfare policy in transition: redefining the social contract for poor citizen families with children. *Focus*. 2000; 21(2):44–50.

103. Lyter D. *Education and Job Training Build Strong Families*. Washington, DC: Institute for Women's Policy Research; 2002.

104. O'Neill K, Primus W. Recent data trends show welfare reform to be a mixed success: Significant policy changes should accompany reauthorization. *Review of Policy Research*. 2005; 22(3):301–324.

105. Kendal A, Olson CM, Frongillo EA Jr. Relationship of hunger and food insecurity to food availability and consumption. *J Am Diet Assoc*. 1996; 96:1019–1024.

106. Wilde P, Nord M. The effect of food stamps on food security: A panel data approach. *Review of Agricultural Economics*. 2005; 27(3):425–432.

107. Sonya J, Jahns L, Laraia L, Haughton B. Lower risk of overweight in school-aged food insecure girls who participate in food assistance. *Arch Pediatr Adolesc Med*. 2003; 157:780–784.

108. Frank-Spohrer GC. *Community Nutrition: Applying Epidemiology to Contemporary Practice*. Long Beach, CA: Aspen; 1996.

109. Economic Research Service, U.S. Department of Agriculture. Food and Nutrition Assistance Programs. Available at: http://www.ers.usda.gov/Briefing/FoodNutritionAssistance. Accessed August 8, 2005.

110. Economic Research Service, U.S. Department of Agriculture. Food Stamp Program. Available at: http://www.ers.usda.gov/Briefing/FoodStamps. Accessed August 11, 2005.

111. Nord M. Economic Research Service, U.S. Department of Agriculture. Food stamp participation and food security. *Food Rev*. 2001; 24:13–19.

112. Wilde P. Strong economy and welfare reforms contribute to drop in food stamp rolls. *Food Rev*. 2001; 24:2–7.

113. Zedlewski SR. Family economic resources in the post-reform era. *Future Child*. 2002; 12:120–145.

114. Rowe G. *Assessing the New Federalism: Welfare Rules Data Book*. Washington, DC: Urban Institute; 2000.

115. Food Research and Action Center. Federal Food Programs: Characteristics of Food Stamp Households. Available at: http://www.frac.org/html/federal_food_programs/programs/fspcharacteristics.html. Accessed August 11, 2005.

116. Bartlett S, Burstein N, Andrews M. Food Stamp Program Access Study: Eligible Nonparticipants. Available at: http://www.ers.usda.gov/publications/efan03013/efan03013-2/efan03013-2fm.pdf. Accessed August 11, 2005.

117. Economic Research Service, U.S. Department of Agriculture. Food Stamp Program: Food Stamp Nutrition Education (FSNE). Available at: http://www.ers.usda.gov/Briefing/FoodStamps/fsne.htm. Accessed July 26, 2006.

118. Clemson University. About Food Stamp Nutrition Education. Available at: http://www.clemson.edu/fsne/about_fsne.php. Accessed July 26, 2006.

119. Anding J, Fletcher RD, Van Laanen P, Supak C. The food stamp nutrition education program's impact on selected food and nutrition behaviors among Texans. *Journal of Extension*. 2001; 39(6):1–10.

120. Perez-Escamilla R, Rerris AM, Haldeman L, et al. Food stamps are associated with food security and dietary intake of inner-city preschoolers from Hartford, Connecticut. *J Nutr*. 2000; 130:2711–2717.

121. Campbell MK, Morreale HL, Farrell D, Carbone E, Brasure M. A tailored multimedia nutrition education pilot program for low-income women receiving food assistance. *Health Educ Res*. 1999; 14(2):257–267.

122. Food and Nutrition Service. Food Distribution Programs. Available at: http://www.fns.usda.gov/fdd. Accessed August 9, 2005.

123. Food and Nutrition Service. Commodity Supplemental Food Program. Available at: http://www.fns.usda.gov/fdd/programs/csfp/pfs-csfp.pdf. Accessed August 9, 2005.

124. Food and Nutrition Service. Food Distribution Program on Indian Reservations. Available at: http://www.fns.usda.gov/fdd/programs/fdpir/pfs-fdpir.pdf. Accessed August 9, 2005.

125. Food and Nutrition Service. The Emergency Food Assistance Program. Available at: http://www.fns.usda.gov/fdd/programs/tefap/pfs-tefap.pdf. Accessed August 9, 2005.

126. Food and Nutrition Service. Nutrition Services Incentive Program. Available at: http://www.fns.usda.gov/fdd/programs/nsip. Accessed August 9, 2005.

127. Food and Nutrition Service. Disaster Manual. 2004. Available at: http://www.fns.usda.gov/fdd/programs/fd-disasters/CommodityDisasterManual.pdf. Accessed August 9, 2005.

128. Grosvenor M, Smolin L. *Nutrition: From Science to Life*. Fort Worth, TX: Harcourt College; 2002.

129. Food and Nutrition Service. School Meals. Available at: http://www.fns.usda.gov/cnd. Accessed August 10, 2005.

130. Food and Nutrition Service. National School Lunch Program. Available at: http://www.fns.usda.gov/cnd/Afterschool/default.htm. Accessed August 10, 2005.

131. National Youth Sports Program. The National Youth Sports Program. Available at: http://www.nyscorp.org/nysp/home.html. Accessed August 10, 2005.

132. Food and Nutrition Service. Child and Adult Care Food Program. Available at: http://www.fns.usda.gov/cnd/Care/CACFP/cacfpfaqs.htm. Accessed August 10, 2005.

133. U.S. Department of Agriculture. Child and Adult Care Food Program. Available at: http://www.fns.usda.gov/pd/ccsummar.htm. Accessed August 4, 2006.

134. Food and Nutrition Service. Women, Infants, and Children. Available at: http://www.fns.usda.gov/wic/factsheets.htm. Accessed August 10, 2005.

135. Food and Nutrition Service. WIC Farmers' Marker Nutrition Program. Available at: http://www.fns.usda.gov/wic/WIC-FMNP-Fact-Sheet.pdf. Accessed August 10, 2005.

136. U.S. Department of Agriculture. Expanded Food and Nutrition Education Program (EFNEP). Available at: http://www.csrees.usda.gov/nea/family/in_focus/youthdev_if_efnep.html. Accessed July 26, 2006.

137. Cooperative State Research, Education, and Extension Service. Food, Nutrition, & Health. Available at: http://www.csrees.usda.gov/nea/food/food.html. Accessed July 28, 2006.

138. Edelstein S. *Nutrition in Public Health: A Handbook for Developing Programs and Services*. 2nd ed. Sudbury, MA: Jones and Bartlett; 2006.

139. Montgomery S, Wells W. Fiscal Year 2005 Impact and Review of the Expanded Food and Nutrition Education Program. Available at: http://www.csrees.usda.gov/nea/food/efnep. Accessed February 22, 2008.

140. Area Agency on Aging. The Elderly Nutrition Program. Available at: http://www.aoa.gov/press/fact/alpha/fact_elderly_nutrition.asp. Accessed January 2, 2007.

141. National Library of Medicine, National Institutes of Health. Nutrition for Seniors. Available at: http://www.nlm.nih.gov/medlineplus/nutritionforseniors.html. Accessed August 4, 2006.

142. Food and Nutrition Service. Senior Farmers' Market Nutrition Program. Available at: http://www.fns.usda.gov/wic/SeniorFMNP/SeniorFMNPoverview.htm. Accessed August 10, 2005.

CHAPTER 5

Private and Government Healthcare Systems

LEARNING OBJECTIVES
- Differentiate between private and government healthcare systems in the United States.
- Discuss the eligibility and services criteria for Medicare and Medicaid.
- Discuss the different types of group insurance.
- List the different types of current health coverage status.
- Discuss the impact of the Personal Responsibility and Work Opportunity Reconciliation Act (PRWORA).

Introduction

In the United States, a wide variety of healthcare providers are available to give comprehensive healthcare to individuals who can afford it. In 2005, total U.S. expenditure on healthcare was $2 trillion, and spending is expected to increase to $2.9 trillion in 2009.[1] However, healthcare services are unevenly distributed. Even some individuals who have access to employer-sponsored *health insurance* are unable to obtain coverage due to the high cost of *premiums* and rising healthcare costs.[2] In 2006, employer health insurance premiums increased by 7.7 percent, which may be one of the reasons why about 47 million Americans are uninsured.[3,4] The United States spends a great deal of money on acute care and insufficient amounts on the promotion of health and prevention of diseases. One of the major goals of Healthy People 2010 is to increase the quality and years of healthy life. This goal can be accomplished by increasing funding for health promotion, disease prevention, and care for people with chronic illnesses and by providing health insurance to the poor.

Poverty limits access to healthcare, leading to poorer *health status*. People in the lowest income households are more likely than those in higher income households to report their health status as fair or poor.[5]

Poor health and physical and mental disabilities can lead to food insecurity by limiting the ability to acquire and prepare food and by affecting nutrient needs.[5] For instance, research shows a higher incidence of iron deficiency anemia in low-income children,[6] and that the incidence of heart disease, cancer, hypertension, and obesity increases with decreasing income.[7,8] In the United States, health insurance coverage is generally classified as either private (non-government) coverage or government-sponsored coverage. The following discussion highlights healthcare economics terms that community nutritionists should be able to recognize.

Healthcare Coverage vs. Uninsured

The National Center for Health Statistics defines health insurance as a broad term that includes both public and private payers who cover medical expenditures incurred by a defined population in a variety of settings.[9] The total number of people with health insurance in 2004 was 247.3 million.[10] In the United States, the risk of becoming uninsured increases significantly for those earning low wages (the working poor); for the unemployed, especially young adults because they have higher rates of unemployment; and when employers are unable to provide or

<table>
<tr><td colspan="3">**TABLE 5.1** The Rate of Healthcare Coverage in 2005–2006[10,12]</td></tr>
</table>

Health Insurance Coverage	2005	2006
People without health insurance coverage	15.3%	15.8%
People covered by employment-based health insurance	60.2%	59.7%
People covered by government health insurance programs	27.3%	27.0%
People covered by Medicaid	13.0%	12.9%
People covered by Medicare	13.7%	13.6%
Uninsured European Americans	10.1%	10.8%
Uninsured African Americans	19.0%	20.5%
Uninsured Hispanics	32.3%	34.1%
Uninsured Asian Americans	17.2%	15.5%

Source: U.S. Census Bureau. Health Insurance Coverage in 2005. Available at: http://www.census.gov/hhes/www/hlthins/hlthin06.html. Accessed April 25, 2007.

TABLE 5.2 The Number and Percentage of People with Health Insurance Coverage

Year	Uninsured Millions	Uninsured Percentage	Medicaid/SCHIP Percentage	Job-Based Insurance Percentage
2005	46.6	15.9	13.0	59.5
2004	45.8	15.7	12.9	59.8
2003	45.0	15.6	12.4	60.4
2002	43.6	15.2	11.6	61.3
2001	41.2	14.6	11.2	62.6
2000	39.8	14.2	10.6	63.6

Source: Center on Budget and Policy Priorities. The Number of Uninsured Americans Continued to Rise in 2004. Available at: http://www.cbpp.org/8-30-05health.htm. Accessed January 10, 2006.

offer *insurance* to workers. These people generally do not qualify for Medicaid because it is for the low-income elderly, children, blind/disabled people, pregnant women, single parents, or unemployed parents (in some states). Employed adults are not eligible for Medicaid regardless of income unless they are blind, disabled, or pregnant.[11] **Table 5.1** presents the rate of healthcare coverage in 2005, and **Table 5.2** presents the trend of declining health insurance coverage.

Private Health Insurance

The majority of private healthcare expenses are incurred by individuals receiving treatment and are paid by private insurers making payments

The risk of becoming uninsured increases significantly for those earning low wages.

on behalf of the client/enrollee.[11] But the use of healthcare is not a rare event. For instance, it was reported that during 2004, an estimated 910.9 million individuals visited physicians' offices in the United States, an overall rate of 315.9 visits per 100 persons. In contrast, uninsured persons (as measured by self-pay and charity visits) had a much lower number of visits to physicians' offices placing them at a disadvantage for disease prevention and early diagnosis.[13,14]

The concept of insurance is to combine the healthcare experiences of many enrollees in order to reduce expenses for any one individual to a manageable prepayment amount. There are different types of insurance plans and organizations. This section will discuss some of the plans and organizations clients may have.

Employment-Based Plans

Employment-based health insurance is coverage offered through one's own employment or a relative's employment. It may be offered by an employer or by a union. Traditionally, a person enrolled in the healthcare delivery system by contracting directly with a healthcare provider for individual care based on fee-for-service, also known as direct-purchase plans.[15] However, in recent years, more physicians are contracting for all or part of their practices with managed healthcare organizations,

health insurance A broad term that includes both public and private payers who cover medical expenditures incurred by a defined population in a variety of settings.

premium A periodic payment required to keep an insurance policy requirement.

health status The condition of an individual's physiological and psychological state, and his or her interaction with the environment.

insurance A plan in which individuals and organizations who are concerned about potential risks will pay premiums to an insurance company, who subsequently will reimburse them if there is loss.

employment-based health insurance Coverage offered through one's own employment or the employment of a relative.

mainly independent practice associations (IPAs), *health maintenance organizations (HMOs)*, and preferred provider organizations (PPOs). These are all prepaid group practice plans that offer healthcare services through groups of medical practitioners.

Direct-Purchase/Fee-for-Service Plans

Fee-for-service plans are the traditional type of healthcare policy. The physician sets a price for each type of service delivered, and then the client or insurance company pays the fee. This type of health insurance provides the most preference to doctors and hospitals. The client can choose any doctor he or she wishes and can change doctors at any time. The client can use any hospital in any part of the country. With fee-for-service, the insurer only pays for part of the doctor and hospital bills. The client pays a monthly fee called a premium. The main concern about the fee-for-service plan is that it encourages unnecessary care (lab tests, procedures, etc.).

The *Medicare* system is based on fee-for-service for paying physicians. The physician payment mechanism for Medicare has been modified. Medicare pays an individual physician an amount that does not exceed the 75th percentile of charges by all physicians in a community. (This is termed the "prevailing" fee.[16])

There are two kinds of fee-for-service coverage: basic and major medical. Basic covers some hospital services and supplies, such as X-rays and prescribed medicine. Basic coverage also pays the cost of surgery, whether it is performed in or out of the hospital, and for some doctor visits. Major medical insurance covers the cost of long-term, high-cost illnesses or injuries plus whatever basic did not cover. Some policies combine basic and major medical insurance coverage into one plan. This is sometimes called a comprehensive plan. It is important for clients to check their policy to make sure they have both kinds of protection. Insurance coverage can be purchased from commercial insurance companies such as Blue Cross Blue Shield.[11,16]

Group Contract Insurance

The group contract health insurance system was developed because of the need for hospitals and physicians to make their products and services affordable to ordinary people in the United States. With unmanaged care (fee-for-service) payments, healthcare providers had the opportunity to increase the number of single services they delivered in order to increase their profit. The more fees paid, the greater the revenue generated for the provider (physician, hospital, etc.) and the greater the cost to the insurer (private or public). This was a cause for concern because of rising health service costs in the last quarter of the twentieth century. Unmanaged care also caused employers to reduce their coverage and shift costs to employees by making the employees pay a larger share of the premiums, higher deductibles, and higher co-payments.[17] This was a concern to the government (Medicare and Medicaid) and to employers because they typically used fee-for-service as their primary payment approach. Increasingly, however, they are using managed care in the hope that it will provide the quality and quantity of care needed to ensure people's health and well-being as well as control costs.[18]

Managed Care

Managed care is a system that manages the cost and delivery of healthcare services, the quality of that healthcare, and access to care. It is based on the belief that healthcare costs can be controlled by "managing" the way in which healthcare is delivered. Enrollees have a financial incentive to use participating providers that agree to provide a wide range of services to them. Providers may be paid on a prenegotiated basis (as with health maintenance organizations, point-of-service plans, and preferred provider organizations).[19]

Managed care influences how much healthcare clients can use. Almost all plans have some type of managed care program to help control costs. For example, if a client needs to go to the hospital, one form of managed care requires that the client receive approval from the insurance company before being admitted because the insurance company wants to make sure that the hospitalization is needed. The hospital cost may not be covered if approval is not obtained.[11]

Health Maintenance Organizations

Health maintenance organizations (HMO) are prepaid health plans. The goal of an HMO is to provide affordable, well-organized healthcare by allowing clients to prepay (**capitation** payment) on a regular monthly basis for all services provided by the practice, including physicians' visits, hospital stays, emergency care, surgery, lab tests, X-rays, and therapy for all members and their families. The HMO arranges for this care either directly in its own group practice or through physician and other healthcare professionals under contract.[20] Typically, the client's choice of physicians and hospitals is limited to those that have agreements with the HMO to provide care. However, exceptions are made in emergencies or when medically necessary.

There may be a small co-payment for each office visit, such as $15 for a doctor's visit or $50 for hospital emergency room treatment. The client's total medical costs will likely be lower and more predictable in an HMO than with fee-for-service health insurance. Because HMOs receive a fixed fee for the coverage of medical care, it is in their interest to make sure the client receives basic healthcare for problems before they become serious. HMOs typically provide preventive care, such as office visits, immunizations, well-baby checkups, mammograms, and physicals. The range of services covered varies among HMOs, so it is important to compare available plans. Some services, such as outpatient mental healthcare, often are provided only on a limited basis. Conventional HMOs employ a staff of physicians, nurses, and other healthcare professionals who earn a salary and consequently have no

---

health maintenance organization (HMO) A managed care company that organizes and provides healthcare for its enrollees for a fixed prepaid premium.

fee-for-service plans The traditional type of healthcare policy; the physician sets a price for each type of service delivered, and then the patient or his or her insurer pays this price.

Medicare A federal entitlement program of medical and healthcare coverage for the elderly and disabled, and persons with end-stage renal disease, governed by Title XVIII of the federal Social Security Act, and consisting of two parts: Part A for institutional and homecare, and Part B for medical care.

managed care A system that seeks to manage the cost of healthcare, the quality of that healthcare, and access to care; it is based on the belief that healthcare costs can be controlled by "managing" the way in which healthcare is delivered.

capitation A payment method in which each provider, such as an HMO, receives a flat annual fee for each individual, regardless of how often services are used.

incentive to provide unnecessary expensive treatments.[17] They can be located at one or more locations in the client's community as part of a prepaid group practice known as the **staff model**. Another type, known as the **group model**, consists of independent groups of physicians who contract with an HMO to provide services to enrollees.

Individual practice associations (IPAs) are made up of private physicians in private offices who provide services to HMO members as well as clients with other forms of insurance. The HMO clients can select a physician from a list of participating physicians that make up the IPA network. In the network type of IPA, the HMO contracts with a number of multi-specialty physician groups to provide services to enrollees. Often, these physician groups also deliver services to non-HMO clients.[11,21]

Point-of-Service Plans

Many HMOs offer an option known as a **point-of-service (POS)** plan. It offers enrollees the option of receiving services from participating or nonparticipating providers. The benefits package is designed to encourage the use of participating providers through higher **deductibles** and/or partial reimbursement for services provided by nonparticipating providers. The primary care physicians in a POS plan usually make referrals to other providers in the plan. However, members can refer themselves outside the plan and still get some coverage.[16] If the physician makes a referral out of the network, the plan pays all or most of the bill. However, if the client refers him- or herself to a provider outside the network (and the service is covered by the plan), the co-payment and deductibles would increase significantly.[11]

Preferred Provider Organizations

A **preferred provider organization (PPO)** is a combination of traditional fee-for-service and an HMO. Similar to an HMO, clients use the physicians and hospitals that have agreed to give discounts to their insurer. The incentive is either a lower insurance premium or a waiver of cost-sharing requirements. Like an HMO, a PPO requires that the clients choose a primary care physician to monitor their healthcare. Most PPOs also cover preventive care. This typically includes visits to the physician, well-baby care, immunizations, and mammograms. If the client decides to choose a physician that is not part of the plan, the client will pay a larger portion of the bill (and also fill out claims forms to be reimbursed for medical expenses). Some people like this option because it does not require network care. For example, if the client's physician is not a part of the network, he or she will not be required to change physicians to join a PPO.[11,16] Healthcare expenditures in the U.S. totaled $2 trillion in 2005.[22]

Government Health Insurance/Public Insurance

Government health insurance includes plans funded by governments at the federal, state, or local level. The major categories of government health insurance are Medicare, Medicaid, and the State Children's Health Insurance Program (SCHIP). The Centers for Medicare and Medicaid Services (CMS), a federal agency, administers these programs. These plans provide a medical safety net for the poor, elderly, disabled, and some uninsured individuals.[23]

The Medicare Program

Medicare, Title XVIII of the Social Security Act, is the designated health insurance for the aged and disabled. Part of the Social Security Amendments of 1965, the Medicare legislation provides hospital and medical insurance to elderly persons, permanently and totally disabled persons, and people with end stage renal disease (ESRD). The Medicare program is administered by the Centers for Medicare and Medicaid Services (CMS), a division of the Department of Health and Human Services. The following groups also are eligible for Medicare benefits: persons entitled to Social Security or Railroad Retirement disability cash benefits for at least 24 months, and certain non-covered aged persons who elected to pay a premium for Medicare coverage.[24] The Medicare, Medicaid, and SCHIP Benefits Improvement and Protection Act of 2000 (Public Law 106-554) allowed persons with amyotrophic lateral sclerosis (Lou Gehrig's disease) to waive the 24-month waiting period.

Medicare has traditionally consisted of two parts: hospital insurance (HI), also known as Part A, and supplementary medical insurance (SMI), also known as Part B (see **Table 5.2**). A third part of Medicare, sometimes known as Part C, is the Medicare Advantage program, which was established as the Medicare + Choice program by the Balanced Budget Act (BBA) of 1997 (Public Law 105-33). Later, it was renamed and modified by the Medicare Prescription Drug, Improvement, and Modernization Act (MMA) of 2003.[25,26]

The MMA also established a fourth part of Medicare: a new prescription drug benefit, known as Part D, which became available in 2004. Part D activities are handled within the SMI trust fund, but in an account separate from Part B. It is important to note that SMI and Part B are different, since SMI now consists of both Part B and Part D. The purpose of the two separate accounts within the SMI trust fund is to ensure that funds from one part are not used to finance the other.[26]

When Medicare began on July 1, 1966, about 19 million people were enrolled. In 2004, almost 42 million people were enrolled in one or both of Parts A and B of the Medicare program, and about 5 million of them chose to participate in a Medicare Advantage plan.[27,28]

In 2004, total federal spending was about $2 trillion. Medicare spending was $265 billion (including offsets), or 12 percent of the total. Spending on Social Security totaled 21 percent ($492 billion), while defense spending accounted for 19 percent ($436 billion). **Figure 5-1** presents Medicare spending as part of the federal budget.[22,27,28]

---

staff model An HMO that employs providers directly and the providers see members/enrollees in the HMO's own facilities.

group model An HMO that contracts with a medical group for the provision of healthcare services.

individual practice association (IPA) A type of healthcare provider organization composed of a group of independent practicing physicians who maintain their own offices and band together for the purpose of contracting their services to HMOs. An IPA may contract with and provide services to both HMO and non-HMO plan participants.

point-of-service plan (POS) A healthcare plan that offers enrollees the option of receiving services from participating or nonparticipating providers.

deductible The amount an individual must pay out-of-pocket, usually yearly on a calendar-year basis, before insurance will begin to cover expenses.

preferred provider organization A network of providers who agree to deliver services for a reduced fee; the providers generally incur no financial risk. The financial burden is on the patient rather than the providers.

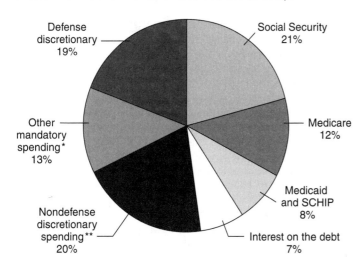

FIGURE 5-1 Medicare Spending as a Share of the Federal Budget, FY 2004

* Includes other retirement and disability programs, unemployment compensation, and farm price supports; also includes offsetting receipts.

** Includes funding for homeland security, transportation, education, and public health.

From: Office of Management and Budget, Budget of the U.S. Government, FY 2006.

Part A Coverage

Part A is generally provided automatically, and free of premiums, to persons age 65 or over who are eligible for Social Security or Railroad Retirement benefits, whether they have claimed these monthly cash benefits or not. Also, workers and their spouses with a sufficient period of Medicare-only coverage in federal, state, or local government employment are eligible beginning at age 65. Equally, individuals who have been entitled to Social Security or Railroad Retirement disability benefits for at least 24 months, and government employees with Medicare-only coverage who have been disabled for more than 29 months, are entitled to Part A benefits.[22,27,28]

Part A coverage also is provided to insured workers with ESRD (and to insured workers' spouses and children with ESRD), as well as ineligible aged and disabled beneficiaries who voluntarily paid a monthly premium for their coverage. In 2005, Part A provided protection against the costs of hospital and specific other medical care to about 42 million people (35 million aged and 7 million disabled enrollees). Part A benefit payments totaled $180 billion in 2005.[22,27,28]

Part B Coverage

In 2005, Part B provided protection against the costs of physician and other medical services to about 40 million people (34 million aged and 6 million disabled). Part B benefits totaled $150.3 billion in 2005. Part B covers physicians' and surgeons' services, including some covered services furnished by chiropractors, podiatrists, dentists, and optometrists. Also covered are the services provided by the following Medicare-approved practitioners who are not physicians: certified registered nurse anesthetists, clinical psychologists, clinical social workers (other than in a hospital), physician assistants, and nurse practitioners and clinical nurse specialists in collaboration with a physician.[22,27]

In 2002, Medicare started to pay qualified dietitians who enrolled in the Medicare program as providers, whether they provide medical nutrition therapy (MNT) services in an independent practice setting, hospital outpatient department, or any other setting. Medicare does not pay dietitians for hospital inpatients or individuals in a skilled nursing facility.[29,30] Medicare will pay dietitians (enrolled as Medicare MNT providers) for services to Medicare beneficiaries with type 1 diabetes, type 2 diabetes, gestational diabetes, non-dialysis kidney disease, and post–kidney-transplant status using specified codes. Referral from a physician for MNT is required.[29,31-33]

The insurance coverage for MNT services plays a significant role in the primary, secondary, and tertiary levels of prevention and in the maintenance of diabetes, cardiovascular diseases, and other diet-related health conditions. For example, primary prevention addresses lifestyle risk factors; the control of blood cholesterol levels is a secondary preventive measure that can slow the onset and progression of heart disease. As for tertiary prevention, heart disease becomes more manageable with intense MNT. Sheils et al.[34] estimated the costs and savings associated with providing the entire Medicare population with coverage for MNT. Results showed that MNT was associated with reduced utilization of hospital services by 9.5 percent for patients with diabetes and 8.6 percent for patients with cardiovascular disease. In addition, utilization of physician services decreased by 23.5 percent for MNT users with diabetes and 16.9 percent for MNT users with cardiovascular disease.[34] The researchers concluded that overall, after an initial period of implementation, coverage for MNT can result in a net reduction in health services utilization and cost. Also, research studies show that diet and exercise can prevent or delay the development of diabetes.[35,36] See **Box 6-1** in Chapter 6 for highlights of the success of the American Dietetic Association in obtaining Medicare coverage for some MNT services.

Coverage Gaps

Although Medicare provides extensive benefits, there are significant gaps in coverage. These gaps include Medicare deductibles, *co-payments*, excess charges by doctors who do not accept Medicare assignments, and medical services and supplies that Medicare does not cover. Additional services that are not covered by Medicare include long-term nursing care, custodial care, and certain other healthcare needs, such as dentures and dental care, eyeglasses, and hearing aids. Medicare Supplemental Insurance, also known as *Medigap*, was developed to provide extra protection beyond Medicare by filling some of the gaps in Medicare coverage.[37] Medigap is a type of private insurance coverage that may be purchased by an individual enrolled in Medicare to cover some needed services that are not covered by Medicare.

Part D

In 2003, the Medicare Prescription Drug Improvement and Modernization Act added a prescription drug benefit that became available in 2006. Part D provides subsidized access to prescription drug insurance coverage on a voluntary basis, upon payment of a premium, to individuals entitled to Part A or enrolled in Part B, with premium and cost-sharing subsidies for low-income enrollees. Beneficiaries may enroll in either a stand-alone prescription drug plan (PDP) or an integrated Medicare Advantage plan that offers Part D coverage.[37] Part D coverage includes most Food and Drug Administration (FDA)–approved prescription drugs.[38]

The Medicaid Program

Title XIX of the Social Security Act is a federal/state entitlement program that pays for medical assistance for certain low-income individuals and families. This program, known as **Medicaid**, became law in 1965 as a cooperative venture jointly funded by the federal and state governments (including the District of Columbia and the Territories) to assist states in providing medical assistance to eligible low-income persons. Medicaid is the largest source of funding for medical and health-related services for poor people. Within broad national guidelines established by federal statutes, regulations, and policies, each state must:[39,40]

- Establish its own eligibility standards
- Determine the type, amount, duration, and scope of services
- Set the rate of payment for services
- Administer its own program

Medicaid policies for eligibility, services, and payment are complex and vary among states of similar size or geographic proximity. Therefore, a person who is eligible for Medicaid in one state may not be eligible in another state, and the services provided by one state may differ considerably in amount, duration, or scope from services provided in a similar or neighboring state. In addition, state legislatures may change Medicaid eligibility, services, and/or reimbursement during the year.[39]

Basis of Eligibility

Medicaid does not provide medical assistance for all poor persons. Under the broadest provisions of the federal statute, Medicaid does not provide healthcare services even for very poor persons unless they are in one of the following designated groups. Individuals are usually eligible for Medicaid if they:[39]

- Meet the requirements for the Aid to Families with Dependent Children (AFDC) program that were in effect in their own state on July 16, 1996.
- Are six years old or younger and have a family income at or below 133 percent of the Federal Poverty Level (FPL). See **Table 4.9** in Chapter 4 for the Federal Poverty Guidelines.
- Are pregnant with a family income below 133 percent of the FPL. (Services to these women are limited to those related to pregnancy, complications of pregnancy, delivery, and postpartum care.)
- Are Supplemental Security Income (SSI) recipients. (Some states use more restrictive Medicaid eligibility requirements that predate SSI.)
- Are recipients of adoption or foster care assistance under Title IV of the Social Security Act.
- Belong to a special protected group (typically individuals who lose their cash assistance due to earnings from work or from increased Social Security benefits, but who may keep Medicaid for a period of time).
- Are born after September 30, 1983, are currently under the age of 19, and are in families with incomes at or below the FPL.

The Personal Responsibility and Work Opportunity Reconciliation Act (PRWORA)

The Personal Responsibility and Work Opportunity Reconciliation Act of 1996 (Public Law 104-193) is known as the "welfare reform" bill. It made restrictive changes regarding eligibility for SSI coverage that impacted the Medicaid program. For example, legal resident aliens and other qualified aliens who entered the United States on or after August 22, 1996, are ineligible for Medicaid for 5 years. Medicaid to resident aliens can continue only if these persons can be covered for Medicaid under some other eligibility status (with the exception of emergency services, which are mandatory).[39,40]

In addition, welfare reform repealed the open-ended federal entitlement program known as Aid to Families with Dependent Children (AFDC) and replaced it with Temporary Assistance for Needy Families (TANF), which provides states with grants to be spent on time-limited cash assistance. TANF generally limits a family's lifetime cash welfare benefits to a maximum of 5 years and permits states to impose a wide range of other requirements as well, in particular those related to employment.[41] However, welfare reform had a significant negative impact on Medicaid coverage before pregnancy among eligible participants, which resulted in a small decline in their first-trimester prenatal care initiation.[42] Under welfare reform, persons who would have been eligible for AFDC generally are still eligible for Medicaid.[39,43]

State Children's Health Insurance Program (SCHIP)

The **State Children's Health Insurance Program (SCHIP)**, Title XXI, was initiated by the Balanced Budget Act (BBA) of 1997. The federal government created the SCHIP program to cover individuals who have incomes too high to qualify for state medical assistance but who cannot obtain private insurance. All states participate, but some do not cover dental. In addition to allowing states to design or expand an existing state insurance program, SCHIP provides more federal funds for states to expand Medicaid eligibility to include children who are currently uninsured. With certain exceptions, those who qualify are:[39,43,44]

- Children in low-income families who would not qualify for Medicaid (based on the plan that was in effect on April 15, 1997)
- Eligible children under the age of 19 whose state provides 12 months of continuous Medicaid coverage (without reevaluation)

Medicaid, Title XIX of the Social Security Act

Title XIX of the Social Security Act allows considerable flexibility within the states' Medicaid plans. However, some federal requirements are mandatory if federal matching funds are to be received. A state's Medicaid program must offer medical assistance for certain basic services to most categorically needy populations. **Box 5-1** presents services generally provided by the state Medicaid programs. This chapter's Successful Community Strategies feature presents a

co-payment A specified amount that an insured individual must pay for a specified service or procedure (e.g., $20 for an office visit).

Medigap A type of private insurance coverage that may be purchased by an individual enrolled in Medicare to cover some needed services that are not covered by Medicare Parts A and B (i.e., "gaps").

Medicaid A joint federal/state/local program of healthcare for individuals whose income and resources are insufficient to pay for their care; it is governed by Title XIX of the federal Social Security Act, and is administered by the states. Medicaid is the major source of payment for nursing home care of the elderly.

State Children's Health Insurance Program (SCHIP) A federal program that covers individuals who have incomes too high to qualify for state medical assistance but who cannot obtain private insurance. All states participate, but some do not cover dental.

Box 5-1 **Services Provided by State Medicaid Programs**

- Inpatient hospital services
- Outpatient hospital services
- Prenatal care
- Vaccines for children
- Physician services
- Nursing facility services for persons age 21 or older
- Family planning services and supplies
- Rural health clinic services
- Home healthcare for persons eligible for skilled-nursing services
- Laboratory and X-ray services
- Pediatric and family nurse practitioner services
- Nurse-midwife services
- Early and periodic screening, diagnosis, and treatment (EPSDT) services for children under age 21

success story of lowering infant mortality by integrating WIC and Medicaid.

Balanced Budget Act

The Balanced Budget Act included a state option known as Programs of All-inclusive Care for the Elderly (PACE). PACE provides an alternative to institutional care for individuals age 55 or older who require a nursing facility level of care. The PACE team (an interdisciplinary team consisting of professional and paraprofessional staff) offers and manages all health, medical, and social services and mobilizes other services as needed to provide preventative, rehabilitative, curative, and supportive care. This care, provided in day health centers, homes, hospitals, and nursing homes, helps the person maintain independence, dignity, and quality of life. Regardless of source of payment, PACE providers receive payment only through the PACE agreement and must make available all items and services covered under both Titles XVIII and XIX, without amount, duration, or scope limitations and without application of any deductibles, co-payments, or other cost sharing. The individuals enrolled in PACE receive benefits solely through the PACE program.[39,45] **Table 5.3** presents a comparison of the Medicare and Medicaid programs. **Figure 5-2** presents the payments by type of service.

TABLE 5.3 **Comparison of the Medicare and Medicaid Programs**

Feature	Medicare	Medicaid
Obtain information	Local Social Security Administration office	State welfare office
Recipients	People who are 65 years old, are disabled, or have permanent kidney failure	Certain low-income people, including children; the aged, blind, and/or disabled; and those eligible to receive federally assisted income
Type of program	Insurance	Insurance
Government affiliation	Federal	All states
Availability	All states	All states
Financing of hospital insurance	Medicare Trust Fund, mandatory payroll deductions (1.45 percent for employed persons; 2.9 percent for self-employed); recipient deductibles; and trust fund interest	Federal and state governments
Financing of medical insurance	Recipient premium payments: Part A: if eligible, none or $206 to $375 per month or Part B: $78.20 per month; and general revenue of the U.S. Treasury	Federal (contributes about 50 to 80 percent to the state) and state governments
Types of coverage	Inpatient and outpatient hospital services; skilled nursing facilities; home health services; mental health treatment; kidney dialysis; hospice care; physician services; and medical and health services equipment and supplies	Inpatient and outpatient hospital services; prenatal care; vaccines for children; physician, dental, and nurse midwifery services; skilled nursing facility services for persons 21 years of age or older; family services; rural health clinic services; diagnosis; treatment of children under 21 years of age; and nutrition services
Eligibility	Part A: if the recipient or spouse worked for at least 10 years in Medicare-covered employment and is a citizen or permanent resident of the United States; or Part B: all Part A enrollees who elect to pay the monthly Part B premium of $78.20 per month	Low-income persons, infants, and pregnant women with family incomes below 133 percent of the poverty level; those 65 years or older; disabled individuals; and the blind

From: Stanhope M, Lancaster J. *Community and Public Health Nursing.* 5th ed. New York: Mosby; 2000. Reprinted with permission.

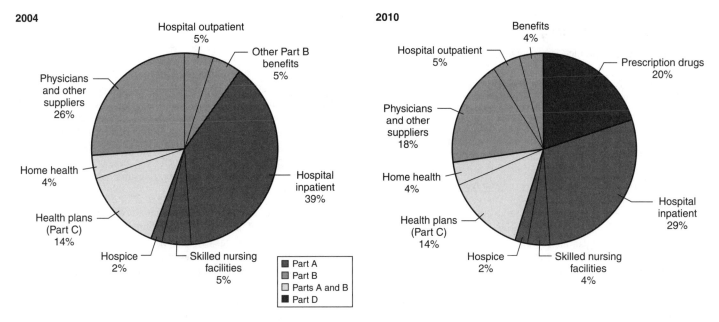

FIGURE 5-2 Medicare Benefit Payments, by Type of Service, FY 2004 (Actual) and FY 2010 (Projected)

Note: Figure does not include administrative expenses. Amount for FY 2004 excludes Part D low-income subsidy payments.

Source: The Henry J. Kaiser Family Foundation. *Section 6 Medicare Spending. Medicare Chartbook*, 3rd ed. (#7284): Congressional Budget Office, Medicare Fact Sheet, March 2005. Available at: http://www.kff.org/medicare/duals.cfm. Accessed February 27, 2008. Reprinted with permission.

Successful Community Strategies

Integrating WIC with Medicaid and Reducing Infant Mortality in Illinois[46]

In 2002, the Illinois infant mortality rate was 7.4 deaths for every 1,000 live births. The Illinois Department of Human Services designed a program to reduce the state's infant mortality rate by merging federal and state funds. It integrated the Special Supplemental Nutrition Program for Women, Infants, and Children (WIC) with two state-funded programs: Family Case Management (FCM) and Targeted Intensive Prenatal Case Management (TIPCM). The WIC (federal funds) and the state funds were used to leverage federal matching funds through the Medicaid program. These programs serve more than 40 percent of all infants born in Illinois every year and about 90 percent of Medicaid-eligible infants. The department supplements these statewide programs with targeted initiatives for women who have a higher chance of giving birth prematurely. Integration of these programs allowed them to operate more

efficiently. For example, staff members of many local health departments were trained to provide both WIC and FCM services. The success of the coordinated program can be summarized as follows:

- The proportion of WIC-eligible children with health insurance increased to 89.9 percent.
- The proportion of fully immunized 1-year-olds in WIC increased to 86.8 percent.
- The proportion of fully immunized 2-year-olds in WIC increased to 76.4 percent.
- The proportion of infants in WIC who were breastfed increased to 61.4 percent.
- The proportion of infants in WIC who continue to breastfeed through 6 months of age increased to 30.5 percent.
- The proportion of children in FCM who received at least three well childcare visits

during the first year of life increased to 57.9 percent.
- For 6 years in a row, infants born to Medicaid-eligible pregnant women who participated in WIC or FCM were in better health than those born to Medicaid-eligible women who did not participate in either program:
  - The rate of premature birth was 60 to 70 percent lower.
  - The rate of infant mortality was 50 to 70 percent lower.
  - Medicaid expenditures for healthcare in the first year of life were 30 to 50 percent lower.
- Participation in WIC and FCM saved Illinois an average of $200 million each year in Medicaid expenses.

Chapter Summary

- Private health insurance is coverage by a health plan provided through an employer or union or purchased by an individual from a private health insurance company.
- Traditionally, a person can enroll in a healthcare delivery system by contracting directly with a healthcare provider for individual care based on fee-for-service, also known as direct-purchase plans.
- Medicare pays individual physicians an amount that does not exceed the 75th percentile of charges by all physicians in a community (termed the "prevailing" fee). The main concern about fee-for-service plans is that they encourage unnecessary care (lab tests, procedures, etc.).
- Managed care influences how much healthcare clients use.
- In some HMOs, physicians are salaried and they all have offices in an HMO building at one or more locations in the client's community as part of a prepaid group practice. This is known as a staff model.
- Although Medicare provides extensive benefits, there are gaps in coverage. Some of these gaps include Medicare deductibles, co-payments, long-term nursing care, custodial care, and certain other healthcare needs, such as dentures and dental care.
- Medicaid became law in 1965 as a cooperative venture jointly funded by the federal and state governments (including the District of Columbia and the Territories) to assist states in providing medical assistance to eligible low-income persons.
- Welfare reform repealed the open-ended federal entitlement program known as Aid to Families with Dependent Children (AFDC) and replaced it with Temporary Assistance for Needy Families (TANF), which provides states with grants to be spent on time-limited cash assistance.
- The federal government created the State Children's Health Insurance Program (SCHIP) to cover individuals whose families have incomes too high to qualify for state medical assistance but who cannot obtain private insurance.

Critical Thinking Activities

The United States does not have a nationwide system of health insurance that assures access to healthcare. Therefore, many people are without health insurance or are underinsured. Which level of prevention and segment of the population (e.g., children, older adults, pregnant and lactating women, etc.) should the government guarantee healthcare services for, and why?

- Discuss as a group the aspect of managed care that should be of the most concern to a consumer and why.
- Determine your own insurance coverage.
- Evaluate two research articles about nutrition services covered through Medicare and/or Medicaid.

Case Study 5-1

Justina, a community dietitian in Chicago, was asked to evaluate the nutritional status of and provide nutrition counseling to older persons in a community health center program where the majority of clients were experiencing nutrition-related health conditions such as hypertension and diabetes. Before carrying out the activities, she read a research article by Ackermann et al.[47] that explored whether lifestyle interventions could be offered in a way that allows a return on investment for private health insurers while remaining attractive for consumers, employers, and Medicare. The results of the research showed that providing a lifestyle intervention at age 50 years could prevent 37 percent of new cases of diabetes before age 65, at a cost of $1,288 per quality-adjusted life year (QALY; a way of measuring both the quality and the quantity of life lived) gained. The researchers concluded that cost-sharing strategies for offering lifestyle interventions for eligible people between ages 50 and 64 could provide financial return on investment for private payers and long-term benefits for Medicare.[47] Justina conducted the nutrition assessment, which showed that:

- 30 percent of the participants were underweight, had poor appetites, and had fluid intakes of less than one liter per day.
- 60 percent of the participants' fruit and vegetable intake was below the recommended amount.
- 80 percent of the participants consumed less than 1,000 kcal daily.
- 60 percent of the participants qualified for Medicare.
- 40 percent had managed care health insurance.

Justina provided diet instruction to help the clients improve their nutrients and fluid intake. She also suggested that they enhance their diet with dietary supplements and keep a record of food intake. On follow-up about 3 weeks later, dietary intake showed improvement (food records). At the 6-week follow-up, the clients had gained more than 10 pounds and were regularly consuming two to three servings of dietary supplements in addition to their regular meals. Their fruit and vegetable intake increased by two to three servings daily. Justina's services were paid for by Medicare and managed care because Justina was a Medicare medical nutrition therapy provider.

Activities

- Determine the eligibility criteria for Medicare and Medicaid.
- Evaluate the nutritional status of older persons participating in a congregate meal program.
- Determine the types of nutrition-related health conditions that can qualify for Medicare.
- Plan a nutrition education class for older persons on how to reduce the incidence of cancer, osteoporosis, and heart disease using current research information/articles.
- Teach older individuals who are not enrolled in the Medicare program about the eligibility criteria for Medicare and Medicaid.

References

1. Catlin A, Cowan C, Heffler S, et al. National health spending in 2005: the slowdown continues. *Health Aff*. 2006; 26(1):142–153.
2. Baicker K, Chandra A, Skinner J. Geographic Variation in Health Care and the Problem of Measuring Racial Disparities. *Perspect Bio Med*. 2005; 48(1):S42–S53.
3. The Henry J. Kaiser Family Foundation. *Employee Health Benefit 2006 Annual Survey*. Available at: http://www.kff.org/insurance/7527. Accessed April 27, 2008.
4. The National Coalition on Health Care. Health Insurance Cost. Available at: http://www.nchc.org/facts/cost.shtml. Accessed April 2007.
5. Heflin CM. Food insufficiency and women's mental health: findings from a 3-year panel of welfare recipients. *Soc Sci Med*. 2005; 61(9):1971–1982.

6. Ali NS, Zuberi RW. The relationship of socio-demographic factors with iron deficiency anemia in children of 1–2 years of age. *J Pakistan Med Assoc.* 2001; 51(3):130–132.

7. Massing MW, Rosamond WD, Wing SB. Income, income inequality, and cardiovascular disease mortality: relations among county populations of the United States, 1985 to 1994. *South Med J.* 2004; 97(5):475–484.

8. Cohen S, Signorello L, Gammon M, Blot W. Obesity and recent mammography use among black and white women in the Southern Community Cohort Study (United States). *Cancer Causes Control.* 2007; 8(7):765–773.

9. National Center for Health Statistics. Health Insurance Coverage. Available at: http://www.cdc.gov/nchs/datawh/nchsdefs/healthinsurancecov.htm. Accessed January 8, 2006.

10. U.S. Census Bureau. People with or without Health Insurance Coverage by Selected Characteristics: 2004 and 2005. Available at: http://www.census.gov/hhes/www/hlthins/hlthin03/hi03t5.pdf. Accessed March 7, 2007.

11. Kovner AR, Jonas S. *Healthcare Delivery in the United States.* 7th ed. New York: Springer; 2002.

12. Center on Budget and Policy Priorities, Poverty and hardship affect tens of millions of Americans. Available at: http://www.cbpp.org/12-20-07pov.pdf. Accessed February 23, 2008.

13. National Center for Health Statistics. Ambulatory Health Care Data. Available at: http://www.cdc.gov/nchs/about/major/ahcd/adata.htm#Physician. Accessed April 29, 2007.

14. National Center for Health Statistics. Ambulatory care visits to physician offices, hospital outpatient departments, and emergency departments: United States 2001–2002. *Vital Health Stat, 2006.* Available at: http://www.cdc.gov/nchs/about/major/ahcd/adata.htm#Physician. Accessed February 23, 2008.

15. Enthoven AC. Employment-based health insurance is failing: now what? *Policy J Health Sphere.* 2003; 3:237–249.

16. Kovener A, Jonas S. *Healthcare Delivery in the United States.* 8th ed. New York: Springer; 2005.

17. Schneider MJ. *Introduction to Public Health.* Sudbury, MA: Jones and Bartlett; 2006.

18. Hitchcock J, Schubert PE, Thomas SA. *Community Health Nursing.* 2nd ed. Clifton Park, New York: Thomson Delmar Learning; 2003.

19. Relman AS. Restructuring the U.S. Health Care System. Available at: http://www.issues.org/19.4/relman.html. Accessed March 7, 2007.

20. National Center for Health Statistics. Health Maintenance Organization (HMO). Available at: http://www.cdc.gov/nchs/datawh/nchsdefs/hmo.htm. Accessed February 23, 2008.

21. The Henry J. Kaiser Family Foundation. Trends and Indicators in the Changing Health Care Marketplace. Available at: http://kaiserfamilyfoundation.org/insurance/7031/ti2004-glossary-set.cfm. Accessed March 7, 2007.

22. The Henry J. Kaiser Family Foundation. Medicare at a Glance—Fact Sheet. Available at: http://www.kff.org/medicare/1066.cfm. Accessed April 27, 2008.

23. Centers for Medicare and Medicaid. Overview. Available at: http://www.cms.hhs.gov/MedicaidGenInfo/01_Overview.asp. Accessed March 9, 2007.

24. Social Security Online. Entitlement to Hospital Insurance Benefits. Sec. 226. [42 U.S.C. 426]. Available at: http://www.ssa.gov/OP_Home/ssact/title02/0226.htm. Accessed March 9, 2007.

25. Megellas M. Medicare modernization: The new prescription drug benefit and redesigned Part B and Part C. *Bayl Univ Med Cent Proc.* 2006; 19(1):21–23.

26. Cox ER, Jernigan C, Coons SJ, Draugalis JL. Medicare beneficiaries' management of capped prescription benefits. *Med Care.* 2001; 39(3):296–301.

27. Centers for Medicare and Medicaid Services. Brief Summaries of Medicare & Medicaid. Available at: http://www.cms.hhs.gov/MedicareProgramRatesStats/02_SummaryMedicareMedicaid.asp. Accessed April 29, 2007.

28. Centers for Medicare and Medicaid Services. Research, Statistics, Data, & Systems. Available at: http://www.cms.hhs.gov/home/rsds.asp. Accessed April 29, 2007.

29. Michael P. Impact and components of the Medicare MNT benefits. *J Am Diet Assoc.* 2001; 101:1140–1141.

30. Hager MH. Medicare reform opens door for preventive nutrition services. *J Am Diet Assoc.* 2004; 104(6):887–889.

31. Philip S. Nutrition support teams: an evidence-based practice. *Nutri Clin Pract.* 2006; 21(1):62–67.

32. Ochs M. New Medicare changes to expand MNT access in 2002. *J Am Diet Assoc.* 2002; 102:30.

33. Boyle M. *Community Nutrition in Action: An Entrepreneurial Approach.* Belmont, CA: Thomson Wadsworth; 2003.

34. Sheils JF, Rubin R, Stapleton DC. The estimated costs and savings of medical nutrition therapy: the Medicare population. *J Am Diet Assoc.* 1999; 99(4):428–435.

35. Harvard Health Publications. Simple changes in diet can protect you against friendly fire. What you eat can fuel or cool inflammation, a key driver of heart disease, diabetes, and other chronic conditions. *Harvard Heart Lett.* 2007; 17(5):3.

36. Daubenmier JJ, Weidner G, Sumner MD, et al. The contribution of changes in diet, exercise, and stress management to changes in coronary risk in women and men in the multisite cardiac lifestyle intervention program. *Ann Behav Med.* 2007; 33(1):57–68.

37. Rice T, Desmond KA, Fox PD. Does open enrollment control premiums? A case study from the Medigap market. *Inquiry.* 2004; 41(3):291–300.

38. Kilian J, Stubbings J. Medicare part D: selected issues for pharmacists and beneficiaries in 2007. *J Managed Care Pharm.* 2007; 13(1):59–65.

39. Centers for Medicare and Medicaid Services. Medicare and Medicaid. Available at: http://www.chcf.org/documents/insurance/HealthCareCosts07.pdf. Accessed April 27, 2008.

40. Berkowitz E. Medicare and Medicaid: the past as prologue. *Health Care Fin Rev.* 2005; 27(2):11–23.

41. Ozawa MM, Yoon HS. "Leavers" from TANF and AFDC: how do they fare economically? *Soc Work.* 2005; 50(3):239–249.

42. Gavin N, Adams K, Manning W, Raskind-Hood C, Urato M. The impact of welfare reform on insurance coverage before pregnancy and the timing of prenatal care initiation. *Health Serv Res.* 2007; 42(4):1564–1588.

43. American Academy of Pediatrics. 2006 Pediatric Medical Cost Model. Available at: http://www.aap.org/research/pedmedcostmodel.cfm. Accessed March 9, 2007.

44. Dubay L, Guyer J, Mann C, Odeh M. Medicaid at the ten-year anniversary of SCHIP: looking back and moving forward. *Health Aff.* 2007; 26(2):370–381.

45. Centers for Medicare and Medicaid Services. HHS. Medicare and Medicaid programs of all-inclusive care for the elderly (PACE) program revisions. Final rule. *Fed Reg.* 2006; 71(236):71243–71337.

46. Illinois Department of Human Services. The Reduction of Infant Mortality in Illinois. Available at: http://www.dhs.state.il.us/page.aspx?item=33703. Accessed February 23, 2008.

47. Ackermann RT, Marrero DG, Hicks KA, et al. An evaluation of cost sharing to finance a diet and physical activity intervention to prevent diabetes. *Diabetes Care.* 2006; 29(6):1237–1241.

CHAPTER

6

Public Policy and Nutrition

LEARNING OBJECTIVES

- Describe how dietitians can become involved in setting policy at the local level.
- Identify tools the government can use to influence policy.
- Describe the United States' legislative process.
- Define the policymaking process.
- List the strategies that can be used to develop policy.
- Describe the major federal agencies that administer nutrition programs.

Introduction

The U.S. government has created policies whose goal is to improve the general health of the public through dietary means. These policies include increasing the purchasing power of the poor, distributing surplus commodities to low-income families, and providing meals to school children and the elderly.[1] Four components form the foundation of U.S. nutrition *policy*: nutrition assistance, nutrition education, nutrition information (labeling), and nutrition research. Each of these four components is vital to promoting health, protecting against disease, and combating the obesity epidemic. Dietetic professionals can influence the food, nutrition, and health policy agenda by supporting individuals' appropriate food choices, delivering high quality nutrition programs and services, and becoming involved with the regulatory process.[2] One example of successful policy change at the local level is the Child and Adolescent Trial for Cardiovascular Health (CATCH) study, presented in this chapter's Successful Community Strategies feature.

This chapter discusses the U.S. legislative process, policymaking processes and strategies, and the link among nutrition monitoring, nutrition research, and nutrition policy.

Legislation and Public Policy

The government can use different tools to influence policies and the lives of citizens. Some of the tools include taxes, tax incentives, price supports for commodities, financial support, and services such as education.[4] Laws are tools that the government uses to form policies. In the United States, Congress is the main legislative body that sets policy and supplies the basic legislation that governs the people. Dietitians or public health professionals can influence the policies that affect people by providing testimony regarding the consequences of food insecurity, lack of nutrition education or nutrition services, or unavailable medical nutrition therapy to legislators who may not have the medical background or in-depth knowledge of people's needs at the local level. Also, dietitians can participate in the legislative process by asking members of Congress to sponsor a bill. For these reasons, all healthcare providers need in-depth knowledge and understanding of how a bill becomes a law.[5]

How a Bill Becomes a Law

The three branches of the federal government are: executive, judicial, and legislative. The executive branch consists of the president and presidential cabinet. The judicial branch, or court system, interprets the laws and settles legal disagreements. Congress is the legislative branch, and its major function is making laws. The U.S. Congress consists of the House of Representatives and the Senate.[6] The legislative branch enacts laws that initiate, modify, authorize, and appropriate funds for all programs and services that the federal government administers.[7] In Congress, most action happens in committees or subcommittees.[6,8] Several committees, such as the Committee on Agriculture, Nutrition, and Forestry and the Committee on Appropriations, consider food, nutrition, and health issues.[8] The legislative process is the same for both federal and state legislation because each level has a Senate and a House of Representatives.[9]

Standing committees are permanently established to create and approve legislation to authorize programs and to supervise program implementation.[8] The majority of standing committees also recommend authorized levels of funds for government operations and for new and existing programs within their jurisdiction. The federal Senate and House of Representatives have a number of standing committees with jurisdiction over food, nutrition, and health-related programs:[7]

policy A framework for making decisions that guide actions to help the public.

standing committees Permanently established committees that create and approve legislation, authorize programs, and oversee program implementation.

Senate:

- *Committee on Agriculture, Nutrition, and Forestry:* Child nutrition and other food programs
- *Committee on Appropriations:* Program funding
- *Committee on Finance:* Medicare and Medicaid programs
- *Committee on Foreign Relations:* International hunger
- *Committee on Labor and Human Resources:* Department of Health and Human Services programs—elderly nutrition, maternal and child health, and food labeling

Successful Community Strategies

Child and Adolescent Trial for Cardiovascular Health (CATCH)[3]

Dietetics professionals who become involved in setting policy at the local level can make a significant impact on the health of individuals in the community, as demonstrated by the CATCH intervention study. The purpose of this study was to assess the outcomes of health behavior interventions, focusing on the elementary school environment, classroom curricula, and home programs for the prevention of cardiovascular disease.

Twenty-eight ethnically diverse third- through fifth-grade students in public schools located in California, Louisiana, Minnesota, and Texas participated in the intervention. At the school level, two primary end points were changes in the fat content of food service lunch offerings and the amount of moderate-to-vigorous physical activity

in the physical education programs. At the level of the individual student, serum cholesterol change was the primary end point and was used for power calculations in the study. Twenty-eight additional schools received the dietary and physical activity intervention as well as family education.

Results showed that in the intervention school lunches, the percentage of energy intake from fat was significantly lower (from 38.7 percent to 31.9 percent) than in control lunches (from 38.9 percent to 36.2 percent). The intensity of physical activity in physical education classes increased significantly during the CATCH intervention in the intervention schools compared with the control schools. Self-reported daily energy intake from fat among students in the intervention schools decreased significantly (from 32.7 percent to 30.3 percent)

compared with students in the control schools (from 32.6 percent to 32.2 percent). Intervention students reported more daily vigorous activity than control students (58.6 minutes vs. 46.5 minutes). Blood pressure, body size, and cholesterol measures, however, did not change significantly between treatment groups.

The findings of the study imply that the CATCH intervention was able to modify the fat content of school lunches, increase moderate-to-vigorous physical activity in physical education, and improve eating and physical activity behaviors in children. These changes were attributed to the policy modification in the food selections offered in the school cafeteria and the content of the physical education classes.

House of Representatives:

- *Committee on Agriculture:* Food programs
- *Committee on Appropriations:* Program funding
- *Committee on Education and Labor:* Child and elderly nutrition programs
- *Committee on Energy and Commerce:* Food labeling
- *Committee on Ways and Means:* Medicare and Medicaid

A bill is a type of proposal used to introduce legislation. Before a bill is signed into law, both houses of Congress must approve it. However, it is very rare for both sides to pass an identical bill.[8] When the two chambers pass a bill that is similar but not identical, the differences between the versions of the bill passed by the House and the Senate are reconciled by a conference committee appointed from members of the relevant House and Senate committees. So, these joint committees have representation from both the House and the Senate.[7] Once the conferees agree on identical language, the bill is sent back to both the House and Senate for approval.[10]

After the bill has passed through the appropriate committees, it goes to the president or state governor for a signature. If the president or governor signs the bill, it becomes law and serves as the basis for financing federal or state agency operations.[7] (See **Box 6-1** for an example of a bill sponsored by the American Dietetic Association [ADA] that was approved and signed into law.) However, if the president or governor disapproves of the bill, he or she can veto it. When that happens, the only way for the bill to become law is for both the House and the Senate to vote by a two-thirds majority to override the veto.[9] Also, if the president refuses to sign the bill within 10 days after Congress has adjourned at the end of its 2-year life span, the bill dies; this is called a "pocket veto." **Figure 6-1** outlines the process a bill undergoes before passage into law.

$\mathcal{B}$ox 6-1 Highlights of the American Dietetic Association's Success with the Legislative Process[4,11–24]

An issue often requires many years before it reaches a critical mass in public support to enable a policy change. The American Dietetic Association (ADA) campaigned and obtained support for **medical nutrition therapy (MNT)**. MNT is the use of specific nutrition services to treat an illness, injury, or condition, and it involves two phases: 1) detailed assessment of a person's medical, psychosocial, and dietary histories and a physical examination and 2) treatment, which includes nutrition therapy, counseling, and the use of specialized nutrition supplements.

Since the 1980s, ADA's government affairs program and other health-related associations have worked diligently to justify and advocate for MNT. ADA's main legislative goal has been to obtain Medicare reimbursement for MNT services provided by registered dietitians. In 1992, ADA began its MNT campaign by publishing a position paper proposing development of healthcare policy that guarantees affordable and accessible healthcare services for all Americans. In addition, ADA proposed that nutrition assessment, therapeutic nutrition services, and intervention be included as an essential part of any healthcare reform legislation.

ADA structured a grassroots lobbying network and campaigned among ADA members to accomplish its goal. These efforts helped to increase the visibility of the dietetics profession on Capitol Hill and to lobby Congress to support MNT. It formed coalitions with other health-related organizations to develop a uniform position on healthcare reform. The president of ADA testified at a hearing by the Health Subcommittee of the House Ways and Means Committee on Medicare and budget reconciliation issues on behalf of the Association. In addition, ADA members wrote letters to legislators and met with Washington lobbyists and important members of Congress. ADA also used advertisements to educate consumers and policy makers about the benefits of nutrition services and potential impact of MNT.

Finally, the Medical Nutrition Therapy Act (H.R. 2247 and S. 1964) was introduced during the 104th Congress with the House version having 91 co-sponsors and the Senate version having 4 co-sponsors. Unfortunately, both bills expired when Congress adjourned. However, ADA was not discouraged because the bill received significant support that encouraged ADA to continue its efforts. ADA renewed its effort by introducing the Medicare Medical Nutrition Therapy Act of 1997 (H.R. 1375 and S. 597) in the 105th Congress on April 17, 1997. This started a new endeavor to obtain a majority of congressional members as co-sponsors of the legislation by March 1998. The efforts for the passage of legislation to include MNT as part of the healthcare reform continued during the following 2 years with the help of the Honorable John E. Ensign, who introduced the bill in the House saying, "[it] will help to save Medicare and, most importantly, to save lives."

After 8 years of effort, on December 15, 2000 Congress finally passed a Medicare Part B MNT provision as part of the Benefits Improvement and Protection Act (P.L.106 to 554 [H.R. 566]). On December 21, 2000, President Clinton signed legislation (Public Law 106-554) that included the provision for creating a new Medicare MNT benefit that was limited to patients with diabetes or kidney disease (predialysis). ADA President Jane White acknowledged the importance of the MNT victory, stating, "As we consider the significance of this victory, we can say without reservation that our work to bring recognition to dietetic professionals working in all settings is producing results. The ability of dietetic professionals to serve in the food and healthcare systems is growing in meaningful ways."

The implementation process for MNT benefits started as soon as President Clinton signed the legislation. The final rules that direct the application of the MNT benefits were developed by the Centers for Medicare and Medicaid Services (CMS) of the U.S. Department of Health and Human Services (DHHS) and were published in the *Federal Register* in November 2001. This process determined the payment levels, provider qualifications, and other coverage details. On January 1, 2002, registered dietitians started to register as Medicare providers and provide services to program beneficiaries.

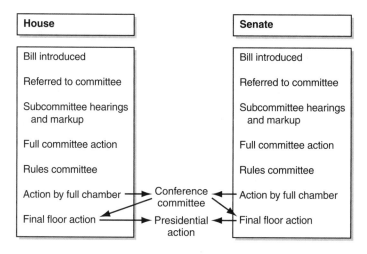

FIGURE 6-1 How a Bill Becomes a Law: Typical Path to Passage of Legislation
Source: Lyons W, Scheb II JM, Richardson LE. *American Government Politics and Political Culture*, p. 360, Figure 12-2. Copyright 1995 by West Publishing Company. Reprinted with permission.

Implementing and Enforcing Nutrition Policy in the United States

As soon as legislation is passed and signed into law, implementation and enforcement of the law become the responsibility of the agency in the executive branch to which it is assigned. The president heads the executive branch.[8] Most of the laws enacted that affect nutrition, food, and health are passed to the U.S. Department of Agriculture (USDA) or the Department of Health and Human Services (DHHS) for implementation in public health services. Therefore, after the law is passed, administrative bodies, such as the USDA interpret the law and provide the detailed regulations or rules that set the policy into effect.[25] Sometimes the regulations are called *secondary legislation*. The total volume of this activity is huge, confirmed by the size of the *Federal Register*. The *Federal Register* contains all regulations and proposed regulations and is published weekly. The **Code of Federal Regulations (CFR)** is a comprehensive summary of all regulations currently in operation. For example, when the Special Supplemental Nutrition Program for Women, Infants, and Children (WIC) program started, the details of the regulations were published in the *Federal Register* on July 11, 1973, about 9 months after Congress passed the law.[4] New laws and amendments to the existing law were enacted over time to increase the amount of money budgeted for the WIC program; the laws and amendments specify how the program should be implemented and approve the continuation of the program for additional budget years.[26,27]

Box 6-2 shows an example of the *Federal Register* notice describing the USDA's Food and Nutrition Service announcement of annual adjustments to the Income Eligibility Guidelines to be used in determining eligibility for free and reduced-price meals or free milk for the period from July 1, 2005 through June 30, 2006.

U.S. Food and Drug Administration

The U.S. Food and Drug Administration (FDA) is a scientific, regulatory, and public health agency that oversees items accounting for 25 cents of every dollar spent by consumers. At some levels, the FDA may be the most well known of the agencies to the general public. The FDA's policies and work affect the lives of almost every American every day because this agency is mainly responsible for determining that the food supply is safe and wholesome. Its jurisdiction encompasses items such as:[28]

- Human and animal drugs
- Therapeutic agents of biological origin
- Medical devices and radiation-emitting products for consumer, medical, and occupational use
- Cosmetics
- Animal feed

The FDA's jurisdiction also covers food products, including:[28]

- Labeling
- Safety of all food products (except meat and poultry)
- Bottled water

The agency has grown from a single chemist in the U.S. Department of Agriculture in 1862 to a staff of about 9,100 employees including chemists, pharmacologists, physicians, microbiologists, nutritionists, veterinarians, pharmacists, lawyers, and many others. The agency scientists evaluate applications for new human drugs and biologics, complex medical devices, food and color additives, infant formulas, and animal drugs. Also, the FDA monitors the manufacture, import, transport, storage, and sale of about $1 trillion worth of products yearly, which costs taxpayers about $3 per person. Investigators and inspectors visit more than 16,000 facilities a year and arrange with state governments to help increase the number of facilities checked. Although the U.S. food supply is among the safest in the world, foodborne illness has been estimated to cause about 76 million illnesses, 325,000 hospitalizations, and 5,000 deaths a year.[29,30] The FDA is also responsible for the safety of 80 percent of all food consumed in the United States—the entire food supply except for meat, poultry, and some egg products, which are regulated by the USDA.

The FDA plays a significant role in protecting the nation's food against bioterrorism. Under the Bioterrorism Preparedness and Response Act of 2002, the FDA developed regulations that require all of the more than 400,000 domestic and foreign food facilities to register with the FDA. This allows the FDA to address quickly high-risk situations. Also, the new rules require importers to tell the FDA in advance about food shipments; this improves the FDA's ability to detect suspected food and require food companies to keep better records so any contamination can be traced back to its source.[31] The law not only strengthens the FDA's authority to detain suspect food, but also allows for more grants to the states to help inspect food facilities.[28]

Additionally, the Total Diet Study (TDS) is the FDA's ongoing market basket survey in which about 280 core foods (TDS foods) in the U.S. food

---

medical nutrition therapy A service provided by a registered dietitian or nutrition professional that includes counseling, nutrition support, and nutrition assessment and screening to improve people's health and quality of life.

Federal Register A weekly publication that contains all regulations, proposed regulations, and the Code of Federal Regulations (CFR).

secondary legislation The action of administrative bodies such as the USDA interpreting the law and providing the detailed regulations or rules that set a policy into effect after a law is passed.

Code of Federal Regulations (CFR) A comprehensive summary of all regulations currently in force.

$\mathcal{B}$ox 6-2 **A Portion of a Proposed Rule Published by the Department of Agriculture's Food and Nutrition Service**[33]

Federal Register: March 18, 2005 (Volume 70, Number 52)

Notices

Pages 13160–13163

From the *Federal Register Online* via GPO Access (wais.access.gpo.gov)

(DOCID: fr18mr05-35)

Department of Agriculture

Food and Nutrition Service

Child Nutrition Programs—Income Eligibility Guidelines

Agency: Food and Nutrition Service, USDA.

Action: Notice.

Summary: This Notice announces the Department's annual adjustments to the Income Eligibility Guidelines to be used in determining eligibility for free and reduced-price meals or free milk for the period from July 1, 2005 through June 30, 2006. These guidelines are used by schools, institutions, and facilities participating in the National School Lunch Program (and Commodity School Program), School Breakfast Program, Special Milk Program for Children, Child and Adult Care Food Program, and Summer Food Service Program. The annual adjustments are required by section 9 of the Richard B. Russell National School Lunch Act. The guidelines are intended to direct benefits to those children most in need and are revised annually to account for changes in the Consumer Price Index.

supply are collected and analyzed to determine levels of various contaminants and nutrients in those foods. Four market baskets are usually collected each year, one in each of four geographic regions of the United States (i.e., West, North Central, South, and Northeast). For each market basket, samples of each TDS food are collected from grocery stores and fast food restaurants in three cities within the region, prepared for consumption, and analyzed to measure the levels of selected contaminants and nutrients. The list of TDS foods is updated from time to time to reflect changing eating patterns in the United States. The target population is all age groups: infants, young children, male and female teenagers, male and female adults, and male and female older persons.[32] For more information on TDS visit the USDA website.

The authority and funding for many public health nutrition programs originate in Washington, DC, but agency administrators and local and state government officials can authorize additional funds and programs to address observed community needs. Many policies originate at the program level as the nutritionist and agency administrators develop their strategies, operational plans, and protocols for delivering

nutrition services and write grant proposals for innovative new programs. The two departments that are important for nutrition purposes at the federal level are the DHHS and the USDA.

Department of Health and Human Services

The Department of Health and Human Services (DHHS) administers the majority of public health and nutrition programs. It is the second largest federal agency in regard to dollar amount received from the federal budget for its programs. Its organizational chart is shown in **Figure 6-2**. The DHHS is the U.S. government's principal agency for protecting the health of all Americans and providing essential human services, especially helping vulnerable populations (low-income families and individuals) help themselves. Its mission is to protect and advance the health of the American people. The department includes more than 300 programs covering a wide variety of activities, including the following:[34]

- Health and social science research
- Disease prevention, including immunization services
- Food and drug safety
- Medicare (health insurance for elderly and disabled Americans) and Medicaid (health insurance for low-income people)
- Health information technology
- Financial assistance and services for low-income families
- Improvement in maternal and infant health
- Head Start (preschool education and services)
- Faith-based and community initiatives
- Child abuse and domestic violence prevention
- Substance abuse treatment and prevention
- Services for older Americans, including home-delivered meals
- Comprehensive health services for Native Americans
- Medical preparedness for emergencies, including potential terrorism

The DHHS's Medicare program is the nation's largest health insurer, handling more than 1 billion claims per year. Medicare and Medicaid together provide healthcare insurance for one in four Americans. The Social Security Act established both Medicare and Medicaid in 1965. The Social Security Administration (SSA) was responsible for Medicare while the Social and Rehabilitation Service (SRS) administered federal assistance to the state Medicaid programs. SSA and SRS were agencies in the Department of Health, Education, and Welfare (HEW). To effectively coordinate Medicare and Medicaid, the Health Care Financing Administration (HCFA) was created under HEW in 1977. In 1980, HEW was divided into the Department of Education and the Department of Health and Human Services. In 2001, HCFA was renamed the Centers for Medicare and Medicaid Services (CMS).

The difference between Medicare and Medicaid is that Medicare is a federal health insurance program that provides funds for medical costs to people who are 65 years of age or older, some people under 65 with disabilities, and people with permanent kidney failure. Medicaid is health insurance for low-income families funded jointly by the federal and state governments (including the District of Columbia and the Territories) to provide partial or full payment of medical costs for categories of individuals and families of any age who are too poor to pay for the care.[35] See Chapter 5 for detailed information on Medicare and Medicaid.

The DHHS works closely with state and local governments, and many DHHS-funded services are provided at the local level by state or county agencies or through private sector grantees. Eleven operating

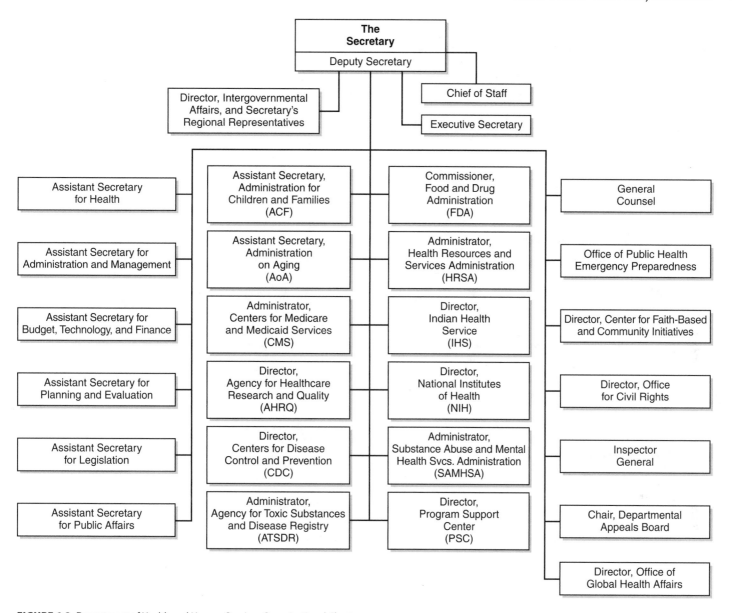

FIGURE 6-2 Department of Health and Human Services Organizational Chart

Adapted from: Department of Health and Human Services website. Available at: http://www.dhhs.gov/about/index.html. Accessed February 27, 2008.

divisions, including eight agencies in the U.S. Public Health Service and three human services agencies, administer the department's programs. The fiscal year 2005 budget for DHHS was $581 billion, and it employed 67,444 people. Some of these agencies and their services are presented in **Table 6.1**. This table does not represent an exhaustive list of nutrition education activities conducted by the federal government.

U.S. Department of Agriculture

The USDA is another federal agency involved in healthcare, predominantly through administering the Food and Nutrition Service (FNS) programs. Its organizational chart is presented in **Figure 6-3**. "The mission of the USDA is to provide leadership on food, agriculture, natural resources, and related issues based on good public policy, the best available science, and efficient management."[34] The FNS oversees a

variety of food assistance activities. It collaborates with state and local government welfare agencies to provide food stamps to low-income persons and to increase their food purchasing power. Other programs include School Breakfast and Lunch Programs, WIC, and grants to states for nutrition education training. In addition, the USDA also provides the following services:[36]

- Directs the federal anti-hunger effort with the Food Stamp, School Lunch, School Breakfast, and WIC Programs
- Responsible for the nation's 192 million acres of national forests and rangelands
- Plays a significant role as the conservation agency, encouraging voluntary efforts to protect soil, water, and wildlife on the 70 percent of America's lands that are in private hands

TABLE 6.1	**Federal Agencies Involved in Public Health Service**[8,37–40]

U.S. Department of Health and Human Services		
Acronym	**Definition**	**Services**
ODPHP	Office of Disease Prevention and Health Promotion	• Coordinates federal health promotion and disease prevention activities. It publishes *Healthy People, Promoting Health/Preventing Disease: Objectives for the Nation*, and the *Surgeon General's Report on Nutrition and Health* • Coordinates the development and implementation of the National Health Objectives for the Years 2000 and 2010
FDA	Food and Drug Administration	• Regulates food, drugs, cosmetics, and other products • Prescribes nutrition labeling on food product packages
NIH	National Institutes of Health	• Manages nutrition research and education programs
• NHLBI	National Heart, Lung, and Blood Institute	• Administers the National Cholesterol Education Program (NCEP) and the National High Blood Pressure Education Program (NHBPEP)
• NCEP	National Cholesterol Education Program	• Provides services and publications to educate the public about diseases of the heart
• NCI	National Cancer Institute	• Takes leadership in research on innovative interventions, nutrition education, and cancer prevention
• NIA	National Institute on Aging	• Leads national programs on research on the biomedical, social, and behavioral aspects of the aging process; the prevention of age-related diseases and disabilities; and the promotion of a better quality of life for all older Americans
• NCCAM	National Center for Complementary and Alternative Medicine	• Explores complementary and alternative medical practices in the context of rigorous science, which involves training NCCAM researchers and disseminating authoritative information
CDC	Centers for Disease Control and Prevention	• Administers nutrition monitoring and other nutrition surveillance activities
NCHS	National Center for Health Statistics	• Administers the periodic National Health and Nutrition Examination Surveys (NHANES) and publishes and disseminates the data
CCDPHP	Center for Chronic Disease Prevention and Health Promotion	• Administers the preventive health services block grant, which covers screening and referral for many chronic diseases, manages pediatric and pregnancy surveillance programs, and administers the Behavioral Risk Factor Survey (BRFS), which includes some nutrition questions
OHDS	Office of Human Development Services—includes the Administration on Aging (AoA)	• Administers meal programs for the elderly under Title III of the Older Americans Act (OAA)
ACF	Administration for Children and Families	• Administers the Head Start Program, which provides health, food, and nutrition education for children and their parents
CMS	Centers for Medicare and Medicaid Services	• Medicare—provides insurance coverage for health services for older Americans; regulations cover nutrition and dietetic services in hospitals, nursing homes, home health agencies, hospices, and other facilities that meet the Medicare conditions of participation • Medicaid—administered through state agencies and funds health services for economically low-income individuals and the disabled; regulates the Early Periodic Screening, Diagnosis, and Treatment (EPSDT) program for children through partnership with states
HRSA	Health Resources and Services Administration	• Administers the maternal and child health block grant through the Division of Maternal and Child Health Resources Development • Fosters public health nutrition programs at the state and local levels by providing expert consultation through its central and regional offices, training materials, and funding for continuing education and graduate training of public health nutritionists • Administers grants for research and for innovative projects including Special Projects of Regional and National Significance and funds for community health centers, migrant health, rural health, AIDS education, and allied health professions training

TABLE 6.1	(Continued)	

	U.S. Department of Agriculture	
Acronym	Definition	Services
USDA	U.S. Department of Agriculture	• Responsible for food and agriculture programs
• HNIS	Human Nutrition Information Services	• Administers the nutrition-monitoring activities of the USDA, including the Nationwide Food Consumption Survey (NFCS), the Continuing Survey of Food Intakes by Individuals (CSFII), and the Nutrient Data Bank CSFII, which has now merged with NHANES
		• Produces a variety of educational materials related to the U.S. Dietary Guidelines for Americans
• FNS	Food and Nutrition Service	• Administers the National School Lunch Program, National School Breakfast Program, Summer Feeding Program, Child Care Food Program, WIC, Commodity Supplemental Food Program, and Nutrition Education and Training Program (NETP)
• FSIS	Food Safety and Inspection Service	• Regulates the safety of meat and poultry products and some aspects of food labeling related to those products

	Other Federal Departments	
FTC	Federal Trade Commission	• Regulates the content of food advertisements and truth-in-labeling laws
DE	Department of Education	• Responsible for working with states in relation to public education
		• Responsible for educational programs for handicapped children; Public Law 99-457, the Education of the Handicapped Amendments of 1986, integrated health services into early intervention programs for infants and children with special needs
		• Nutrition services are listed as one of the health services, with nutritionists designated as part of the early intervention team
DT	Department of the Treasury	• Regulation of the sale and labeling of alcoholic beverages by the Bureau of Alcohol, Tobacco, and Firearms

- Provides housing, modern telecommunications, and safe drinking water to rural America
- Responsible for the safety of meat, poultry, and egg products
- Conducts research in human nutrition and new crop technologies that allows the production of food and fiber using less water and pesticides
- Ensures open markets for U.S. agricultural products
- Provides food aid to people in need overseas

The Policymaking Process

It is important for public health/community nutritionists to know the definition of policy before they can effectively initiate or change policies. "Policy is a framework that directs the actions to be followed by an individual, an organization, a government, or communities to meet the needs of society and individuals."[8,41] Public policies exercise a significant impact on societal behavior; they materialize when science, economics, social, and political circumstances induce government response and direction to meet a need or solve a problem.[8,41] Public policies are interpreted and implemented by public and private entities.[42] There are different types of public policies, including the following, that can impact food, nutrition, and health:

- *Agricultural policy* influences the quantity and quality of the food supply and the costs of foods in the grocery store.[43-45]

- *Health policy* is enacted to achieve a preferred health outcome, either for an individual, a family, a group, a community, or society as a whole.[46] One example of health policy is ensuring adequate healthcare (immunization, flu shots, prenatal care, etc.) for low-income families.
- *Environmental policy* influences consumer food intake patterns. For example, the public may perceive potential carcinogenic pollutants in foods, water, and the like as a major health problem; therefore, an effective public policy may be developed to reduce the risk of public exposure to these pollutants.
- *Science policy* influences funding priorities for research and for development of new food products. For example, a nutritionist may receive funding to conduct research activities that can reduce the incidence of colon cancer or develop a low-calorie food item.
- *Socioeconomic policy* influences food assistance programs for low-income individuals, creates eligibility criteria, and affects food costs.
- *Educational policy* influences nutrition education programs and the capability of consumers, both youth and adults, to make educated food choices.[43]

Policies that are meticulously devised can guarantee consistent actions and prevent impulsive decisions. Mission statements, position

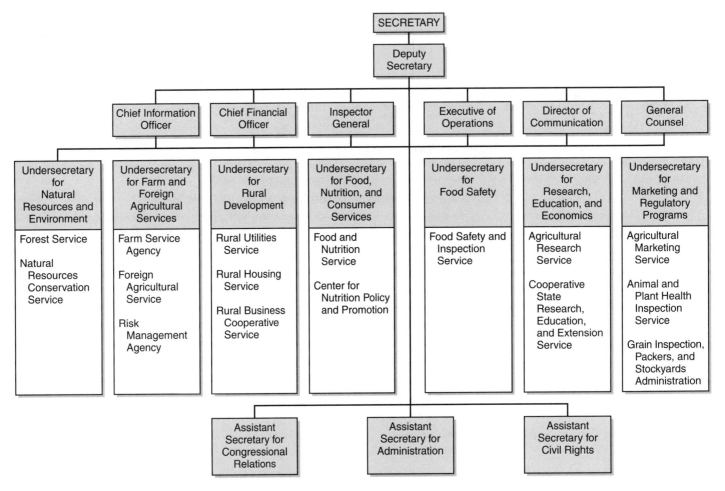

FIGURE 6-3 Department of Agriculture Organizational Chart
Adapted from: U.S. Department of Agriculture website. Available at: http://www.usda.gov. Accessed March 6, 2008.

papers, procedure manuals, protocols, office rules, and written memoranda from administrators or program managers communicate policies within an organization.[8,44]

Policymaking Strategies

It is important for community/public health nutritionists to select the most effective strategies for a successful policy. The following outline some strategies for securing approval of a policy.[8,44]

Strategy 1: Prepare a Scientific/Evidence Base

Start by studying the issue, the target audience, and the environment thoroughly; be prepared to answer questions regarding the issues. Identify the need for the policy or legislation. Review related literature on the issue using credible professional journals such as the *Journal of the American Dietetic Association*.

Strategy 2: Develop Broad Support

Form an alliance with various groups such as researchers, healthcare professionals, educators, farmers, consumers, religious groups, men's and women's groups, and individuals who can assist and support the issue.

It is important to be proactive, and network with nutrition experts, influential citizens in the community, friends of decision-makers, and respected community groups with policy power, including the League of Women Voters, Chambers of Commerce, parent teacher associations, and local affiliates of voluntary health agencies, such as the American Heart Association and the American Diabetes Association.

Strategy 3: Analyze the Opposition

Policymakers need to hear strong factual arguments that refute the opponent's position. A constructive response to the opposition's arguments may contribute to the success of the policy. For example, at the local level, the discussion of whether to fluoridate drinking water in Lincoln, Nebraska, to prevent dental decay in children triggered some opposition by older adults who did not see the benefit to them. But the counterargument was that fluoridation of the water also may prevent osteoporosis in older adults.

Strategy 4: Develop Alternative Approaches or Compromise Positions

Listen to and analyze the opposition's viewpoint and provide an alternative solution. For example, the desire to increase nutrition service to the Hispanic community may trigger some opposition from other community members due to the increase in costs. An alternative approach or compromise might be to find volunteers from the Hispanic community who can serve as interpreters or provide other activities that can help reduce the cost of providing services to their community. Another alternative approach might be providing tax advantages to private healthcare providers such as physicians so they can significantly reduce their fees to low-income Hispanic women who need prenatal care or other healthcare services.

Strategy 5: Estimate Needed Resources

It is important to determine the expenses involved in carrying out a legislative campaign. The expenses must be paid, so the nutritionist or policy maker must solicit the support of community members who are interested in the issue, such as special interest groups. They can help by identifying resources or contribute in-kind to the campaign. Some examples of costs are funds for media coverage, travel to various sites related to the issue, and telephone bills. It also is essential to identify the main individuals who will maintain contact with the policy makers.

Strategy 6: Adopt Successful Strategies from Others

It is very helpful for the policy maker to identify and learn the successful strategies used by other healthcare professionals and interest groups. This step will reduce costs and save time. Review existing/established policy constantly to ensure that it is addressing the objectives of the program.

Strategy 7: Set a Clear Direction Before Starting

Establish points for possible compromise early. In the early stage of policy formation, the direction may not be completely clear, so be amenable to changes that may be necessary during the process. Work closely with the individuals that are responsible for implementing the program and those affected by the policy.

State and Local Policy

State health agencies may provide services through district or regional offices in states where there are no official local public health agencies. State governments are responsible for the health of their citizens.[8,47] State government policymaking structures and processes are comparable to those of the federal government. At the state level, government officials depend on state community/public health nutritionists as their experts on the nutritional status of their community.[8]

The local authorities who make policies may be executives, elected officials, federal agencies, welfare workers, public health nurses, community nutritionists, and other people working in government agencies. The population segments within rural counties that would have distinct viewpoints and interests relating to nutrition and health also may make policies. The following are many ways community nutritionists can influence policymaking processes at the grassroots level:[8,48,49]

- Evaluate the community's food, nutrition, and health needs, and present these findings to program directors, agency administrators, and boards.
- Propose programs using need assessments results.
- Supervise and report their agency's progress in meeting nutritional objectives.
- Establish policies, procedures, and protocols for nutrition services for their agency.

- Adopt national model standards for their nutrition services.
- Talk with people in the local school, such as the Parent Teacher Association, the principal, teachers, and parents. Get them excited about the potential to make healthy changes in the district.
- Contact the American Dietetic Association ActionNet for help. Visit their website at http://www.eatright.org/cps/rde/xchg/ada/hs.xsl/advocacy_767_ENU_HTML.htm. It serves as a local and national contact with members of Congress.

The local political structures in the United States are diverse, so community nutritionists need to examine the structures of their local governments. Many states have strong county governments with elected boards of commissioners or supervisors who pass ordinances and approve the county budget.[8] They may have a local informant, a tribal head, a director of a highly visible voluntary not-for-profit health organization, or a chamber of commerce director. In some situations the county government is responsible for public health services. The county commissioners typically appoint the county manager and the county's Board of Health. In large cities, a city council transmits local ordinances, budgets local revenues, and appoints the city Board of Health. An elected mayor or appointed city manager administers the daily activities of the city.[8,50] The county or city Board of Health appoints the chief health official, who may or may not be a health professional. The chief health official is responsible for local public health policy. A nutritionist can advise the chief health official and the Board of Health on nutrition policy.

How Dietitians Can Become Involved in Local and National Public Policy

There are many ways that dietitians can become involved in public policy, although it seems like an overwhelming task to some individuals. The ADA periodically issues "Action Alerts" that call for members to send letters or e-mails to their senators or representatives. If the time and resources are available, people can become more involved in public policy work by volunteering as an ADA *legislative network coordinator (LNC)* or a *grassroots liaison (GRL)* for a state or district. LNCs are elected by each state affiliate and they organize and mobilize ADA members at the state level to become involved in federal public policy issues.[51] LNCs are the main liaisons between the state affiliate and ADA government relation's staff. GRLs, which represent each federal congressional district, are appointed or elected by state affiliates to serve as the principal communicator between ADA members and their congressperson. Also, the Public Policy Workshop (PPW) provided by the ADA each spring in Washington, DC, is a very good opportunity for dietitians. They can learn more about advocacy and can have the opportunity to visit the offices of the senator or representative from their state.

If the community nutritionist does not feel comfortable writing a congressperson or does not have time to volunteer locally or attend the PPW, he or she can support the ADA's public policy agenda by contributing to the ADA's political action

legislative network coordinator (LNC) An elected state affiliate member of the American Dietetic Association (ADA) who organizes and mobilizes ADA members at the state level to become involved in federal public policy issues.

grassroots liaison (GRL) A position in the American Dietetic Association (ADA) that is appointed or elected by the state affiliate to serve as the primary communicator between ADA members and their congressperson.

political action committee (PAC)
A group of individuals united by similar interests/issues.

committee (ADAPAC). A *political action committee (PAC)* is a group of individuals united by similar interests. PACs represent corporations, trade associations, ideological groups, labor unions, or member associations. The purpose of a PAC is to help elect candidates whose views support the group's mission or goals. Its function is to keep the lines of communication open between policy makers and the interest group's membership. In 1971, a campaign finance reform law legitimized PACs by granting them the status and legal authority to collect funds from individuals and make federal campaign contributions.[49,52]

The ADAPAC attempts to influence the policymaking process and its outcome. "It serves as a collective voice for dietitians by supporting candidates for federal office who are willing to support the ADA's mission, vision, and principles."[51] Most importantly, "ADAPAC increases ADA's visibility and access to public policy makers, consequently increasing the power of dietetics professionals' views on important legislative issues."[51] ADAPAC is non-partisan and solicits only ADA members for donations. A five-person Board of Directors appointed by the ADA president directs ADAPAC. The ADAPAC Board selects candidates for contributions based on whether they are in a position to assist the ADA on priority issues. In the 2000 election cycle, the ADAPAC was one of the top 20 contributors among healthcare professional PACs.[51]

Initiating Policy

Community nutritionists can unite with political leaders and concerned citizens to propose a policy change for nutrition-related issues. Some examples of issues that may need policy change in the community are food safety, obesity, funding for school lunch and breakfast programs, and food security. If the community nutritionist decides to seek change for any issue, for example, food insecurity in the community, it is important to understand that there are three basic components to follow: process, projects, and policy.[53]

The process component involves building participation through community planning and collaboration. This can be accomplished by defining the community to be served, conducting a community-based needs assessment (see Chapter 2), building links with diverse groups, using the key informant process of gathering local data, developing comprehensive strategies, and incorporating a long-term strategic design.[53] The community assessment data can be presented in public meetings, legislative hearings, or other forums. An ongoing surveillance system can be developed to monitor hunger, malnutrition, obesity, diabetes, diet-related health problems, and utilization of food assistance programs.

The nutritionist and other community members can design projects, such as community gardens, farmers' markets, and food-related enterprise developments, to meet different objectives. For instance, they can work to increase the production and marketing of locally grown foods and expand lower-income persons' access to high quality, nutritious foods. They can use data gathered by extension educators as discussion pieces to engage the community in a dialogue about health priorities, capacities, and future directions.[50]

Finally, government policies need to be assessed to determine whether they act as barriers or enablers to community food security projects.[53] **Table 6.2** presents different ways a community nutritionist can influence public policy at the grassroots level.

TABLE 6.2	Ways a Community Nutritionist Can Influence Public Policy at the Grassroots Level	
How to Influence Policy	**Actions**
Express your opinions.	• Present ideas at public meetings.
	• Write a letter to the editor of a newspaper, magazine, or scientific journal.
	• Testify at hearings at a local or state level (present oral and written information).
Be a political actor/cultivate public officials.	• Campaign for political office.
	• Sponsor a referendum.
	• Initiate a campaign to bring an issue to the attention of the general public or policy makers.
	• Participate in a local advisory board that can influence the political process in the community.
	• Organize a collection of signatures for a petition to be sent to your state legislature or city council.
	• Help fundraise for a local politician.
Participate in a PAC.	• Donate to the ADAPAC.
Network/build coalitions.	• Collaborate with the American Diabetic Association, American Heart Association, and American Cancer Society in the local area to address different health issues.
	• Talk with people in the local schools, such as the Parent Teacher Association, principals, teachers, and parents.
	• Talk with people in the community including nurses, social workers, other healthcare professionals, the mayor, campaign workers, businesses, special interest groups, church groups, and women's clubs.
Lobby.	• Advocate blocking passage of legislation that does not promote the ADA's mission. Use personal contacts, letters, fax messages, telephone calls, and e-mails to express viewpoints.
	• Advocate for passage of legislation that promotes the ADA's mission.

The Links Among Nutrition Monitoring, Nutrition Research, and Nutrition Policy

Nutrition monitoring supplies information for public policy decisions and scientific research. Nutrition monitoring and examination information are used to determine dietary habits, identify high-risk population groups to plan public health intervention programs, and initiate food assistance awareness efforts; establish the national health agenda and evaluate progress towards achieving national health objectives;[54,55] establish guidelines for the prevention, detection, and management of nutritional conditions;[56–62] and evaluate the impact of nutrition initiatives for military feeding systems.[63] Data also are used to monitor food production and marketing programs and their impact on the food supply.[54,55]

Research, monitoring, and policy are intertwined through a complex set of interrelationships.[56] As shown in **Figure 6-4**, nutrition monitoring is vital to policymaking and research.[63,64] Monitoring provides information and a database for public policy decision making and establishes research priorities.[65,66] In an equally important role, nutrition research provides data for policymaking and for identifying nutrition-monitoring data needs.[56,65,67]

Emerging Policy Issues in the United States

In the late twentieth and early twenty-first centuries, the American Dietetic Association's main legislative goal was to obtain Medicare reimbursement for medical nutrition therapy (MNT) services provided by registered dietitians. On January 1, 2002, registered dietitians began to register as Medicare providers and started providing services to program beneficiaries. Other significant ADA public policy efforts over the years led to the passage of the Nutrition Labeling and Education Act (NLEA), which established mandatory nutrition labeling for packaged foods. This enabled consumers to make more informed and healthier food product choices in the context of their daily diet. The NLEA also required that the FDA issue regulations that establish standards to define serving size.[68,69]

In 2005, the ADA took a new approach to Medicare MNT. Representative Fred Upton and Senator Larry Craig restructured their legislation to give the Centers for Medicare and Medicaid Services (CMS) the authority to expand future coverage to any disease, disorder, or condition where MNT is cost-effective using its National Coverage Determination (NCD) process. The NCD process determines the extent to which Medicare will cover specific services, procedures, or technologies on a national basis.[70] This bill does not mandate any expansion of the current MNT benefits; rather, it merely provides the CMS the authority to broaden MNT coverage through the NCD process. The MNT benefits could be expanded to cover conditions such as hypertension, dyslipidemia (abnormal blood lipids), prediabetes, obesity, or HIV/AIDS if there is evidence that nutrition intervention is effective. It allows the CMS to review the science behind recommendations to further expand the benefits without having to get Congressional approval.[71]

Obesity

In July 2004, DHHS announced a new Medicare coverage policy "that would remove barriers to covering anti-obesity interventions if scientific and medical evidence demonstrated their effectiveness in improving Medicare beneficiaries' health outcomes."[71,72] Even with Medicare's new policy toward obesity, MNT cannot qualify as an anti-obesity intervention without specific Congressional approval. However, if the ADA's new bill is enacted the CMS can review MNT evidence outcomes and make a determination as to whether coverage would be "reasonable and necessary."[70]

Prediabetes

Another example of why a broader MNT benefit is important and can be cost-effective is in the treatment of prediabetes. In March 2002, DHHS estimated that 16 million people suffer from prediabetes. DHHS-supported research shows that most people with prediabetes will likely develop diabetes within a decade unless they make modest changes in their diet and level of physical activity.[73–75] A cost analysis study published in March 2004 predicts that lifestyle intervention (including diet) is more cost-effective than drugs in preventing prediabetes progression to diabetes.[70,76]

HIV/AIDS

The nutritional management of persons infected with HIV poses a unique challenge. Malnutrition and wasting are vital issues in medical care plans as HIV-infected persons survive life-threatening infections through the use of effective medical therapies. Aggressive nutrition support can delay or reverse wasting in many cases, and there is evidence that maintaining lean body mass may prolong the life of HIV-infected individuals.[77] Researchers have established that deficiencies of energy, protein, and micronutrients negatively affect the immune

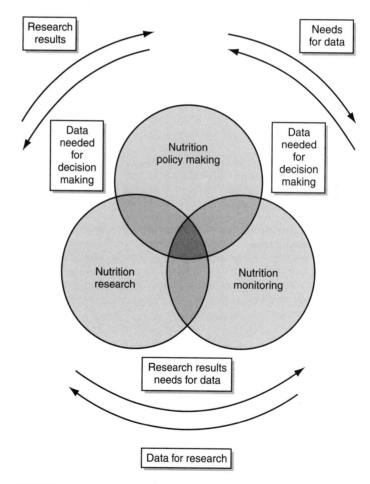

FIGURE 6-4 Overlapping of Nutrition Monitoring, Policy Making, and Research
From: U.S. Department of Health and Human Services, U.S. Department of Agriculture. Research Triangle Institute. *Final Report: Sampling Designs and Population Descriptors of Nationwide Food Consumption Surveys.* Triangle Park, NC: Research Triangle Institute for DHHS and USDA; July 1991.

system and other normal body functions.[78] In addition, the medications taken by patients with HIV induce diabetes-like states, high blood cholesterol, and a fat storage disorder called lipodystrophy, which are best treated with MNT intervention.[70,79] In 2006, Congress passed a 3-year reauthorization of the Ryan White CARE Act, the largest federal program specifically for people with HIV and AIDS, which paid new attention to the unique dietary needs of patients.[80] With passage of the MNT bill (Public Law 106-554), a registered dietitian can do that counseling for approved conditions or diseases. Dietitians are paid at a rate of 85 percent of what a physician would charge for the same service, so the bill will result in a net savings to Medicare.[71]

The American Dietetic Association's public policy agenda is established in recognition of the broad interests of ADA members. Priorities are established in areas where the association can work proactively on issues where dietetics professionals can make a unique contribution to the policy debate. **Box 6-3** presents the ADA's 2008 public policy agenda.

Some of the issues in **Box 6-3** will be decided in Washington, DC, some in individual states, some in private businesses and insurance companies, and some in hometowns. For instance, the Child Nutrition Reauthorization Act 2004 (Public Law 108-265) that was passed in June 2004 required each school district in the country to develop a wellness policy to take effect by fall of 2006. This law required that, at a minimum, the wellness policies must:[79]

- Include goals for nutrition education, physical activity, and other school-based activities designed to promote student wellness in a manner that the local educational agency determines appropriate
- Include nutrition guidelines for all foods available on the school campus during the school day

---

Box 6-3 The American Dietetic Association's 2008 Public Policy Agenda[71,81]

- Medical nutrition therapy—to cover hypertension, dyslipidemia, prediabetes, and possibly obesity
- Healthy aging in the reauthorization of the Older Americans Act (OAA) and in state initiatives relating to nutrition care
- Local "wellness" policies for schools
- Disease prevention and disease management
- Reimbursement
- Research and funding for nutrition initiatives across the board

---

- Involve parents, students, and representatives of the school food authority, the school board, school administrators, and the public in the development of local wellness policies

The USDA was responsible for sending information about the implementation process to all the districts. In turn, all local districts were required to submit their wellness policy to the USDA by June 30, 2006, for implementation in the fall of 2006. **Box 6-4** presents an example of existing state and school district policies regarding school-based activities, and **Box 6-5** presents sources of information on federal legislation

---

Box 6-4 An Example of Existing State and School District Policies Regarding School-Based Activities[85]

School District of Marshfield, Wisconsin, School Nutrition Policy

The School District of Marshfield included a school-based activities policy in its mission. This district-wide nutrition policy encouraged all members of the school community to create an environment that supports lifelong healthy eating habits. The policy emphasized that all the decisions made in all school programming must reflect and encourage positive nutrition messages and healthy food choices. Presented below is the policy of the School District of Marshfield:

1. Provide a positive environment and appropriate knowledge regarding food.
   - Ensure that all students have access to healthy food choices during school and at school functions.
   - Provide a pleasant eating environment for students and staff.
   - Allow a minimum of 20 minutes for students to eat lunch and socialize in the designated cafeteria area.
   - Enable all students, through a comprehensive curriculum, to acquire the knowledge and skills necessary to make healthy food choices for a lifetime.

2. When using food as a part of class or student incentive programs, staff and students are encouraged to utilize healthy, nutritious food choices.
3. When curricular-based food experiences are planned, staff and students are encouraged to seek out good nutrition choices whenever appropriate.
4. Reduce student access to foods of minimal nutritional value.
   - In keeping with contractual obligations to the National School Lunch/Breakfast Programs, ensure the integrity of the School Lunch Program by prohibiting food and beverage sales that are in direct conflict with the Lunch/Breakfast Programs.
   - Encourage the practice of good nutrition by reducing the sale or distribution of foods of minimal nutritional value through a 4-year plan that focuses on:
     - Reducing access to non-nutritional foods
     - Educating students about healthy foods

Box 6-5 Sources of Information on Federal Legislation and Regulations

Congressional Handbook: Directory of members of Congress and Senate (annual). U.S. Chamber of Commerce, Legislative Action Department, 1615 H Street NW, Washington, DC 20062. Available at: https://usch.bachcsi.com/products.php.

Congressional Quarterly, Inc.: Documents related to legislative, executive, and judicial branch activities. Congressional Quarterly, Inc., 1414 22nd Street NW, Washington, DC 20037. Available at: http://www.loc.gov/flicc/svcdir/cq.html.

Congressional Yellow Book: Comprehensive directories of Congress and federal agencies. Washington Monitor, Inc., 1301 Pennsylvania Avenue NW #1100, Washington, DC 20004. Available at: http://www.leadershipdirectories.com/products/cyb.htm.

Federal Register, Congressional Register: Congressional and agency reports. Superintendent of Documents, Government Printing Office, Washington, DC 20402. Available at: http://www.gpoaccess.gov/fr/index.html and http://www.copyright.gov/statements.html.

House and Senate Bills: From offices of members of Congress or the Senate:

House Document Room
H-226, U.S. Capitol
Washington, DC 20515

Senate Document Room
SH B-04
Hart Senate Office Building
Washington, DC 20515

Available at: http://www.gpoaccess.gov/bills/index.html and http://www.senate.gov/pagelayout/legislative/d_three_sections_with_teasers/bills.htm.

Directory of Health Organization. Specialized Information System (SIS): Specialized Information System: NLM/NIH, 2 Democracy Plaza, Suite 510, 6707 Democracy Boulevard MSC 5467, Bethesda, MD 20892. Available at: http://dirline.nlm.nih.gov.

National Journal: The Weekly on Politics and Government, The Almanac of American Politics (annual): National Journal, Inc., 17320 M Street NW, Washington, DC 20036. Available at: http://nationaljournal.com.

Reports of Congressional Audits of Federal Programs: General Accounting Office, Information Handling and Support Facility, Document Handling and Information Service Component, P.O. Box 6015, Gaithersburg, MD 20877. Available at: http://www.gao.gov.

Adapted from: Kaufman M. *Nutrition in Promoting the Public's Health: Strategies, Principles, and Practice.* Sudbury, MA: Jones and Bartlett; 2007.

---

and regulations. Policies were written at the school district level. Dietitians' involvement in this process can be but are not limited to:[81,83,84]

- Talking with people in their community about becoming involved
- Finding out who is in charge of food services for the district
- Finding out if the district food service director is not a registered dietitian, and offering to serve on the wellness policy committee as a nutrition advisor

- Finding out if the food service director is a registered dietitian, and if not, talking to him or her about volunteering time to serve on the advisory committee for the district

Table 6.3 presents how local districts can create and implement a local wellness policy, and **Table 6.4** presents how schools can evaluate the progress of the school's physical education policies.

TABLE 6.3   How Local Districts Can Create and Implement a Local Wellness Policy

Step	Action
Do the initial homework.	• Identify and review existing state laws and guidelines about education, health, and/or agriculture; other school districts' policies; and your local district policies that address wellness topics before meetings start. For example, compare local wellness policies with the requirements of Section 2004 of the Child Nutrition and WIC Reauthorization Acts of 2004.
	• At a minimum, your school district's new wellness policies must be in compliance with the federal statutory requirements, plus all relevant state and district requirements.
	• The process may vary from one district to another. The school district superintendent's office will be helpful if you are not familiar with your district's procedures.

(continues)

TABLE 6.3   **(Continued)**

Step	Action
Identify a policy development team.	• Anyone can initiate a process to create a new policy or adopt an existing policy. The law requires: • Parents. • Students. • Representatives of the school food authority. • The school board. • School administrators. • The public (make sure everyone who will be affected by the policy is involved). • It is important to collaborate with any existing efforts in the school or community. If your school district is already working on student wellness issues and has an existing infrastructure, such as a school health council, a coordinated school health program, a local Team Nutrition team, or staff involved in the Carol M. White Physical Education Program (PEP), these people can assist in the development of the policy. • The following are some resources to assist schools and school districts in establishing a new team, if needed, or in building on existing teams and partnerships. • North Carolina's *Effective School Health Advisory Councils—Moving from Policy to Action*. • *Promoting Healthy Youth, Schools, and Communities: A Guide to Community-School Health Councils* from the American School Health Association (at cost). • *Improving School Health: A Guide to School Health Councils*, a PDF from the American Cancer Society. • *Team Nutrition Resources* from the USDA.
Assess the district's needs.	• Assess the current situation and the nutrition and physical activity needs of the students before making plans to develop policies. • Look for data on the education and health status of young people in your particular state. Web resources include: • The CDC's data on *Obesity Trends*. • The CDC's *Youth Risk Behavior Surveillance System*. • Action for Healthy Kids' *State Profiles for Action*. • The following tools may help you assess your schools' existing policies, programs, and areas that need improvement: • *Changing the Scene Improvement Checklist* is a simple checklist to help you assess the situation in your school and to help you focus on exactly what needs to be done. The State of Michigan modified this improvement checklist to measure progress as actions are taken. • *School Health Index: A Self-assessment and Planning Guide* is the CDC's self-assessment and planning guide that includes physical activity and healthy eating. This tool enables schools to identify the strengths and weaknesses of nutrition and physical activity policies and programs and develop an action plan for improvement. • *Keys to Excellence: Standard of Practice for Nutrition Integrity* is a guide published by the School Nutrition Association (SNA) that identifies the elements of a quality school nutrition program. This publication provides an easy-to-use evaluation form for assessing school meal programs' quality and tracking progress. • *It's Time for Your School's Physical Education Check-Up* is a checklist of physical activity measurements, created by the National Association for Sport and Physical Education (see **Table 6.5**).
Draft a policy.	• Based on your needs assessment, draft the initial policy statements. • Address nutrition education, physical activity, other school-based activities that promote student wellness, nutrition guidelines for all foods available on each campus, and a plan for measuring implementation, as required by Public Law 108-265, Section 2004. For more information about the components that must appear in the wellness policy, see the USDA's *Health Wellness Policy Requirements*. • To save time, consider adapting or adopting another district's or organization's existing policy to meet the needs of your school district. Check out the USDA's *Examples: Local Wellness Policies* for some ideas, available at http://teamnutrition.usda.gov/Healthy/wellnesspolicy_examples.html.

TABLE 6.3	(Continued)

Step	Action
Draft a policy. (*cont.*)	• Additionally, some state agencies that administer school meal programs offer guidance to assist local districts to create and implement local wellness policies.
	• Also check with professional associations and organizations for model school wellness policies and useful resources. The non-governmental organizations that are acting as collaborators on the local wellness policy can be a good resource.
	• The goals that are set for nutrition education and physical activity, the nutrition guidelines, and other school-based activities must be developed in recognition of both the school district's goals and the current school wellness status.
	• The goals should be realistic and attainable.
	• Propose several policy options from which decision makers can choose. The local school board or superintendent may be interested to know the financial implications of each policy option, particularly in regard to nutrition guidelines for foods sold in vending machines or school stores. The examples of success stories where schools improved their nutritional quality of foods offered and maintained revenue can be found in the USDA and CDC's joint publication *Making It Happen*.
	• Draft a plan for implementing and measuring the new policy while you are drafting the policy itself. For example, you may consider:
	• What indicators will be used to evaluate the progress of implementation?
	• Who will be responsible for monitoring the implementation of the policy?
	• How often will the implementation be evaluated?
	• Keep the school district's decision makers informed about the proposed wellness policy and obtain their support throughout the development process.
	• For more information on the policy development process, the following resources are available to assist you:
	• The USDA's Local Wellness Policy web pages can help you draft policies specifically targeting nutrition education, physical activity, and nutrition guidelines for all foods available on school campuses during the school day, and other school-based activities designed to promote student wellness.
	• *Fit, Healthy, and Ready to Learn* is a school health policy guide developed by the National Association of State Boards of Education that provides sample policies on healthy eating, physical activity, and other topics.
	• *Changing the Scene: Improving the School Nutrition Environment—A Guide to Local Action* was developed by the USDA's Team Nutrition in collaboration with 16 education, health, and nutrition organizations to help schools take action in improving their nutrition environment.
	• *CDC Guidelines for School Health Programs to Promote Lifelong Healthy Eating* identifies the school-based strategies most likely to be effective in promoting lifelong healthy eating among young people.
	• *CDC Guidelines for School and Community Programs to Promote Lifelong Physical Activity Among Young People* identifies the strategies most likely to be effective in helping young people adopt and maintain a physically active lifestyle.
Build awareness and support.	• It is important to obtain support from schools and your community in order for the policy to be smoothly adopted and widely implemented. Student involvement also is an important component of building awareness and support. Use the resources from the USDA in *Changing the Scene* to help educate various audiences about your policy initiative, available at http://teamnutrition.usda.gov/Resources/changing.html.
	• Recruit local media to spread awareness of the district's needs and community leaders to speak out in favor of the proposed solutions.
	• Be prepared for challenges that may arise and ensure all spokespeople for the policy are providing a consistent message.
	• When dealing with the education community, it is helpful to identify the potential benefits the policy can have on student learning and academic achievement.
	• *Making It Happen* contains many success stories of districts that built broad local support for school health policy goals. This is available at http://teamnutrition.usda.gov/Resources/makingithappen.html.

(*continues*)

TABLE 6.3	(Continued)

Step	Action
Adopt the policy.	• In most, if not all, school districts, the district board of education (the school board or school committee) must approve the wellness policy before it can be implemented. • A public hearing or presentation might be necessary. The district superintendent's office can describe the usual process and advise you on how matters are brought before the board. • Team members will have a better understanding of board procedures if they have attended board meetings prior to presenting the policy proposal. • Prepare a persuasive and concise case in support of the policy and provide supportive background information. • Invite and involve policy supporters (such as parents, school nurses, and other community members) to attend the board meeting to voice their support and/or make a presentation on behalf of the proposed policy. • For help with this process, see USDA's PowerPoint presentation *Welcome to Wellness: Putting School Nutrition Legislation into Practice*. Also, check out the School Nutrition Association's PowerPoint presentation *Talking to Your School Administrators: An Overview of the Local Wellness Policy*.
Implement the policy.	• Implementation requires good planning and management skills, the necessary resources, consistent oversight, and widespread school staff and local community agreement. • Implementation can occur all at once or may be phased in over time. Your team is in the best position to determine which approach is likely to be most effective in your district. • The attitude of all school personnel, from individuals serving the food, to the personnel who stock vending machines, students, coaches, teachers, and administrators, can have a significant effect on the response to the policy. A positive attitude toward new foods, new physical activity options, or other changes from everyone in the school community can make a big difference. • Marketing can be an important tool for policy implementation. Consider how marketing principles of product, price, placement, and promotion can work to help with policy implementation. • *Implementation Tools and Resources* provides links to specific examples of programs and activities that are helping schools fulfill their wellness policy goals. These links, available at http://teamnutrition.usda.gov/Healthy/wellnesspolicy_tools.html, can help you start thinking about creative ways to implement the policies and provide resources to ease the burden of creating new curricula and learning devices.
Maintain, measure, and evaluate the effort.	• Designate one or more persons with operational responsibility for ensuring that the school is meeting the policy. • A sustained effort by each district is necessary to assure that new policies are faithfully implemented. • Periodically assess how well the policy is being managed and enforced. • Reinforce the policy goals with school staff if necessary. • Be prepared to update or amend the policy as the process moves on. • The school district or individual schools should celebrate policy success milestones (and the district team can do the same).

TABLE 6.3	(Continued)

Step	Action
Maintain, measure, and evaluate the effort. (*cont.*)	• Evaluation and feedback are very important in maintaining a local wellness policy.
	• Document any financial impact to the school foodservice program, school stores, or vending machine revenues.
	• It also is important to assess student, parent, teacher, and administration satisfaction with the new policies.
	• A good evaluation plan does not need to be extensive, formal, or put additional undue burdens on staff that is involved in the process.
	• Through the evaluation process, you will be able to answer some basic questions that are very important to policy makers, students, school staff, parents, and the general public:
	• What changes to nutrition education, physical activity, the nutritional quality of foods available to students, and other aspects covered by the policy occurred in each school as a result of the district wellness policy? For example:
	• Did the number of students participating in nutrition education change?
	• Did the students have a different number of minutes of physical activity?
	• Did any of the campuses change available food options?
	• Did participation in the National School Breakfast or Lunch Program change?
	• Did the policy and implementation address the issues identified in the needs assessment? For example:
	• Is it making a difference?
	• What's working?
	• What's not working?
	• How can the impact of the policy be increased to enhance its effect on student health and academic learning?
	• For more information on the evaluation process, the following resources are among those available to assist you:
	• *Evaluation Primer: An Overview of Education Evaluation.* This material is excerpted from *Understanding Evaluation: The Way to Better Prevention Programs.*
	• *Evaluating Community Programs and Initiatives* (Chapters 36–39 of the Community Toolbox), developed by the University of Kansas Work Group on Health Promotion and Community Development. This document contains information on developing a plan for evaluation, methods for evaluation, and using evaluation to understand and improve the initiative.
	• *Framework for program evaluation is a CDC publication, MMWR. 1999; 48(No. RR-11).* This outlines steps and standards for effective program evaluation.
	• *Criteria for Evaluating School-Based Approaches to Increasing Good Nutrition and Physical Activity,* by Action for Healthy Kids. This outlines an array of issues to consider when evaluating school-based programs.

Source: U.S. Department of Agriculture. Food and Nutrition Service/Team Nutrition. Available at: http://www.fns.usda.gov/tn/Healthy/wellnesspolicy_steps.html. Accessed October 19, 2007.

TABLE 6.4	**Your School's Physical Education Check-Up: How Are You Doing?**	
1.	Is physical education taught by a qualified teacher with a degree in physical education?	Yes/No
2.	Do students receive formal instruction in physical education: a) for a minimum of 150 minutes per week (elementary) and 225 minutes per week (middle and high)? OR b) at least 3 class periods per week for all grades the entire school year?	Yes/No
3.	Is the physical education class size similar to other content areas to ensure safe, effective instruction?	Yes/No
4.	Is there adequate equipment for every student to be active?	Yes/No
5.	Is technology incorporated on a regular and continuing basis?	Yes/No
6.	Are indoor and outdoor facilities safe and adequate (so that physical education classes need not be displaced by other activities)?	Yes/No
7.	Is there a written mission statement and sequential curriculum based on state and/or national standards for physical education?	Yes/No
8.	Are formative and summative assessments of student learning included in the physical education program, and are they related to meaningful content objectives?	Yes/No
9.	Does the program provide for maximum participation for every student (e.g., inclusion, no elimination games, all students active at once, developmentally appropriate activities, etc.)?	Yes/No
10.	Does the program help to systematically develop the physical, cognitive, and social-emotional aspects of each student?	Yes/No
11.	Do physical education teachers regularly participate in physical education professional development activities and have memberships in related professional organizations?	Yes/No
12.	Do physical education teachers receive student health information and have a plan for handling emergencies?	Yes/No
13.	Are there regular periodic evaluations of teacher performance by the administrators of the physical education program?	Yes/No
14.	Do physical education teachers communicate with each other and parents on a frequent basis?	Yes/No
15.	Do physical education teachers seek feedback for improvement from students, peers, and parents as a means for program evaluation and improvement?	Yes/No

How Did You Do?

If you answered "Yes" to all of the questions on the Physical Education Check-Up, your school may qualify for the NASPE STARS national recognition program for quality physical education programs. For more information, visit http://www.naspeinfo.org. If you answered "No" to one or more of the questions on the Physical Education Check-Up, please utilize this Action Plan for Quality Physical Education (see **Table 6.5**) to get you started improving your school physical education program. The National Association for Sport Physical Education (NASPE) has the necessary physical education standards, the opportunity to learn standards, and the appropriate instructional practices and assessment tools to help you.

Source: Reprinted with permission from Physical Education Program Checklist (2004) with permission from the National Association for Sport and Physical Education (NASPE), 1990 Association Drive, Reston, VA 20191-1599. *Tools for Observing Physical Education*. Available at: http://www.aahperd.org/naspe/template.cfm?template=observePE/main.html. Accessed October 19, 2007.

TABLE 6.5 **Action Plan for Quality Physical Education**

Criteria	Action	Short-Term Objectives/Goals	Long-Term Objectives/Goals	Criteria Met
List any questions with a "No" response from the physical education check-up.	How do you propose to change this to a "Yes" response? List action steps here.	List specific goals for the first 1–3 years.	List specific goals for the next 3–5 years. Place the date of success here.	Place the date of success here.

Source: Reprinted with permission from the National Association for Sport and Physical Education (NASPE), 1990 Association Drive, Reston, VA 20191-1599. *How Did You Do?* Available at: http://www.aahperd.org/naspe/pdf_files/2004PEchecklist.pdf. Accessed October 19, 2007.

Chapter Summary

- Many laws and regulations passed by local, state, and national officials affect the nutrition programs and nutritional status of citizens where these healthcare providers work.
- The U.S. Congress consists of the House of Representatives and the Senate. The legislative branch enacts laws that initiate, modify, authorize, and appropriate funds for all programs and services administered by the federal government.
- Most of the laws enacted that affect nutrition, food, and health are passed to the U.S. Department of Agriculture (USDA) or the Department of Health and Human Services (DHHS) for implementation.
- DHHS and USDA are the two federal departments important for nutrition issues.
- The government can use tools such as taxes, tax incentives, and price supports for commodities to influence policy.
- Agricultural policy initiates the nutrition policy process because it influences the quantity and quality of the food supply and the costs of foods in grocery stores.
- Individuals and organizations can testify at congressional hearings and make recommendations to modify a specific program.
- Dietetics professionals can take the lead in prevention programming because their training as counselors and educators provides skills that make them multitalented members of coalitions.
- Community nutrition professionals develop and refine leadership abilities through experience and reflection.
- Leadership refers to the influence that nutritionists exert on improving clients' health, whether clients are individuals, families, groups, or entire communities.
- Nutrition management refers to the way nutritionists manage resources when providing services.

Critical Thinking Activities

- Plan a letter writing campaign.
- Determine the legislative process for your local government.
- Determine how to network with other health professionals to influence a bill.
- Talk to local school districts and gather information about how they are implementing local wellness policies.

Case Study 6-1

Two federal bills related to early intervention for pregnant women and the regulation of weight loss product fraud are at the committee level. These issues are very important because not all pregnant women receive adequate prenatal care. Also, Americans are becoming increasingly victimized by weight loss product fraud, and many of the people using these products believe that the products' claims are regulated by the government. Reports show that:[86]

- 34 percent of the public has used weight loss products with unproven claims
- 63 percent are using them to try to improve their personal health
- 54 percent think that the FDA approves these products' safety

- 46 percent think that the FDA approves these products for efficacy
- 37 percent believe that these products are safer than prescription or over-the-counter medications

Angelina Okoro, a public health nutrition professor, collaborated with Omari, a community nutritionist, to increase the awareness of these bills because their passage is very important to the practice of community and public health nutrition. Therefore, they enlisted students enrolled in a community nutrition class to carry out some of the activities.

Activities

- Divide into groups and write letters with other community and public health professionals to influence this legislation.
- Compare and contrast two grassroots approaches Omari used in the previous bill in addressing these problems.
- Identify city council members, the president of the Chamber of Commerce, the director of family services, the mayor, a religious leader, and other community leaders who can help you accomplish your goals.
- Create a list of questions that would help these leaders understand the major strengths and problems of the community regarding these issues.

References

1. Stewart W. The use of government to protect and promote the health of the public through nutrition. *Fed Proc*. 1979; 38(12):2557–2559.

2. Borra ST, Earl R, Gilbride JA. At a crossroads: ADA and public policy. *J Am Diet Assoc*. 2002; 102(4):464–466.

3. Luepker RV, Perry CL, McKinlay SM, et al. Outcomes of a field trial to improve children's dietary patterns and physical activity. The Child and Adolescent Trial for Cardiovascular Health. CATCH collaborative group. *JAMA*. 1996; 275:768–776.

4. Boyle M. *Community Nutrition in Action: An Entrepreneurial Approach*. 4th ed. Belmont, CA: Thomson Wadsworth; 2005.

5. Mahan SS. *Krause's Food, Nutrition, and Diet Therapy*. 11th ed. Philadelphia, PA: Saunders; 2003.

6. Endres JB. *Community Nutrition Challenges and Opportunities*. Columbus, OH: Prentice Hall; 1999.

7. The Library of Congress. *How Our Laws Are Made*. Available at: http://thomas.loc.gov/home/lawsmade.toc.html Accessed April 27, 2008.

8. Kaufman M. *Nutrition in Promoting the Public's Health: Strategies, Principles, and Practice*. Sudbury, MA: Jones and Bartlett; 2007.

9. Stoker J. Influencing the legislative process: how a bill becomes a law. *Home Healthcare Nurse*. 2003; 21(5):299.

10. Owen A, Splett PL, Owen GM. *Nutrition in the Community: The Art and Science of Delivering Services*. 4th ed. New York: McGraw-Hill; 1999.

11. American Dietetic Association. Position of the American Dietetic Association: affordable and accessible health care services. *J Am Diet Assoc*. 1992; 92:746–748.

12. American Dietetic Association. White paper on health care reform. *J Am Diet Assoc*. 1992; 92:749.

13. American Dietetic Association. ADA's lobbying efforts focus on health care reform. *J Am Diet Assoc*. 1993; 93:754.

14. American Dietetic Association. ADA continues push for medical nutrition therapy, improved child nutrition programs, and labeling of dietary supplements. *J Am Diet Assoc*. 1994; 94:721.

15. Stewart WH. The use of government to protect and promote the health of the public through nutrition. *Fed Proc.* 1979; 38(12):2557–2559.

16. American Dietetic Association. Health care reform initiatives stress grass-roots lobbying and coalition-building. *J Am Diet Assoc.* 1993; 93:528.

17. American Dietetic Association. ADA mobilizes grassroots action to secure Medicare coverage for medical nutrition therapy. *J Am Diet Assoc.* 1996; 96:1241.

18. Smith R. Summary of medical nutrition therapy 2005–2006. *J Am Diet Assoc.* 2006; 106(3):358–361.

19. American Dietetic Association. New ADA campaign seeks more cosponsors for Medicare Medical Nutrition Therapy Act: update on child/elderly bills. *J Am Diet Assoc.* 1997; 12:1372–1373.

20. Ensign JE. Remarks on introducing the Medical Nutrition Therapy Act of 1997 in the House of Representatives. *Congressional Record.* April 17, 1997: E696.

21. American Dietetic Association. New ADA campaign seeks more cosponsors for Medicare Medical Nutrition Therapy Act; update on child/elderly bills. *J Am Diet Assoc.* 1997; 97:1372.

22. American Dietetic Association's Public Relations Team. *Improving Health and Saving Health-Care Dollars: Medical Nutrition Therapy Works.* Chicago, IL: American Dietetic Association; 2002.

23. Michael P. Impact and components of the Medicare MNT benefits. *J Am Diet Assoc.* 2001; 101:1140–1141.

24. Winterfeldt E. Influencing public policy. *Topics Clin Nutr.* 2001; 16:8–16.

25. Pastors J, Warshaw H, Daly A, Franz M, Kulkarni K. The evidence for the effectiveness of medical nutrition therapy in diabetes management. *Diabetes Care.* 2002; 25:608–613.

26. U.S. Department of Agriculture. Center for Nutrition Policy and Promotion. Available at: http://www.cnpp.usda.gov. Accessed January 3, 2007.

27. Austin JE, Hitt C. *Nutrition Intervention in the United States.* Cambridge, MA: Vallinger; 1979.

28. U.S. Food and Drug Administration. FDA's Counterterrorism Role. Available at: http://www.fda.gov/oc/bioterrorism/role.html. Accessed August 8, 2006.

29. Spake A. FDA eyes bigger role on imported food. *U.S. News World Rep.* 1998; 125(13):38.

30. Mead PS, Slutsker L, Dietz V, et al. Food-related illness and death in the United States. *Emerg Infect Dis.* 1999; 5(5):607–625.

31. U.S. Food and Drug Administration. Administrative detention of food for human or animal consumption under the Public Health Security and Bioterrorism Preparedness and Response Act of 2002. Final rule. *Fed Reg.* 2004; 69(108):31659–31705.

32. U.S. Food and Drug Administration. Total Diet Study. Available at: http://www.cfsan.fda.gov/~comm/tds-toc.html. Accessed August 8, 2006.

33. U.S. Government Printing Office. *Federal Register.* Available at: http://www.gpoaccess.gov/fr/index.html. Accessed March 10, 2008.

34. U.S. Department of Health and Human Services. About DHHS. Available at: http://www.dhhs.gov/about/index.html. Accessed May 13, 2005.

35. Center for Medicare Advocacy, Inc. Differences Between Medicare and Medicaid. Available at: http://www.medicareadvocacy.org/medicaid_diff.vs.medicare.htm. Accessed April 27, 2008.

36. U.S. Department of Agriculture. About USDA. Available at: http://www.usda.gov/wps/portal/!ut/p/_s.7_0_A/7_0_1OB?navtype=MA&navid=ABOUT_USDA. Accessed May 13, 2005.

37. National Institutes of Health. NIH Is the Nation's Medical Research Agency—Making Important Medical Discoveries That Improve Health and Save Lives. Available at: http://www.justnutri.com/national_institutes_of_health.html. Accessed April 27, 2008.

38. Centers for Disease Control and Prevention. About the CDC. Available at: http://www.cdc.gov/about. Accessed March 10, 2008.

39. U.S. Department of Agriculture. Food and Nutrition Service. Available at: http://www.fns.usda.gov/fsnep. Accessed January 7, 2007.

40. U.S. Department of Health and Human Services. HHS: What We Do. Available at: http://www.hhs.gov/about/whatwedo.html. Accessed March 10, 2008.

41. Sims LS. Public policy in nutrition: a framework for action. *Nutr Today.* 1993; 28(2):10–20.

42. Birkland TA. *An Introduction to the Policy Process: Theories, Concepts, and Models of Public Policy Making.* Armonk, NY: M.E. Sharpe; 2001.

43. Chapman N. Consensus and coalitions—key to nutrition policy development. *Nutr Today.* 1987; 22(5):22–29.

44. Policy Hub. Better Policy Making. Available at: http://www.nationalschool.gov.uk/policyhub/better_policy_making. Accessed March 7, 2008.

45. Spasoff RA. The role of nutrition in healthy public policy. *Rapport.* 1989; 4:6–7.

46. Stanhope M, Lancaster J. *Community and Public Health Nursing.* 5th ed. New York: Mosby; 2000.

47. Institute of Medicine. *Committee for the Study of the Future of Public Health. The Future of Public Health.* Washington, DC: National Academy Press; 1988.

48. Samour P, Ochs M. Growing policy with grassroots activism. *J Am Diet Assoc.* 2004; 104(12):1786–1787.

49. White JV, Hughes BAF. If dietetics is your profession, public policy is your business. *J Am Diet Assoc.* 2001; 101(2):172.

50. Wright ML. Building local knowledge for developing health policy through key informant interviews. *J Extension.* 2002; 40(1).

51. Watts ML. How dietitians can make a difference through political action. *J Am Diet Assoc.* 2002; 102(9):1226–1227.

52. Federal Election Commission. Federal Campaign Finance Law. Available at: http://www.fec.gov/law/feca/feca.shtml. Accessed March 10, 2008.

53. McCullum CC. Use of a participatory planning process as a way to build community food security. *J Am Diet Assoc.* 2002; 102(7):962–967.

54. U.S. Department of Health and Human Services. *Healthy People 2000, National Health Promotion and Disease Objectives.* PHS Publication No. 91-50212. Washington, DC: Author; 1991.

55. U.S. Department of Health and Human Services. *Healthy People 2010: Conference Edition in Two Volumes.* Washington, DC: Author; 2000.

56. Berdanier C, Feldman E, Flatt W, St. Jeor S. *Handbook of Nutrition and Food.* Washington, DC: CRC Press; 2002.

57. Chobanian A, Bakris G, Black H. Seventh report of the joint national committee on prevention, detection, evaluation, and treatment of high blood pressure. *Hypertension.* 2003; 42:1206.

58. Ricardo U, Kain J. The epidemiological transition: need to incorporate obesity prevention into nutrition programmes. *Pub Health Nutr.* 2002: 5:223–229.

59. Flaskerud J, Winslow B. Conceptualizing vulnerable populations: health-related research. *Morbidity and Mortality Weekly Report.* 1998; 47(2):69–78.

60. National Institutes of Health. *Optimal Calcium Intake.* Bethesda, MD: Author; 1994.

61. U.S. Department of Health and Human Services. *The Surgeon General's Report on Nutrition and Health.* PHS Publication No. 88-50210. Washington, DC: Author; 1988.

62. National Research Council. *Diet and Health. Implications for Reducing Chronic Disease Risk.* Washington, DC: National Academy Press; 1989.

63. Committee on Military Nutrition Research. Food and Nutrition Board, Institute of Medicine. *Military Nutrition Initiatives.* Washington, DC: Institute of Medicine; 1991.

64. Woteki RR, Briefel CJ, Klein PF, et al. Nutrition monitoring: summary of a statement from an American Society for Nutritional Sciences Working Group. *J Nutr.* 2002; 132:3782–3783.

65. Sims L. *Research Aspects of Public Policy in Nutrition Generating Research Questions to Determine the Impact of Nutritional, Agricultural, and Health Care Policy and Regulations on the Health and Nutritional Status of the Public. The Research Agenda for Dietetics Conference Proceedings.* Chicago, IL: American Dietetic Association; 1993.

66. Frankle RT, Owen AY. *Nutrition in the Community*. 4th ed. St. Louis, MO: Mosby; 1999.

67. Radimer K. National nutrition data: contributions and challenges to monitoring dietary supplement use in women. *J Nutr*. 2003; 133:2003S–2007S.

68. Smith RE, Patrick S, Michael P, Hager M. Medical nutrition therapy: the core of ADA's advocacy efforts (part 1). *J Am Diet Assoc*. 2005; 105(5):825–834.

69. American Dietetic Association. Final food labeling regulations. *J Am Diet Assoc*. 1993; 93(2):146–148.

70. Goldfarb B. Pushing for CMS coverage of medical nutrition therapy. *DOC News*. October 1, 2005; 2(10):1.

71. American Dietetic Association. Medicare Medical Nutrition Therapy Act of 2005. Available at: http://www.eatright.org/Public/GovernmentAffairs/98_9015.cfm. Accessed May 13, 2005.

72. Smith RE. Passing an effective obesity bill. *J Am Diet Assoc*. 2006; 106(9): 1349–1353.

73. Kanaya AM, Narayan KM. Prevention of type 2 diabetes: data from recent trials. *Prim Care*. 2003; 30(3):511–526.

74. Dalgaard M. Effects of one single bout of low-intensity exercise on postprandial lipemia in type 2 diabetic men. *Brit J Nutr*. 2004; 92(3):469–476.

75. Smith RE, Patrick S, Michael P, Hager M. Medical nutrition therapy: the core of ADA's advocacy efforts (part 2). *J Am Diet Assoc*. 2005; 105(6):987–996.

76. Keers JC, Groen H, Sluiter WJ, Bouma J, Links TP. Cost and benefits of a multidisciplinary intensive diabetes education programme. *J Eval Clin Pract*. 2005; 11(3):293–303.

77. Nerad J, Romeyn M, Silverman E, et al. General nutrition management in patients infected with human immunodeficiency virus. *Clin Infect Dis*. 2003; 36(Suppl):S52–S62.

78. Lanzillotti JS, Tang AM. Micronutrients and HIV disease: a review pre- and post-HAART. *Nutr Clin Care*. 2005; 8(1):16–23.

79. Tinnerello D. HIV and nutrition. *Body Positive*. 1998; 11(9):24.

80. Watts ML. Ryan White CARE Act reauthorization: opportunities for patients and dietetics professionals. *J Am Diet Assoc*. 2004; 104(11):1661–1662.

81. Ochs M, Samour P. Growing policy with grassroots activism. *J Am Diet Assoc*. 2004; 104(12):1786–1787.

82. Reeves RS. Translating nutrition policies and messages into healthier children: ADA's role. *J Am Diet Assoc*. 2006; 106(1):19.

83. Food Research Analysis Center. Current News and Analyses: Congress Enhances WIC Food Package Definition and Creates Review Requirements. Available at: http://www.frac.org/html/federal_food_programs/cnreauthor/WIC_Food_Package.html. Accessed January 6, 2007.

84. Stang J, Taft Bayer C, Flatt MM. Position of the American Dietetic Association: child and adolescent food and nutrition programs. *J Am Diet Assoc*. 2006; 106(9):1467–1475.

85. U.S. Department of Agriculture, Food and Nutrition Service. Healthy Schools. Available at: http://teamnutrition.usda.gov/Healthy/wellnesspolicygoals_schoolbased.html. Accessed August 6, 2006.

86. American Dietetic Association. Advocacy and the Profession: ADA Policy Initiatives and Advocacy Report. Available at: http://www.eatright.org/cps/rde/xchg/ada/hs.xsl/advocacy.html. Accessed April 27, 2008.

CHAPTER 7

Public Health Nutrition: An International Perspective

CHAPTER OUTLINE

- Introduction
- Overview of World Hunger
- Current Nutrition Issues in Developing and Developed Countries
- Malnutrition, Food Insecurity, and Hunger
- Women's Contribution to Food Security
- Causes of Hunger and Malnutrition
- Solving World Hunger and Malnutrition
- Global Initiatives
- Emergency Relief Efforts
- Refeeding Severely Malnourished Individuals
- The Role of Community Nutritionists

LEARNING OBJECTIVES

- Compare the prevalence of under- and overnutrition in developing and developed countries.
- Discuss the effects of undernutrition on children.
- Discuss factors that contribute to world hunger and malnutrition.
- Define food security.
- Describe women's role in preventing food insecurity.
- Identify how children become infected with human immunodeficiency virus (HIV).
- Discuss current international nutrition issues in developing and developed countries.
- Provide feeding guidelines during emergency relief periods.
- Discuss the different types of emergency feeding programs.
- Describe appropriate feeding methods for severely malnourished individuals.

Introduction

Food supplies have increased significantly, especially in higher income ***developed countries***, that have enough to feed their population for at least the next few decades.[1,2] However, many ***developing countries*** experience hunger and malnutrition. It is expected that some low-income and food-insecure countries will experience lack of food in the next decade unless their population growth is matched with increased agricultural production and a growth in purchasing power.[3]

The lack of food supply leads to undernutrition. The number of chronically undernourished people declined because many countries are using modern technologies to increase food supply. However, this number still represents about 800 million people.[1] The food supply of those individuals who are chronically undernourished is less than 2,000 calories per day.[4] The latest estimates indicate that about 826 million people are undernourished, 792 million of whom are in developing countries and 34 million of whom are in developed countries.[5] The countries with the highest rates of undernutrition lack the financial resources to provide government-funded food assistance programs, such as those found in the United States.

The food assistance programs in the United States were described in earlier chapters. These include children's School Lunch and Breakfast Programs, childcare and eldercare food programs, food assistance programs for older adults such as congregate meals, and the Special Supplemental Nutrition Program for Women, Infants, and Children (WIC) that supplies low-income pregnant women and mothers with nourishing food.

Overview of World Hunger

The most recent data show that 94 percent of the 842 million people who are chronically hungry in the world are from developing countries.[5] Many developed countries, such as most European countries, Japan, Australia, New Zealand, and the United States, have enough food to provide their population with 3,400 calories per person per day. In contrast, the lowest income countries such as Angola, Chad, Mozambique, and Somalia have an average daily supply of less than 1,800 calories per person.[6,7]

In 1960, India, China, and other Asian countries had similar problem of hunger, but now they are among the most successful at increasing food production and consumption. Food shortages, both chronic and acute, now mainly occur in sub-Saharan Africa.[8] In Asian countries, modern technologies are used to increase food supply and family planning programs help reduce population growth. In addition, rural, agricultural economic growth generated increased incomes for the rural poor, stabilized food prices, and increased non-agricultural economic growth, which contributed to a reduction in chronic food shortages in Asia.[8] According to the Food and Agriculture Organization (FAO) of the United Nations, the number of Asians who were chronically undernourished decreased by half in the last twenty years from 40 percent in 1970 to 19 percent in 1990. In China specifically, the rate of extreme poverty decreased from 33 percent in 1990 to 16.6 percent in 2001.[9]

The gap between the rich and the poor is increasing, which is one factor that contributes to chronic undernutrition and hunger. The range between the rich and the poor in Australia, Sweden, the United King-

FIGURE 7-1   Global Map Showing Levels of Hunger

Source: Weissmann D. *2006 Global Hunger Index: A Basis for Cross-Country Comparisons*. Issue Brief 47. Washington, DC: International Food Policy Research Institute. Reproduced with permission from the International Food Policy Institute, http://www.ifpri.org. The brief from which this map comes from can be found at http://www.ifpri.org/pubs/ib/ib47.pdf.

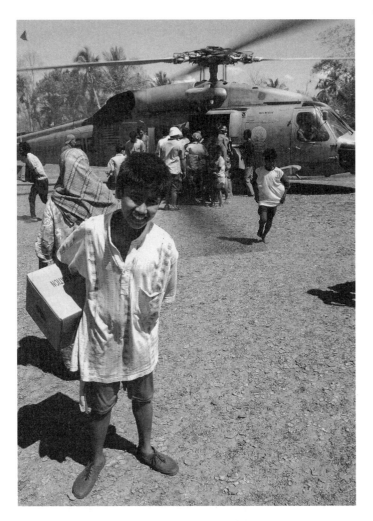

A large supply of high-quality foods can prevent malnutrition.

dom, and the United States has increased over the last two decades. In the United States, about 12.6 percent of Americans, including 17.6 percent of children, live at or below the poverty level.[10] The International Food Policy Research Institute (IFPRI) has warned that at the threshold of the twenty-first century, widespread poverty, hunger, and malnutrition threaten to undermine global economic, social, political, and environmental conditions. It has been reported that the richest 20 percent of the world's population share a global income that is 86 times that of the poorest 20 percent.[11,12] In addition, industrialized countries hold 97 percent of all patents, and global corporations hold 90 percent of all technology and product patents, which makes it more difficult for developing countries to compete in the global market.[13]

During the past decade, budget deficits in many developing countries have caused governments to re-examine their polices. Many countries relaxed their agricultural markets and eliminated production and marketing controls in an effort to stimulate production. The elimination of retail price controls increased prices for domestically grown foods. Also, devaluations of exchange rates made imported foods more expensive, further increasing prices for domestically grown foods.[14] These countries' policy changes made food less affordable for many and increased nutritional vulnerability for their citizens. Rising food

prices in many developing countries have not been matched by an increase in purchasing power. For example, per capita income declined between 1980 and 1992 by 2.7 percent per year in North Africa and the Near East and by 1.1 percent per year in sub-Saharan Africa. Per capita income growth in Latin America remained flat during that period. Asia was the only region with impressive performance—per capita income grew 3.3 percent per year in South Asia and 6.2 percent per year in East Asia.[15,16] Decreasing per capita incomes are not unique to developing countries. Developed countries also experience recessions. The concern about the performance in developing countries is their low income base and the toll such declines take from those low bases. In 1992, about 140 million people in the world earned less than 50 U.S. cents a day, and about 1.4 billion earned less than $1 U.S. a day. In 2006, worldwide, 1.3 billion people lived on less than $1 a day; 3 billion lived on under $2 a day, 1.3 billion had no access to clean water; 3 billion had no access to sanitation; and 2 billion had no access to electricity.[17] **Figure 7-1** presents a global map showing the levels of hunger.

Current Nutrition Issues in Developing and Developed Countries

The habit of consuming diets that are high in energy, saturated fat, cholesterol, and sodium and low in fiber has contributed to increases in nutrition-related chronic health conditions. Regardless of the prevalence of undernutrition in developing countries, overnutrition and its complications are emerging as major health concerns.[18] Nutrition-related chronic diseases either are appearing or are already established in every country around the world.[19,20] The incidences of chronic diseases are increasing while infectious diseases remain a common problem in countries where urbanization is happening rapidly.[21,22]

Rapid urbanization also has contributed to a dietary change in many developing countries. It is estimated that 40 percent of the population of the developing world lived in cities in the year 2000, and 50 percent will be urban dwellers by 2015.[23] In 1990, seven of the world's "megacities" (population of more than 10 million) were in developing countries, and six more were added between 1990 and 2000. The urban environment is usually more favorable to good nutritional status in children, but urbanization has some disadvantages, including reduced breastfeeding rates and duration, household *food insecurity* linked to the cash economy for very poor urban families, and increases in obesity associated with sedentary lifestyles.[24,25]

It has been estimated that over the next decade, about 30 to 40 countries will remain in the lowest income bracket with high incidences of infectious childhood diseases, undernutrition, and high fertility.[26] The major problems continue to be diarrheal diseases, acute respiratory illnesses in young children, HIV

developed countries Countries that have reached a stage of economic development characterized by the growth of industrialization. The amount of money made by the population (national income) is enough to pay for schools, hospitals, and other services (domestic savings).

developing countries Countries that have not reached the stage of economic development characterized by the growth of industrialization. The amount of money made (national income) is less than the amount of money needed to pay for schools, hospitals, and other services (domestic savings).

food insecurity The inability to obtain sufficient food for any reason.

infection, measles, tetanus, polio, malaria, micronutrient deficiencies, parasitic diseases, and reproductive mortality.[27] In areas such as sub-Saharan Africa and South Asia, nutrition and health education need to focus on the establishment of a basic primary healthcare infrastructure: breastfeeding, maternal nutrition, *immunization* against vaccine-preventable diseases, control of diarrheal diseases, and family planning. An analysis of trends in childhood undernutrition in the 15-year period between 1970 and 1995 showed a 15.5 percent reduction in the rates of underweight children due to an improvement in formal nutrition education, national food availability, and basic sanitation and health services.[28]

In a group of moderately higher income countries in East Asia, Latin America, and the Middle East infectious diseases, malnutrition, and reproductive health problems remain high while rapid urbanization, industrialization, and economic development are causing new health problems including occupational injuries and preventable chronic diseases.[29,30]

In high-income countries, diet-related chronic diseases dominate the public health nutrition agenda. Problems of undernutrition and access to food primarily affect lower income groups. In the United States and the United Kingdom, obesity and its complications also are prevalent among poorer segments of the population. So-called "diseases of affluence" are actually diseases of poverty in some of the richer countries.[31,32]

Nations in Eastern Europe and the former Soviet Union present special cases. These have been categorized as "industrialized, non-market economies."[33] They have passed through demographic, epidemiologic, and nutrition transitions, but are undergoing an epidemic of high mortality from preventable causes among young adults.[34] These include high alcohol consumption, trauma, poisoning, respiratory diseases (often secondary to smoking), and complications of pregnancy and childbirth. Also, the very high cost of foods contributed to dietary and nutritional problems, such as inadequate fruit and vegetable intake; micronutrient deficiencies in some groups, including iodine deficiency disease; and undernutrition in the elderly.[35–37]

Malnutrition, Food Insecurity, and Hunger

Food security means "access at all times by all people to an adequate amount of safe, nutritious, and culturally appropriate foods for active and healthy lives."[38] A significant number of people are food insecure or hungry worldwide. The Food and Agriculture Organization (FAO) reported that over 840 million people in the world do not have enough to eat.[39] More than half of all child deaths worldwide are associated with *malnutrition*.[40,41] Malnutrition is poor nutritional status due to dietary intake either above or below the optimal level. Micronutrient deficiencies are especially widespread. In the developing countries, about 20 percent of the population suffer from iodine deficiency, about 25 percent of children have a subclinical vitamin A deficiency, and more than 40 percent of women are anemic.[42,43]

The Effect of Hunger and Malnutrition on Health

Hunger is defined as a condition in which people lack the basic food intake needed to provide them with the energy and nutrients for fully productive, active lives.[44] In developing countries, hunger and poverty are more prevalent than acute hunger caused by *famine*, which is a widespread lack of access to food due to a disaster, drought, political conflict, or war that causes a collapse in the area's food production and marketing systems. Approximately, 33 percent of children less than 5 years of age in developing countries are stunted (malnourished based on height for age), signifying long-term, cumulative effects of inadequate nutrition and/or poor health conditions.[45] Approximately, 27

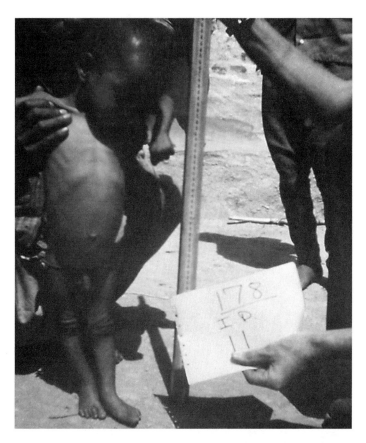

Marasmic kwashiorkor is a condition in which there is a deficiency of both calories and protein with severe tissue wasting, a loss of subcutaneous fat, and dehydration.

percent of children in developing countries ages 3 to 5 years are wasted (malnourished based on weight-for-age).[45] Impairment of growth can have both immediate and long-term negative effects on a child's health, impairing their ability to learn and their potential for future achievement, and increasing their risk for developing chronic diseases later in life. The United Nations International Children's Emergency Fund (UNICEF) stated that the mortality rate of those under 5 years is a good measure of the mother's knowledge of many important public health services, such as immunization; the availability of prenatal and other health services; income; the availability of food, clean water, and safe sanitation; and the overall safety of the child's environment.[46] **Table 7.1** shows the percentage of undernourished children under the age of 5 in various regions of the world.

Good nutrition is an essential part of good health. An extensive network of food assistance programs provides nutritious foods daily to millions of U.S. citizens.[47] One of every six Americans receives food assistance of some kind at a total cost of almost $33 billion per year.[48] Despite that, the programs are not fully successful in preventing hunger, even among those who receive their benefits. In the United States from 2003 to 2004, the prevalence of food insecurity increased from 11.2 percent to 11.9 percent and the prevalence of food insecurity with hunger increased from 3.5 percent to 3.9 percent.

Inadequate food intake and infection operate in a vicious cycle that accounts for the high morbidity and mortality rate in developing countries. When children's dietary intake is inadequate, their immune

TABLE 7.1	Regional Summaries[a] of Percentage of Undernourished Children Under Age 5 (1996–2005)		
Region	**Moderate and Severely Underweight**	**Moderate and Severely Wasting**	**Moderate and Severely Stunting**
Sub-Saharan Africa	28	9	37
East and South Africa	27	7	4
West and Central Africa	28	10	35
Middle East and North Africa	16	8	24
South Asia	45	14	44
East Asia and the Pacific	15	—	19
Latin America and the Caribbean	7	2	15
CEE/CIS[b] and the Baltic states	1	3	14
Developing countries	27	10	31
Least developed countries	35	10	42
World	25	9	30

[a]Data refers to the most recent year available during the period specified in the column heading.

[b]Central and Eastern Europe/Commonwealth of Independent States.

Sources: United Nations Children's Fund. *The State of the World's Children 2007.* New York: UNICEF; 2007. Available at: http://www.unicef.org/sowc07/statistics/tables.php. Accessed March 12, 2008; And from Struble MB, Aomari LL. Position of the American Dietetic Association: Addressing world hunger, malnutrition, and food insecurity. *J Am Diet Assoc.* 2003; 103:1046–1057. Copyright Elsevier (2003). Reprinted with permission.

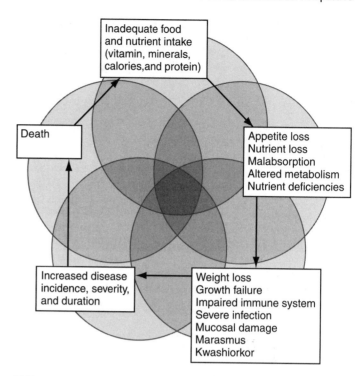

FIGURE 7-2   Inadequate Dietary Intake and the Cycle of Disease[55,56]

system defenses decrease, causing higher incidence, severity, and duration of diseases. In turn, many diseases suppress appetite and increase nutrient loss, thus continuing the cycle. **Figures 7-2** and **7-3** present the inadequate dietary intake/disease cycle and the effect of malnutrition on child mortality, respectively.[49]

In addition to causing human suffering, hunger and malnutrition have negative effects on cognitive development, growth, and health.[50-52] Hunger and malnutrition also have negative effects on labor productivity and a nation's development. According to the World Bank, the global loss of social productivity in one year alone, caused by three overlapping types of malnutrition—nutritional *stunting* and wasting, iodine deficiency disorders, and deficiencies of iron and vitamin A—is equivalent to 46 million years of productive, disability-free life.[53,54] Hence, a significant effort to eliminate hunger could yield positive benefits for individuals, nations, and the world community.

Women's Contribution to Food Security

Women contribute significantly to prevent food insecurity and malnutrition worldwide, especially in developing countries.[57] However, this contribution is overlooked and mostly uncompensated. Women represent 50 percent of the adult population, make up one-third of the official labor force, perform nearly two-thirds of all working hours, receive only one-tenth of the world's income, and own less than 1 percent of property.[58] To illuminate the roles of women in national and international development, the United Nations declared the United Nations Women's Decade from 1975 to 1985. This recognition contributed to an appreciation of rural women as energizers of any nation's economy, especially in countries whose economies are agriculture-based, such as developing countries.[59]

Poverty has become a women's issue. In the United States, almost 28 percent of households with children headed by single women live below the poverty level. Seven out of 10 hungry people in the world are women and girls, yet they receive only about half of the available food aid and often use

immunization Injection of a killed or inactivated organism into the body to stimulate the immune system to develop antibodies against an active disease-causing organism.

food security To have access to an adequate amount of food at all times that is safe, nutritious, and culturally appropriate for an active and healthy life.

malnutrition Poor nutritional status due to dietary intake either above or below the optimal level.

famine Widespread lack of access to food due to a disaster or war that causes a collapse in the food production and marketing systems.

stunting A decrease in linear growth rate that is an indicator of inadequate nutrient intake in children.

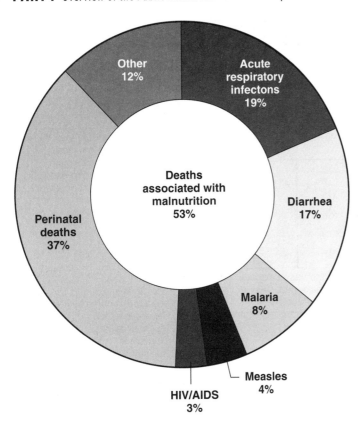

FIGURE 7-3 The Effects of Malnutrition on Child Mortality

Source: Müller O, Krawinkel M. Malnutrition and health in developing countries. *Can Med Assoc J.* 2005;173(3):279–286. Reprinted with permission.

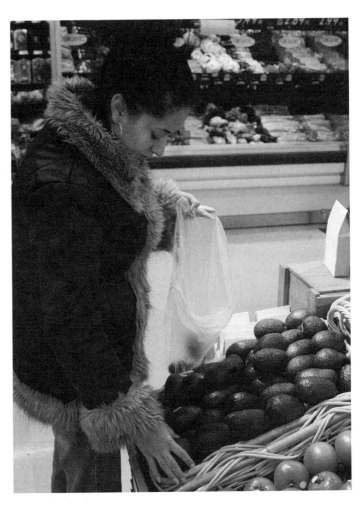

Good dietary practices start at the grocery store.

it to feed their children as well as themselves. Even starving women are more likely to give food they receive to their hungry children first. In Asia and Africa, about 60 to 80 percent of women are engaged in farming, have less access to jobs in a formal labor market, have fewer opportunities to enroll in primary and secondary schools, and have fewer opportunities to own and control land and housing. In one-third of households worldwide, women are the sole breadwinners.[60,61] Malnourished women in poverty bear sickly infants who cannot resist the diseases of poverty, and many die within the first years of life.[62] One child in six is born underweight, and 10 million die by age 5, half from malnutrition-related causes.[63]

In the United States, President Clinton signed the Personal Responsibility and Work Opportunity Reconciliation Act in 1996, initiating a major reform of the U.S. welfare system. One of the main objectives of the reform was to move mothers permanently from welfare to employment. Data show that less-educated mothers are disproportionately represented in occupations with low wages and high rates of ***nonstandard work schedules*** (irregular days, rotating hours or days, weekend days, and regular evening or night hours). Many of these women who work nonstandard hours do so mainly because of the labor market rather than from personal choice. In addition, job characteristics rather than family characteristics are more likely to cause employment during nonstandard times.[64,65] Thus, less-educated mothers are drawn into working nonstandard hours by a lack of options. The most common occupations held by these women include cashiers, nursing aids, and waitresses, and at least 40 percent of them work nonstandard hours. Welfare reform has created a group called the "working poor," people who are employed, but earn low wages that cause food insecurity and homelessness, which affects children as well as adults.[66]

Caregiving is a major role for women throughout their lives. About 72 percent of unpaid family caregivers are women, the majority of whom are middle-aged daughters or daughters-in-law.[65] For many women, caring for family members is informal care that they provide in addition to paid employment outside the home. Mothers assume the primary responsibility for the health and illness of their young families, wives often care for their aging and ill husbands, and daughters and daughters-in-law care for aging parents or in-laws. Unfortunately, in today's society, the role of the caregiver is devalued. In a family with three or more children, women spend about 90 hours a week in paid and unpaid work, while men typically spend only 60 hours.[64] The added responsibility and financial strain of the caregiver role can lead to caregiver burden and increased stress.

nonstandard work schedule
Persons who work irregular hours, irregular days, rotating hours or days, weekend days, and regular evening or night hours.

Maternal and women's health issues are critical to examine from a global perspective. Ninety-nine percent of deaths during childbirth occur in developing countries, and most of them are preventable. Infectious diseases, blood loss, and unsafe abortions account for most of the deaths.[67,68] In the developing countries, an estimated 529,000 women died during pregnancy and childbirth in 2000, and many millions more suffered with treatment. Annual maternal mortality rates vary widely among the regions of the world; it is low in Latin America (22,000), but very high in Africa (251,000) and Asia (253,000).[69] In many of the poor African countries, one mother dies from pregnancy complications and delivery per every 100 live births.[70,71] One of the goals of the World Bank and the United Nations is called the Millennium Development Goals (MDGs). The purpose of MDGs is to promote poverty reduction, education, maternal health, and gender equality; to combat child mortality, AIDS, and other diseases; and to reduce maternal death rates by three-quarters by 2015. Information on MDGs can be obtained on the United Nations Development Programme website at http://www.undp.org/mdg.

Prevalence of HIV/AIDS in Women and Children

In addition to hunger, poverty, and malnutrition, women and children also experience a high rate of HIV infection. In 2005, about 700,000 children under 15 became infected with human immunodeficiency virus (HIV), mainly through mother to child transmission (MTCT). MTCT occurs when an HIV-positive woman passes the virus to her baby. This can occur during pregnancy, labor and delivery, or breastfeeding. Without treatment, about 15 to 30 percent of babies born to HIV-positive women will become infected with HIV during pregnancy and delivery, and about 5 to 20 percent will become infected through breastfeeding.[72]

HIV is responsible for the development of AIDS, a devastating illness that was first recognized in 1981.[73] A retrovirus, HIV infects a cell and uses an enzyme called reverse transcriptase to transcribe the viral genome onto the cell's DNA, resulting in viral replication by the infected cell.

A three-fold strategy is needed to prevent babies from acquiring HIV from their infected mothers:[74,75]

- Prevent HIV infection among prospective parents.
- Avoid unwanted pregnancies among HIV-positive women.
- Prevent the transmission of HIV from HIV-positive mothers to their infants during pregnancy, labor and delivery, and breastfeeding. This can be achieved through the use of antiretroviral drugs, safer feeding practices, and other interventions.

At the end of 2005, women accounted for 48 percent of all adults living with HIV worldwide and for 59 percent in sub-Saharan Africa. Young people (15 to 24 years old) accounted for half of all new HIV infections worldwide. About 6,000 become infected with HIV every day. Estimates of the global HIV and AIDS epidemic at the end of 2005 is presented in **Box 7-1**.

It is the position of the American Dietetic Association and Dietitians of Canada that efforts to optimize nutritional status, including medical nutrition therapy and nutrition-related education, should be components of the total healthcare provided to people infected with HIV.[76]

Nutrition Education and Counseling for Those with HIV/AIDS
Specific counseling guidelines and recommendations address the following areas, as appropriate, for the client with HIV/AIDS:[76–78]

Box 7-1 Estimates of the Global HIV and AIDS Epidemic at the End of 2007

	Estimate	Range
Total people living with HIV	33.2 million	30.6 to 36.1 million
Adults living with HIV	30.8 million	28.2 to 33.6 million
Women living with HIV	15.4 million	13.9 to 16.6 million
Children under 15 years living with HIV	2.5 million	2.2 to 2.6 million
Total people *newly infected* with HIV	2.5 million	1.8 to 4.1 million
Adults living with HIV	2.1 million	1.4 to 3.6 million
Children under 15 years living with HIV	420,000	350,000 to 540,000
Total AIDS deaths	2.5 million	1.8 to 4.1 million
Adults	1.7 million	1.6 to 2.1 million
Children under 15 years	300,000	310,000 to 380,000

From: Joint United Nations Programme on HIV and AIDS (UNAIDS), World Health Organization (WHO). 2007 AIDS Epidemic Update. Available at: http://www.unaids.org/en/KnowledgeCentre/HIVData/EpiUpdate/EpiUpdArchive/2007/default.asp.asp. Accessed March 12, 2008. Reproduced with kind permission of UNAIDS.

- Providing a healthful eating plan and principles to ensure adequate nutrient intake using recommended foods and amounts.
- Enforcing food and water safety issues, including food shopping, storage, preparation, and dining away from home.
- Integrating perinatal nutrition and breastfeeding recommendations for HIV-infected mothers of newborn children. Ensure access to infant formula and food as an alternative to breastfeeding.
- Considering cultural and ethnic beliefs related to diet and food.
- Establishing nutrition strategies for symptom management, such as anorexia, early satiety, swallowing problems, nausea and vomiting, diarrhea, food intolerances, and other barriers to food intake.
- Observing food–medication interactions, including meal timing for optimal medication efficacy and supplementation and foods to emphasize or avoid unwanted interactions (such as reduced medication absorption, nutrient depletion, or altered laboratory values).
- Reconciling psychosocial and economic issues that may prevent appropriate nutrient intake, including referral and access to community resources that help support nutrition and health-related parenting classes or other support groups.
- Establishing alternative feeding methods (supplementation, tube feeding, or parenteral nutrition) or special diets, individual vitamin and mineral supplementation, and other complementary nutrition practices.
- Seeking additional therapies that support nutrition, including physical activity and exercise; medications for symptom management, inflammation, and hormonal modulation; and disease management.

- Establishing strategies for treatment of altered fat metabolism and deposition, including diet and exercise, lipid-lowering medication, glycemic control, hormonal normalization, and anabolic medications.
- Conducting community-based nutrition research to determine how many individuals with HIV/AIDS need to participate in home-delivered meal programs.

Causes of Hunger and Malnutrition

Poverty is the major cause of hunger and malnutrition. The causes of poverty include lack of resources, unequal income distribution around the world and within specific countries, and conflict. There are an estimated 1.3 billion poor people in developing countries that live on $1 U.S. a day or less.[79,80] Of these, an estimated 798 million suffer from chronic hunger, which means that their daily intake of calories is not enough for them to lead active and healthy lives.

Conflict is another cause of hunger and poverty and, subsequently, malnutrition. The United Nations High Commissioner for Refugees (UNHCR) reported that as of July 5, 2005, there were 4,772,000 refugees.[81] The incidence of malnutrition is widespread at the early stages of refugee emergencies, which increases the risk of disease and death.[63] The causes of hunger and malnutrition comprise a wide variety of problems that include, but are not limited to:[63,82]

- Maternal undernutrition
- Iodine, vitamin A, iron, and zinc deficiencies
- Diarrhea, HIV, and other infectious diseases
- Inadequate infant and child feeding practices
- Female time constraints
- Limited household income and agricultural production
- Food insecurity
- Environmental degradation and urbanization

The United Nations Children's Fund (UNICEF) developed and promoted an inclusive conceptual framework of causes of malnutrition to organize scientific knowledge and to develop coherent strategies for addressing hunger and malnutrition. This framework is presented in **Figure 7-4**.

Solving World Hunger and Malnutrition

Solving world hunger is a daunting task. It involves controlling population growth, increasing food production and economic opportunity, and providing for and maintaining adequate, culturally acceptable food and nutritional supplies for a large and diverse population. Also, the solutions involve economic policies that promote sustainable agriculture, technological advancement, education, maintaining the global ecosystem, and legislative measures. In addition, the input of politicians, nutrition scientists, economists, and the food industry is essential to solving the problem of world hunger and malnutrition.

Another way to decrease world hunger is to maintain the world's food supply for the long term by developing policies that promote sustainable agriculture. Three general areas of concern inspire the concept of sustainable agriculture:[83–85]

- *Economic concerns* (economic justice) to increase or maintain the number, quality, and long-term economic possibility of farming and other agricultural business opportunities in a community or region. This would foster the continued existence of owner-operated farms and the long-term profitability of agriculture by embedding local agricultural and food production into the community.

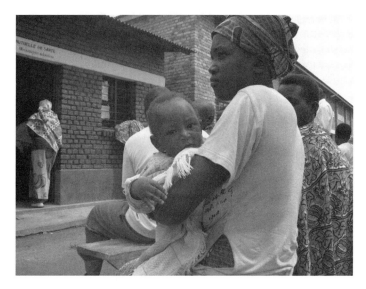

Women and children are most affected by HIV/AIDS.

- *Environmental concerns* to increase, rather than diminish, the integrity, diversity, and long-term productivity of both the managed agricultural ecosystem and the surrounding natural ecosystems. This would reduce the undesirable impact of agriculture on land, water, and wildlife resources.
- *Public welfare concerns* to increase rather than threaten the health, safety, and aesthetic satisfaction of agricultural producers and consumers. This would increase food quality and reduce human exposure to toxic chemicals. Linking these efforts explicitly to sustainable agriculture and promoting more engagement between ecologically oriented farmers and their communities could stimulate more economic and political support for these farmers and help them and their communities to achieve greater sustainability.

In addition to sustainable agriculture, sufficient energy and adequate nutrients in the diet ensure the nutritional health of a population. If the foods and crops that are grown or imported do not meet all nutrient needs, the quality of the diet will be poor and malnutrition will occur. Nutrification of foods may be the solution to this problem. *Nutrification* is the process of adding one or more nutrients to commonly consumed foods with the goal of increasing the nutrient intake.[86] The foods selected for nutrification should be those the majority of the population consumes.

Global Initiatives

A major focus of health and nutrition policies and programs in developing nations is to prevent undernutrition by improving food security, the availability of health services, and economic status. A problem facing international development agencies is how to promote economic growth and at the same time prevent the undesirable effects of nutrition transition. *Nutrition transition* is a shift in dietary habit from a diet high in complex carbohydrates and fiber to a diet higher in fat, saturated fat, and sugar; this occurs as incomes increase. To address growing concerns about this problem, individual countries have developed public health campaigns and policies that also include strategies to prevent overnutrition and promote healthy lifestyles.[87]

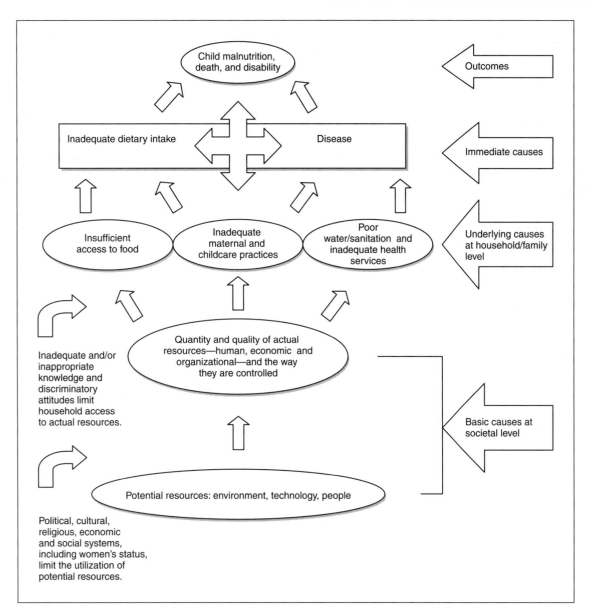

FIGURE 7-4   The United Nations Children's Fund Conceptual Framework for the Causes of Malnutrition

Source: United Nations Children's Fund. Strategy for improved nutrition of children and women in developing countries. UNICEF policy review. New York: Author; 1990. Available at: www.tulane.edu/~panda2/Analysis2/nutrdata/causes_of_malnutrition.htm. Accessed March 28, 2007. Reprinted with permission.

International campaigns also target the prevention and control of chronic diseases. Some of these programs include the World Health Organization International Code of Marketing of Breast-Milk Substitutes (WHO Code), which aims to protect and promote breastfeeding. Data collected between 1990 and 2000 show that exclusive breastfeeding in developing countries increased among infants less than 4 months (from 46 percent to 53 percent) and among infants older than 6 months (from 34 percent to 39 percent).[88] Another program is Interhealth, developed by WHO. Each country involved in Interhealth must assess its nutritional behaviors and intakes, physical activity levels, blood pressures, blood cholesterol levels, and other chronic disease risk factors, such as smoking, alcohol consumption, and obesity. Then they must implement strategies to reduce these risk factors, monitor trends in mortality, and evaluate the success of their programs. Programs directed toward feeding people are emphasized in countries where chronic disease rates are low and infectious disease rates

nutrification The process of adding one or more nutrients to commonly consumed foods in an attempt to increase their nutrient content.

nutrition transition A shift in dietary habit from a diet high in complex carbohydrates and fiber to a diet higher in fat, saturated fat, and sugar; this occurs as incomes increase.

Women contribute to food security worldwide.

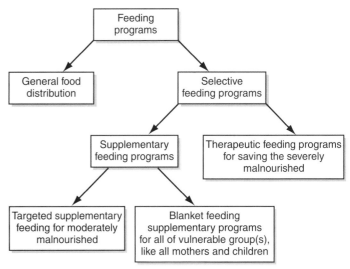

FIGURE 7-5 The Types of Feeding Programs

Source: Mason J. History of food and nutrition in emergency relief: lesson on nutrition of displaced people. *J Nutr.* 2002;132:2096s–2103s. Reprinted with permission.

and undernutrition are high. For countries with high chronic disease risks, nutrition recommendations similar to the *Dietary Guidelines for Americans* encourage maintenance of appropriate body weight; decreased consumption of total fat, saturated fat, cholesterol, and sodium; increased consumption of fiber-rich foods and complex carbohydrates; and moderate alcohol intake.[89,90]

Emergency Relief Efforts

Emergency food and feeding programs have existed throughout history. References to this are seen in Babylonian records and the Old Testament (such as the Joseph story). However, in the past century, relief efforts have been continuous. Several organizations have been established to anticipate immediate and future disasters and address ongoing situations. Several countries have organized emergency response agencies for domestic relief, and international agencies have been established by international agreements to address transnational emergency concerns. In addition, many nongovernmental organizations are interested in and conducting relief services.[91]

Persistent high mortality rates among refugee populations were observed in the last two decades. Studies show that the problem of extremely high mortality rates for populations in camps persists for months after people's arrival at the camps.[92,93] Logically, even if the initial high death rates could not be avoided, once people are in camps and in touch with assistance, the continuing large numbers of deaths should be preventable.

Food Supplies

Estimates of overall food supplies provided to refugee camps, accumulated in the mid-1990s, showed that in many cases the supplies were inadequate; for example, in one survey, about a quarter of the camps were receiving less than 1,000 kcal/person/day and almost all were receiving less than 2,000 kcal.[94] In many camps, the mortality rate was extraordinarily high. It was determined that a camp would not have a normal mortality rate if the inhabitants received below 1,500 kcal/day. In 1989, a "minimal level" of 1,900 kcal/person/day replaced the 1,000 kcal/person/day standard.[95]

More realistic estimates of energy requirements of around 2,000 kcal/person/day are now in force. In 1995, the U.S. National Academy of Sciences Committee recommended a minimum of 2,100 kcal/

person/day.[96] This level was endorsed by UNHCR and the World Food Programme (WFP) in 1997.[97] In 2000, the WHO recommended 2,100 kcal/person/day with a range of 1,900 to 2,300 kcal/person/day.[98]

Types of Emergency Food Programs

Ensuring an adequate general food supply during a disaster is a major public health priority. Two common types of programs are general and selective. Selective programs are of two types: 1) therapeutic feeding programs for treatment of the severely malnourished and 2) supplementary feeding programs. **Figure 7-5** presents the types of feeding programs.

Supplementary feeding programs often are targeted either toward the moderately malnourished alone or toward the moderately malnourished plus other groups. When the supplementary feeding becomes wide enough, it is then referred to as a blanket supplementary feeding program; this type of program covers the needs of a specified vulnerable group (e.g., all mothers and young children).[99]

Therapeutic feeding programs are now well established. They began by treating children in experimental wards and continued with the transference of expensive hospital diets to refugee situations.[100] Casein was used instead of milk products alone because of concerns for lactose intolerance, but the need to have available and inexpensive mixtures minimized the concern.[99] Therefore, the procedure of frequent feeding with high-energy milk-based diets was successfully introduced into refugee situations in the 1970s. In fact, the procedures described by the WHO in 2000[45] are practically the same as those used 22 years earlier.[101]

One early example of a therapeutic diet was reported by Mason et al.[102] They found that very rapid nutritional catch-up could be achieved using a simple dry skim milk/sugar/oil/micronutrient mix, fed in a milk-like preparation. The formula concentration is 1 kcal/g at an intake of 150 kcal/kg body weight/day in refugee setting. The growth rates were such that children could recover within a few weeks, and the mortality rates, even under the difficult circumstances of a refugee camp, were not as high as those in a hospital setting. However, mortality rates of 10 to 20 percent have persisted for many years, and the next stages of treatment for severe malnutrition should involve reducing this mortality and at the same time maintaining high recovery rates.[103]

Oral Rehydration Therapy (ORT)

Oral rehydration therapy (ORT) has been very helpful in reducing the mortality rate in malnourished individuals. As mentioned earlier, the relationship between malnutrition and infection is cyclical. Infection predisposes children to malnutrition, which impairs the immune defense system and, subsequently, predisposes children to infection.[104] Diarrhea also is a major cause of childhood malnutrition and death, and it is common during emergency feeding periods (due to infections). Diarrheal illnesses are persistent worldwide, and they have a large impact in developing countries. Children under the age of 5 are affected most, suffering from over 3 million deaths a year due to dehydration associated with diarrheal illness. ORT involves the replacement of fluids and electrolytes lost during an episode of diarrheal illness.[105] WHO estimates that over 1 million deaths are prevented annually by ORT.[106] WHO and UNICEF are the principal sponsors of global rehydration projects.[107] These projects involve the development and distribution of prepackaged solutions, combined with education efforts for instruction in home preparation and delivery. There is some variation among packaged solutions, but the principal ingredients are glucose, sodium, and potassium. The UNICEF recipe for a simple homemade solution contains 5 cupfuls of boiled water, 8 teaspoons of sugar, and 1 teaspoon of salt, resulting in 1 liter of solution. In addition, fruit juices, coconut water, and other indigenous solutions can adequately substitute for oral rehydration solution.

Other Types of Emergency Foods

The foods that are provided during emergency situations are mostly unprocessed grains, although processed foods are critical for meeting micronutrient needs and helping in situations where local processing capability is absent. Processed foods that are distributed in significant quantities include wheat flour, bulgur wheat, cornmeal, vegetable oil (usually from soybeans), and various forms of soy-fortified cereals and cereal blends. All of these processed grains are fortified with micronutrients.[89]

Foods of interest designed for young children include blended foods, corn–soy blends (CSB), and wheat–soy blends (WSB). These are the richest sources of micronutrients for emergency feeding programs. The micronutrient premixes consist of 17 minerals and vitamins important to the growth and health of young children and other physiologically vulnerable groups, such as pregnant and lactating women.[89]

The U.S. Department of Agriculture (USDA) and U.S. Agency for International Development (USAID) developed these foods with assistance from the National Institutes of Health (NIH).[108] They intended to compliment the supply and acceptance of dry milk as a protein source, which was widely distributed and a common U.S. agricultural surplus.

The protein source provided during an emergency must be of high biologic value and easily digested. Cow's milk is mostly available, but as mentioned earlier, some clinicians worry about the possibility of lactose malabsorption in severely malnourished people. However, cow's milk is typically well tolerated and assimilated by severely malnourished children and can be safely promoted. Goat's, ewe's, buffalo's, and camel's milk also can be used.[109,110] Human, mare's, and donkey's milk have very low protein concentrations. Cow's dried skimmed milk has very low energy density, which must be restored by adding sugar and/or vegetable oil. Eggs, meat, fish, soy isolates, and some vegetable protein mixtures also are sources of protein.[110]

Introduction of Traditional Foods

Other foods, especially those available at home, can gradually be introduced into the diet in combination with the high-energy, high-protein formulas. This procedure should be carried out when edema is not present, skin lesions are improved, the client is active and interacts with the environment, the appetite is restored, and adequate rates of catch-up growth have been achieved. Local traditional foods can then be used in appropriate combinations in addition to the liquid formula.[111,112] This information is presented in **Box 7-2**. The foods can be served as separate dishes or the parts can be mashed or blended and fed as paps/custards to infants and young children.

Refeeding Severely Malnourished Individuals

Refeeding syndrome may develop in severely malnourished clients during the first week of nutritional repletion.[114-116] During refeeding, extracellular fluid volume expands rapidly and often causes dependent edema. This is due to increased sodium intake combined with sodium retention caused by the effect of insulin stimulated by the increased carbohydrate consumption. Low sodium diet during refeeding can reduce this aspect of the syndrome.[117] The specific changes in body composition due to refeeding are determined by the existing metabolic state, body composition, and most importantly, the composition of the refeeding diet.[118-120] The following criteria have been observed:[121-123]

- A diet high in sodium and carbohydrate predisposes the client to increases in extracellular volume and edema.
- A low-protein, high-energy refeeding diet produces fat gain without an increase in lean tissue mass.
- A high-protein diet (e.g., 2 g/kg body weight/day) can stop ongoing nitrogen losses, even when energy balance is negative.
- A high-energy, high-protein diet will replete both fat and lean tissue stores at a rate that can be predicted with reasonable accuracy from the resulting energy and nitrogen balances, both of which can be measured or estimated.

Box **7-2 Appropriate Combination of Foods**[113]

- One part of a dry legume or its flour (e.g., black beans, soybeans, kidney beans, cowpeas) and three parts of a dry cereal or flour (e.g., corn, rice, wheat). Fat or oil should be added to the mashed or strained legume during or after cooking in amounts equal to the weight of the dry legume or flour and to the cereal preparations in amounts of 10 to 30 mL (2 to 6 teaspoons) oil/100 g dry cereal product, depending on the type of preparation.
- Four parts of a dry cereal (e.g., rice or wheat) and one part of fresh fish, fowl, or meat. Fat or oil should be added in amounts equal to 20 to 40 percent of the dry weights.

Variety is important to good dietary practice (shown here: soy, wheat, and corn).

- Malnourished patients with limited mobility will increase their central protein stores, which confer an important benefit, but they cannot be expected to gain muscle mass unless their muscles are exercised. Therefore, physical activity is a factor because it increases energy needs and, more importantly, exercises muscles.

Generally, the best steps in refeeding severely malnourished individuals are normalizing fluid and electrolyte parameters and maintaining them, continuing supplementation, and providing a mixed diet at the maintenance energy level to establish tolerance and avoid the refeeding syndrome.[112]

Mortality

The mortality rate of refugees in hospitals due to severe malnutrition has not changed in about 40 years. Currently it is at about 20 to 40 percent,[124] despite the fact that under refugee camp conditions, mortality rates of 5 to 10 percent are achieved.[125] This mortality rate is due to poor case management of edematous protein energy malnutrition (PEM).[126] It has been reported that low mortality is attainable with adequate treatment, and in some centers, it is as low as 4 to 6 percent for both edematous and non-edematous forms.

Refugees and Famine Relief

The methods for treating clients *en masse*, or without highly trained nursing staff, have not been adopted in resource-poor settings. The lack of a clear method to manage refugees may contribute to malnutrition and, subsequently, the high mortality rate associated with refugee camps. The humanitarian movement during the Biafran war of independence in Nigeria used dietary methods that were mostly experimental five decades ago. During this time, the Medicines sans Frontiers (MSF; Doctors without Borders) was formed; the International Committee of the Red Cross (ICRC) added a nutrition department; and the Oxford Committee for Famine Relief (Oxfam) expanded and

Successful Community Strategies 🏠🏠🏠🏠

Fighting Malnutrition in Senegal and Madagascar[127]

Two successful large-scale community nutrition projects in Africa used a contracting approach in rural and urban areas to prevent malnutrition. The two case studies were the Secaline project in Madagascar and the Community Nutrition Project in Senegal. Both projects were very similar in the types of services they provided and in combining private administration with public finance.

In Senegal, the Community Nutrition Project (CNP) started in 1996 in poor peri-urban areas and served 100,000 children up to 3 years of age, plus 131,000 women in 14 cities. The Madagascar (Secaline) project started in 1994, and this project was similar to that of CNP, but it aimed at rural areas in two of the most vulnerable regions of the country, serving 241,000 children under 5 years

of age and their mothers in 534 villages for over 4 years. Both projects were executed outside the Ministry of Health but followed the national health policy. In Senegal, the project was managed by Agetip, a non-governmental organization (NGO) that works on the principles of delegated contract management and which signed a convention with the government to execute the project. The Inter-ministerial National Commission against Malnutrition, located within the Presidency of the Republic, closely monitored this project. In Madagascar, a project staff was linked to the office of the prime minister, whose workers managed the project. Agetip and Secaline's project units managed contracts for the government, monitored them, and were fully responsible for project implementation and results.

Children stayed in the program for 6 months in Senegal and 4 months in Madagascar. Both projects provided the following services at the community level:

- Monthly growth monitoring of the children
- Weekly nutrition and health education sessions for women
- Referral to health services for unvaccinated children, pregnant women, severely malnourished children, and sick beneficiaries
- Home visits to follow up on beneficiaries who were referred or who did not go to the services
- Food supplementation to malnourished children (in Senegal, a flour mix made of local ingredients; in Madagascar, locally

Intervention relief during emergency periods can save lives.

formed an effective nutrition department. These three organizations and their advisors developed the *K-mix 2* diet. The diet that UNICEF was advocating for treatment of severe malnutrition in 1996 is the K-mix 2 diet that was developed during the Biafran war 27 years earlier.[92] Hence, it is important to update the method in which refugees are managed.

Internet resources for more information about hunger and malnutrition can be found at http://nutrition.jbpub.com/communitynutrition. Also available online are the nutritional characteristics of wheat–soy blends and corn–soy blends and formulations for high-protein, high-energy liquid foods.

The Role of Community Nutritionists

Community nutritionists can play important leadership roles in preventing hunger and malnutrition at the international level. They also can collaborate with policy makers, government and community leaders, health departments, anti-hunger organizations, and community-based organizations, including emergency food providers, to reduce food insecurity, hunger, and subsequently malnutrition.

To assist in preventing the causes of poverty and malnutrition, community nutritionists need to work directly with the poor and do field work. There are three possible levels of involvement in fieldwork for community nutritionists. First, nutritionists can seek community participation in a given project. Second, they can raise awareness of the situation among the population. Finally, they can help mobilize the masses to effectively empower the poor. Because village/local problems are often not the governments' problems, the nutritionist must convert local needs into concrete issues so that a course of action can be mapped out. In addition, the nutritionist can use part of the goals that the USDA's Community Food Security Initiative developed to reduce hunger in half by 2015. These goals include, but are not limited to:[127]

- Improve coordination between existing anti-hunger programs.
- Increase public awareness of the causes and consequences of food insecurity.
- Highlight innovative community solutions to hunger.

Successful Community Strategies presents successful community efforts to reduce malnutrition.

bought non-manufactured food)
- Improved access to water stand pipes (in Senegal) or referral to a social fund for income-generating activities (in Madagascar)

In urban Senegal these services were provided in a rented building called the Community Nutrition Center (CNC), while in rural Madagascar, they were provided in a thatch and bamboo structure.

Impact on the Nutritional Status of Children

In both projects malnutrition rates decreased rapidly among the children reached by the projects. In Madagascar, the project's coverage rate in the targeted zones increased from 50 percent to 87 percent by September 1997, while malnutrition rates among beneficiary children diminished significantly.

In Senegal, a similar trend was observed, and a community-based study in one city confirmed with two cross-sectional surveys that malnutrition rates decreased throughout all the neighborhoods. The study showed that after 17 months of project implementation, severe malnutrition disappeared among children of 6 to 11 months, and moderate malnutrition among those of 6 to 35 months decreased from 28 to 24 percent. The impact seems directly linked to the project as there was no significant change in socioeconomic characteristics between the baseline and impact studies, and also because the study showed that malnutrition rates were lower among children who participated in the project previously compared to those who never participated. For example, the rate of malnutrition was 23 percent among children of 12 to 17 months who participated in the previous project, compared to 30 percent of those who did not participate in the project.

These projects illustrate that contracting out is a feasible option for organizing large-scale prevention programs. These projects show strong indications of success in terms of reducing malnutrition and increasing community involvement. When choosing this type of option, a government can tap available private local human resources through contracting out, rather than delivering those services using public sector resources.

Chapter Summary

- Nutrition-related chronic diseases are either appearing or are already established in every country around the world.
- It has been estimated that, over the next decade, about 30 to 40 countries will remain in the lowest income bracket with high incidences of infectious childhood diseases, undernutrition, and high fertility.
- The International Food Policy Research Institute (IFPRI) warned that at the threshold of the twenty-first century, widespread poverty, hunger, and malnutrition threaten to undermine global economic, social, political, and environmental conditions.
- In addition to human suffering, hunger and malnutrition have negative effects on cognitive development, growth, and health.
- Food security means access at all times by all people to adequate amounts of safe, nutritious, and culturally appropriate food for an active and healthy life.
- Ninety-nine percent of maternal deaths occur in developing countries, and most of them are preventable.
- Women represent 50 percent of the adult population, make up one-third of the official labor force, perform nearly two-thirds of all working hours, receive only one-tenth of world income, and own less than 1 percent of the world's property.
- The refeeding syndrome may develop in severely wasted clients during the first week of nutritional repletion.
- The specific changes in body composition induced by refeeding are determined by the existing metabolic state, body composition, and, most importantly, the composition of the refeeding diet.
- The mortality rate in hospitals from severe malnutrition has not changed in about 40 years. Currently, it is at about 20 to 40 percent, despite the fact that under refugee camp conditions mortality rates of 5 to 10 percent are achieved.

Critical Thinking Activities

- Choose three to four countries and compare the rate of income per capita for each country.
- Identify the different types of grains grown in three different countries and discuss how these grains can be utilized to prevent malnutrition. Prepare a blend of grains that will provide adequate calories and protein.
- Choose a country and determine the labor force composition.
- Interview a welfare-to-work mother and determine the advantages and disadvantages of working instead of being on welfare. Determine the possibility of obtaining a job that does not have a nonstandard work schedule for her.
- Prepare a low-cost meal (lunch) on a $1 U.S. budget.
- Read and summarize an article on food insecurity, world hunger, and relief efforts.
- Determine the nutrient content of a blended diet for the management of malnutrition.
- Brainstorm how to solve world hunger.

Case Study 7-1

Five undergraduate students who enrolled in a community nutrition course were assigned to appeal to businesses and churches in the community for foods to feed homeless persons. They also were asked to prepare and serve at least two meals to feed men, women, and children in a homeless shelter and to read about food insecurity, world hunger, and various relief organizations' efforts to help undernourished people in developing countries. Some of the assigned international relief organizations included Catholic Charities USA, UNICEF, USAID, and WHO. After they had completed the assignments, the students became concerned about the high rate of hunger and malnutrition in developing countries. Although they are college students who cannot afford to make significant monetary contributions to relief organizations, they decided to contribute in other ways. They wrote letters to their state representatives and senators about proposing policies that would reduce world hunger. They also involved their friends in creating awareness of the prevalence of hunger and malnutrition in the world.

Activities

- List at least five ideas for campus-wide programs to increase awareness of global hunger and nutrition issues during World Food Day, October 16.
- Select two areas in the world (Asia, Africa, Europe, etc.) where hunger and undernutrition are major problems. List and discuss the causes of undernutrition in these areas. Discuss the solutions that are in place or proposed to solve these problems.
- Volunteer at a local soup kitchen or homeless shelter once a month.
- Someone dies of hunger everyday. Go to http://www.thehunger-site.com and click on Click Here to Give—It's Free to send a meal to someone in need. This site is affiliated with the UN World Food Program, which tracks the number of clicks and then sends a bill to one of its corporate or nonprofit sponsors.
- Go to the Power to End Hunger website at http://www.action. org to learn how to speak powerfully about ending world hunger, and then write to your senator or representative.

References

1. Missiaen M, Shapouri S. Food shortages in developing countries continuing. *Food Rev.* 1995; 18:24–31.
2. Johnson DG. Population, food, and knowledge. *Am Econ Rev.* 2000; 90(1):1–15.
3. Alexandratos N. Countries with rapid population growth and resource constraints: issues of food, agriculture, and development. *Popul Devel Rev.* 2005; 31(2):237–258.
4. Ge KY, Chang SY. Definition and measurement of child malnutrition. *Biomed Environ Sci.* 2001; 14(4):283–291.
5. Food Insecurity and Vulnerability Information Mapping System. What Is Meant by Food Insecurity and Vulnerability? Available at: http://www.fivims.net/static. jspx?lang = en&page = overview. Accessed March 14, 2007.
6. Putnam J, Allshouse J, Scott Kantor L. U.S. per capita food supply trends: more calories, refined carbohydrates, and fats. *Food Rev.* 2002; 25(3):1–15.
7. U.S. Department of Agriculture, Economic Research Service. Food Security Assessment, 2005. GFA-2017. Available at: http://www.ers.usda.gov/ publications/GFA17/GFA17.pdf. Accessed March 15, 2007.
8. Herdt RW. Food shortages and international agricultural programs. *Crit Rev Plant Sci.* 2004; 23(6):505–517.
9. United Nations. *Review of the first United Nations Decade for the Eradication of Poverty (1997–2006).* E/CN.5/2006/3. 2006. Available at: http://www.un.org/ esa/socdev/csd/csocd2006.htm. Accessed March 13, 2008.
10. U.S. Department of Agriculture, Foreign Agricultural Service. Discussion Paper on Domestic Food Security. Available at: http://www.fas.usda.gov/icd/summit/ discussi.html. Accessed March 14, 2007.

11. Journey to Forever. Community Development. Available at: http://journeytoforever.org/community2.html. Accessed July 4, 2006.

12. Joachim von Braun M, Rosegrant W, Pandya-Lorch R, et al. *New Risks and Opportunities for Food Security Scenario Analyses for 2015 and 2050*. Washington, DC: International Food Policy Research Institute; 2005. Available at: http://www.ifpri.org/2020/dp/dp39/2020dp39.pdf. Accessed March 13, 2008.

13. United Nations Development Programme. *Human Development Report 2000*. New York: Oxford University Press; 2000.

14. United Nations Conference on Trade and Development. *The Least Developed Countries Report 2002: Escaping the Poverty Trap*. New York: United Nations; 2002.

15. Hartwig de Haen KS, Prakash S, Prabhu P. The world food economy in the twenty-first century: challenges for international co-operation. *Dev Pol Rev*. 2003; 21(5–6):683–696.

16. Pinstrup-Andersen P. The future world food situation and the role of plant diseases. *Plant Health Instructor*. St. Paul, MN: American Phytopathological Society; 2001.

17. Global Issues. Causes of Poverty: Poverty Facts and Stats. April 2006. Available at: http://www.globalissues.org/TradeRelated/Facts.asp. Accessed July 5, 2006.

18. Shi Z, Lien N, Kumar BN, Dalen I, Holmboe-Ottesen G. The sociodemographic correlates of nutritional status of school adolescents in Jiangsu Province, China. *J Adolesc Health*. 2005; 37(4):313–322.

19. Smith SC, Jackson R, Pearson TA. Principles for national and regional guidelines on cardiovascular disease prevention. *Circ*. 2004; 109:3112–3121.

20. Soowon K, Symons M, Popkin B. Contrasting socioeconomic profiles related to healthier lifestyles in China and the United States. *Am J Epidemiol*. 2004; 159:184–191.

21. Vorster H, Bourne LT, Venter CS, Oosthuizen W. Contribution of nutrition to the health transition in developing countries: a framework for research and intervention. *Nutr Rev*. 1999; 57:341–349.

22. McMichael AJ. Environmental and social influences on emerging infectious diseases: past, present and future. *Philos Trans R Soc Lond B Biol Sci*. 2004; 359(1447):1049–1058.

23. Cohen B. Urbanization in developing countries: current trends, future projections, and key challenges for sustainability. *Tech Soc*. 2006; 28:63–80.

24. Mendez MA, Monteiro CA, Popkin BM. Overweight exceeds underweight among women in most developing countries. *Am J Clin Nutr*. 2005; 81(3):714–721.

25. Smith LC, Ruel MT, Ndiaye A. Why is child malnutrition lower in urban than rural areas? Evidence from 36 developing countries. Available at: http://www.ifpri.org/DIVS/FCND/dp/papers/fcndp176.pdf. Accessed March 15, 2007.

26. Black R, Morris S, Bryce J. Where and why are 10 million children dying every year. *Lancet*. 2003; 361(9376):2226–2234.

27. Caulfield LE, de Onis M, Blossner M, Black RE. Undernutrition as an underlying cause of child deaths associated with diarrhea, pneumonia, malaria, and measles. *Am J Clin Nutr*. 2004; 80(1):193–198.

28. Smith L, Haddad L. *Explaining Child Malnutrition in Developing Countries: A Cross-Country Analysis*. Washington, DC: International Food Policy Research Institute; 2000.

29. Ruel MT. Urbanization in Latin America: constraints and opportunities for child feeding and care. *Food Nutr Bull*. 2000; 21(1):12–24.

30. Barba CVC, Rabuco LB. Overview of ageing, urbanization, and nutrition in developing countries and the development of the reconnaissance project. Available at: http://www.unu.edu/Unupress/food/V183e/ch03.htm. Accessed March 15, 2007.

31. Banks J, Marmot M, Oldfield Z, Smith JP. Disease and disadvantage in the United States and in England. *JAMA*. 2006; 295(17):2037–2045.

32. Taylor WC, Poston WSC, Jones L, Kraft MK. Environmental justice: obesity, physical activity, and healthy eating. *J Health Polit Policy Law*. 2006; 31(1):S30–S54.

33. Babetskii I, Babetskaia-Kukharchuk O, Raiser M. How deep is your trade? Transition and international integration in Eastern Europe and the former Soviet Union. *J Econ Lit*. 2003; 83:1–23.

34. Popkin B. An overview on the nutrition transition and its health implications: the Bellagio meeting. *Public Health Nutr*. 2002; 5(1A):93–103.

35. Tamara M, Brennan P, Boffetta P, Zaridze D. Russian mortality trends for 1991–2001: analysis by cause and region. *BMJ*. 2003; 327:7964.

36. Döbróssy L. Epidemiology of head and neck cancer: magnitude of the problem *Cancer Metastasis Rev*. 2005; 24(1):9–17.

37. Shahar D, Shai I, Vardi H, Shahar A, Fraser D. Diet and eating habits in high and low socioeconomic groups. *Nutr*. 2005; 21(5):559–566.

38. Coates J, Frongillo EA, Lorge Rogers B, Webb P, Wilde PE, Houser R. Commonalities in the experience of household food insecurity across cultures: what are measures missing? *J Nutr*. 2006; 136:1438S–1448S.

39. United Nations Food and Agriculture Organization. *The State of Food Insecurity in the World 2002*. Rome, Italy: United Nations Organization; 2002.

40. Caulfield LE, Richard SA, Black RE. Undernutrition as an underlying cause of malaria morbidity and mortality in children less than five years old. *Am J Trop Med Hyg*. 2004; 71(2 Suppl):55–63.

41. Mulholland EK, Adegbola RA. Bacterial infections—a major cause of death among children in Africa. *N Engl J Med*. 2005; 352:75–77.

42. Black R, Morris R, Bryce J. Where and why are 10 million children dying every year? *Lancet*. 2003; 361:2226–2234.

43. Jackson RT, Pellet PL. Introductory observations: the region, nutrition, and health. *Ecol Food Nutr*. 2004; 43:3–16.

44. Struble MB, Aomari LL. Position of the American Dietetic Association: addressing world hunger, malnutrition, and food insecurity. *J Am Diet Assoc*. 2003; 103:1046–1057.

45. Cole M, Neumayer E. The impact of poor health on total factor productivity. *J Develop Studies*. 2006; 42(6):918–938.

46. United Nations Children's Fund. *The State of the World's Children 2001*. New York: UNICEF; 2001.

47. Nord M, Andrews M, Carlson S. *Household Food Security in the United States, 2002*. Washington, DC: U.S. Department of Agriculture; 2003.

48. U.S. Department of Agriculture. Briefing Room 2000. Available at: http://www.usda.gov. Accessed March 13, 2008.

49. Podewils L, Mintz E, Nataro J, Parashar U. Acute, infectious diarrhea among children in developing countries. *Semin Pediatr Infect Dis*. 2004; 15(3):155–168.

50. Pelletier D, Frongillo EA. Changes in child survival are strongly associated with changes in malnutrition in developing countries. *J Nutr*. 2003; 133:107–119.

51. Beaton GH, Martorell R, Aronson KJ, et al. *Effectiveness of Vitamin A Supplementation in the Control of Young Child Morbidity and Mortality in Developing Countries*. Nutrition Policy Discussion Paper No. 13. Geneva, Switzerland: Administrative Coordinating Committee, Subcommittee on Nutrition; 1993.

52. Vozoris N, Tarasuk VS. Household food insufficiency is associated with poorer health. *J Nutr*. 2003; 133:120–126.

53. Kouhkan A, Pourpak Z, Moin M, Reza M, Reza D, Alizadeh S. A study of malnutrition in Iranian patients with primary antibody deficiency. *Iranian J Allergy Asthma Immunol*. 2004; 3(4):189–196.

54. Djazayery A. Regional overview of maternal and child malnutrition: trends, interventions and outcomes. *Eastern Mediterranean Health J*. 2004; 10(6):731–736.

55. Müller O, Krawinkel M. Malnutrition and health in developing countries. *Can Med Assoc J*. 2005; 173(3):279–284.

56. Andrew T, Watson F. *Malnutrition and Infection*. Geneva, Switzerland: Administrative Coordinating Committee, Subcommittee on Nutrition; 1989.

57. Kotzé DA. Role of women in the household economy, food production and food security: policy guidelines. *Outlook Agriculture*. 2003; 32(2):111–121.

58. Hindin MJ. Women's input into household decisions and their nutritional status in three resource-constrained settings. *Public Health Nutr*. 2006; 9(4):485–493.

59. Fonchingong CC. Negotiating livelihoods beyond Beijing: the burden of women food vendors in the informal economy of Limbe, Cameroon. *Int Soc Sci J*. 2005; 57(184):243–253.

60. Ganguli I, Terrell K. Institutions, markets and men's and women's wage inequality: evidence from Ukraine. *J Coop Econ.* 2006; 14:1–33.

61. Gupta GR, Malhotra A. Empowering Women through Investments in Reproductive Health and Rights. Available at: http://www.packard.org/assets/files/population/program%20review/pop_rev_gupta.pdf. Accessed March 16, 2007.

62. Oldewage-Theron WH, Dicks EG, Napier CE, Rutengwe R. A community-based integrated nutrition research programme to alleviate poverty: baseline survey. *Public Health.* 2005; 119(4):312–320.

63. World Health Organization. Nutrition Risk Factors. Available at: http://www.who.int/bulletin/volumes/86/3/en/index.html. Accessed March 13, 2008.

64. American Psychological Association. Working Mothers: Happy or Haggard? Available at: http://www.apa.org. Accessed March 13, 2008.

65. Robinson K. Family care giving: who provides the care, and at what cost? *Nurs Econ.* 1997; 15(2):243.

66. Furness BW, Simon SP, Wold CM, Asarian-Anderson J. Prevalence and predictors of food insecurity among low-income households in Los Angeles County. *Public Health Nutr.* 2004; 7:791–794.

67. Mutharayappa R. Reproductive morbidity of women in Karnataka. *J Health Manage.* 2006; 8(1):23–50.

68. Radda G, Michael T, Meade D. Suicide rates in China. *Lancet.* 2002; 359:2274–2282.

69. UNICEF. Maternal Mortality. Available at: http://childinfo.org/areas/maternalmortality. Accessed August 14, 2006.

70. United Nations Organization for Economic Co-operation and Development International Monetary Fund, World Bank. *A Better World for All.* Washington, DC: Communication Development; 2000.

71. Hill K, Arifeen SE, Koenig M, Al-Sabir A, Jamil K, Raggerse H. How should we measure maternal mortality in the developing world? A comparison of household deaths and sibling history approaches. *Bull World Health Org.* 2006; 84:173–180.

72. De Cock KM, Fowler MG, Mercier E, et al. Prevention of mother-to-child HIV transmission in resource-poor countries: translating research into policy and practice. *JAMA.* 2000; 283(9):1175–1182.

73. Chin J. *Control of Communicable Diseases Manual.* 17th ed. Washington, DC: American Public Health Association; 2000.

74. United Nations Joint Programme on HIV/AIDS, World Health Organization. Questions & Answers III—Selected Issues: Prevention and Care; Available at: http://www.UNAIDS_Bangkok_press/docs/QA_PartIII_en.doc. Accessed May 5, 2008.

75. Duerr A, Hurst S, Kourtis AP, Rutenberg N, Jamieson DJ. Integrating family planning and prevention of mother-to-child HIV transmission in resource-limited settings. *Lancet.* 2005; 366(9481):261–263.

76. Fields-Gardner C, Ayoob K. Position of the American Dietetic Association and Dietitians of Canada: nutrition intervention in the care of persons with human immunodeficiency virus infection. *J Am Diet Assoc.* 2000; 100:708–717.

77. Nerad J, Romeyn M, Silverman E, et al. General nutrition management in patients infected with human immunodeficiency virus. *Clin Infect Dis.* 2003; 36:S52–S62.

78. Kraak VI. Home-delivered meal programs for homebound people with HIV/AIDS. *J Am Diet Assoc.* 1995; 95(4):476–481.

79. World Bank. Global Monitoring. Available at: http://www.worldbank.org. Accessed March 13, 2008.

80. World Hunger Education Service. World Hunger Facts 2008 Available at: http://www.worldhunger.org/articles/Learn/world%20hunger%20facts%202002.htm. Accessed June 29, 2006.

81. United Nations High Commissioner for Refugees. Refugee Populations, New Arrivals and Durable Solutions in 84, Mostly Developing, Countries. Available at: http://www.unhcr.ch. Accessed March 13, 2008.

82. Grosvenor B, Smolin L. *Nutrition from Science to Life.* New York: Harcourt; 2002.

83. William NM. Green chemistry and the path to sustainable agriculture. *Am Chem Soc.* 2004; 887:7–21.

84. Fish R, Seymour S, Watkins C. Sustainable farmland management as political and cultural discourse. *Geograph J.* 2006; 172(3):183–189.

85. Brodt S, Feenstra G, Kozloff R, Klonsky K, Tourte L. Farmer-community connections and the future of ecological agriculture in California. *Agriculture Human Values.* 2006; 23:5–88.

86. Koplan JP, Jeffrey P, Puska P, Cahill K, Huttunen J. Improving the world's health through national public health institutes. *Bull World Health Org.* 2005; 83(2):154–157.

87. Labbok MH, Blanc A, Clark D, Terreri N. Trends in exclusive breastfeeding: findings from the 1990s. *J Human Lactation.* 2006; 22(3):272–276.

88. Birch M, Miller S. Humanitarian assistance: standards, skills, training, and experience. *BMJ.* 2005; 330(7501):1199–1201.

89. Marchione T. Foods provided through U.S. government emergency food aid programs: policies and customs governing their formulation, selection and distribution. *J Nutr.* 2002; 132:2104s–2111s.

90. James R, Hargreaves M, Collinson A, Kahn K, Clark D, Tollman SM. Childhood mortality among former Mozambican refugees and their hosts in rural South Africa. *Int J Epidemiol.* 2004; 33(6):1271–1278.

91. Thomas JL, Luke C, Adam K, Kuiper HK, Beyrer C. Mortality rates in conflict zones in Karen, Karenni, and Mon states in eastern Burma. *Trop Med Int Health.* 2006; 11(7):1119–1127.

92. Golden M. The development of concepts of malnutrition. *J Nutr.* 2002; 132:2117s–2122s.

93. U.S. Department of Health and Human Services, Public Health Service. Famine-affected, refugee, and displaced populations: recommendations for public health issues. *MMWR.* 1992; 41(RR-13):1.

94. Posner B, Quatromoni P, Franz M. Nutrition policies and interventions for chronic disease risk reduction in international settings: the INTERHEALTH Nutrition Initiative. *Nutr Rev.* 1994; 52:179–187.

95. National Academy of Sciences. *Estimated Mean per Capita Energy Requirements for Planning Emergency Food Aid Rations.* Washington, DC: National Academy Press; 1995.

96. United Nations High Commission for Refugees, World Food Programme. *Guidelines for Estimating Food and Nutrition Needs in Emergencies.* Geneva, Switzerland: Author; 1997.

97. World Health Organization. *The Management of Nutrition in Major Emergencies.* Geneva, Switzerland: Author; 2000.

98. Ville de Goyet SJ, Geijer U. *The Management of Nutrition Emergencies in Large Population.* Geneva, Switzerland: World Health Organization; 2004.

99. Mason J. History of food and nutrition in emergency relief: lesson on nutrition of displaced people. *J Nutr.* 2002; 132:2096s–2103s.

100. Spiegel PB, Salama P, Maloney S, van der Veen A. Quality of malnutrition assessment surveys conducted during famine in Ethiopia. *JAMA.* 2004; 292(5):613–618.

101. Mason J, Hay R, Leresche J, Peel S, Darley S. Treatment of severe malnutrition in relief. *Lancet.* 1974; 2:332–335.

102. World Health Organization. *Management of Severe Malnutrition: A Manual for Physicians and Other Senior Health Workers.* Geneva, Switzerland: Author; 1999.

103. Bhatia R, Thorne-Lyman A. Food aid in emergencies and public health nutrition. *Forum Nutr.* 2003; 56:391–394.

104. Centers for Disease Control and Prevention. Managing acute gastroenteritis among children: oral rehydration, maintenance, and nutritional therapy. *MMWR.* 2003; 52(RR16):1–16.

105. World Health Organization. Protecting, Promoting, and Supporting Breastfeeding. The Management of Bloody Diarrhea in Young Children. 1994. Available at: http://www.who.int/child-adolescent-health/New_Publications/CHILD_HEALTH/WHO_CDD_94.49.htm. Accessed March 19, 2007.

106. World Health Organization. *Oral Rehydration Salts (ORS): A New Reduced Osmolarity Formulation.* Geneva, Switzerland: Author; 2002.

107. Senti F. Guidelines of the nutrient composition of processed foods. *Cereal Sci Today.* 1972; 17:157–161.

108. Grant C, Rotherham B, Sharpe S. Randomized, double-blind comparison of growth in infants receiving goat milk formula versus cow milk infant formula. *J Paediatr Child Health.* 2005; 41(11):564–568.

109. Brewster DR. Critical appraisal of the management of severe malnutrition: complications. *J Paediatr Child Health.* 2006; 42(10):583–593.

110. Kukuruzovic H, Brewster DR. Milk formulas in acute gastroenteritis and malnutrition: a randomized trial. *J Paediatr Child Health.* 2002; 38(6):571–577.

111. Colecraft EK, Esi K, Marquis GS, et al. A longitudinal assessment of the diet and growth of malnourished children participating in nutrition rehabilitation centres in Accra, Ghana. *Public Health Nutr.* 2004; 7(4):487–494.

112. Shils M, Olson JA, Shihe M, Ross CA. *Modern Nutrition in Health and Disease.* 9th ed. Baltimore, MD: Lippincott Williams & Wilkins; 1999.

113. Flesher ME, Archer ME, Katharine KA, et al. Assessing the metabolic and clinical consequences of early enteral feeding in the malnourished patient. *J Parenter Enteral Nutr.* 2005; 29(2):108–117.

114. Hearing SD. Refeeding syndrome. *BMJ.* 2004; 328:908–909.

115. Fotheringham J, Jackson K, Kersh R, Gariballa SE. Refeeding syndrome: life-threatening, under diagnosed, but treatable. *QJM.* 2005; 98:318–319.

116. Tsintzas K, Jewell K, Kamran M, et al. Differential regulation of metabolic genes in skeletal muscle during starvation and refeeding in humans. *J Physiol.* 2006; 575(Pt 1):291–303.

117. Camilla H, Mølgaard C, Michaelsen KF. Cow's milk and linear growth in industrialized and developing countries. *Ann Rev Nutr.* 2006; 26:131–173.

118. Kerruish KP, O'Connor J, Humphries IR, et al. Body composition in adolescents with anorexia nervosa. *Am J Clin Nutr.* 2002; 75(1):31–37.

119. Hoppe C, Mølgaard C, Juul A, Michaelsen KF. High intakes of skimmed milk, but not meat, increase serum IGF-I and IGFBP-3 in eight-year-old boys. *Eur J Clin Nutr.* 2004; 58(9):1211–1216.

120. Thapar N, Sanderson IR. Diarrhea in children: an interface between developing and developed countries. *Lancet.* 2004; 363(9409):641–653.

121. Amadi B, Mwiya M, Chomba E, et al. Improved nutritional recovery on an elemental diet in Zambian children with persistent diarrhoea and malnutrition. *J Tropic Pediatr.* 2005; 51(1):5–10.

122. Manary MJ, Yarasheski KE, Smith S, Abrams ET, Hart CA. Protein quantity, not protein quality, accelerates whole-body leucine kinetics and the acute-phase response during acute infection in marasmic Malawian children. *Brit J Nutr.* 2004; 92(4):589–595.

123. Ashworth A, Chopra M, McCoy D, et al. WHO guidelines for management of severe malnutrition in rural South African hospitals: effect on case fatality and the influence of operational factors. *Lancet.* 2004; 363(9415):1110–1115.

124. Brewster DR. Critical appraisal of the management of severe malnutrition: 1. Epidemiology and treatment guidelines. *J Paediatr Child Health.* 2006; 42(10):568–574.

125. Jahoor F, Badaloo A, Reid MA, Forrester T. Protein kinetic differences between children with edematous and nonedematous severe childhood undernutrition in the fed and postabsorptive states. *Am J Clin Nutr.* 2005; 82(4):792–800.

126. National Center for Appropriate Technology. Available at: http://www.ncat.org. Accessed March 13, 2008.

127. Mark T, Diallo I, Ndiaye B, Rakotosalama J. Successful contracting of prevention services: fighting malnutrition in Senegal and Madagascar. *Health Pol Planning.* 1999; 14(4):382–389.

PART II
Nutrition Interventions for
Vulnerable Populations

CHAPTER

8

Nutrition During Pregnancy and Infancy

CHAPTER OUTLINE
- Introduction
- Progress Report Toward Healthy People 2010 Objectives
- Physiologic Events of Pregnancy and Mother's Health
- Preconception Health
- Factors That Can Influence the Outcome of a Pregnancy
- Diet-Related Complications of Pregnancy
- Nutrition Assessment During Pregnancy
- Adolescent Pregnancy
- Physical Activity During Pregnancy
- Nutrition in Infancy
- Nutrient Needs During Infancy
- Nutrition-Related Health Concerns During Infancy
- Methods of Feeding Infants
- Breastfeeding/Lactation
- Management and Techniques for Successful Breastfeeding
- Supplemental Nutrition Programs During Pregnancy, Infancy, and Lactation

LEARNING OBJECTIVES
- Identify stages of development for the fetus.
- List the maternal weight gain recommendations.
- Discuss the nutritional complications of pregnancy.
- Identify common nutrition issues that affect infants.
- Identify different screening and assessment methods for infants.
- Discuss the nutritional needs of infants and pregnant and lactating women.
- Discuss the benefits of breastfeeding.
- List the guidelines for successful breastfeeding
- List the food assistance programs and services available for children and pregnant women.

Introduction

A mother's previous life experiences, general health and fitness, life-long dietary habits, and genetic heritage are part of each pregnancy. A woman's nutritional habits prior to pregnancy are as important to the success of the pregnancy as her diet during the 9 months of gestation.[1] Providing pregnant women with their nutrient needs is a public health priority in the United States and many other countries. This priority is based on the fact that malnutrition during pregnancy has serious, long-term effects on the mother and child. For example, two international studies done by the Institute of Nutrition of Central America and Panama (INCAP) and the Nutrition Collaborative Research Support Program (NCRSP) found that marginal malnutrition during pregnancy caused stunted growth and functional impairments early in life.[2] The consequences of early malnutrition persisted even later in life. The NCRSP study also showed that multiple micronutrient deficiencies were associated with poor growth and function. The researchers' overall conclusion was that attention should be directed to determining the adequacy of micronutrient status during the prenatal period and to develop approaches that can prevent early growth failure. One way for women to prevent birth defects is by maintaining adequate vitamin and mineral intake at least 2 months before pregnancy.

Progress Report Toward Healthy People 2010 Objectives

In the United States, national goals to increase the number of pregnant women who receive *prenatal* care have been established (see **Table 8.1**). Of the 17 maternal and infant health objectives included in Healthy People 2000, progress was made toward the target in eight objectives, and direction was made away from the target in five objectives. Observable gains were made in the areas of decrease in infant deaths, decrease in fetal deaths, increase in breastfeeding, increase in early use of prenatal care, decrease in hospitalization for complications of pregnancy, increase in abstinence from tobacco use during pregnancy, decrease in cesarean sections (particularly repeat cesareans), and increase in screening for fetal abnormalities and genetic disorders. However, no progress was made in the areas of decrease in maternal deaths, decrease in incidence of *fetal alcohol syndrome (FAS)*, and decrease in incidence of *low birth weight*. For the other objectives, progress was mixed. Child health objectives were not included in the Maternal and Infant focus area in Healthy People 2000.[3]

Many of these conditions and risk factors disproportionately affected certain racial and ethnic groups. The disparities between European American and non-European American groups in infant death, maternal death, and low birth weight were wide and, in many cases, growing. Specifically, African American and Hispanic women were less likely than European Americans to participate in early prenatal care. For both African American and European American women, the proportion entering prenatal care in the first trimester rose with maternal age until the late thirties and then began to decline. For example, in 1998, 57 percent of African American women under age 18, compared with 66 percent of European American women of the same age, participated in prenatal care in the first trimester. Among women ages 18 to 24 years, 68 percent of African Americans received care in their first trimester, compared to 76 percent of European American women.[4]

According to the most current review of Healthy People 2010, some progress has been made toward reduction in the *infant mortality rate (IMR)* from 7.2 deaths per 1,000 live births in 1998 to 7.0 per 1,000 in 2002. A decline of 36 percent overall is needed to reach the targeted IMR of 4.5 infant deaths per 1,000 live births in 2010, and even greater declines are required for certain racial/ethnic populations to reach the target. Although a reduction in IMRs was observed in Hispanics, European Americans, and Native Americans, no change was noted for African Americans.

There also was a decrease in the incidence (new cases) of spina bifida from 6 per 10,000 live births in 1996 to 4.8 per 10,000 in 2000. The Healthy People 2010 target is 3 per 10,000 live births. This decline can be attributed to public health awareness programs geared toward educating young women to increase their consumption of folic acid from various sources such as dietary supplements and fortified foods.[5]

Physiologic Events of Pregnancy and the Mother's Health

Maternal nutritional needs are based on the mother's physiologic demands and those of fetal growth and development. Therefore, understanding the physiological changes during pregnancy is important when assessing the nutritional and educational needs of pregnant women. **Table 8.2** briefly reviews the prenatal events that cause the varying nutritional needs of the mother.[6]

During weeks 8 to 40 of gestation the mother reserves additional nutrients in preparation for childbirth and lactation. Optimal nutritional reserves and continuing support are essential at every stage of pregnancy, however. Pregnancy requires an abundant maternal nutrient base, making preconception nutrition essential.

Physiologic and Metabolic Changes in Pregnancy

Many physiologic and biochemical changes occur during a normal pregnancy. Some of the changes are as follows:[7,8]

- Blood volume expands by 50 percent, resulting in a decrease in hemoglobin levels, blood glucose values, and serum level of albumin.
- Increased cardiac output increases oxygen requirements, and the threshold for CO_2 is lowered, which makes breathing more difficult.
- Increased progesterone level relaxes the uterine muscle.
- Gastrointestinal motility diminishes to allow for increased absorption of nutrients.[6]

Pregnancy is a normal physiologic process that is associated with significant changes in every maternal organ system and metabolic pathway. Every single blood and urine measurement of nutrients is significantly altered from nonpregnant values because of these changes. Values change as the pregnancy advances from the first to the third

prenatal (antenatal) Occurring before childbirth.

cesarean section Surgical childbirth in which the infant is delivered through an incision in the woman's abdomen and uterus.

fetal alcohol syndrome The cluster of symptoms seen in an infant or a child whose mother consumed excessive alcohol during pregnancy.

low birth weight (LBW) A birth weight less than 2.5 kg (5.5 lb) at birth; mostly due to preterm birth (born before 37 weeks of gestation).

infant mortality rate (IMR) The death of an infant under 1 year of age, expressed as a rate per 1,000 live births.

TABLE 8.1	**Healthy People 2010 Maternal and Infant Health Objectives**			
HP 2010 Objective Number	**Healthy People 2010 Objective**	**Baseline (Year)**	**Progress Review (2002)**	**2010 Target**
16.1c	Reduce infant mortality (i.e., within 1 year of birth) to no more than 4.5 per 1,000 live births.	7.2 (1998)	7.0	4.5
	a. African Americans	13.8 (1998)	13.8	4.5
	b. Hispanics	5.8 (1998)	5.6	4.5
	c. Native American/Alaskan Natives	9.3 (1998)	8.6	4.5
16.4	Decrease the number of maternal deaths to 3.3 per 100,000 live births.	9.9 (1999)	8.9	3.3
	a. African American women	25.4 (1999)	24.7	3.3
16.6	Increase the number of pregnant women who receive prenatal care in the first trimester of pregnancy.	83% of live births (1998)	84%	90%
16.10 a and b	Reduce low birth weight to an incidence of no more than 5 percent of live births and very low birth weight to no more than 0.9% of live births.	7.6% (1998) 1.4% (1998)	7.8% 1.5%	5.0% 0.9%
	African American infants			
	(a) Low birth weight	13.0% (1998)	13.3%	5.0%
	(b) Very low birth weight	3.1% (1998)	3.1%	0.9%
16.13	Increase the percentage of healthy full-term infants who are put down to sleep on their backs.	35% (1996)	66% (2000)	70%
16.15	Reduce the occurrence of spina bifida and other neural tube defects to 3 per 10,000 live births.	6 (1996)	4.8	3
16.17a	Increase abstinence from alcohol use by pregnant women to 94 percent.	86% (1996–1997)	90.9%	94%
16.17c	Increase abstinence from tobacco use by pregnant women to at least 99 percent.	87% (1998)	89%	99%
16.17d	Increase abstinence from illicit drugs (cocaine and marijuana) by pregnant women to 100 percent.	98% in (1996–1997)	Data not available	100%
16.18	Reduce the occurrence of fetal alcohol syndrome to no more than 0.12 per 1,000 live births.	0.67 (1993)	Data not available	0.12
16.19a	Increase the number of mothers who breastfeed their babies in the early postpartum period to at least 75 percent.	64% (1998)	70%	75%
16.19b	Increase the proportion that breastfeed for 5 to 6 months after birth to at least 50 percent.	29% (1998)	33%	50%
19.12c	Reduce the incidence of iron deficiency to less than 7 percent for ages 12 to 49 years.	11% (1988–1994)	12%	7%
19.13	Reduce the incidence of anemia in low-income pregnant women in the third trimester to 20 percent.	29% (1996)	33% (2001)	20%

Source: National Center for Health Statistics, Department of Health and Human Services. *Healthy People Progress Review*. Hyattsville, MD: Public Health Service; 2004. Available at: http://www.cdc.gov/nchs/hphome.htm#Healthy%20People%202010. Accessed March 13, 2008.

trimester, to delivery, and then returns toward normal during the postpartum period. The major physiologic changes are:[7,8]

- A 50 percent expansion of plasma volume with a 20 percent increase in hemoglobin mass
- Increasing levels of estrogen and progesterone as well as other placenta-related hormones
- Increase in red blood cell volume
- Increase in body water

- Increase in renal glomerular filtration rate
- Increase in respiratory tidal volume

These changes have impact on maternal lipids, cholesterol, carotene, and vitamin E, and on blood clotting factors. The first major physiologic changes include decreased biochemical levels of substances in the blood such as albumin and hemoglobin during pregnancy, which returns to normal within 8 to 10 weeks postpartum. The second is the estrogen-progesterone placental hormone changes that cause lipid levels to increase during pregnancy and return to baseline levels postpartum.[7,9]

The mother also must adapt to progressive increases in cardiac output to a peak at 28 weeks, accumulation of body water, and changes in renal, respiratory, gastrointestinal, and genitourinary functions. These physiologic adaptations during pregnancy alter the blood levels of many nutritional components.

In general, nutrients that are water-soluble (such as vitamin C, folic acid, vitamin B_6, and vitamin B_{12}) decrease as serum albumin and ferritin levels decrease and white blood cells increase.[7,9,10] In addition, urinary

TABLE 8.2	**Nutrients Needs Throughout Fetal Growth and Development**		
Stages of Development	**Events and Types of Tissue Development**	**Major Nutrients Needed**	**Dietary Reference Intake/Day (19–50 years)**
First stage: 1–2 weeks after fertilization of the egg. The first stage of fetal development is the implantation stage.	The special cells develop within 9–10 days.	Calories	—
	The ***trophoblast*** attaches the ovum to the uterine wall and supplies nutrients to the embryo.	Protein	60 g
		Iron	27 mg
	The trophoblast later becomes the placenta.	Calcium	1,000 mg
	Rapid fetal development and growth.	Folic acid	600 µg
		Thiamin	1.4 mg
		Riboflavin	1.4 mg
		Niacin	18 mg
		Vitamin C	85 mg
		Vitamin D	5 µg
		Vitamin A	770 µg
Second stage: 2 to 8 weeks after fertilization. Differentiation of major organs and tissues.	Cell differentiation occurs to develop the embryo.	Calories	*340 kcal extra per day
	Three basic layers of tissue form and develop into three different organs (ectoderm, mesoderm, and endoderm).	Protein	60 g
		Iron	27 mg
	Ectoderm (outer layer) becomes the brain, nervous system, skin, and hair.	Calcium	1,000 mg
	Mesoderm (middle layer) produces all the bones, voluntary muscles, and all parts of the cardiovascular and excretory systems.	Folic acid	600µg
		Thiamin	1.4 mg
	Endoderm (inner layer) forms all the glands and all parts of the respiratory and digestive systems.	Riboflavin	1.4 mg
		Niacin	18 mg
		Vitamin C	85 mg
		Vitamin D	5 µg
		Vitamin A	770 µg
Third stage: 8–40 weeks (term).	Intensive maternal physiologic growth occurs.	Calories	*452 kcal extra per day
		Protein	60 g
		Iron	27 mg
		Calcium	1,000 mg
		Folic acid	600 µg
		Thiamin	1.4 mg
		Riboflavin	1.4 mg
		Niacin	18 mg
		Vitamin C	85 mg
		Vitamin D	5 µg
		Vitamin A	770 µg

*Pregnant women need extra kilocalories per day.

Data from: Williams SR. *Nutrition and Diet Therapy*. 7th ed. St. Louis, MO: Mosby; 1993.

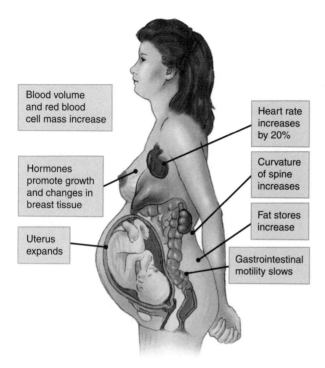

Maternal changes during pregnancy.

Women with chronic diseases such as diabetes should be evaluated about their effect on pregnancy and should receive the best therapy for a better pregnancy outcome.[15]

The Importance of Folate

Preconception folate status is an important concern because inadequate folate very early in the pregnancy can cause ***neural tube defects (NTD)*** including spina bifida and anencephaly.[15,16] Women of childbearing age should be aware of the importance of folate on ***fetus*** development.

In the United States, about 4,000 pregnancies each year are affected by the incidence of NTDs.[17] Daily intake of 400 μg of folic acid throughout the period before and after conception could prevent 50 to 70 percent of the incidences.[18] Krishnaswamy and Madhavan Nair reported that the incidence of NTDs could be cut in half if all women have an adequate folate intake during the preconception period.[19]

Women can obtain enough folate by consuming a good basic diet and a fortified breakfast cereal (e.g., Smart Start, Total, or Product 19) or a regular breakfast cereal (e.g., Cheerios, corn flakes, or raisin bran). Prior to cereal fortification, mean total folate intake in U.S. women was about 250 μg per day.[17] Cereal fortification is estimated to increase folate intake in most women by an average of 80 μg per day. Efforts to prevent birth defects should include more than cereal fortification, but also include other folate sources such as orange juice, cooked asparagus, lentils, and lettuce. Vegans and other strict vegetarians also should take a supplement of vitamin B_{12} because their diets contain no animal products, which are the main source of B_{12}. Low folate and vitamin B_{12} levels are independent risk factors for NTDs.[17,20] **Table 8.3** provides more information about the Dietary Reference Intake (DRI) recommendations for specific nutrients before and during pregnancy. **Box 8-1** presents a case study on preconception health.

> **trophoblast** The outer layer of embryonic ectoderm that nourishes the embryo or develops into fetal membranes with nutritive functions.
>
> **phenylketonuria (PKU)** An inherited error in phenylalanine metabolism, most commonly caused by a deficiency of phenylalanine hydroxylase, which converts the amino acid phenylalanine to tyrosine.
>
> **neural tube defect** Developmental abnormality resulting in anencephaly (absence of a brain) or spina bifida (spinal-cord or spinal-fluid bulge through the back); related to folic acid deficiency.
>
> **fetus** The developing infant from 8 weeks after conception until birth.

excretion of the end products of folate, niacin (N'methylnicotinamide), and pyridoxine metabolism, and of intact riboflavin increases. In contrast, the serum levels of several fat-soluble nutrients such as carotene and vitamin E (tocopherol) increase as much as 50 percent during pregnancy; however, vitamin A levels seem unchanged.[7]

Public health and community nutritionists need to interpret the laboratory results of pregnant clients against gestational norms, not against the nonpregnant female standards. It also may be necessary to conduct biochemical assessments throughout gestation.[10]

Preconception Health

Preconception counseling is a type of preventive medicine that consists of risk assessment, health promotion, and intervention. Therefore, it may be the most critical aspect of prenatal care for the prevention of birth defects. All women of childbearing age should be considered at risk for birth defects and be advised about preventive activities. This includes folic acid supplementation, rubella and hepatitis B immunization, avoiding tobacco use, alcohol use, and substance abuse, following instructions for appropriate nutrition and weight gain, avoiding pesticides, and undergoing genetic carrier screening (e.g., ***phenylketonuria [PKU]***, sickle cell anemia, etc.), depending on ethnicity. Genetic screening is important because about 3,000 to 4,000 U.S.-born women of childbearing age have had babies with PKU but without severe mental retardation thanks to the strict medical nutrition therapy they received during pregnancy.[11-13] Infants are at very high risk for mental retardation if women with PKU do not maintain a low phenylalanine diet during pregnancy. PKU is an inherited disorder in phenylalanine metabolism, primarily caused by a deficiency of phenylalanine hydroxylase, which converts the amino acid phenylalanine to tyrosine. Blood phenylalanine levels before and throughout the pregnancy must be maintained to prevent an undesirable outcome.[14]

SPINE AFFECTED BY SPINA BIFIDA

Skin on back
Spinal fluid
Spinal cord
Vertebra

Spina bifida is a neural tube defect.

TABLE 8.3			**Nutrient Requirements Before and During Pregnancy**		
Nutrient	**Pregnant**	**Non-Pregnant**	**Importance in Pregnancy**	**Risk Factors for Deficiency**	**Concerns**
Iron	27 mg	14–18 y: 15 mg 19+ y: 18 mg	• Iron "costs" of pregnancy are approximately 1 g. • Needed for maternal red blood cells. • Incorporated into the placenta and the developing fetus. • Anemia raises maternal cardiac workload and may place the fetus at risk for preterm birth.	• Pregnancy • Heavy menstrual blood loss prior to conception • Frequent blood donation • Multiple gestations • Vegetarian diet • Low intake of Vitamin C • Chronic aspirin use	• Few women can meet the demand for iron with diet alone. • Encourage vitamin C intake to enhance absorption of iron. • Milk, coffee, and tea inhibit iron absorption and should not be consumed with iron supplements.
Folate (DFE)	600 μg	400 μg	• Essential for cell metabolism and replication. • Needed for hemoglobin synthesis. • Plays role in DNA and RNA synthesis. • Deficiencies present with elevated homocysteine levels and macrocytic anemia.	• Diet poor in foods that supply folic acid: add fortified whole grain bread and cereal, legumes, leafy vegetables, fruit, and yeast • Cigarette smoking • Alcohol abuse • Oral contraceptive use • Malabsorption syndrome	• Teach the importance of adequate folic acid intake to lower the risk of neural tube defects. • Supplementation should begin prior to conception because closure of the neural tube occurs by the 28th day of gestation.
Vitamin C	18 y: 80 mg 19+ y: 85 mg	14–18 y: 65 mg 19+ y: 75 mg	• Promotes collagen synthesis for use in connective tissue. • Has antioxidant properties. • Assists in the absorption of other nutrients and drugs.	• Poor dietary intake • Cigarette smoking • Drug and alcohol abuse • Aspirin use • Oral contraceptive use	• No known link of deficiency to pregnancy outcome. • Transports easily to the fetus; high doses during pregnancy may cause dependency and scurvy symptoms in babies.
Vitamin B$_6$	1.9 mg	14–18 y: 1.2 mg 19+ y: 1.3 mg	• Required for protein, lipid, and carbohydrate metabolism. • Helps form nonessential amino acids and neurotransmitters. • Theories suggest a potential link between B$_6$ and problems related to pregnancy: nausea and vomiting, preeclampsia, and depression.	• Inadequate dietary intake	• Pregnant women may need help to evaluate scientific claims of a role for B$_6$ supplementation. • Although fetal growth increases B$_6$ needs during pregnancy, no clear evidence exists to support its use in treating problems related to pregnancy.
Thiamin Riboflavin Niacin (NE)	1.4 mg 14 mg 18 mg	14–18 y: 1.0 mg 19+ y: 1.1 mg 14–18 y: 1.0 mg 19+ y: 1.1 mg 14 mg	• These B complex vitamins function primarily to release energy from cells. • Deficiencies harm fetuses in animal studies but similar effects in humans have not been identified.	• Women in the U.S. take insufficient quantities of thiamin and riboflavin from dietary sources to meet needs during pregnancy.	• Thiamin and riboflavin have a low potential for toxicity. • High doses of nicotinic acid (a form of niacin) may cause flushing and gastrointestinal problems at high doses.

TABLE 8.3 (Continued)

Nutrient	Pregnant	Non-Pregnant	Importance in Pregnancy	Risk Factors for Deficiency	Concerns
Vitamin B_{12}	2.6 μg	2.4 μg	• Needed for normal cell division and protein synthesis.	• History of gastric resection or malabsorption • Strict vegetarian diet	• Supplementation is normally not necessary during pregnancy. • Monitor for signs of deficiency in vegans. • Nontoxic, but the effects of high doses on the fetus are not known.
Pantothenic acid	6 mg	5 mg	• Regulates adrenal activity, essential for gluconeogenesis and carbohydrate and lipid metabolism.	• Deficiency is rare; needs may increase with malabsorption.	• Supplementation is generally not needed during pregnancy.
Vitamin A (RAE)	14–18 y: 750 μg 19+ y: 770 μg	700 μg	• Poor maternal vitamin A status in undernourished populations increases preterm birth, intrauterine growth, retardation, and low birth weight.	• Deficiency is rare in the U.S. but widespread in developing countries. • Fat malabsorption.	• Excess vitamin A causes a variety of fetal abnormalities in animals. • Inform women of reproductive age to avoid high doses of vitamin A, including the derivative found in some acne medications.
Vitamin D*	5.0 μg	5.0 μg	• Regulates the use of calcium in mother and baby. • Deficiencies are linked to neonatal hypocalcemia and maternal osteomalacia.	• Northern climates with low exposure to sunlight • Darkly pigmented skin • Low intake of vitamin D–fortified milk	• Supplementation is not needed during pregnancy if milk consumption is adequate. • Toxicity may cause excess calcium absorption in fetus.
Vitamin E	15 mg	15 mg	• Acts primarily as an antioxidant. • Deficiency is associated with spontaneous abortion in animals but human effects are not clear.	• Fat malabsorption • Impaired bile secretion or pancreatic function	• Deficiencies are common among premature infants but this may not reflect maternal vitamin status.
Vitamin K*	14–18 y: 75 μg 19+ y: 90 μg	14–18 y: 75 μg 19+ y: 90 μg	• Essential for blood clotting. • Transfer of maternal vitamin K to the fetus is limited.	• Fat malabsorption • Long-term antibiotic therapy	• Most newborns in the U.S. receive vitamin K by injection shortly after birth.
Calcium*	14–18 y: 1,300 mg 19+ y: 1,000 mg	14–18 y: 1,300 mg 19+ y: 1,000 mg	• Essential for formation of fetal skeleton and teeth.	• Diet lacking in milk products	• Supplement pregnant women who do not consume dairy foods.
Phosphorous	14–18 y: 1,250 mg 19+ y: 700 mg	14–18 y: 1,250 mg 19+ y: 700 mg	• Essential for formation of fetal skeleton and teeth.	• Deficiency is rare because phosphorous is found in a variety of foods.	• Studies suggest that an imbalance of phosphorous and calcium causes leg cramps during pregnancy.
Magnesium	14–18 y: 400 mg 19–30 y: 350 mg 31 y: 360 mg	14–18 y: 360 mg 19–30 y: 310 mg 31 y: 320 mg	• Used for tissue growth and cell metabolism.	• Deficiency is rare because magnesium is widely distributed in food. • Absorption increases when intake is low.	• Routine supplementation during pregnancy is not necessary.

(continues)

TABLE 8.3 *(Continued)*

Nutrient	Pregnant	Non-Pregnant	Importance in Pregnancy	Risk Factors for Deficiency	Concerns
Iodine	220 μg	150 μg	• Acts as an essential component of thyroid hormones. • Iodine deficiency causes cretinism in newborns. • Also may cause more subtle cognitive and developmental impairments.	• Deficiency is not prevalent in the United States.	• Pregnant women should use iodized salt to avoid deficiency. • Excessive doses may cause congenital goiter.
Zinc	14–18 y: 12 mg 19+ y: 11 mg	14–18 y: 9 mg 19+ y: 8 mg	• Used in forming DNA and RNA. • In animal models, deficiency causes fetal malformation; human studies show poor pregnancy outcomes with zinc deficiency.	• Deficiency may occur in women taking iron supplementation for anemia.	• Suggest zinc supplementation for pregnant women taking more than 30 mg of iron daily. • Excessive zinc has been associated with preterm labor and stillbirth.

Dietary Reference Intakes: recommended intakes of vitamins and minerals for individuals. DFE, dietary folate equivalent; NE, niacin equivalents; RAE, retinol activity equivalents, α-tocopherol.

Note: Values are presented as Recommended Dietary Allowance (RDA), which are set to meet the needs of 97 to 98 percent of individuals in a group. Nutrients followed by * are listed as adequate intake (AI), indicating that some uncertainty exists regarding the percentage of individuals covered by this intake.

Source: Worthington PH. *Practical Aspects of Nutritional Support: An Advanced Practice Guide*. Philadelphia, PA: Saunders; 2004. Reprinted with permission.

Box **8-1 Case Study on Preconception Health**

Angela, a 22-year-old college student, visited the student health center with complaints of stress, heavy menstrual blood loss, and tiredness. During the nutrition assessment with the university dietitian, she disclosed that she does not like to drink milk or eat other dairy products. She likes to drink coffee (brewed, regular), at least five cups a day, and eats breakfast only on weekends. The psychosocial evaluation revealed that Angela works 30 hours a week as a bartender in a local pub where smoking is allowed and lives in an apartment with her recently unemployed husband, Andrew. Both Angela and her husband are full-time students. They have discussed starting a family after graduating from college, but their parents want grandchildren now. They currently are not practicing any birth control methods. Further interviews revealed that Angela has minimal knowledge of preconception nutrition; she consumes a diet of take-out foods that is high in fat, sodium, and sugar with infrequent consumption of fresh fruits or vegetables. She drinks three or four cans of beer on weekends with Andrew and smokes one pack of cigarettes a week. She does not do any physical activity because she is very busy and does not like to exercise. Their yearly income is below 130 percent of the U.S. poverty guideline.

Activities
- Explain the benefits of following the MyPyramid food guide and provide Angela with a pamphlet containing the Dietary Guidelines.
- Teach her how to follow MyPyramid.
- Encourage her to stop smoking and to start some physical activity. Explain the benefits of physical activity and quitting smoking.
- Explain the effects of inadequate folate and iron intake and relate them to preconception care.
- Encourage Angela to participant in the Food Stamp and/or WIC programs. Explain the function and eligibility criteria of both programs.

Adequate preconception nutrition is essential to a successful pregnancy.

Factors That Can Influence the Outcome of a Pregnancy

Many factors affect the health of a mother and her fetus and require special sensitive counseling.[6] These factors include, but are not limited to, socioeconomic status, age and parity of the mother, inadequate prenatal care, use of illegal or over-the-counter medications, prenatal ketosis, caffeine, alcohol, cigarette smoking, and pica. These and other factors are discussed in the following sections. **Box 8-2** lists the modifiable practices or conditions that are harmful to the developing fetus.

Low Socioeconomic Status

Community and public health nutritionists need to pay close attention to low-income or poor women and young girls. Some of the socioeconomic situations that can cause problems during pregnancy include inadequate healthcare, poor health practices, and lack of education.[21]

Community nutritionists should refer low-income pregnant women to government programs such as the Special Supplemental Nutrition Program for Women, Infants, and Children (WIC), the WIC Farmers' Market Nutrition Program (FMNP), and other state and federal programs so they can get help with food, housing, and health insurance (Medicare or Medicaid). The WIC program provides vouchers for specified nutritious foods along with nutrition education to low-income

pregnant or postpartum women, infants, and children less than 5 years of age who are nutritionally at risk. The FMNP can play an important role in reducing nutrition-related complications in low-income pregnant women.[22] It builds on the WIC program by providing additional vouchers to selected WIC recipients to help them buy fresh produce at local farmers' markets. This can reduce nutrition-related problems such as iron deficiency anemia and NTD.

Age and Parity

Pregnancy at very early or later age of the reproductive cycle creates high-risk situations. The obstetric history of a woman is expressed in terms of number and order of pregnancies, or the gravida status. But a pregnant 15-year-old or younger is at high risk because she has not completed her own growth; therefore, adequate weight gain and the quality of her diet are essential and need special attention.[23] However, a primigravida (first pregnancy) older than 35 years also needs special attention because of the complications that are associated with bearing children later in the reproductive cycle. These complications include, but are not limited to, hypertension, either preexisting or pregnancy-induced, obesity, diabetes, and having a child with Down syndrome.[6]

In addition, having children too close together can deplete a mother's nutritional stores, making each successive pregnancy a higher risk.[6] Infants born less than a year apart are more likely to be born with a low birth weight than those further apart in age. In Zhu et al.'s study, the risks of low birth weight, preterm birth, or small size for gestational age were higher for infants conceived fewer than 6 months apart compared to those conceived 18 to 23 months apart.[24] Both shorter and longer interpregnancy intervals were associated with higher risks. Infants conceived 18 to 23 months after a live birth had the lowest risk.[24] This risk was more prevalent among younger and Hispanic women. Community and public health nutritionists should pay close attention to these risk factors, especially in women who have other risk factors (e.g., use of tobacco or alcohol, and those at a younger or older maternal age).

Inadequate Prenatal Care

Inadequate, absent, or delayed prenatal care are associated with potential negative pregnancy outcomes. The negative outcomes include anemia, gestational diabetes, nutritional deficiencies in the fetus; for mothers suffering from chronic diseases, such as hypertension or diabetes, the risk of fetal damage can increase.[25,26] Prenatal care includes physical examinations, lab tests, nutritional counseling, and regular checkups, which can help detect preexisting conditions and possible complications, as well as help women know what to expect during their pregnancy. Lack of prenatal care can cause a woman to deliver a low-birth-weight baby, and the baby is more likely to die during the first 4 weeks of life than a normal-birth-weight infant.[27] The ideal time to start prenatal care is before conception. Yet, about 20 percent of women in the United States receive no prenatal care in the first trimester.[7]

Illegal or Over-the-Counter Drug Use

Drug use, both recreational and medicinal, also poses numerous problems.[28] The use of over-the-counter medication poses potential adverse effects. For example, over-the-counter medications (OTC) contain both active and inactive ingredients (colorings, sweeteners, flavorings, and preservatives) that are often combined, which may cause unfavorable interactions.[29] The most frequently used OTC medications are cold remedies that typically contain 15 inactive ingredients plus active

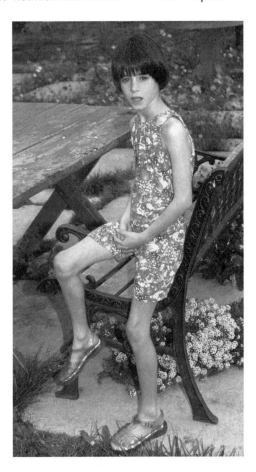

Consumption of alcohol during pregnancy may cause irreversible brain damage, mental retardation, and facial abnormalities.

ingredients, any of which could have interactions.[30] Pregnant women are discouraged from using OTC medications without medical advice. However, in a retrospective study of 2,752 mothers who gave birth to normal infants, results showed that two-thirds of these mothers used OTC medication one and one-half times more often than prescribed medication.[31] Results also showed that the use of OTC medications correlated positively with multiple illnesses, higher socioeconomic status, and European American women. In another study, pregnant women also reported that they used between 2.3 and 2.6 OTC medications during pregnancy.[32,33]

In addition, megadosing with basic nutrients such as vitamin A during pregnancy may cause fetal damage. In particular, drugs made from vitamin A compounds—retinoids such as Accutane or etretinate that are prescribed for severe acne—are harmful to the fetus. Reports show that they have caused spontaneous abortions of malformed infants by women who conceived during such acne treatment.[6,34]

The use of street drugs is especially hazardous, exposing the developing fetus to the risks of addiction and possibly AIDS due to the mother's use of contaminated needles. Cocaine has the most devastating consequences for the developing fetuses.[35,36] As cocaine use has become more common, the number of infants born to cocaine-using women has increased.[37] Maternal use of cocaine during pregnancy is linked to preterm birth, low birth weight, and other physical malformations in newborns. Community nutritionists should explain to pregnant women that exposure of the fetus to cocaine disrupts the development of the brain and nervous system and may reduce interactive behaviors and responses to environmental stimuli.[38]

Caffeine During Pregnancy and Lactation

Information on the effects of caffeine consumption during pregnancy on the fetus is mixed. The Food and Drug Administration (FDA) recommendation for pregnant women is to avoid caffeine or to consume it sparingly because caffeine can enter into the bloodstream through the placenta, and the developing fetus has a limited ability to metabolize it. Caffeine is also known to decrease the availability of calcium, iron, and zinc.[39] It can affect fetal heart rate and breathing.[40] The recommendation is to limit intake to one cup of coffee or 12 ounces of caffeinated beverages per day. **Table 8.4** shows the caffeine content per serving of some common foods.[39,41] Caffeine does pass into breast milk; therefore, consumption during lactation also should be limited.

Alcohol and Cigarette Smoking

Consumption of alcohol during pregnancy may cause irreversible brain damage, growth retardation, mental retardation, facial abnormalities, and vision abnormalities.[42] Results of one research study showed that excessive consumption of alcohol affects fetal development and causes fetal alcohol syndrome (FAS), irreversible damage to the brain, and mental and physical retardation in the fetus.[42] Community nutritionists should discourage the use of alcohol during pregnancy and explain to clients that FAS is preventable by abstaining from alcohol during pregnancy.

Dietitians should explain that alcohol does not increase milk volume and that chronic consumption can inhibit the milk ejection reflex. The American Academy of Pediatrics (AAP) recommends that the breastfeeding mother should avoid drinking alcohol because it can pass to the baby through the breast milk. However, AAP recommends that if breastfeeding mothers choose to drink alcohol, they should do so just after breastfeeding rather than just before. The allowable alcohol consumption while breastfeeding is no more than 2 to 2.5 ounces of liquor, 8 ounces of wine, or 2 cans of beer on any day.[43]

Cigarette smoking is responsible for 20 to 30 percent of all low-birth-weight deliveries in the United States and increases the risk of infant mortality.[3] Carbon monoxide and nicotine from smoking increase fetal carboxyhemoglobin, reduce placental blood flow, and limit the oxygen supply to the fetus. Also, women who smoke cigarettes are at risk of delivering low-birth-weight infants.

Pica

Pica is a persistent compulsive consumption of nonfood items. It is an unusual type of craving that is more common during pregnancy. Pica is more common in African American than Caucasian women, in rural rather than urban women, and in women with a family history of the practice.[44] It is a recognized complication of pregnancy because it contributes little or no nutritional value. Pica occurs worldwide, and it is found in both genders and in all ages and races. It is of special concern because pregnant women and their children may absorb toxic substances, such as lead, from the material they consume. Fecal impaction and parasite infections (from ingested soil) also may occur in women and children who experience pica.[45]

Pica is classified into four categories distinguished by the substance consumed: *Geophagia* is the consumption of earth and clay, *amylophagia* is the consumption of starch, and *pagophagia* is excessive

TABLE 8.4	Caffeine Content of Selected Foods Per Serving		
Food Name	**Serving Portion**	**Caffeine Content (mg)**
Candy, semisweet chocolate	1 oz	17.58
Candy, sweet chocolate	1 oz	18.71
Cocoa powder, unsweetened	1 Tbsp	12.42
Coffee, brewed, regular	6 fl oz	103.24
Coffee, brewed, espresso	6 fl oz	377.54
Coffee, instant, regular, prepared	6 fl oz	57.28
Coffee, instant, decaffeinated, prepared	6 fl oz	1.79
Coffee, instant, cappuccino flavor, prepared	6 fl oz	74.88
Coffee, instant, French flavor, prepared	6 fl oz	51.03
Coffee, instant, mocha flavor, prepared	6 fl oz	33.84
Cola beverage, regular	12 fl oz	37.00
Cola beverage, diet	12 fl oz	49.70
Ice cream, chocolate	0.5 cup	40.92
Milk, chocolate	8 fl oz	5.00
Tea, brewed	6 fl oz	35.60
Tea, instant, unsweetened, prepared	6 fl oz	23.14
Tea, instant, unsweetened, lemon flavored, prepared	6 fl oz	19.64

Source: The U.S. Department of Agriculture Nutrient Database for Standard Reference, release 11-1; and The Nutrition Coordinating Center, University of Minnesota, Nutrition Data System for Research, database version 38. *Table Caffeine Content of Selected Common Foods per Serving*. The Nutrition Coordinating Center, University of Minnesota; 2007. Reprinted with permission.

$\mathcal{B}$ox 8-2 Modifiable Practices That Are Harmful to the Developing Fetus[47,48]

- Drinking alcohol (causes birth defects)
- Heavy use of aspirin (causes bleeding)
- Using illegal drugs such as cocaine or using over-the-counter medications (causes birth defects)
- Smoking (causes low-birth-weight infants and other problems)
- Inadequate diet such as few or no fruits and vegetables or dairy products or a great deal of high-fat and -sugar food (may cause anemia, birth defects, obesity, etc.)
- Excessive vitamin A intake (above 10,000 IU [3,000 RAE/day]) and megadose use of other nutrient supplements (may cause birth defects)
- Excessive caffeine intake—more than one cup of coffee or 12 ounces of caffeinated beverages per day, such as Coca-Cola, tea, chocolate, and coffee (affects fetal heart rate and breathing, can cause low-birth-weight infants)

eating of ice. The fourth (miscellaneous) category includes consumption of ash, chalk, antacids, paint chips, baking soda, mothballs, wax, charcoal, burnt matches, hair, and other substances.[46]

The origin of this practice is not well understood. The nutritional hazards most frequently linked with pica are lead poisoning and iron deficiency anemia, but it is not clear whether pica is a cause of these problems.

Mother and Father's Health

Adequate nutrient intake is important for a successful pregnancy. During pregnancy, eating healthfully is essential for a positive outcome for both the fetus and the mother. Pregnant women should be encouraged to plan their food intake using the dietary food guide presented in **Table 8.5**.

Community nutritionists also should advise fathers-to-be to consider their eating and other habits. Limited evidence suggests that men who consume too few fruits and vegetables containing vitamin C or who drink too much alcohol in the weeks before conception may sustain damage to their sperm's genetic material. This damage can cause birth defects in future children.[49] Also, if they practice eating nutritiously, it can encourage the mother-to-be to eat nutritiously.

Maternal Weight Gain During Pregnancy

Appropriate weight gain during pregnancy is necessary for a successful pregnancy outcome. For this reason, health professionals have adopted the Institute of Medicine (IOM) guidelines regarding weight gain. A review found that the best pregnancy outcomes were obtained when the weight-gain guidelines (shown in **Table 8.6**) were followed.[52] Weight gain below the recommendations was associated with a risk of preterm delivery and low birth weight; those above the suggested range had a higher risk of cesarean delivery and excessive postpartum weight retention.

Although African American women are at greater risk of delivering low-birth-weight babies, an empiric evaluation of the IOM's pregnancy weight-gain guidelines by race does not support a recommendation that these women should strive for weight gains in the upper half of the IOM recommended range[53] because the data show questionable benefits in the reduction of risk for low-birth-weight babies.

Obese women have a greater risk of pregnancy complications, including *gestational diabetes*, hypertensive disorders, cesarean deliveries, and postoperative morbidity. Infants of obese women also may be at greater risk for perinatal death.[54,55]

Rate of Weight Gain

The recommendation for pregnancy weight gain is to gain a total of 3 to 5 pounds during the first trimester and 1 pound per week for the second and third trimesters. In 1996, the Maternal Weight Gain Expert Group

pica The practice of eating nonfood items such as dirt, laundry starch, or clay.

gestational diabetes Diabetes that appears during pregnancy.

| TABLE 8.5 | Diet Planning Guide for Pregnant, Lactating, and Non-Pregnant Women[a,50,51] |

Food Groups	Non-pregnant Women	Pregnant or Lactating Women	1,600 Calories	2,000 Calories	2,600 Calories	3,100 Calories	Serving Sizes	Examples of Foods	Major Source Of
Grains[b]	6–11 servings	7 to 11 (7+) servings	6 servings	7–8 servings	10–11 servings	12–13 servings	1 slice bread / 1 oz dry cereal / ½ cup cooked rice, pasta, or cereal	Whole wheat bread, English muffin, pita, bagel, cereals, grits, oatmeal, crackers, unsalted pretzels, and popcorn	Energy and fiber
Vegetables	3–5 servings	4–5 (5+) servings	3–4 servings	4–5 servings	5–6 servings	6 servings	1 cup raw leafy vegetables / ½ cup cooked vegetables / 6 oz vegetable juice	Tomatoes, potatoes, carrots, green peas, squash, broccoli, turnip greens, collards, kale, spinach, artichokes, green beans, lima beans, and sweet potatoes	Rich sources of potassium, magnesium, and fiber / Vitamin A & C
Fruits	2–4 servings	3–4 (4+) servings	4 servings	4–5 servings	5–6 servings	6 servings	6 oz fruit juice / 1 medium fruit / ¼ cup dried fruit / ½ cup fresh, frozen, or canned fruit	Apricots, bananas, dates, grapes, oranges, orange juice, grapefruit, grapefruit juice, mangoes, melons, peaches, pineapples, prunes, raisins, strawberries, and tangerines	Important sources of potassium, magnesium, vitamin C, and fiber
Dairy products, low-fat or fat-free dairy foods	2 servings	3–4 (4+) servings	2–3 servings	2–3 servings	3 servings	3–4 servings	8 oz milk / 1 cup yogurt / 1 ½ oz cheese	Fat-free or low-fat milk, fat-free or low-fat buttermilk, fat-free or low-fat regular or frozen yogurt, and low-fat and fat-free cheese	Major sources of calcium, vitamin D, and protein
Meats, poultry, fish	2–3 servings	3 (3+) servings	1–2 servings	2 or less servings	2 servings	2–3 servings	3 oz cooked meat, poultry, or fish	Select only lean; trim away visible fats; broil, roast, or boil instead of frying; remove skin from poultry	Rich sources of protein, vitamin D, and magnesium
Nuts, seeds, legumes	2–3 servings (¼ cup of cooked dry beans or peas equals 1 ounce of products in the meat and beans group)	3 (3+) servings	3–4 servings/ week	4–5 servings/ week	1 serving	1 serving	⅓ cup or 1½ oz nuts / 2 Tbsp or ½ oz seeds / ½ cup cooked dry beans or peas	Almonds, filberts, mixed nuts, peanuts, walnuts, sunflower seeds, kidney beans, and lentils	Rich sources of energy, magnesium, potassium, protein, and fiber

[a]This plan is based on 1,600, 2,000, 2,600, and 3,100 calories. The number of daily servings in a food group and amounts vary to accommodate a participant's caloric and nutritional needs or food preferences. This table can help in planning menus and food selection in homes, restaurants, and grocery stores.

[b]Whole grains are recommended for most servings to meet fiber recommendations.

[c]Equals ½ to 1¼ cups, depending on cereal type. Check the product's Nutrition Facts Label.

[d]Fat content changes serving counts for fats and oils. For example, 1 Tbsp of regular salad dressing equals 1 serving; 1 Tbsp of low-fat dressing equals ½ serving; 1 Tbsp of fat-free dressing equals 0 servings.

TABLE 8.6	Recommended Range of Weight Gain for Pregnant Women[56,57]				
Prepregnancy Weight-for-Height Body Mass Index (BMI)	Weight Category	Total Weight Gain (Pounds)	Total Weight Gain (Kilograms)	Weight Gain First Trimester (Pounds)	Weight Gain Second and Third Trimesters (Pounds Week)
< 19.8	Underweight	28–40	12.5–18.0	5.0	1.07
19.8–26.0	Normal weight	25–35	11.5–16.0	3.5–5.0	0.97–1.0
26.0–29.0	Overweight	15–25	7.0–11.5	2.0	0.67
> 29.0	Obesity	15–25	7.0		0.50

*The range for women with twins is 35 to 45 pounds (16.0–20.5 kilograms). The range for women with triplets is 45 to 55 pounds (20.5 to 25.0 kilograms). Young adolescents (< 2 years after **menarche**) and African American women should strive to gain at the upper end of the range. Short women (less than 62 inches tall [< 157 cm]) should strive to gain at the lower end of the range. Weight gain varies widely, and these values are suggested only as guidelines for identifying individuals whose weights may be too high or low for health.

of the National Academy of Sciences suggested a weight gain of 1.5 pounds per week for normal weight women during the second half of a twin pregnancy.[57]

The weight gain of pregnant women consists of water, protein, and fat. The measurements of maternal water gain may predict birth weight better than measurements of composite weight gain. The total amount of weight gained, the composition of gain, and the rate of energy metabolism differ among healthy pregnant women. **Table 8.7** presents typical weight-gain distribution.[39] Many women express concern regarding the weight they gain during pregnancy; community nutritionists should advise them that only a small amount of fat is stored and that the stored fat will be a source of energy for breastfeeding.

Pregnant women should avoid dieting to lose weight because pregnancy is an anabolic state that requires additional calories to support the growth and metabolic activity of the fetus, *placenta*, and maternal tissues. In addition, pregnancy uses calories to build maternal fat stores that supply the energy needed to meet the metabolic demands of late pregnancy and lactation.[58] Women's energy needs increase 340 kcal/day during the second trimester and 452 kcal/day during the third. This extra energy can be obtained from milk, vegetables, and grains.

menarche The onset of menstruation (monthly bleeding); normally happens between 10 and 15 years of age.

placenta An organ that forms inside the uterus early in pregnancy. The placenta transfers oxygen and nutrients from the mother's blood to the fetus; fetal wastes are removed through the placenta, and it releases hormones that maintain the pregnancy.

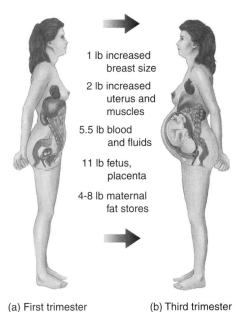

1 lb increased breast size

2 lb increased uterus and muscles

5.5 lb blood and fluids

11 lb fetus, placenta

4–8 lb maternal fat stores

(a) First trimester   (b) Third trimester

Components of maternal weight gain.

TABLE 8.7	Typical Weight Distribution During Pregnancy		
Source		Pounds	Kilograms
Amniotic fluid		2.0–2.6	4.4–5.7
Fetus		7.0–8.5	15.4–18.7
Fat/breast tissue stores for breastfeeding		1.0–4.0	2.2–8.8
Increased blood volume		4.0–5.0	8.8–11.0
Increased weight of uterus		2.0	4.4
Maternal fat stores		4.0–7.0	8.8–15.4
Placenta		2.0–2.5	4.4–5.5
Extra tissue fluid		3.0–5.0	6.6–11.0
Total		**25–35**	**55–77**

Source: Berdanier CD, Feldman EB, Flatt WP. *Handbook of Nutrition and Food*. Washington, DC: CRC Press; 2002. Reprinted with permission.

Box **8-3   The Effects of Prenatal Ketosis**[38,59]

The fetal brain uses **ketone bodies** poorly. Crash diets or fasting for more than 12 hours during pregnancy is not advisable. A pregnant woman can develop significant ketosis after only 20 hours of fasting. Eating about 100 g of carbohydrates every day prevents ketosis. Even non-pregnant women usually eat twice this amount. Community nutritionists should discourage mothers from skipping meals or dieting, especially during pregnancy.

Box **8-4   Remedies for Nausea and Vomiting**[6,38]

- Eat small, frequent meals.
- Eat dry/cold foods.
- On waking, arise slowly.
- Chew gum or suck on hard candies.
- Take prenatal vitamins and iron supplements on a full stomach or at a time of day when feeling well.
- Avoid caffeine.
- Eat combinations of foods that are salty and tart.
- Avoid spicy foods, acidic foods, and strong odors.
- Sniff lemon.

Energy needs during the first trimester are the same as for nonpregnant women.[6,38]

Dietitians working with pregnant women should explain to their clients that adequate weight gain reduces the risk of low-birth-weight infants and that crash diets may cause prenatal **ketosis** and slow down the fetus's brain development (see **Box 8-3**). They should encourage their clients to plan their food intake using the dietary guidelines presented in **Table 8.5**.

Diet-Related Complications of Pregnancy

Several complications of pregnancy may impact nutritional status. Some of these include nausea and vomiting, *hyperemesis gravidarum* (severe nausea, dehydration, and vomiting during pregnancy), constipation, and gestational diabetes.

Nausea and Vomiting/Morning Sickness

Approximately 70 percent of pregnant women experience nausea during the first 14 to 16 weeks of pregnancy, and 37 to 58 percent of them experience vomiting. This is due to the hormonal changes that occur early in pregnancy. The incidents range from mild queasiness to unbearable nausea. Many women complain that smells—mainly cooking smells—make them sick. The remedies for this condition may include diet changes, the use of ginger extract, increased fluids, and reassurance.[58,60] **Box 8-4** provides suggestions that may help to combat nausea.

Heartburn, Constipation, and Hemorrhoids

Heartburn is a burning sensation in the lower esophagus near the heart. This is common during pregnancy because a hormone produced by the placenta, progesterone, relaxes the muscles in both the uterus and the intestinal tract. This often causes heartburn as stomach acid flows back into the esophagus.[49] The remedies are to not lie down after eating, to eat less fat so the foods pass more quickly from the stomach into the small intestine, and to avoid spicy foods.

Constipation is common in pregnancy due to decreased motility of the gastrointestinal tract caused by the relaxing hormone of the placenta (progesterone). Iron supplementation also increases the incidence of constipation, as do low fiber and low fluid intake. The recommendation is to consume 20 to 30 grams of dietary fiber daily, perform exercise regularly, and eat dried fruits, such as dried apricots and plums.[61,62]

Straining during elimination can lead to hemorrhoids, and it may be necessary to reevaluate the need for and dose of iron supplementation and the dietary patterns of the client.[63]

Anemia

Blood volume increases during pregnancy; this leaves proportionately fewer red blood cells in a pregnant woman's bloodstream.[64] The lower ratio of red blood cells to total blood volume is a condition known as physiological anemia. It is a normal response to pregnancy; however, anemia also may result from inadequate iron stores and a low dietary iron intake, and may be a condition that requires medical attention.[65]

In some cases, iron-deficient women have normal hemoglobin values. However, such women do not have iron stores to draw from during illness, injury, or pregnancy. The consequences of iron deficiency are iron deficiency anemia and low blood volume. Iron deficiency anemia at the beginning of pregnancy is linked to a risk of preterm delivery and low-birth-weight infants.[66,67] In addition, iron deficiency during pregnancy is very dangerous because it increases the risk of maternal and infant death significantly and may contribute to low iron status in the infant. Iron deficiency has been attributed to low scores on intelligence, language, gross motor development, and attention tests in affected children at the age of 5 years.[66,68,69]

Pregnant women should be encouraged to eat iron-rich foods such as lean red meat, fish, poultry, dried fruits, and iron-fortified cereals. It has been reported that meat and ascorbic acid–rich fruits increase nonheme iron absorption. Whole grain cereals, unleavened whole grain breads, legumes, tea, and coffee should be consumed separately from iron-fortified foods and iron supplements because they reduce iron absorption.[66,67,70]

Pregnancy-Induced Hypertension

Another serious disorder whose symptoms may include high blood pressure, edema, and protein in the urine is pregnancy-induced hypertension. In very severe form, kidney failure, convulsions, and even death of the mother and fetus may occur. In its mild forms it is known as preeclampsia, and in severe forms as *eclampsia*. The exact cause is not known, but calcium, magnesium sulfate supplements, and bed rest may lower the risk of preeclampsia.[71]

Gestational Diabetes Mellitus

Gestational diabetes mellitus (GDM) is glucose intolerance during pregnancy. Individuals who were diagnosed as diabetic before pregnancy are not classified as having gestational diabetes. Screening for gestational diabetes is recommended between 24 and 28 weeks of pregnancy using a 50 g, 1-hour oral glucose challenge.[72]

GDM occurs in about 3 to 4 percent of all pregnancies, resulting in approximately 135,000 cases annually in the United States, but it disappears at the end of the pregnancy. Women who have had gestational diabetes mellitus are at increased risk for developing type 2 diabetes later, however. Some studies have reported that about 40 percent of women with a history of GDM were subsequently diagnosed as having diabetes.[73] The risk factors for GDM include pregnancy after age 30, obesity, previous congenital abnormalities, previous stillbirth, and family history of type 2 diabetes.[73] The major concerns for the fetus of gestational diabetic individuals are high birth weight (9 pounds at term or in the 90th *percentile* in weight for gestational age), hypoglycemia at birth, and increased incidence of obesity.

Foodborne Illness During Pregnancy

Pregnant women are at high risk for foodborne illness.[74,75] The most common causes of diarrhea during pregnancy are several food- or waterborne pathogens such as bacteria, protozoa, or viruses including the *Salmonella* species, *Helicobacter pylori*, *Shigella*, *Escherichia coli* (*E. coli* O157:H7), and *Cryptosporidium*.[76] Hepatitis A also is a food- or waterborne pathogen of concern. During pregnancy, listeriosis, caused by *Listeria monocytogenes*, can result in premature delivery, stillbirth, or infection in the newborn.[77] *Toxoplasma gondii* is a protozoan that can be passed from the mother to the fetus and can result in infant death or mental retardation.[78] The following are guidelines for pregnant women to avoid foodborne illnesses:[77-81]

- Do not consume unpasteurized juices, raw sprouts, or raw (unpasteurized) milk products.
- Avoid raw or undercooked meat, poultry, eggs, fish, or shellfish.
- Cook leftovers and ready-to-eat food (e.g., hot dogs) until steaming hot, and avoid homemade cheese, cheese purchased from street vendors, and soft cheeses such as Brie, feta, blue, and Camembert to avoid listeriosis.
- To avoid toxoplasma, wash hands thoroughly after handling cat feces and cleaning the cat litter box.
- Handle all foods safely by washing hands with warm soapy water, and cook food thoroughly.

The Food and Drug Administration also advises pregnant women to avoid consuming large fish, including shark, swordfish, king mackerel, and tilefish, because these fish accumulate unsafe levels of methylmercury.[82] A moderate amount (6 to 12 ounces or less per week) of other fish (tuna steaks, halibut, snapper, canned albacore, or chunk white tuna) may be safe during pregnancy. Pregnant women should contact their state or local health departments for more information or advisories on fish caught or sold in their local markets.

See **Box 8-5** for additional risk factors in pregnancy.

Nutrition Assessment During Pregnancy

Nutrition assessment is an essential component of the nutritional care of a pregnant woman. It provides the foundation for planning a woman's education, individualized care, and direction throughout the pregnancy, which is necessary for a positive outcome for both the mother and baby. The nutrition assessment during pregnancy addresses the three stages of gestation and the postpartum stage. Preferably, the first prenatal visit should be a follow-up of the preconception visit. However, preconception visits are not yet common. The assessment performed during the first prenatal visit is influenced by the stage of gestation.[39,56]

Nutrition assessment during pregnancy should include the use of the Nutritional Risk Tool provided in **Table 8.8** that shows a quantitative method for assessing a client's diet.[39] The client's usual intake is determined for each of the food groups (meats and alternatives, dairy, bread and cereal, fruits and vegetables) and the score is tallied. A client with less than 80 points is at nutritional risk. Clients with a score less than 50 should receive dietary counseling. The dietitian also should determine whether the client has problems such as nausea, vomiting, lactose intolerance, constipation, or cravings for nonfood items. In addition, **Table 8.9** can be used to assess for risk factors and referral for counseling and nutrition intervention

Box 8-5 Pregnancy Risk Factors[82,83]

Risk Factors Present at the Onset of Pregnancy
- Age < 15 years or > 35 years
- Frequent pregnancies: three or more during a 2-year period
- Poor obstetric history or poor fetal performance
- Poverty
- Abuse of nicotine, alcohol, or drugs
- Therapeutic diet required for a chronic disorder
- Weight < 85 percent or > 120 percent of standard weight
- Level of education (less than high school education)

Risk Factors Occurring During Pregnancy
- Low hemoglobin or hematocrit: Hgb < 12 g; Hct < 35 mg/dl
- Inadequate weight gain: Any weight loss or weight gain of < 1 kg (2 lb)/month after the first trimester
- Excessive weight gain: > 1 kg (2 lb)/wk after the first trimester
- Late prenatal care
- Genetic make-up

ketone bodies The compounds, such as acetone and diacetic acid, formed when fat is metabolized incompletely.

ketosis The physical state of the human body when ketone bodies are elevated in the blood and present in the urine; one example is diabetic ketoacidosis.

hyperemesis gravidarum Excessive vomiting that produces weight loss and dehydration during pregnancy.

eclampsia Advanced pregnancy-induced hypertension (PIH) that is characterized by convulsions.

percentile Classification of a measurement of a unit into divisions of 100 units.

<table>
<tr><td colspan="2">

TABLE 8.8 **Nutritional Risk Score (Massachusetts Department of Health)**

</td></tr>
</table>

Foods Usually Eaten	Amount
Meat or alternatives = Meats, fish, poultry (fresh or processed), liver, eggs, nuts, peanut butter, legumes	_____ servings
1 oz = 5 points	_____ oz of meat, fish, cheese
Maximum score = 40 points	_____ oz alternate
Milk (type _____) 1 unit = 5 points	_____ fluid
1 unit = 8 fl oz.	_____ cups
Cheese[ab] (type _____)	_____ oz
Maximum score = 15 points	
Bread[c] **and cereal** = whole grain, enriched, others	_____ servings
Maximum score = 15 points	
Fruits and vegetables = citrus and/or vitamin C–rich vegetables, green and yellow vegetables, all others, including potato	_____ servings _____ servings _____ servings
vitamin A vitamin C	_____ serving
1 unit = 5 points 1 unit = 5 points	
2 units = 15 points 2 units = 15 points	
Supplements[d] (type _____)	_____ amount
Other foods and beverages	

Total score: more than 80 = no risk, less than 80 = risk, less than 50 = high risk

[a]Cheese in excess of the 3 units scored in milk; 1 oz cheese equals 1 unit.

[b]Maximum of 3 oz scored.

[c]Unit = 1 slice of bread or 1 oz cereal. Less than 3 units = 0, 3 units = 5 points, 4 units = 10 points, 5 units = 15 points.

[d]Not given a score.

From: Kennedy ET. A prenatal screening system for use in a community-based setting. *J Am Diet Assoc.* 1986; 86:1372–1375. Copyright Elsevier (1986). Reprinted with permission.

<table>
<tr><td colspan="3">

TABLE 8.9 **Risk Factors for Prenatal Nutritional Risk**

</td></tr>
</table>

Risk Factor	Low Risk	High Risk
Is the client preadolescent, adolescent, or less than 3 years postmenarche?	No	Yes
Is the client economically disadvantaged or does the client have a limited income for food?	No	Yes
Does the client have a history of anemia or is anemic (hematocrit < 32 mg/percent during pregnancy)?	No	Yes
Is the client's BMI < 19.8 or > 26.1?	No	Yes
Does the client have a history of fad dieting or restrictive eating?	No	Yes
Does the client have an illness or medication that will interfere with absorption; is she HIV+?	No	Yes
Does the client use tobacco, alcohol, or drugs?	No	Yes
Does the client practice pica (consume ice, starch, clay, or other substances in large amounts)?	No	Yes
Does the client experience nausea and/or vomiting?	No	Yes
Is the client lactose intolerant?	No	Yes
Is weight gain 0.8–1.0 lb/wk?	No	Yes
Does the client stay within the weight gain range recommended for her prepregnancy BMI?	No	Yes
Is weight gain < 15 lbs or > 45 lbs?	No	Yes

From: Berdanier CD, Feldman EB, Flatt WP. *Handbook of Nutrition and Food.* Washington, DC: CRC Press; 2002. Reprinted with permission.

programs.[39] The techniques for assessing a pregnant woman's needs are outlined in **Table 8.10** and may include personal history (demographic, social, etc.), dietary assessment, clinical observations and physical examination, anthropometry, and laboratory data. These criteria may be used for assessing and monitoring nutritional status, planning care, and promoting the health of pregnant women.

Adolescent Pregnancy

In the United States, about 1 million adolescent girls between the ages of 12 and 19 become pregnant each year.[84] Many teenage women, es-

pecially the youngest ones, have not had time to store the nutrients needed to support their own rapid growth and development, much less store nutrients needed to support pregnancy and a developing fetus. Adolescents have more miscarriages, premature births, stillbirths, and low-birth-weight infants than adult women.[85,86] Undoubtedly, teenage pregnancy is a major public health problem.

The personal and societal impact of teenage pregnancy in the United States is huge; an estimated 84 percent of teenage pregnancies are unintended (i.e., they occur sooner than desired or are not wanted at the time).[87] Research shows that post-neonatal mortality rates were higher for mothers aged 12 to 17 years after adjusting for socioeconomic and other known risk factors. The high post-neonatal mortality rate observed in this study was attributed to increased risk of accidental and infectious deaths in these infants. These incidences could be due to maternal maturity and ability to adequately supervise these developing infants. Results also showed that participation in WIC and Medicaid was helpful in reducing the neonatal mortality rate.[88]

More than 70 national health and social welfare organizations support age-appropriate comprehensive school health-education programs to reduce teenage pregnancy.[89] These programs counsel abstinence as well as provide teenagers with the knowledge and skills they need to

TABLE 8.10	Criteria for Assessing and Monitoring Nutritional Status During Pregnancy and Postpartum[56,85,86]				
Stages/Visits	**Personal History Data**	**Dietary Assessment**	**Clinical and Physical Examination**	**Anthropometric Assessment**	**Laboratory Measures**
First trimester	Age Medical records: • Review previous obstetrical history • Medical condition • Genetic disorder • Medications/supplements • Number of pregnancy • Parity (number of children born alive) • Breastfeeding experience Socioeconomic status: • Low income • Inadequate access to food Education level Substance abuse Cigarette use Living situation Cultural background Sleep pattern (7 to 8 hours)	Dietary history: Pica practice Lactose intolerance Food allergies and intolerances PKU	General examination of gums, teeth, tongue, eyes, and hair History of pregnancy-induced hypertension (PIH), gestational diabetes, or iron deficiency anemia	Measurements of height, weight, BMI, and skinfold measurements (as needed)	Hemoglobin and hematocrit Screen for anemia, urine analysis for ketone bodies, glucose, and protein levels
Second trimester/ follow-up visits	Review medical records Food assistance programs (WIC, Food Stamp Program, etc.)	Dietary history Additional probing of dietary practice Dietary supplements (iron, folate) and nutrients deficiency	Screen for anemia, dental health Iron, B_{12}, and folate deficiency	Weight gain using BMI measures	Hemoglobin and hematocrit Urinalysis for ketone bodies, protein, and glucose levels
Third trimester/ follow-up visits	Review medical records Food assistance programs (WIC, Food Stamp Program, etc.)	Additional probing of dietary practice Dietary supplements (iron, folate)	Screen for anemia, dental health Iron, folate, and B_{12} deficiency	Rate of weight gain	Hemoglobin and hematocrit Urinalysis for ketone bodies, protein, and glucose levels
Postpartum visits	Review medical records Support at home Assistance with initiating breastfeeding Avoidance of harmful substances Adequate rest	Dietary history Availability of food Review the need for food assistance programs (WIC, Food Stamp, etc.)	Screen for anemia, dental health Iron, folate, and B_{12} deficiency	Weight management method after delivery	Check for postpartum anemia if heavy blood loss occurred at delivery

avoid unplanned pregnancies. In addition to health education efforts, family-planning services for sexually active teenagers are essential for reducing teenage pregnancy.

The pregnant adolescent is viewed as a high-risk individual who is highly susceptible to poor pregnancy outcomes. Identification of pregnant adolescents and management of their problems and concerns should be a primary goal of community health organizations. The following are issues in adolescent pregnancy that influence nutritional well-being and that need to be addressed in intervention strategies:[85]

- *Acceptance of the pregnancy:* The desire to carry out a successful pregnancy and acceptance of responsibility

- *Food resources:* Family meals (timing, quantity, quality) and food assistance (willingness to participate in WIC)
- *Body image:* Degree of acceptance of an adult body, maturity in facing bodily changes throughout pregnancy
- *Living situation:* Acceptance by partners and extended family, financial support, and ethnic group (religious, cultural, and social patterns)
- *Relationship with the father of the child:* Presence or absence of the father, quality of relationship, influence on mother's nutritional habits, tolerance of physical changes in pregnancy, and physical needs of mother and child
- *Peer relationship:* Support from friends and their influence on general lifestyle
- *Nutritional state:* Weight-for-height proportion, tissue stores of nutrients, history of dietary patterns and nutritional status, substance use, and activity patterns
- *Prenatal care:* Initiation of and compliance with prenatal care and dependability on supporting resources.

Physical Activity During Pregnancy

Research shows that physical activity can facilitate labor and reduce psychological stress. Women who remain active during pregnancy report fewer discomforts throughout their pregnancies and gain less weight than those who are not physically active.[90] Studies show that structured exercise three or four times per week during the third trimester produced lower infant birth weights.[39] The odds of a lower infant birth weight were substantially increased for those who exercised five or more times per week and modestly increased for those at the other extreme, who engaged in structured exercise two or fewer times per week.[91] Physical activities during pregnancy should be chosen with care. See **Box 8-6** for physical activity guidelines and the warning signs to stop physical activity.

Nutrition in Infancy

Infancy is defined as the period between birth and 1 year of age. Early infancy from birth to 6 months of age is when the most rapid growth happens. Middle infancy is from 6 to 9 months, when growth slows but is still rapid, and late infancy is 9 to 12 months, when growth slows and babies' maturation and activity allow them to eat a wider variety of foods. The average weight of a healthy term infant is 7.7 lb (3.5 kg).[39] Full-term newborns who weigh less than 5.5 lb. (2.5 kg) are **small for gestational age (SGA)**. Infants lose about 10 percent of their body weight in the first week of life, but both breast-fed and formula-fed infants should regain it within 2 weeks of age. This first year of life is critical for the rapid growth of all major organ systems. This rapid growth rate makes nutrition a critical element of caring for infants. Nutrition during this time influences how an infant will grow and thrive.

The Special Supplemental Nutrition Program for Women, Infants, and Children (WIC) is a federal health, nutrition, and prevention program with a successful record of improving diet and reducing infant mortality and morbidity. The infant mortality rate in the United States has decreased slightly from 6.84 in 2003 to 6.78 in 2004.[92] However, the U.S. IMR remains higher than that of many other industrialized countries. Infant mortality rates vary widely by racial and ethnic group and geographically, with the highest rate among infants born to African American mothers in the largest U.S. cities. It also has been reported that infant mortality rates are higher for infants born preterm or with a low birth weight.[93]

Box 8-6 Guidelines and Warnings for Physical Activity

Activity Guideline

Intensity	Reduce the intensity of exercise by 25 percent.
Heart rate	Do not exceed 140 beats per minute.
Temperature	Do not go above 101 degrees.
Time	Moderate activity should not exceed 30 minutes; intersperse with low-intensity exercise and rest periods.
Position	Avoid lying on back for more than 5 minutes after entering the second trimester.
Frequency	Exercise should be performed consistently at least three times per week and include a warm-up and a cool-down period.

Warning Signs to Stop Physical Activity

- Vaginal bleeding
- Uterine contractions
- Nausea, vomiting
- Dizziness or faintness
- Difficulty walking
- Decreased fetal activity
- Palpitations or rapid heart rate
- Numbness in any part of the body
- Problems with vision

Modified from: Berdanier CD, Feldman EB, Flatt WP. *Handbook of Nutrition and Food.* Washington, DC: CRC Press; 2002. Reprinted with permission.

Nutritionists and other healthcare professionals can use different intervention strategies to help reduce the incidence of infant mortality and improve the health of mothers. For example, the Infant Health and Development Program (IHDP) examined the effect of regular home counseling, free daycare center programs, and participation in a parental support group on more than 1,000 infants and families. The mothers of 377 infants received the 3-year intervention; the control group was closely monitored and mothers were referred to all appropriate community services. Results showed that the intervention made a significant difference in the development of the premature and low-birth-weight infants and their mothers. The intervention group infants had significantly higher IQs, fewer behavioral problems, and no major illness; in addition, their mothers were less depressed and less likely to smoke compared to the control group. After 5 years, the differences between the intervention and control groups lessened.[94]

Physical Growth and Development Assessment

Community and public health dietitians use anthropometric measurements as well as **growth charts** to monitor children's growth and development. Infants double their birth weight by 4 to 6 months and gain about 5 to 7 ounces a week. They typically triple their birth weight in 1 year.[95,96] Body weight is measured with an electronic scale or a beam balance without detachable weights. Infants gain about 1 inch per month from birth to 6 months and gain one-half inch per month from 6 to 12 months. They typically increase their *length* by 50 percent in their first year.[95,96] The measurement of length requires two examiners using a calibrated length board with a fixed headpiece and movable footboard.

Head circumference is measured with a narrow flexible steel or paper tape applied to the head above the eye ridges and encircling the most prominent parts of the forehead and the back part of the head or skull. A maximum of three measurements are used to determine the maximal circumference.

Normal growth is a strong indicator of nutritional adequacy and the overall health of an infant. During routine checkups throughout childhood and adolescence, nutritionists and other healthcare professionals measure weight, height (or length), and head circumference and plot these values on growth charts. Each growth chart consists of a set of curves called percentiles that show the distribution of values for U.S. children based on a certain measurement.[39,59,97] The latest growth charts can be obtained on the Centers for Disease Control and Prevention website at http://www.cdc.gov/growthcharts.

Length and head circumference are more sensitive measures than weight for assessing a baby's growth and nutritional status. Weight alone reflects recent nutritional intake. Head circumference measures brain growth and development. Chronic malnutrition can limit brain growth and is reflected in inadequate gains in head size. Head circumference measurements are more useful in infants and children up to 2 years of age.[97,98]

Introduction to Solid Food

Weaning is the ending of breast- or bottle-feeding and substitution of food for breast milk or infant formula. The American Academy of Pediatrics recommends that solid foods be introduced between the ages of 4 and 6 months.[99] This range allows for differences in growth and development among babies. **Table 8.11** presents suggestions for adequate supplemental foods for infants.

infancy The period between birth and 1 year of age.

small for gestational age (SGA) Full-term newborns who weigh less than 2.5 kg (5.5 lb).

growth chart Charts that plot the weight, length, and head circumference of infants and children as they grow.

length The proper measurement method of infants and children not yet able to stand.

head circumference Measurement of the largest part of an infant's head to determine brain growth.

TABLE 8.11	Age-Specific Introduction of Food[59,100–102]		
Food	**Amounts**		**Age of Introduction**
Breast milk or formula	16–32 oz/day		0–4 months
Iron-fortified baby cereal, rice, barley, oatmeal (start with rice cereal)	1 Tbsp cereal mixed with human milk or formula; gradually increase the amount of cereal to 3–4 Tbsp once or twice a day		4–6 months
Human milk or formula	24–32 oz per day		
Strained or pureed vegetables plus fruits such as mashed bananas, pears, applesauce, and fruit juices	Vegetables, 2 Tbsp twice per day and fruits, 2 Tbsp twice a day; fruit juices 1–2 ounces twice per day		6–8 months
Toast or teething biscuits, iron-fortified cereal	2–4 Tbsp twice per day		
Human milk or formula	24–32 oz per day		
Water	2–4 oz twice per day		
Strained meats	1–2 Tbsp twice a day		6–8 months
Egg yolk, yogurt	1–2 Tbsp per day		6–8 months
Well-cooked, soft, bite-sized pieces of meats	2–3 Tbsp per day		9–10 months
Fruit juices	1–2 oz twice per day		
Vegetables, carrots, banana, applesauce, spinach, squash	2–4 Tbsp twice per day		
Soft breads, infants' cereal, creamed rice, and other finger foods	2–3 Tbsp twice a day		
Human milk or formula	16–32 oz per day		
Water	2–4 oz per day		
Egg white; small tender pieces of meat, chicken, or fish; mild cheese; cooked dried beans	1 oz or ¼ cup twice per day		12 months
Infant cereals, bread, rice, noodles	2–4 servings per day		
Cooked vegetable pieces and all fresh fruits, peeled and seeded	¼ cup twice per day		
Human milk or formula	16–32 oz per day		
Water	2–4 oz per day		

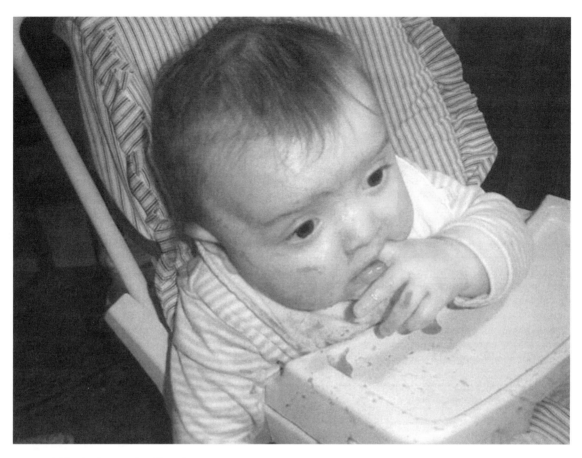

Eating solid foods after months of liquids is enjoyable.

Water

Infants have higher insensible water losses (the continual loss of body water by evaporation from the respiratory tract and diffusion through the skin) as well as a higher overall metabolic rate. They are more susceptible to developing dehydration from vomiting and diarrhea, especially if solute intake is high, as it is in cow's milk. Infants need 1.5 milliliters of water per kilocalorie consumed. Human milk fulfills this need, and properly prepared formula accomplishes the same task. Foods high in protein or electrolytes, such as meat and eggs, may cause dehydration if offered without water.[59] Water should be offered to infants regularly once they are eating solid food (2 to 4 ounces twice a day). **Table 8.12** presents some rules for introducing solid foods.

Nutrient Needs During Infancy

Energy

Because of the rapid growth that occurs during infancy, babies' energy and nutritional requirements are always changing. As mentioned earlier, infants usually double their birth weight by 4 to 6 months and triple it by 1 year.[59,96,100] Infants require about 108 kcal/kg of body weight per day from birth to 6 months, about 650 kcal/day. The recommended amount of calories for infants 6 to 12 months is 98 to 100 kcal/kg body weight, about 850 kcal/day.[100] Infants need a higher energy intake than adults because the resting metabolic rates of infants and their needs for growth and development are very high. A normal infant pulse rate is 120 to 150 beats per minute, and their normal respiratory rate is 30 to 50 breaths per minute.[101] Because of the large proportion of skin surface to body size, temperature regulation takes significant energy. Also, an activity such as crying may double the infant's energy expenditure.[59,101]

Protein

The recommended amount of protein for infants birth to 6 months is about 2.2 g/kg body weight, and for 6 to 12 months is 1.6 g/kg body weight. It is important to include the nine essential amino acids; any deficiency in any of the amino acids can cause growth retardation.[97] The protein in breast milk is easy to digest and contains all the essential amino acids infants need. Human milk contains about 70 percent whey and 30 percent casein (phosphorus-containing proteins). The whey portion of milk consists of soluble proteins that are easily digested. The major whey protein in breast milk is alpha-lactalbumin, which has an amino acid prototype much like that of the body's tissues. The infant's body can absorb it easily and without much processing; infants use it for building tissue.[101] In comparison, cow's milk contains about 18 percent whey and 82 percent casein. Casein forms hard curds in the infant's stomach that they cannot digest or absorb.[97]

Carbohydrates and Fats

Carbohydrates and fats contribute the majority of an infant's energy. The carbohydrate in human milk and in infant formulas made from cow's milk is lactose.[97] Infants digest lactose easily and tolerate it well.

TABLE 8.12	Some Rules for Introducing Solid Foods[39,59,85,97]	

Actions	Alternative Actions
• Introduce one new food at a time for three to five days, and check for reactions such as stomachaches, diarrhea, skin rashes, or wheezing. Then start with the next food.	• If the child rejects it, try the same food later. • Keep diapering areas separate from food preparation areas.
• The best first food is iron-fortified infant rice cereal mixed with breast milk or formula. It provides a good source of iron as well as a good distribution of calories, protein, fat, and carbohydrate. Rice cereal is less likely to cause an allergic reaction than other foods. Offer cereal on a spoon, not in a feeding bottle.	• Delay introduction of allergenic foods such as cow's milk, eggs, peanuts, fish, shellfish, soy, and wheat, especially in families with a strong history of allergies. • Start with one cereal feed daily until the child is taking two meals daily and getting a daily total of ⅓ to ½ cup.
• Avoid adding salt, sugar, and other seasonings or using foods such as hot dogs, canned spaghetti dinners, and canned soups because their high salt content can put an additional load on the infant's kidneys.	• Provide a wide variety of foods. Feeding infants a variety of foods enhances their acceptance of new foods. • Offer cereal on a spoon unless medically indicated by conditions such as esophageal reflux.
• Avoid putting solid foods in the bottle. • Parents should be the first ones to introduce new foods and changes in a child's feeding routine. • Wash all fruits and vegetables, and cook meat until juices run clear and no pink remains. • Infants younger than 12 months of age should not consume honey or corn syrup because these products can cause a potentially fatal form of food poisoning (spores of clostridium). _botulinum_	• Do not force-feed. • Parents should decide and determine how the child will be fed. • Delay introducing foods that the child cannot break down easily in the mouth such as popcorn, nuts, hard candy, hot dogs, and raw fruits and vegetables (such as grapes and carrots) because they can lead to choking, especially in children less than 3 years old. Also avoid peanut butter on bread; it can form a sticky bolus and block the child's airway.

Breast milk contains amylase, which is 40 to 60 times more active than in cow's milk.[102] The lactose in milk supplies galactose, which is important for the formation of brain cells.[101]

Fat is important for the development of the central nervous system and provides most of the infant's energy source. Human milk contains alpha-linolenic acid, an essential omega-3 fatty acid, which can be converted to eicosapentaenoic acid (EPA); and docosahexaenoic acid (DHA). Research shows that visual acuity and learning abilities correlate with the amount of DHA in the retina and brain phospholipids.[103] About 95 to 98 percent of the fat in human milk is absorbed because breast milk contains the enzyme lipase, which begins the digestion process for the infant.

Vitamins and Minerals

Vitamin and mineral needs are usually met if the infant is breastfed by a well-nourished mother or receives well-prepared infant formula. Infant formula is fortified with all essential vitamins and minerals according to guidelines established by the AAP and enforced by the FDA.

Vitamin B_{12} is needed for the division of cells and normal folate metabolism. Recent research with vegan women showed that they produced milk containing only one-fourth to one-third as much vitamin B_{12} as women consuming a mixed diet.[104] Another research study reported vitamin B_{12} deficiencies in strict vegetarian breastfeeding mothers, which caused severe neurological deterioration in 4- to 8-month-old infants.[105] Mothers who included meat, fish, and dairy products in their diets produced milk that was adequate in vitamin B_{12}.[97] However, compared to meat, cow's milk alone is not a good source of B_{12}.

Vitamin D is important for calcium absorption and mineralization of bone. However, human breast milk contains more vitamin C and less vitamin D than cow's milk. The vitamin D precursor in breast milk can be converted to vitamin D in the infant's skin if the infant is exposed to sunlight. Therefore, Vitamin D deficiency may be a concern for infants who are not exposed to sunlight.[97,101]

Infants need the same minerals as other human beings. The two-to-one calcium-to-phosphorus ratio of breast milk is ideal for calcium absorption, and both of these minerals, along with magnesium, support the rate of growth expected in a human infant. Calcium is needed for tooth development, muscle contraction, nerve irritability, blood coagulation, and heart muscle action. Infants can absorb about 67 percent of the calcium in breast milk, compared to 25 percent of the calcium in cow's milk.[102]

Another mineral that is important for the formation of hemoglobin and mental and psychomotor development is iron.[106,107] An infant's fetal iron stores are depleted 4 to 6 months after birth. Therefore, solid food additions at this time will help supply the iron the infant needs. Iron-fortified cereal, eggs, and later meat will achieve this task. Iron-fortified formula and foods were found to reduce the incidence of iron deficiency anemia in children from homeless families enrolled in WIC.[108,109]

Breast milk contains less iron than cow's milk, but infants absorb about 49 percent of it compared to about 10 percent from cow's milk. Iron absorption from breast milk is better because it contains less protein and phosphorus and more lactose and vitamin C.[102] The bioavailability of zinc in breast milk is about 60 percent, compared to 43 to 50 percent in cow's milk and 27 to 32 percent in infant formulas.[49,110]

Nutrition-Related Health Concerns During Infancy

Community nutritionists, parents, and other healthcare professionals need to be observant about feeding practices that may cause health-related problems in infants. Some of the health-related problems are due to improper feeding practices and poor nutrient intakes. For example, mothers may replace human milk or formula with large amounts of fruit juice before 6 months of age; use goat's milk that is low in iron, folate, and vitamin C; and not provide a variety of foods to their infants. Other problems include, but are not limited to, feeding bottle tooth decay, iron deficiency anemia, milk allergies, and failure to thrive.

Feeding Bottle Tooth Decay

Tooth decay during infancy, also known as **dental caries**, is linked to putting infants to bed with bottles filled with milk, juice, or other carbohydrate-rich fluids that nourish decay-producing bacteria. The upper teeth are affected most because the tongue protects the lower teeth. To prevent feeding bottle tooth decay:[97,101]

- Avoid giving a bottle filled with human milk, formula, or juice to quiet the infant or to encourage sleep.
- Encourage the infant to sleep by holding the baby snugly, and creating a gentle, regular motion/rocking. (Other options are reading, or rubbing or patting the infant's back while holding him or her on the shoulder and chest.)
- Clean the infant's gums and teeth twice a day using a washcloth on the gums and a soft toothbrush with water on the teeth.
- Introduce a drinking cup at 6 months and provide juice in a cup instead of a bottle, limiting juice to 4 to 6 ounces per day.
- Use fluoridated water, approximately 0.8 to 1.0 mg/L parts per million (PPM).

Iron Deficiency Anemia

Iron deficiency in infants is not as common as in toddlers. Factors that may cause iron deficiency anemia in infants are inadequate dietary iron intake, too much milk feeding (known as milk anemia), and not enough iron-fortified solid foods.[49,109] The onset of anemia is common in infants after their fourth month when iron stores are depleted, their birth weight has increased, and they are synthesizing new red blood cells daily.[110]

The Pediatric Nutrition Surveillance System (PedNSS) reported that the highest prevalence of anemia in the United States was in children younger than age 2; however, the prevalence decreased as the children grew older. The rate of anemia was high in infants ages 6 to 11 months (16.2 percent) and children ages 12 to 17 months (15.0 percent). The rate of anemia varied among racial and ethnic groups. African American children had the highest rate of anemia (19 percent). The overall prevalence of anemia in children in the United States decreased from 15.8 percent in 1994 to 12.8 percent in 2003.[111]

The Healthy People 2010 objectives (19.12c and 19.13) are to reduce iron deficiency to less than 7 percent among women ages 12 to 49 years and to reduce anemia among low-income pregnant females in their third trimester. The progress data show a decrease of 12 and 33 percent, respectively.

Milk Allergy

The risk of infants developing allergies doubles if a parent or sibling has allergies.[112] An infant may develop a food allergy to the protein in a cow milk–based formula over time. In a healthy infant, protein is broken down during digestion and allergy may result when small groups of two or three amino acids are absorbed in the small intestine. In some cases, the intestinal lining may allow larger chains of amino acids to be absorbed, triggering a reaction.[113]

The absorption of intact protein fragments is the basis for allergic reactions. When this happens with cow milk protein, the infant can be switched to a soy-based formula. In cases where soy formula still produces an allergic reaction, the infant can be switched to a predigested protein formula. About 6 to 8 percent of children fewer than 4 years of age have allergies that started in infancy.[113] The most common allergic reactions are respiratory and skin symptoms, such as wheezing or skin rashes.[114]

Failure to Thrive

Failure to thrive (FTT) is a term used when a decrease in or slow physical growth is observed over time using a national standard growth chart. Although the definitions of FTT vary, most practitioners diagnose FTT when a child's weight-for-age falls below the fifth percentile of the standard National Center for Health Statistics (NCHS) growth chart. Conversely, weight-for-height above the 95th percentile signifies a child who is overweight.[115] FTT is mainly used to describe conditions resulting from failure to obtain or use necessary calories.[115]

Different classification systems have been developed to identify the reasons for FTT in children, such as organic (meaning a diagnosed medical illness is the basis), nonorganic (meaning not based on a medical diagnosis), or a mixed FTT. Nonorganic FTT is generally due to a variety of environmental and psychosocial factors. It is associated with interactions between the primary caregiver and the infant. Any disturbance in the relationship between the primary caregiver and the infant can result in an inadequate provision of food. The following are some of the causes of nonorganic FTT:[111]

- Poor feeding or feeding-skills disorder
- Dysfunctional family interactions and difficult parent–child interactions
- Lack of preparation for parenting and lack of support (e.g., no friends, no extended family)

Organic FTT refers to growth failure due to an acute or chronic disorder known to interfere with normal nutrient intake, absorption, metabolism, or excretion or known to result in increased energy requirements to sustain and promote growth. The following are some examples of the causes of organic FTT:[116]

- Maternal malnutrition, and alcohol, smoking, medications, and infections during pregnancy
- Inborn error of metabolism

In mixed FTT, organic and nonorganic FTT overlap. The physician will determine each of the contributing factors to the child's abnormal growth. Mixed FTT is diagnosed in children who were born prematurely and who have evidence of disproportionate growth failure later in infancy, and in those who have a deformity.[116]

The role of the dietitian is to assess the infant's growth and nutritional adequacy, establish a care plan, and provide follow-up as part of a team approach. The dietitian may work with other health specialists and work on medical or psychological aspects of treatment. One of the goals for the management of FTT is to increase the infant's growth rate. The median expected increase in weight per day for infants is summarized in **Table 8.13**. On average, infants gain 1 kg/month for the first 3 months, 0.5 kg/month from 3 to 6 months, 0.33 kg/month from 6 to 9 months, and 0.25 kg/month from 9 to 12 months. FTT can occur

TABLE 8.13	**Median Daily Weight Gain**	
Age	**Grams**	**Ounces**
0–3 months	26.0–31.0	0.9–1.09
3–6 months	17.0–18.0	0.6–0.63
6–9 months	12.0–13.0	0.42–0.46
9–12 months	9.0	0.32

Modified from: Bassali RW, Benjamin J. Failure to Thrive. Available at: http://www.emedicine.com/PED/topic738.htm. Accessed September 27, 2005.

in all socioeconomic strata, but it is more common in families living in poverty.[117]

Children with FTT will need 150 percent of their recommended daily caloric intake, based on their expected, not actual, weight.[116] In infants, this increased caloric intake may be accomplished by concentrating formula or adding rice cereal to pureed foods. WIC also provides high-calorie milk drinks (e.g., PediaSure). It provides 30 calories per ounce, and one or two cans per day can be used.

Methods of Feeding Infants

Breastfeeding is the preferred method for feeding infants and has advantages over other methods of feeding.[117] However, some mothers may prefer to use formula as opposed to breast milk when feeding their infants. Some formulas are prepared according to ethnic or religious practices. Community nutritionists and healthcare professionals need to monitor these formulas closely. Mothers who are on prescription or illegal drugs also may consider using formula to feed their infants,[118] as may mothers who are HIV positive. Research studies indicate that not all women have the same risk of transmitting HIV to their breastfed infants. The factors that may increase the risk of transmission include early mixed feedings, nipple lesions, and mastitis (inflammation of the breasts).[119,120] Guidelines for formula preparation can be found online at http://nutrition.jbpub.com/communitynutrition.

Breastfeeding/Lactation

Human milk is the best choice for infants. It provides appropriate amounts of energy, nutrients, and **colostrum** that provides protection against infections, and it rarely causes allergic responses. The American Dietetic Association has issued position statements in support of breastfeeding.[121] The La Leche League, an international nonprofit organization, provides encouragement to women who wish to breastfeed.

In the United States, the Healthy People 2010 objective for breastfeeding is to increase the number of mothers who breastfeed their babies in the early postpartum period to at least 75 percent. The progress report shows an increase so far to 70 percent. This Healthy People 2010 breastfeeding goal appears to be within reach; however, considerable work remains to achieve the 50 percent goal for breastfeeding up to 6 months and the new 25 percent goal for breastfeeding at 12 months.[121] Only 31.4 percent of all infants are still being breastfed at 6 months of age and 17.6 percent are being breastfed at 12 months.[122] The greatest benefits of breastfeeding are associated with exclusive breastfeeding

for at least 6 months and continued breastfeeding with complementary foods for at least 12 months.[123,124] In an effort to achieve these goals, federally supported breastfeeding promotion efforts have continued to expand in number and scope, including the national USDA/WIC social marketing campaign for breastfeeding.

Barriers to Breastfeeding

Training new mothers in the hospital on how to initiate breastfeeding has the potential to boost breastfeeding, but the implementation of this practice is limited in some U.S. hospitals.[125] Delayed identification and treatment of lactation problems can lead to morbidity and excessive costs.[126] Several sociocultural factors also contribute to lack of or short-term breastfeeding, including some of the barriers outlined in **Table 8.14**.

There are many ways to facilitate breastfeeding and, therefore, support infant health and the mother–infant bond. Providing home visits during the newborn period can compensate for short hospital stays if personnel with training in assessment and management of lactation perform these visits. Rental of an electric pump or purchase of other

dental caries Tooth decay that results from formula or juice (and even human milk) bathing the teeth as the child sleeps with a bottle in his or her mouth.

colostrum The first fluid secreted by the breast during late pregnancy and the first few days after birth. This thick fluid is rich in immune factors and protein.

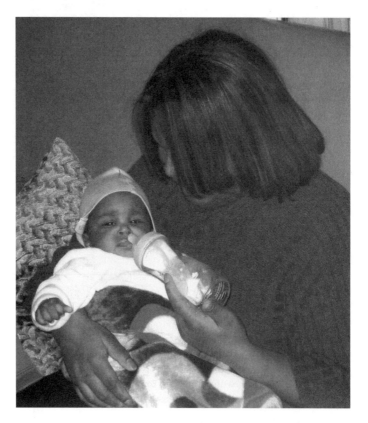

Mothers can use an electric pump to express breast milk. The mother should be instructed to wash her hands and breasts before handling the equipment or pumping. During feeding, the position of the baby and the bottle are both important.

TABLE 8.14	Barriers to Breastfeeding[127,128]

Barriers to Breastfeeding	Possible Solution
Loss of traditional knowledge and support for breastfeeding	• Reposition breastfeeding as a way for a family to establish a special relationship with their child from the very onset of its life.
Lack of generational breastfeeding experience	• Help mothers to breastfeed through mother-to-mother support. • Provide prenatal exposure to human milk. • Make home visits 2 weeks after discharge from the hospital. • Provide postpartum follow-up along with professional intervention. • Provide support from the pregnant woman's mother and healthcare professionals.
Teenage or single motherhood	• Communicate the importance of breastfeeding through family members and peers. • Provide prenatal exposure to human milk. • Provide home visits 2 weeks after discharge from the hospital. • Provide postpartum follow-up along with professional intervention.
Reliance on childcare outside the home	• Healthcare providers should assist mothers in identifying common misperceptions and helping mothers work through them.
Relatively short-term maternity leave	• Companies should institute policies that promote breastfeeding.
Inflexible work hours when returning to work	• Healthcare professionals and mothers should use a variety of methods and a broad range of outlets, including legislative, policy, and organizational development, and the media to promote breastfeeding. • They should use grassroots advocacy, professional training and education, peer counselor programs, and direct marketing and advertising to promote breastfeeding.
Lack of paid breastfeeding or pumping breaks in the workplace	• Employers can contribute to the health of their employees and their families by establishing a policy of support for breastfeeding mothers. • Mothers can rent an electric pump. • Encourage mothers to use break times during the work day to express milk, which can be stored and taken home at the end of the day and used for feedings.
Prolonged separation from the infant	• Employers can provide childcare at the facility. • Managers should ensure it is possible for staff to take breaks as appropriate.
Advertising campaigns that promote early termination of breastfeeding in the first 2 weeks	• Distribute educational materials to reach mothers, friends, and relatives at home and in various environments in which mothers and their friends and relatives obtain infant care information.
Marketing or providing commercial products during hospital discharge that promote maternal–infant separation, undermine maternal confidence, and contribute to early mixed feedings	• Use media as well as grassroots advocacy with a congratulatory tone to stress the importance of breastfeeding. • Provide postpartum follow-up along with professional intervention.

equipment (all of which are frequently not reimbursed by third-party payers) would be a valuable practice. Supportive work environments where mothers can have the infant present or have access to on-site or nearby facilities for time to pump and store milk would enhance the goal to increase the rate of breastfeeding.[127,128] **Box 8-7** presents the advantages of breastfeeding and the benefits of breastfeeding for mothers.

The Mother's Nutritional Needs During Lactation

The nutritional needs for a lactating mother are different from those of a pregnant woman (see the RDA and AI tables at the front of this book). The best approach is to eat a balanced diet using the *Dietary Guidelines for Americans*. The diet should supply at least 1,800 kcal per day. Milk production requires about 800 kcal every day. Based on an average milk secretion of 750 to 800 mL/day in the first 6 months and 600 mL/day in the second 6 months, the additional daily energy requirements become 640 kcal and 510 kcal, respectively. The reason for recommending 500 kcal daily above prepregnancy levels is because the 4 to 6 lb (2 to 3 kg) of fat retained postpartum can provide the remaining energy needed for lactation. Weight loss of 1 to 4 lb per month in the lactating mother is appropriate. Significant weight loss that occurs with severe dieting when an energy intake is less than 1,500 kcal/day greatly reduces milk output.[6,97,128]

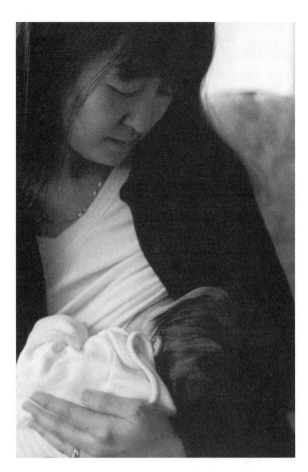

A mother's milk has the needed amounts of fat, sugar, water, vitamins, minerals, and protein for a baby's growth and development. Breastfeeding also helps a mother bond with her baby.

Management and Techniques for Successful Breastfeeding

Early mother–infant contact increases the duration of breastfeeding by as much as 50 percent, and nursing should be initiated immediately after delivery when possible. The guidelines for successful breastfeeding are presented in **Box 8-8**. Monitoring and assessing infant growth is an important part of identifying potential lactation problems. Healthcare professionals should recognize the following signs and symptoms of insufficient milk:[39]

- Infant lethargy and/or irritability
- Jaundice
- Infrequent defecating or urinating
- Failure to gain weight
- Excessive weight loss (7 to 10 percent of birth weight)

Supplemental Nutrition Programs During Pregnancy, Infancy, and Lactation

In the United States, several resources are available to pregnant women. Some of the resources include programs such as the federally funded Commodity Supplemental Food Program (CSFP), WIC, the Food Stamp Program, and other emergency food or financial assistance programs described below, as well as other state and local programs.

Box **8-7 Advantages of Breastfeeding for Infants and Mothers**[38,39,96,102,112,128–132]

Benefits for Infants

- Enhances protection against infectious disease early in life, including infectious diarrhea, lower respiratory tract disease, and middle ear infection
- Reduces overfeeding and decreases the incidence of obesity
- Promotes optimal development of the central nervous system
- Has a low sodium content and a low solute load
- Gathers minerals in breast milk that are bound to protein and are balanced to enhance bioavailability
- Is more economical
- Decreases tendencies towards obesity
- Avoids overfeeding as compared with formula feeding
- Lowers the incidence of constipation
- Provides immunologic protection
- May protect against developing allergies later in life
- Avoids risk of allergies associated with cow's milk protein
- Reduces risk of foodborne illnesses
- Facilitates close contact that fosters the mother–child relationship
- Reduces the need for sterilized equipment and formula preparation
- Provides enzymes that aid digestion and absorption of nutrients
- Decreases insulin-dependent diabetes
- Provides generous amounts of essential fatty acids, especially docosahexaenoic acid, and is nutritionally superior to any alternative
- Contains a powerful antibacterial agent called lactoferrin, which binds iron and keeps it from supporting the growth of harmful bacteria and fungi in the infant's intestinal tract

Benefits for Mothers

- Lactation amenorrhea
- Can help regulate maternal weight or fat loss
- Protects against premenopausal breast cancer and ovarian cancer
- Results in more optimal blood glucose profiles in women with gestational diabetes
- Lowers the risk of ovarian cancer by inhibiting ovulation

An example of a successful state-sponsored program promoting prenatal care is BabyCal, a public awareness and education campaign that has been carried out by the California Department of Health Services since 1991. The BabyCal outreach program used a statewide network of community-based support organizations (CBSO), along with a focused media campaign involving pop music and television personalities, to

- Examine the breasts and nipples for any potential problems.
- Inquire about the availability of prenatal breastfeeding classes.
- Seek breastfeeding support groups such as the La Leche League and local lactation consultants.
- Ensure appropriate positioning and latch-on to avoid breast soreness and/or engorgement.
- Schedule early follow-up visits at home or in a clinic setting.
- Nurse the baby at least 8 to 12 times in 24 hours (every 2 to 3 hours).
- Baby should have 4 to 6 wet diapers per day during days 2 to 4.
- Baby should have 6 to 8 wet diapers of light yellow urine per day after day 4.
- Baby should have 4 to 6 stools per day by the first week.
- Baby should sleep at least 2 hours after a feeding.
- Feedings should last at least 10 minutes per breast, but generally not more than 20 minutes per breast.
- The feeling of fullness in the breast signifies change from colostrum to milk.

reach low-income expectant mothers with messages stressing prenatal care, a healthy lifestyle during pregnancy, and the importance of infant immunization.[133]

In addition, the CBSO used various other methods to carry out the BabyCal program. For instance, they conducted health fairs to reach the majority of participants and developed wallet-sized pocket calendars to help expectant mothers keep track of their prenatal appointments. The BabyCal campaign continually explored unique opportunities to support its CBSO network. For example, for BabyCal's 10th birthday campaign, they introduced a 60-minute videotape designed to help CBSO educate pregnant women on the importance of prenatal care, healthy behaviors, and the availability of state programs that could help their clients pay for prenatal care services. The BabyCal program increased the rates of participation in prenatal care programs and over the past decade reduced statewide infant mortality by 15 percent.[133]

Clients screened and found to be at nutritional risk can be referred to various federal and state assistance programs, many of which are described in the following sections.

Commodity Supplemental Food Program (CSFP)

The Commodity Supplemental Food Program (CSFP) is a federal food assistance program that works to prevent malnutrition and improve the health of low-income pregnant and breastfeeding women, other new mothers up to 1 year postpartum, infants, and children up to age 6 by supplementing their diets with nutritious USDA commodity foods.[134] The population served by CSFP is similar to WIC, but CSFP also serves

elderly people and provides food rather than the food vouchers that WIC participants receive. Eligible people may not participate in both programs at the same time.[134]

The USDA purchases food and makes it available to state agencies and Indian Tribal Organizations (ITO). It also provides funds for administrative costs. State agencies that administer CSFPs are typically departments of health, social services, education, or agriculture. State agencies store the food and distribute it to public and nonprofit private local agencies for distribution to the recipients.[134]

Food packages include a variety of foods, such as infant formula and cereal; non-fat dry and evaporated milk; juice; farina; oats; ready-to-eat cereal; rice; pasta; egg mix; peanut butter; dry beans or peas; canned meat, poultry, or tuna; and canned fruits and vegetables. The most current list of foods is available at www.fns.usda.gov/fdd/programs/csfp.

Special Supplemental Nutrition Program for Women, Infants, and Children (WIC)

WIC provides food, nutrition counseling, and access to health services to low-income women, infants, and children.[135] It was established as a pilot program in 1972 and made permanent in 1974. The Food and Nutrition Service of the USDA administers WIC at the federal level.

The WIC program is funded as part of the Child Nutrition Program legislation to provide nutrition education and to improve the nutritional status of pregnant and lactating women and children up to 5 years of age for low-income families. WIC regulations require that income and nutritional-risk eligibility criteria be used to certify program participants. Although nutritional-risk criteria are established by each state agency, federal regulations recommend that the individual has medical-based (low hemoglobin levels) or dietary-based (poor diet) indicators of poor nutritional status.[136]

The program involves cash grants to state health departments and comparable agencies that make available supplemental foods and nutrition education through participating health clinics. It is intended to assist low-income persons who are at high risk medically. Studies have shown that WIC participants had lower medical costs for themselves and their babies, longer gestation periods, and higher birth weights. Lower infant mortality, improved children's diets, and decreased incidences of iron deficiency anemia in children also were observed.[137,138]

Only 65 percent of people eligible to participate in WIC receive services because of lack of funding. WIC can collaborate with other agencies to provide nutrition education and improve the participants' diets. Successful Community Strategies highlights the success stories of collaborative efforts. **Table 8-15** presents nutritional risk criteria for WIC.

WIC Farmers' Market Nutrition Program

The WIC Farmers' Market Nutrition Program (FMNP) provides vouchers redeemable for fresh fruits and vegetables at farmers' markets. The purpose of FMNP is to increase the awareness and use of farmers' markets to selected participants in the WIC program in addition to their regular WIC benefits. A study entitled Project FRESH examined the effects of the FMNP program on attitudes about buying, preparing, and eating fruits and vegetables; redemption of vouchers; and the number of fruit and vegetable servings consumed. Results showed that FMNP coupons had a direct effect on increasing fruit and vegetable consumption behavior. The maximum impact of the intervention was achieved through a combination of education and vouchers. This study demon-

TABLE 8.15	Nutritional Risk Criteria for Special Nutrition Program for Women, Infants, and Children[56,97,139–141]

Women	Infants
Nutritional Risks	
Pregnant women and breastfeeding women determined to be at nutritional risk because of a nutrition-related medical condition (low hematocrit or hemoglobin). Also, underweight (BMI < 19 kg, low maternal weight gain < 0.45 kg/month), or overweight prenatal or postpartum weight gain.	Infants and children determined to be at nutritional risk because of a nutrition-related medical condition.
Failure to meet the dietary guidelines or inappropriate nutrition practices (eating disorder, pica).	Infants up to 6 months of age whose mothers participated in WIC or could have participated and had a serious medical problem.
Pregnant or breastfeeding women at nutritional risk because of an inadequate dietary pattern.	Infants and children at nutritional risk because of an inadequate dietary pattern.
Alcohol, drug or tobacco use.	
Dietary deficiencies that impair or endanger health.	Low-birth-weight or preterm infants.
Non-breastfeeding, postpartum women with any nutritional risk.	Abnormal pattern of growth (short, underweight, overweight).
Individuals at nutritional risk only because they are homeless or migrants, and current participants who, without WIC foods, could continue to have medical and/or dietary problems.	Failure to thrive (low head circumference, underweight, etc.).
Under the age of 18.	
High parity and young age.	
Pregnancy Complications	
Poor pregnancy outcomes (preterm delivery, low-birth-weight infant)	
Miscarriage or still birth	
Infant with congenital defect	
Gestational diabetes	
Neonatal death	
Health Conditions	
Cancer	
Depression	Low hematocrit or hemoglobin (after 6 months of age)
Diabetes	High blood lead levels
Eating disorders (bulimia, anorexia nervosa)	Food allergies
Gastrointestinal disorders	Fetal alcohol syndrome
HIV/AIDS	Inborn errors of metabolism (PKU, galactosemia, etc.)
Infectious diseases	
Pregnancy-induced hypertension	Otitis media
Renal diseases	
Thyroid disorders	
Urinary tract infections	

strated that incentives, such as vouchers, might encourage increased fruit and vegetable intake, especially in low-income populations.[143]

Title V Maternal and Child Health Program

Title V of the Social Security Act provides federal support to strengthen the states' ability to promote, improve, and deliver maternal and child health (MCH) services and programs for children with special health-care needs (CSHCN), mainly in rural areas and areas of severe economic distress.[144] When the Social Security Act was passed in 1935, the federal government, through Title V, pledged to support states' efforts to extend and improve health and welfare services for mothers and children. Although specific initiatives may vary among the states and jurisdictions using Title V funds, all programs must work to accomplish the activities listed in **Box 8-9**.[145]

The Maternal and Child Health Bureau (MCHB) is a part of the Health Resources and Services Administration (HRSA) of the U.S. Department of Health and Human Services (DHHS) and it administers the Title V program. Some of the MCHB responsibilities include, but are not limited to:[145]

- Coordinating the MCH Formula Grants to States program
- Promoting coordination at the federal level of the activities authorized under Titles V and XIX of the act, especially early and

Box 8-9 Activities Covered by Title V Funds[145]

- Create services to decrease infant mortality and promote maternal, infant, and child health.
- Increase the number of children who are immunized against disease.
- Increase the number of children in low-income households who receive assessments and follow-up diagnostic and treatment services.
- Provide comprehensive perinatal care for women.
- Provide preventive and childcare services, including long-term care services for children with special healthcare needs and rehabilitation services for blind and disabled children under 16 years of age who are eligible for Supplemental Security Income.
- Facilitate the development of comprehensive, family-centered, community-based, culturally competent, coordinated systems of care for children with special healthcare needs.
- Provide nutrition assessment, dietary counseling, nutrition education, and referral to food assistance programs for infants, preschool, and school-age children.

periodic screening, diagnosis, and treatment programs (EPSDT); related activities funded by the Departments of Agriculture and Education; and health block grants and categorical health programs, such as immunizations, administered by DHHS

- Administering the two types of discretionary grants: Special Projects of Regional and National Significance (SPRANS) and Community Integrated Service Systems (CISS)

Another federally funded program that is administered through the MCHB is the Healthy Start Program (HSP). This program began in 1991 to reduce the high rate of infant mortality, especially in U.S. minority groups. For example, the preliminary national infant mortality rates in 2004 were 13.6 per 1,000 live births for African Americans, 8.45 for Hispanic origin and American Indian, and 5.66 for European Americans; the overall U.S. infant mortality rate was 6.78 per 1,000 live births. The high rate of infant mortality is due to limited availability of prenatal care.[146]

The HSP is designed to break down barriers to care by providing accessible, culturally competent, and, in some communities, mobile clinics to minority groups. The program addresses the clients' basic health as well as prenatal care needs and makes referrals for depression or substance abuse screenings. Through Healthy Start, women learn how to improve their overall health by not smoking or drinking before, during, and after pregnancy. Healthy Start also works within communities by providing resources, such as job employment services, to assist families in finding employment. This program provides services to about 96 communities in 36 states, the District of Columbia, and Puerto Rico.[146]

Community Health Center

The MCHB also administers the Community Health Center (CHC), which is designed to provide health services and related training to medically underserved areas. The CHC program was launched by the Office of Economic Opportunity in 1966 and was subsequently authorized by Section 330 of the Public Health Service Act. Priority for funding was given to medically underserved areas, particularly those with high infant mortality rates, older populations, and shortages of healthcare personnel. CHCs exist in areas where economic, geographic, or cultural barriers limit access to primary healthcare for a substantial portion of the population, and they tailor services to the needs of the community.[144]

The main health services include physicians' services, diagnosis, treatment, diagnostic X-rays, laboratory services, and emergency medical care. It provides family-oriented primary preventive services including prenatal and postpartum care, well-child care, children's eye and ear examinations, immunizations, preventive dental services, voluntary family planning services, health education, and nutrition assessments. CHCs provide links to welfare, Medicaid, substance abuse treatment, the WIC program, and related services. It also provides pharmacy services as well as related services such as health education, transportation, translation, and prenatal services.[147]

Food Stamp Program

Another program that provides assistance to low-income families is the Food Stamp Program (FSP). The FSP was established in 1964 to supple-

Successful Community Strategies 🏠🏠🏠

WIC and EFNEP Collaborative Work[142]

The Cook County Expanded Food and Nutrition Education Program (EFNEP) in Chicago partnered with WIC. The purpose of this project was to provide nutrition education to WIC participants and increase clients' fruit and vegetable consumption. They accomplished this goal by partnering with the Cook County jail. The Cook County EFNEP provided seeds and gardening expertise to the prisoners. Then WIC bought the produce from the Chicago Farmer's Market. EFNEP then provided food demonstrations and recipes in the WIC Food Centers throughout the summer. The WIC participants were very receptive to the foods and were eager to try the foods on their own. This project also made a significant positive impact on the prisoners.

ment the food-buying power of low-income individuals and families. Monthly allotments of vouchers (link card) are provided for approved food items in approved grocery stores. The Food Stamp Program is an entitlement program, which means that clients who meet eligibility criteria are entitled to receive assistance. Eligibility and allotments are based on income, household size, assets, housing costs, work requirements, and other factors. To qualify for the FSP, households must have gross incomes below 130 percent of the official poverty level and only net income is required for households with elderly people or individuals with disabilities.[148] See Chapter 4 for an overview of the Food Stamp Program.

Personal Responsibility and Work Opportunities Reconciliation Act of 1996 (PRWORA)

The mid-1990s was a period of welfare reform. Many states had waivers of the rules for the cash welfare program, Aid to Families with Dependent Children (AFDC), before major welfare reform legislation was enacted in 1996. The Personal Responsibility and Work Opportunities Reconciliation Act of 1996 (PRWORA) removed the entitlement of recipients to AFDC and replaced that with a new block grant to states called Temporary Assistance to Needy Families (TANF).[149]

Although the Food Stamp Program was reauthorized in the 1996 Farm Bill, major changes to the program were enacted through PRWORA. Some of the changes include, but are not limited to:[149]

- Placing a time limit on food stamp receipts of 3 out of 36 months for able-bodied adults without dependents (ABAWD) who are not working at least 20 hours a week or participating in a work program
- Reducing maximum allotments by setting them at 100 percent of the change in the Thrifty Food Plan (TFP), from 103 percent of the change in the TFP.

In May 2002, the Food Security and Rural Investment Act of 2002 was enacted, including reauthorization of the Food Stamp Program. Major changes to food stamps included:[148]

- Restoration of eligibility for food stamps to qualified aliens who have been in the United States at least 5 years
- Restoration of eligibility for immigrants receiving certain disability payments and for children, regardless of how long they have been in the country
- Adjusting the standard deduction to vary by household size and indexing each year for inflation
- Replacing enhanced funding for states with low error rates with a performance bonus system based on several different measures of performance
- Providing states with several options to simplify the program, including aligning the definition of income and/or resources to that used in TANF or Medicaid, adopting a simplified reporting system, and providing transitional benefits for clients leaving TANF

Electronic Benefits Transfer (EBT)

Households used to receive food stamp monthly allotments in the form of vouchers from state welfare or human services agencies that were redeemable for food at authorized grocery stores. However, since October 2002, benefits are issued to recipients in an electronic form known as the EBT card (Electronic Benefits Transfer card), which is similar to a bankcard. Electronic Benefits Transfer allows a recipient to authorize transfer of their government benefits from a federal account to a retailer account to pay for products received. The EBT keeps an electronic record of all transactions and makes fraud easier to detect. EBT is currently being used in many states to issue food stamps and other benefits.[150]

The Food Stamp Nutrition Education Program (FSNEP) or the Family Nutrition Program)

The Food Stamp Nutrition Education Program (FSNEP) started in 1986. Funding for the program is provided by the Food Stamp Program administrative budget. To qualify for the funds, participating states are required to provide 50 percent matching funds. The major goal is to improve the diet and nutrition-related skills of food stamp recipients and their families. **Box 8-10** presents some of the FSNEP objectives.[149]

Nutrition Assistance Program (NAP) in Puerto Rico, American Samoa, and the Commonwealth of the Northern Marianas Islands

The Nutrition Assistance Program (NAP) in Puerto Rico, American Samoa, and the Commonwealth of the Northern Marianas Islands provides food and nutrition assistance to low-income individuals through block grants to territory administrative agencies. The territories provide cash or checks to eligible participants. The Nutrition Assistance Program replaced the Food Stamp Program in Puerto Rico in 1982. The same program started in the Northern Marianas in 1982 and in American Samoa in 1994.[139,149]

Food Distribution Program on Indian Reservations (FDPIR)

The Food Distribution Program on Indian Reservations (FDPIR) began in the 1930s. It originally was known as the Needy Family Program and was the major type of food assistance program for all low-income individuals in the United States until early 1970s when the Food Stamp Program was expanded.[139] The FDPIR provides monthly supplemental food packages to low-income households living on Indian reservations and to eligible American Indian households living in approved areas near reservations. The USDA commodities consist of canned meats and fish products; vegetables, fruits, and juices; dried beans; peanuts or

---

Box **8-10 Food Stamp Nutrition Education Program Objectives**[149]

- Improved self-sufficiency of food stamp recipients
- Decreased reliance on emergency food resources
- Increased skills in food budgeting and meal planning
- Improved diet for the entire family
- Increased consumption of fruits and vegetables
- Increased variety of food choices
- Improved food preparation skills
- Improved knowledge of safe food practices
- Increased physical activity
- Increased promotion of healthy lifestyles for youth as outlined in the *Dietary Guidelines for Americans*

peanut butter; milk, butter, and cheese; pasta, flour, or grains; adult cereals; corn syrup or honey; and vegetable oil and shortening. The participants may decide each month whether they will participate in the Food Stamp Program or the Food Distribution Program. The majority of participants on reservations prefer the Food Distribution Program due to a lack of access to grocery stores.[139]

Temporary Emergency Food Assistance Program (TEFAP)

The Temporary Emergency Food Assistance Program (TEFAP) provides commodity foods to emergency kitchens (often referred to as soup kitchens), homeless shelters, and similar organizations that serve meals to low-income individuals. Eligibility criteria are set between 130 and 150 percent of the poverty line for some states.[151] In many states, food stamp participants are automatically eligible for TEFAP. The types of foods the USDA purchases for TEFAP distribution vary depending on the preferences of each state and agricultural market conditions.

Cooperative Extension Program, Expanded Food and Nutrition Education Program

The Cooperative Extension Program provides hands-on training in homes and community settings for the people of each community, usually through a state university. This program is funded under the USDA and operated in each U.S. state and territory. It has offices at the state land-grant universities and a network of local or regional offices. One component of the Cooperative Extension Program is the Expanded Food and Nutrition Education Program (EFNEP), which provides education tailored to low-income families.[152]

Medicaid and Early and Periodic Screening, Diagnosis, and Treatment (EPSDT)

The Early and Periodic Screening, Diagnosis, and Treatment (EPSDT) service is Medicaid's comprehensive and preventive child health program for individuals under the age of 21. It was established in 1969 by an amendment to Title XIX of the Social Security Act (Medicaid). The Deficit Reduction Act (PL 109-171) of 2005 (enacted February 2006) gave states the option to modify their approach to delivery of services to children enrolled in Medicaid. DRA gave states the option to restructure their approach to benefits under Medicaid without federal waiver

and to extend Medicaid to underinsured, moderate-income children with serious disabilities.[153]

The EPSDT was defined by law as part of the Omnibus Budget Reconciliation Act of 1989 (OBRA 89) legislation and includes periodic screening, vision, dental, and hearing services. The EPSDT program consists of two mutually supportive operational components: 1) assuring the availability and accessibility of required healthcare resources, and 2) helping Medicaid recipients and their parents or guardians effectively use these resources. These components enable Medicaid agencies to manage a comprehensive child health program of prevention and treatment and to seek out eligible clients and inform them of the benefits of prevention and the health services and assistance available. It also enables them to assess the child's health needs through initial and periodic examinations and evaluations and to assure that the health problems found are diagnosed and treated before they become more complex and their treatment more expensive.[154] Children can be referred for nutrition intervention for growth retardation, iron deficiency anemia, cardiovascular disease, obesity, and other nutrition-related conditions.[154] Nutrition counseling for these problems is reimbursable. Brochures from the state agency promote EPSDT services and inform clients about how to obtain health and nutrition information and services for children who need them. Following are elements to remember when working with clients:[154]

- **Early**: Identify problems early, starting at birth
- **Periodic**: Check children's health at periodic, age-appropriate intervals
- **Screening**: Conduct physical, mental, developmental, dental, hearing, vision, and other screening tests to detect potential problems
- **Diagnosis**: Perform diagnostic tests to follow up when a risk is identified
- **Treatment**: Treat the problems observed

In addition, the OBRA of 1986 (PL 99-509) and 1987 (PL 100-203) gave states the option to expand Medicaid coverage and to determine the income eligibility to provide health services to pregnant women, infants, and children up to age 5 with poor medical conditions. The new provisions of Medicaid now provide funding for nutrition assessment, counseling, and education.[136] Table 4.10 in Chapter 4 presents a list of federally funded food assistance programs.

Chapter Summary

- A mother brings to gestation her previous life experiences, diet, general health and fitness, lifelong dietary habits, and genetic heritage.
- Preconception nutritional status is more important than the mother's diet during the 9 months of gestation.
- Adequate vitamin and mineral intake at least 8 weeks before conception and during pregnancy can help prevent birth defects such as neural tube defects.
- Infant mortality rates (IMRs) can be used to monitor pregnancy outcomes in the population.
- Pregnant and breastfeeding mothers should not drink alcohol or ingest any substance that will harm the infant (tobacco, illegal drugs, etc.).
- Obese women have a greater risk for pregnancy complications, especially gestational diabetes, hypertensive disorders, cesarean deliveries, and postoperative morbidity.
- Pregnant women found to be at nutritional risk can be referred to a nutritionist and to the Special Supplemental Food Program for Women, Infants, and Children (WIC).
- Physical activity is important during pregnancy because research shows that being active can facilitate labor and reduce psychological stress.
- Infants have higher energy requirements than adults because of their rapid growth rate.
- Failure to thrive may be queried when an infant's weight for age falls below the fifth percentile of the standard National Center for Health Statistics (NCHS) growth chart.
- Human milk contains all the essential amino acids and nutrients an infant needs.
- The greatest benefits of breastfeeding are associated with exclusive breastfeeding for at least 6 months and continued breastfeeding with complementary foods for at least 12 months.
- In the United States, the Centers for Disease Control and Prevention (CDC) advises women who are HIV positive not to breastfeed.
- Programs such as WIC, the Commodity Supplemental Food Program, and the Food Stamp Program are available to low-income pregnant women.

Critical Thinking Activities

- Examine health statistics and demographic data to identify the rate of infant mortality and maternal mortality in your geographic area. What resources and agencies are available in the area to support pregnant and lactating women? What services are available from federal, state, and local sources?
- Determine the eligibility criteria for women and infants' food assistance programs.
- Working with other students, make appointments with key persons in the WIC Farmers' Market Nutrition Program, social welfare agencies, and Cooperative Extension Expanded Food and Nutrition Education Program to find out what each agency offers, how clients can access the services, who is eligible, how the agency receives funding, and what methods are used to evaluate the agency's ability to meet the needs of its target.
- Identify nutritionists in the community who work with pregnant and lactating women and other vulnerable groups. Invite these nutritionists to come to a class meeting to share their experiences. What constitutes a typical workday? What are the rewards and challenges of working with vulnerable populations? How do they deal with the frustrations and challenges of their work? What advice might they offer to students working with a vulnerable group? How are they involved in political advocacy related to vulnerable populations?
- Imagine a nutritionist working with a vulnerable population making a home visit to a family in an impoverished neighborhood. How have their life experiences and education prepared them (or not) for working in an impoverished neighborhood? What are their expectations? Write and discuss ideas with classmates.
- Discuss welfare reform with other students. How does the welfare system work? Who receives welfare? Who is eligible for benefits? What are the strengths and weaknesses of welfare reform in America? What are the financial and personal costs of welfare reform? Identify federal and state senators and representatives for your community. Where do they stand on the issue of welfare reform? How would they restructure the welfare system?

Case Study 8-1

Amy is a 17-year-old female at 24 weeks' gestation. She is attending high school and lives with the father of her baby. During her health checkup at the community center clinic, she complained of feeling tired most of the time. A blood sample was drawn and analyzed; her hemoglobin level was 8.5 mg/dl and hematocrit was 30 percent. The normal hemoglobin value is 12 to 16 g/dl and hematocrit 37 to 47 percent. Typically, many physiologic and biochemical changes occur during pregnancy but Amy's blood values were lower than the usual physiologic changes that occur during pregnancy. Amy indicated that she is still smoking because she is worried about gaining too much weight. She has only visited the community center clinic twice since she found out she was pregnant, and she has stopped taking her prenatal vitamins because one of her friends told her that the vitamins could make her constipated. She continues to wear the clothes she wore before the pregnancy even though the clothes are tight on her. The nurse at the clinic referred Amy to the local WIC program for more assessment.

Additional assessment showed that Amy's weight-for-height (BMI) was less than 18.5. The dietitian assessed Amy's dietary intake using a 24-hour recall and the Nutritional Risk Score (see **Table 8.8**). Her 24-hour recall showed a lack of some of the essential nutrients such as protein, iron, folate, calories, and some vitamins. Amy's Nutritional Risk Score was less than 50. Her daily caloric intake was 1,000 kcal per day. She likes to drink espresso, at least 4 cups a day. Amy's present income is at 185 percent of the U.S. poverty guidelines.

Activities

- As a group, design a nutrition education program to explain to Amy the importance of prenatal care visits to monitor the growth of the fetus and to prevent maternal complications such as anemia and spina bifida.
- Encourage her to take her prenatal care supplements and explain that the best way to avoid constipation is to eat foods that are high in fiber, such as fruits and vegetables, and ask her to

drink plenty of water. Provide her with a list of fiber-rich foods. Encourage moderate exercise such as brisk walking or riding a bicycle, provide her with a list containing different types of physical activity, how long each activity should take, and the amount of calories expanded for each activity.

- Ask Amy to stop smoking cigarettes because it can cause growth retardation and sudden infant death syndrome (SIDS). Show pictures/diagrams of the effect of cigarette smoking on the lungs, fetus, and any other body tissues.
- Encourage her to participate in group or peer support sessions; this may help her feel less socially isolated.
- Explain to her that it is *not* safe to lose weight during pregnancy because it can reduce the infant's growth and cause maternal complications such as anemia.

Further Action

- Do a more thorough assessment to determine why Amy is missing her appointments.
- Consider other factors affecting food choices, such as appetite, food preferences, access to food, food markets, transportation, storage facilities in the home, and cooking skills when making an assessment for Amy.
- Determine socioeconomic factors that influence eating practices such as income, ethnic food traditions, taboos, cravings, educational achievement, housing, and family situation.
- Determine what food practices she should continue and which need to be changed.
- Find out how capable and interested Amy is in changing her food choices.
- Determine the assistance that she needs to overcome her problems.

References

1. Cucó G, Fernández-Ballart J, Sala J, et al. Dietary patterns and associated lifestyles in preconception, pregnancy and postpartum. *Eur J Clin Nutr.* 2006; 60(3):364–371.

2. Allen LH. Malnutrition and human function: a comparison of conclusions from the INCAP and nutrition CRSP studies. *J Nutr.* 1995; 125(4):S1119–S1126.

3. U.S. Department of Health and Human Services, Public Health Service. *Healthy People 2000: National Health Promotion and Disease Prevention Objectives.* Washington DC: U.S. Government Printing Office; 1990.

4. U.S. Department of Health and Human Services. *Healthy People 2010.* 2nd ed. 2 vols. Washington, DC: U.S. Government Printing Office; 2000. Available at http://www.healthypeople.gov. Accessed March 24, 2008.

5. U.S. Department of Health and Human Services. Maternal, Infant, and Child Health. Progress Review. Available at: http://www.healthypeople.gov/data/2010prog/focus16/Maternal_Progress_Review.pdf. Accessed September 23, 2005.

6. Rodwell Williams S, Schlenker E. *Essentials of Nutrition and Diet Therapy.* 8th ed. St. Louis, MO: Mosby; 2003.

7. Shils ME, Olson JA, Moshe Shike A, et al. *Modern Nutrition in Health and Disease.* 9th ed. Baltimore, MD: Williams and Wilkins; 1999.

8. Huy AT. Biochemical tests in pregnancy. *Aust Prescr.* 2005; 28:98–101.

9. Bruinse HW, van den Berg H. Changes of some vitamin levels during and after normal pregnancy. *Eur J Obstet Gynecol Reprod Biol.* 1995; 61(1):31–37.

10. Ackurt F, Wetherilt H, Loker M, Hacibekiroglu M. Biochemical assessment of nutritional status in pre- and post-natal Turkish women and outcome of pregnancy. *Euro J Clin Nutr.* 1995; 49(8):613–622.

11. Brown A, Fernhoff PM, Waisbren SE. Barriers to successful dietary control among pregnant women with phenylketonuria. *Genet Med.* 2002; 4:84–89.

12. Centers for Disease Control and Prevention. Extending the Successful Prevention of Mental Retardation through Newborn Screening. Available at: http://www.cdc.gov/ncbddd/press/pku.htm. Accessed January 8, 2007.

13. Riskin-Mashiah S. Preconception counseling—for all. *Harefuah.* 2004; 143(7):530–547.

14. Brown AS, Fernhoff PM, Waisbren SE, et al. Barriers to successful dietary control among pregnant women with phenylketonuria. *Genet Med.* 2002; 4(2):84–89.

15. Dietrich M, Brown CJ, Block G. The effect of folate fortification of cereal-grain products on blood folate status, dietary folate intake, and dietary folate sources among adult non-supplement users in the United States. *J Am Coll Nutr.* 2005; 24(4):266–274.

16. Botto LD, Lisi A, Robert-Gnansia E. International retrospective cohort study of neural tube defects in relation to folic acid recommendations: are the recommendations working? *Brit Med J.* 2005; 330(7491):571.

17. Carter H, Petrini JR. Use of vitamins containing folic acid among women of childbearing age—United States, 2004. *MMWR.* 2004; 53(36):847–850.

18. Norsworthy B, Skeaff CM, Adank C, Green TJ. Effects of once-a-week or daily folic acid supplementation on red blood cell folate concentrations in women. *Eur J Clin Nutr.* 2004; 58(3):548–554.

19. Krishnaswamy K, Madhavan Nair K. Importance of folate in human nutrition. *Br J Nutr.* 2001; 85(Suppl 2):S115–S124.

20. Institute of Medicine. *Dietary Reference Intakes for Thiamin, Riboflavin, Niacin, Vitamin B6, Folate, Vitamin B12, Pantothenic Acid, Biotin, and Choline.* Washington, DC: National Academy Press; 1998.

21. Anorlu RI, Oluwole AA, Abudu OO. Sociodemographic factors in anaemia in pregnancy at booking in Lagos, Nigeria. *J Obstet Gynaecol.* 2006; 26(8):773–776.

22. Conrey EJ, Frongillo EA, Dollahite JS, Griffin MR. Integrated program enhancements increased utilization of Farmers' Market Nutrition Program. *J Nutr.* 2003; 133(6):1841–1844.

23. Luke B, Leurgans S. Maternal weight gains in ideal twins outcomes. *J Am Diet Assoc.* 1996; 96(2):178.

24. Zhu BP, Rolfs RT, Nangle BE, Horan JM. The effect of the interval between pregnancies on perinatal outcomes. *New Engl J Med.* 1999; 340:589.

25. Shetty SS, Harrison LH, Hajjeh RA. Determining risk factors for candidemia among newborn infants from population-based surveillance: Baltimore, Maryland, 1998–2000. *Pediatr Infect Dis J.* 2005; 24(7):601–604.

26. Sommers AS, Kenney GM, Dubay L. Implementation of mandatory Medicaid managed care in Missouri: impacts for pregnant women. *Am J Managed Healthcare.* 2005; 11(7):433–442.

27. Wen SW, Tan H, Yang Q, Walker M. Prediction of small for gestational age by logistic regression in twins. *Aust N Z J Obstet Gynaecol.* 2005; 45(5):399–404.

28. Ness RB, Grisso JA, Hirschinger N, et al. Cocaine and tobacco use and the risk of spontaneous abortion. *N Engl J Med.* 1999; 340:333.

29. Tillett J, Kostich L, VandeVusse L. Use of over-the-counter medications during pregnancy. *J Perinat Neonat Nurse.* 2003; 17(1):3–18.

30. Kacew S. Fetal consequences and risks attributed to the use of prescribed and over-the-counter (OTC) preparations during pregnancy. *Int J Clin Pharmacol.* 1994; 32(7):335–341.

31. Buitendijk S, Bracken M. Medication in early pregnancy: prevalence of use and relationship to maternal characteristics. *Am J Obstet Gynecol.* 1991; 165:33–40.

32. Henry A, Crowther C. Patterns of medication use during and prior to pregnancy: the MAP study. *Aust N Z J Obstet Gynecol.* 2000; 40(2):165–172.

33. Rubin J, Ferenez C, Loffredo C. The Baltimore-Washington Infant Study. Use of prescription and non-prescription drugs in pregnancy. *J Clinc Epidemiol.* 1993; 46(6):581–589.

34. Rosa FW, Wilk AL, Kelsey FO. Teratogen update: vitamin A congeners. *Teratol.* 1986; 33(3):355–364.

35. Ogunyemi D, Hernández-Loera GE. The impact of antenatal cocaine use on maternal characteristics and neonatal outcomes. *J Maternal-Fetal Neonatal Med.* 2004; 15(4):253–259.

36. Shankaran S, Das A, Bauer CR. Association between patterns of maternal substance use and infant birth weight, length, and head circumference. *Pediatr.* 2004; 114(2):e226–e234.

37. Zuccato E, Chiabrando C, Castiglioni S. Cocaine in surface waters: a new evidence-based tool to monitor community drug abuse. *Environ Health.* 2005; 4:14.

38. Wardlaw GM, Kessel M. *Perspectives in Nutrition.* 5th ed. New York NY: McGraw-Hill; 2002.

39. Berdanier CD, Feldman EB, Flatt WP. *Handbook of Nutrition and Food.* Washington, DC: CRC Press; 2002.

40. Briggs GG, Freeman RK, Yaffe SJ. *Drugs in Pregnancy and Lactation.* Baltimore, MD: Williams and Williams; 1994.

41. Kaiser LL, Allen L. Position of the American Dietetic Association: nutrition and lifestyle for a healthy pregnancy outcome. *J Am Diet Assoc.* 2002; 102(10):1479–1490.

42. Lundsberg LS, Bracken MB, Saftlas AF. Low-to-moderate gestational alcohol use and intrauterine growth retardation, low birthweight and preterm delivery. *Ann Epidemiol.* 1997; 7:498–508.

43. American Academy of Pediatrics. Parenting Corner: Breastfeeding Q&A. Available at: http://www.aap.org/pubed/ZZZNIUQXQ7C.htm?&sub_cat = 1. Accessed September 11, 2005.

44. Grosvenor M, Smolin L. *Nutrition: From Science to Life.* Fort Worth, TX: Harcourt College Publishers; 2002.

45. U.S. Surgeon General. The Surgeon General's report on nutrition and health. Washington, DC: US Department of Health and Human Services, 1988. DHHS (PHS) Publication No. 88-50210.

46. Crosby W. Pica. *JAMA.* 1976; 235:2765.

47. Ross MP, Brundage S. Preconception counseling about nutrition and exercise. *J S C Med Assoc.* 2002; 98(6):260–263.

48. Eskenazi B, Stapleton AL, Kharrazi M, Chee WY. Associations between maternal decaffeinated and caffeinated coffee consumption and fetal growth and gestational duration. *Epidemiol.* 1999; 10:242–249.

49. Cataldo C, Whitney E, Rolfes S. *Nutrition and Diet Therapy. Principles and Practice.* 6th ed. Belmont, CA: Thomson Wadsworth; 2002.

50. U.S. Department of Health and Human Services, National Institutes of Health, National Heart, Lung, and Blood Institute. Your Guide to Lowering Your Blood Pressure with DASH. NIH Publication No. 06-4082. Available at: http://www.nhlbi.nih.gov/health/public/heart/hbp/dash/index.htm. Accessed January 9, 2007.

51. Karanja NM, Obarzanek E, Lin PH. Descriptive characteristics of the dietary patterns used in the Dietary Approaches to Stop Hypertension Trial. DASH Collaborative Research Group. *J Am Diet Assoc.* 1999; 99(8):S19–S27.

52. Abrams B, Altman SL, Pickett KE. Pregnancy weight gain: still controversial. *Am J Clin Nutr.* 2000; 71(Suppl):S1233–S1241.

53. Schieve LA, Cogswell ME, Scanlon KS. An empiric evaluation of the Institute of Medicine's pregnancy weight gain guidelines by race. *Obstet Gynecol.* 1998; 91:878–884.

54. Scholl TO, Hediger ML, Schall JI, Smith WK. Gestational weight gain, pregnancy outcome, and postpartum weight retention. *Obstet Gynecol.* 1995; 86:423–427.

55. Villamor E, Cnattingius S. Interpregnancy weight change and risk of adverse pregnancy outcomes: a population-based study. *Lancet.* 2006; 368: 1164–1170.

56. Institute of Medicine. *Nutrition During Pregnancy and Lactation: An Implementation Guide.* Washington, DC: National Academies Press; 1992.

57. Suitor CW. *Maternal Weight Gain: A Report of an Expert Work Group.* Arlington, VA: National Center for Education in Maternal and Child Health; 1997.

58. Centers for Disease Control and Prevention. Trends in cigarette smoking among high school students—United States, 1991–1999. *MMWR.* 2000; 49(33):755–758.

59. Worthington P. *Practical Aspects of Nutritional Support: An Advance Practice Guide.* Philadelphia: Saunders; 2004.

60. Borrelli F, Capasso R, AvielloG, Pittler M, Izzo A. Effectiveness and safety of ginger in the treatment of pregnancy-induced nausea and vomiting. *Obstet Gynecol.* 2005; 105:849–856.

61. Klebanoff MA, Levine RJ, DerSimonian R, Clemens JD, Wilkins DG. Maternal serum paraxanthine, a caffeine metabolite, and the risk of spontaneous abortion. *N Engl J Med.* 1999; 341:1639–1644.

62. Louik C, Hernandez-Diaz S, Mitchell A. Nausea and vomiting in pregnancy: maternal characteristics and risk factors. *Paediatric and Perinatal Epidemiology.* 2006; 20: 270–278.

63. Prather CM. Pregnancy-related constipation. *Curr Gastroenterol Rep.* 2004; 6(5):402–404.

64. Casanova BF, Sammel MD, Macones GA. Development of a clinical prediction rule for iron deficiency anemia in pregnancy. *Am J Obstet Gynecol.* 2005; 193(2):460–466.

65. Scholl TO, Reilly T. Anemia, iron and pregnancy outcome. *J Nutr.* 2000; 130:443S–447S.

66. Allen LH. Biological mechanisms that might underlie iron's effects on fetal growth and preterm birth. *J Nutr.* 2001; 131:S581–S589.

67. Allen HL. Anemia and iron deficiency: effects on pregnancy outcome. *Am J Clin Nutr.* 2000; 71(5):S1280–S1284.

68. Williams DR. Racial/ethnic variations in women's health: the social embeddedness of health. *Am J Public Health.* 2002; 92:588–597.

69. Lozoff B, Jimenez E, Smith J. Double burden of iron deficiency in infancy and low socioeconomic status: a longitudinal analysis of cognitive test scores to age 19 years. *Arch Pediatr Adolesc Med.* 2006; 160:1108–1113.

70. American Dietetic Association. Nutrition and Women's Health. Position Paper. Available at: http://www.eatright.org/cps/rde/xchg/ada/hs.xsl/index.html. Accessed March 18, 2008.

71. Belizan JM, Villar J, Gonzalez L, Campodonico L, Bergel E. Calcium supplementation to prevent hypertensive disorders of pregnancy. *New Engl J Med.* 1991; 325:1399–1405.

72. King H. Epidemiology of glucose intolerance and gestational diabetes in women of childbearing age. *Diabetes Care.* 1998; 21(Suppl 2):B9–B13.

73. Gellin B, Broome C, Bibb W, Weaver R, Gaeta S, Mazola L. The epidemiology of listeriosis in the United States—1986. Listeriosis Study Group. *Am J Epidemiol.* 1991; 133:392–401.

74. Voetsch AC, Angulo FJ, Jones TF, Moore MR, Nadon C. Reduction in the incidence of invasive listeriosis in foodborne diseases active surveillance network sites, 1996–2003. *Clin Infect Dis.* 2007; 44:513–520.

75. Bonapace FS, Fisher RS. Constipation and diarrhea in pregnancy. *Gastroenterol Clin North Am.* 1998; 27:197–211.

76. Centers for Disease Control and Prevention. Multistate outbreak of listeriosis: United States, 1998. *MMWR.* 1998; 47(50):1086.

77. U.S. Food and Drug Administration, U.S. Department of Agriculture, U.S. Environmental Protection Agency, Centers for Disease Control and Prevention. Appendix B: Some Important Microbial Pathogens Associated with Foodborne Illness. Food Safety from Farm to Table: A National Food Safety Initiative; Report to the President. Available at: http://www.cdc.gov/foodsafety. Accessed March 18, 2008.

78. U.S. Food and Drug Administration, Center for Food Safety and Applied Nutrition. To Your Health Food Safety for Seniors. Available at: http://www.foodsafety.gov/%7Efsg/sr2.html. Accessed March 18, 2008.

79. Food Safety and Inspection Service. Listeriosis and Pregnancy: What Is Your Risk? Available at: http://www.fsis.usda. Accessed September 27, 2006.

80. U.S. Department of Agriculture, U.S. Department of Health and Human Services. *Dietary Guidelines for Americans.* 5th ed. Home and Garden Bulletin No. 232. Washington, DC: U.S. Department of Health and Human Services, 2000.

81. Evans EC. The FDA recommendations on fish intake during pregnancy. *J Obstet Gynecol Neonatal Nurs.* 2002; 31(6):715–720.

82. Raichel L, Sheiner E. Maternal obesity as a risk factor for complications in pregnancy, labor and pregnancy outcomes. *Harefuah*. 2005; 144(2):107.

83. Brabin B, Prinsen-Geerligs P, Verhoeff F, Kazembe P. Anaemia prevention for reduction of mortality in mothers and children. *Trans R Soc Trop Med Hyg*. 2003; 97(1):36–38.

84. American Academy of Pediatrics, Committee on Adolescence. Adolescent pregnancy—current trends and issues. *Pediatr*. 1999; 103:516–520.

85. Rodwell SW, Worthington-Roberts BS. *Nutrition Throughout the Life Cycle*. 2nd ed. St Louis, MO: Mosby; 1996; p. 374.

86. Trissler RJT. The child within: a guide to nutrition counseling for pregnant teens. *J Am Dietetic Assoc*. 1999; 99:516–520.

87. Centers for Disease Control and Prevention. State-specific pregnancy and birth rates among teenagers: United States, 1991–1992. *MMWR*. 1995; 44(37):676–684.

88. Markovitz B, Cook R, Flick L, Leet T. Socioeconomic factors and adolescent pregnancy outcomes: distinctions between neonatal and post-neonatal deaths? *BMC Public Health*. 2005; 5(79):1471–2458.

89. Kirby D. *No Easy Answers: Research Findings on Programs to Reduce Teen Pregnancy*. Washington, DC: The National Campaign to Prevent Teen Pregnancy; 1997.

90. Clapp JF. The effect of continuing regular endurance exercise on the physiologic adaptations to pregnancy and pregnancy outcome. *Am J Sports Med*. 1996; 24:S28–S29.

91. Campbell MK, Mottola MF. Recreational exercise and occupational activity during pregnancy and birth weight: a case-control study. *Am J Obstet Gynecol*. 2001; 184(3):403–408.

92. National Center of Health Statistics. New CDC Report Shows Record Low Infant Mortality Rate. Available at: http://www.cdc.gov/nchs/pressroom/03facts/lowinfant.htm. Accessed September 19, 2005.

93. Maternal and Child Health Library. Knowledge Path: Infant Mortality. Available at: http://www.mchlibrary.info/KnowledgePaths/kp_infmort.html. Accessed September 19, 2005.

94. Harvard Public Health Review. Bringing Up Baby—Better. Available at: http://www.hsph.harvard.edu/review/review_winter_02/677baby.html. Accessed September 2005.

95. Story M, Holt K, Sofka D, Clark EM, eds. *Bright Futures in Practice: Nutrition Pocket Guide*. Arlington, VA: National Center for Education in Maternal and Child Health, Georgetown University; 2002.

96. Trahms CM, Pipes P. *Nutrition in Infancy and Childhood*. 6th ed. Belmont, CA: WCB/McGraw-Hill; 1997.

97. Insel P, Turner RE, Ross D. *Nutrition 2002 Update*. 5th ed. Sudbury, MA: Jones and Bartlett; 2002.

98. American Academy of Pediatrics. Breastfeeding and the Use of Human Milk. Available at: http://aappolicy.aappublications.org/cgi/content/full/pediatrics%3B100/6/1035. Accessed September 20, 2005.

99. Skinner JD, Carruth BR, Houck K. Transitions in infant feeding during the first year of life. *J Am Coll Nutr*. 1997; 16(3):209–214.

100. Kennedy E, Goldberg J. What are American children eating? Implications for public policy. *Nutr Rev*. 1995; 53:111–126.

101. Lutz C, Prztulski P. *Nutrition and Diet Therapy*. 3rd ed. Philadelphia PA: Davis; 2001.

102. Hamosh M. Digestion in the newborn. *Clin Perinatol*. 1996; 23(2):191–209.

103. Hoffman DR, Birch EE, Castaneda YS. Visual function in breast-fed term infants weaned to formula with or without long chain polyunsaturated fat at 4 to 6 months: a randomized clinical trial. *J Pediatrics*. 2003; 142(6):669–677.

104. Scott JM, Weir DG. Folate composition, synthesis and function in natural materials. *Clin Haematol*. 1976; 3:547–568.

105. Graham SM, Arvela OM, Wise GA. Long-term neurologic consequences of nutritional vitamin B_{12} deficiency in infants. *J Pediatr*. 1992; 121:710.

106. Holst MC. Developmental and behavioral effects of iron deficiency anemia in infants. *Nutr Today*. 1998; 33(1):27.

107. Hurtado EK, Claussen AH, Scott KG. Early childhood anemia and mild or moderate mental retardation. *Am J Clin Nutr*. 1999; 69:115–119.

108. Partington S, Nitzke S, Csete J. The prevalence of anemia in a WIC population: a comparison by homeless experience. *J Am Diet Assoc*. 2000; 100:469–471.

109. Fomon SJ. Infant feeding in the 20th century: formula and beikost. *J Nutr*. 2001; 131:409S–420S.

110. Soh P, Ferguson E, McKenzie J, Homs M, Gibson R. Iron deficiency and risk factors for lower iron stores in 6–24-month-old New Zealanders. *European Journal of Clinical Nutrition*. 2004; 58:71–79.

111. Polhamus B, Dalenius K, Thompson D. *Pediatric Nutrition Surveillance 2003*. Atlanta: U.S. Department of Health and Human Services, Centers for Disease Control and Prevention; 2004.

112. Garcia-Careaga M, Kerner JA. Gastrointestinal manifestations of food allergies in pediatric patients. *Nutr Clin Pract*. 2005; 20(5):526–535.

113. Sicherer SH, Morrow EH, Sampson HA. Dose-response in double-blind, placebo-controlled oral food challenges in children with atopic dermatitis. *J Allergy Clin Immunol*. 2000; 105:582–586.

114. Peroni DG, Piacentini GL, Bodini A, Rigotti E, Pigozzi R, Boner AL. Prevalence and risk factors for atopic dermatitis in preschool children. *Br J Dermatol*. 2008; 158(3):539–543.

115. Krugman SD. Failure to thrive. *Am Fam Physician*. 2003; 68(5):879–884.

116. Bassali RW, Benjamin J. Failure to Thrive. Available at: http://www.emedicine.com/PED/topic738.htm. Accessed September 27, 2005.

117. Laurence RM, Lawrence RA. Breastfeeding: benefits, risks, and alternatives, *Curr Opin Obstet Gynecol*. 2000; 12(6):519–524.

118. Dobson B, Murtaugh, M. Position of the American Dietetic Association: breaking the barrier of breastfeeding. *J Am Diet Assoc*. 2001; 101(10):11213–11220.

119. Embree JE, Njenga S, Datta P. Risk factors for postnatal mother–child transmission of HIV-1. *AIDS*. 2000; 14(16):2535–2541.

120. Coutsoudis A, Pillay K, Kuhn L, et al. Method of feeding and transmission of HIV-1 from mothers to children by 15 months of age: prospective cohort study from Durban. *South Africa AIDS*. 2001; 15(3):379–387.

121. U.S. Department of Health and Human Services. Healthy People 2010. Available at: http://www.health.gov. Accessed March 19, 2008.

122. Ruowei L, Zhen Z, Mokdad A, Barker L, Grummer-Strawn L. Prevalence of breastfeeding in the United States: The 2001 National Immunization Survey. *Ped*. 2003; 111(5):1198–1201.

123. Raisler J, Alexander C, O'Campo P. Breastfeeding: a dose-response relationship? *J Am Public Health*. 1999; 89:25–30.

124. Kramer MS, Chalmers B, Hodnett ED, et al. Promotion of breastfeeding intervention trial (PROBIT): a randomized trial in the Republic of Belarus. *JAMA*. 2001; 285(4):413–420.

125. World Health Organization. *Protecting, Promoting, and Supporting Breastfeeding. The Special Role of Maternity Services. A Joint WHO/UNICEF Statement*. Geneva, Switzerland: WHO/UNICEF; 1989.

126. Cooper WO, Atherton HD, Kahana M, Kotagal UR. Increased incidence of severe breastfeeding malnutrition and hypernatremia in a metropolitan area. *Pediatr*. 1995; 96:957–960.

127. Gielen AC, Faden RR, O'Campo P, Brown CH, Paige DM. Maternal employment during the early period: effects on initiation and continuation of breastfeeding. *Pediatr*. 1991; 87:298–305.

128. Hills-Bonczyk SG, Avery MD, Savik K, Potter S, Duckett LJ. Women's experiences with combining breast-feeding and employment. *J Nurse Midw*. 1993; 38(5):257–266.

129. Kleinman RE. *Pediatric Nutrition Handbook*. 4th ed. Elk Grove, IL: American Academy of Pediatrics; 1998.

130. Zavaleta N, Nombera J. Rojas R. Hambraeus L, Gislason J, Lönnerdal B. Iron and lactoferrin in milk of anemic mothers given iron supplements. *Nutr Res.* 1995; 15(5):681–690.

131. U.S. Department of Health and Human Services. *Blueprint for Action on Breastfeeding.* Washington, DC: Office of Women's Health; 2000.

132. Tamborlane WV. *The Yale Guide to Children's Nutrition.* New Haven, CT: Yale Press; 1997.

133. California Department of Health Services. *New Corporate Partners Support Baby-Cal's Efforts.* Sacramento, CA: California Department of Health Services; 1999.

134 U.S. Department of Agriculture. Commodity Supplemental Food Program. Available at: http://www.fns.usda.gov/fdd/programs/csfp/pfs-csfp.pdf. Accessed April 27, 2005.

135. Krauses K, Mahan K, Escott-Stump S. *Food, Nutrition, and Diet Therapy.* 11th ed. Philadelphia: Saunders; 2003.

136. Kaufman M. *Nutrition in Public Health: A Handbook for Developing Programs and Services.* Rockville, MD: Aspen; 1990.

137. U.S. Department of Agriculture. *Continuing Survey of Food Intakes by Individuals 1994–1996.* Beltsville, MD: U.S. Department of Health and Human Services; 1998.

138. Rose D, Habicht J-P, Devaney B. Household participation in the Food Stamp and WIC programs increases the nutrient intakes of preschool children. *J Nutr.* 1998; 128:548–555.

139. Boyle M. *Community Nutrition in Action: An Entrepreneurial Approach.* 4th ed. Belmont, CA: Thomson Wadsworth; 2005.

140. Institute of Medicine. WIC nutrition risk criteria: a scientific assessment. In: Committee on Scientific Evaluation of WIC Nutrition Risk Criteria Food and Nutrition Board, ed. Washington, DC: National Academy Press; 1996, pp. 356–377.

141. U.S. Department of Agriculture/Food and Nutrition Service. WIC Program Fact Sheet. March 2006. Available at: http://www.fns.usda.gov/wic/howtoapply/eligibilityrequirements.htm. Accessed April 2, 2008.

142. Cooperative State Research Education, and Extension Service, Expanded Food and Nutrition Education Program Impacts. 2005 Success Stories. Available at: http://www.csrees.usda.gov/nea/food/efnep/impacts.html. Accessed April 2, 2008.

143. Anderson JV, Bybee DI, Brown RM, et al. 5 a day fruit and vegetable intervention improves consumption in a low income population. *J Am Diet Assoc.* 2001; 101(2):195–202.

144. U.S. Department of Health and Human Services. *The Report of the Select Panel for the Promotion of Child Health. Better Health for Our Children: A National Strategy. Analysis and Recommendations for Selected Federal Programs.* Vol. 2. DHHS (PHS) 79-55071. Washington, DC: Author; 1981.

145. Health Resources and Services Administration. Understanding Title V of the Social Security Act. Available at: http://mchb.hrsa.gov/about/dsch.htm. Accessed March 17, 2008.

146. U.S. Department of Health and Human Services. HHS Awards $80.5 Million in Healthy Start Grants to Reduce Infant Mortality. Available at: http://www.hhs.gov/news/press/2005pres/20050622.html. Accessed March 19, 2008.

147. Health Resources and Services Administration. Community Health Centers. Available at: http://bhpr.hrsa.gov/kidscareers/community_hc_program.htm. Accessed September 17, 2005.

148. U.S. Department of Agriculture. Food Stamp Program. Available at: http://www.fns.usda.gov/fsp/faqs.htm. Accessed March 19, 2008.

149. U.S. Department of Health and Human Services. Administration for Children and Families. The Personal Responsibility and Work Opportunity Reconciliation Act of 1996. Available at: http://www.acf.dhhs.gov/programs/cse/new/prwora.htm. Accessed March 19, 2008.

150. U.S. Department of Agriculture. Electronic Benefit Transfer (EBT). Available at: http://www.fns.usda.gov/fsp/ebt/default.htm. Accessed April 2, 2008.

151. U.S. Department of Agriculture. The Emergency Food Assistance Program (TEFAP). Available at: http://www.state.nj.us/agriculture/divisions/fn/fooddistrib/tefap.html. Accessed April 2, 2008.

152. U.S. Department of Agriculture. Cooperative State Research, Education and Extension office. Available at: http://www.csrees.usda.gov/Extension/index.html. Accessed March 19, 2008.

153. Rosenbaum S, Wise P. Crossing the Medicaid-private insurance divide: the case of EPSDT. *Health Affairs.* 2007; 26(2):382–393.

154. Peters C. EPSDT: Medicaid's critical but controversial benefits program for children. *NHPF.* 2006; 819:1–24. Available at: http://www.nhpf.org/pdfs_ib/IB819_EPSDT_11-20-06.pdf. Accessed March 19, 2008.

CHAPTER 9

Nutrition in Childhood and Adolescence

LEARNING OBJECTIVES

- Identify the nutritional needs of adolescents and school-age children.
- Discuss common nutrition problems during childhood and adolescence.
- List the diagnostic criteria for eating disorders in adolescents.
- Discuss the contributing factors to childhood overweight and obesity.
- Discuss the causes of malnutrition in children globally and in the United States.
- Discuss the effect television has on children's eating habits.
- Discuss and outline different child nutrition programs.

Introduction

Maintaining the proper physical, social, and cognitive development of children (ages 1 to 11) and adolescents is essential and depends upon adequate energy and nutrient intake. Children and adolescents who lack adequate energy and nutrient intake are at risk for a variety of nutrition-related health conditions, including growth retardation, malnutrition, iron deficiency anemia, poor academic performance, protein–energy malnutrition, development of psychosocial difficulties, and an increased likelihood of developing chronic diseases such as metabolic syndrome, diabetes, heart disease, and osteoporosis during adulthood.[1-5] Children and adolescents who live below the national poverty level are more likely to experience nutrient deficiencies, food insecurity, and hunger.[6,7] In the United States, child nutrition programs subsidize meals served to children and adolescents in schools and other organizations that may help prevent malnutrition. The programs that make up the federal child nutrition programs are the following: Special Supplemental Nutrition Program for Women, Infants, and Children (WIC); National School Lunch Program (NSLP); School Breakfast Program (SBP); Summer Food Service Program (SFSP); and Special Milk Program (SMP). In addition, low-income families are eligible to enroll in the Food Stamp Program (FSP). These programs will be discussed later in this chapter.

Nutrition Status of Children and Adolescents in the United States

The diets of many children and adolescents in the United States are below the recommended dietary standards. A small number of U.S. children eat the recommended amounts of grains, fruits, vegetables, dairy products, and meat or meat alternatives from the MyPyramid.[8] The majority of them consumes calorie-dense snacks and meals, with added sugars and larger portion sizes, which increase the overall amount of caloric intake.[9-12] Children's total fat, saturated fat, and sodium intake generally are above recommended levels.[9,10] Children and adolescents also consume large amounts of beverages that are high in added sugars, such as soft drinks and fruit drinks.[13] These habits can lead to inadequate intakes of essential vitamins and minerals.

Over-consumption of calories and inactivity are major factors contributing to the increased rate of childhood overweight and obesity in the United States.[14] The prevalence of overweight and obesity in children ages 6 to 17 years has doubled in the past 30 years. About 4.7 million children ages 6 to 17 years are seriously overweight or obese.[14,15]

diabetes mellitus A disease caused by insufficient insulin secretion by the pancreas or insulin resistance by body tissues causing high blood glucose level.

Overweight and obesity at any age increase the risk for type 2 *diabetes mellitus*, cardiovascular disease, and severe social and psychological problems.[14,15] Research shows that overweight and obese children with poor nutritional practices tend to have difficulty learning and concentrating and are more likely to be sick and miss school.[16-18] **Table 9.1** provides examples of fruits and vegetables that parents and caregivers can use to feed toddlers and preschoolers.

Healthy People 2010

The goal of Healthy People 2010 is to increase the proportion of adolescents who participate in daily school physical education to 50 percent and to increase the proportion of adolescents who engage in moderate physical activity (> 30 minutes on at least 5 days of the previous 7) and vigorous physical activity that promotes cardiorespiratory fitness on more than 3 days per week for 20 minutes per occasion.[19] Reports show slight progress toward these objectives.[20] **Table 9.2** presents the Healthy People 2010 objectives for children and adolescents progress review.

TABLE 9.1 Food Guide for Toddlers and Preschoolers[25]

Food Group	Servings Per Day	Foods	Toddler Amounts	Preschooler Amounts	Nutrients Supplied
Grains	6	Bread, tortilla pieces, waffle squares, noodles, rice, pasta, etc.	¼–½ slice / ¼ cup	½ slice / ⅓ cup	Carbohydrates, iron, fiber, and thiamin
		Hot cereal (oatmeal, grits)	¼ cup	⅓ cup	
		Cold cereal (ready-to-eat cereal, any variety)	¼ cup	⅓ cup	
Vegetables	3–5	Cooked vegetables (broccoli, peas, sweet potatoes, squash, mushrooms, green beans, winter squash, spinach, etc.)	2 Tbsp	¼ cup	Carbohydrates, magnesium, fiber, carotenoids, vitamin A, and phytochemicals
		Raw vegetables (carrot sticks, tomatoes, etc.)	2 Tbsp	¼ cup	
Fruits	2–4	Fresh fruit (raisins, kiwi slices, berries, strawberries, melon, etc.)	2 Tbsp	¼ cup	Carbohydrates, vitamin C, potassium, fiber, and phytochemicals
		Fruit juice (apple, pineapple, orange, etc.)	¼ cup	½ cup	
		Canned fruit (any variety)	¼ cup	½ cup	
Milk and dairy products	3–4	Milk or yogurt	½ cup	¾ cup	Carbohydrates, protein, vitamin D, calcium, and phosphorus
		Cheese (cheese cubes, cheese sticks)	1 oz	1 ½ oz	
Meat and poultry	2–3	Meat (beef cubes, turkey rollups)	1 oz	1 ½ oz	Protein, vitamin B, iron, zinc, and phytochemicals
		Chicken			
		Turkey			
		Fish (tuna and salmon without bones)	1 oz	1 ½ oz	
		Cooked beans	2 Tbsp	¼ cup	
		Eggs	½ an egg	1 egg	
		Peanut butter	1 Tbsp	2 Tbsp	
		Nuts			

| TABLE 9.2 | Healthy People 2010 Objectives Related to Children and Adolescents |

Healthy People 2010 Objectives Number	Healthy People 2010 Objective	Baseline (Year)	Progress Review (2002)	Healthy People 2010 Target
19.2	Decrease the occurrence of iron deficiency among children:			
	a. 1 to 2 years	9% (1988–1994)	7%	5%
	b. 3 to 4 years	4% (1988–1994)	Not available	1%
19.3	Reduce the proportion of children and adolescents who are overweight or obese.	11% (1988–1994)	16%	5%
19.4	Reduce growth retardation among low-income children, 5 years and younger.	8% (1997)	8%	5%
19.5	Increase the proportion of persons age 2 years or older who consume at least three daily servings of fruit.	28% (1994–1996)	Little or no change	75%
19.6	Increase the proportion of persons age 2 years or older who consume at least three daily servings of vegetables, with at least one-third being dark green or deep yellow vegetables.	3%	No change	50%
19.7	Increase the proportion of persons age 2 years and older who consume at least six daily servings of grain products, with at least three being whole grains.	7%	Little or no change	50%
19.8	Increase the proportion of persons age 2 years or older who consume less than 10% of calories from saturated fat.	Females 2–11 years: 23% 12–19 years: 34% Males 2–11 years: 23–25% 12–19 years: 27% (1994–1996)	No change	75%
19.9	Increase the proportion of persons age 2 years or older who consume no more than 30% of calories from fat.	33%	No change	75%
19.11	Increase the proportion of persons age 2 years or older who meet dietary recommendation for calcium.	46%	Data statistically unavailable	75%
22.6	Increase the number of adolescents who engage in moderate physical activity for at least 30 minutes on 5 or more of the previous 7 days.	27% (1999)	26%	35%
22.7	Increase the proportion of the adolescents who engage in vigorous physical activity that promotes cardiorespiratory fitness 3 or more days per week for 20 or more minutes per occasion.	65% (1999)	65%	85%
22.9	Increase the number of adolescents who participate in daily school physical education.	29% (1999)	32%	50%

Data from: National Center for Health Statistics. Healthy People Tracking the Nation's Health. Available at: www.cdc.gov/nchs/about/otheract/hpdata2010/focusareas/fa16-mich.htm. Accessed October 14, 2005.

Growth and Physical Development and Assessment

The physical growth rate slows down during the preschool and school years after the first year of rapid growth until the pubertal *growth spurt* of *adolescence*.[21] The rate of growth during middle childhood is steady. On average, a 7-year-old child grows about 5 to 6 cm per year in stature and about 2 kg per year in weight, but the increase in weight is about 4 kg per year by 10 years of age. By age 2, children quadruple their birth weight. They gain an average of 4.5 to 6.5 pounds (2 to 3 kg) per year between the ages of 2 and 5.[21] Also between these ages, children grow 2.5 to 3.5 inches (6 to 8 cm) in height per year.[22]

A 1-year-old child has several teeth, and his or her digestive and metabolic systems are functioning at or near adult capability.[21,22] By 1 year of age, most children are walking or beginning to walk. With improved coordination over the next few years, their activity level increases noticeably. Childhood and adolescent eating behaviors are presented later in this chapter. Presented below are some eating behaviors of toddlers:[23,24]

- They can learn to feed themselves independently during the second year of life.

- They can manage to use a cup, with some spilling, at 15 months.
- Two-year-olds prefer foods that can be picked up with their fingers.
- Toddlers tend to be apprehensive of new foods and may refuse to eat them. (Continue to offer the new foods; it takes about 15 times before they will accept them.)
- They tend to play with food and refuse any help from the caregiver/mother.
- Young children are curious about new foods, but may be reluctant to try them.

Using Surveys to Monitor Nutrient Intake

The U.S. Department of Agriculture's Center for Nutrition Policy and Promotion (CNPP) developed the Healthy Eating Index (HEI) to evaluate and monitor the dietary status of the U.S. population. The HEI (see **Table 9.3**) represents different aspects of a healthful diet, and provides

Children should consume a daily total of three cups of milk or the equivalent from other dairy products daily.

an overall picture of the type and quality of foods people eat, their compliance with specific dietary recommendations, and the variety in their diets. The CNPP used the *Dietary Guidelines for Americans*, the Food Guide Pyramid, and the recommendations of the Committee on Diet and Health of the National Research Council to formulate the HEI. The USDA/CNPP is currently revising the HEI so that it conforms to the *2005 Dietary Guidelines*, maximizes variation in individual scores, and standardizes dietary scores.[26,27]

The total HEI score is the sum of the 10 dietary components shown in **Table 9.3**. Each component has a maximum score of 10 and a minimum score of 0; the highest possible overall HEI score is 100. An HEI score over 80 is interpreted as a "good" diet, a score between 51 and 80 is interpreted as a diet that "needs improvement," and a score of less than 51 is interpreted as a "poor" diet.[27]

The data from the 1999–2000 National Health and Nutrition Examination Survey (NHANES) show that children ages 2 to 3 had the highest mean HEI score (75.7) among all children, as well as among all other age/gender groups. The mean score for fruits for children ages 2 to 3 was significantly higher than 11 to 14 year olds' score, 7.3 vs. 2.7; for vegetables their mean score was 6.5, compared to 5.0 for children ages 7 to 10.[28] The likely reasons for the poor quality diet of older children are a diminished parental role in providing nutritious foods, peer pressure, and increased consumption of fast foods.[28]

In the United States, national surveys of dietary intakes are used to determine the types and amounts of food people consume. Wilkinson et al.[29] compared nationally representative USDA surveys of dietary intakes

growth spurt A period of peak growth rate that begins at about ages 10 to 13 years in girls and 12 to 15 years in boys.

adolescence The period of life between 12 and 19 years of age.

TABLE 9.3	Components of the Healthy Eating Index (HEI) and Scoring System			

Food Components	Score Ranges[a]	Criteria for a Maximum Score of 10	Criteria for a Minimum Score of 0
Grain consumption	0–10	6–11 servings[b]	0 servings
Vegetable consumption	0–10	3–5 servings[b]	0 servings
Fruit consumption	0–10	2–4 servings[b]	0 servings
Milk consumption	0–10	2–3 servings[b]	0 servings
Meat consumption	0–10	2–3 servings[b]	0 servings
Total fat intake	0–10	30% or less of energy from fat	45% or more of energy from saturated fat
Saturated fat intake	0–10	Less than 10% of energy from saturated fat	15% or more of energy from saturated fat
Cholesterol intake	0–10	300 mg or less	450 mg or more
Sodium intake	0–10	2,400 mg or less	4,800 mg or more
Food variety	0–10	8 or more different items in a day	3 or fewer different items in a day

[a]People with consumption or intake between the maximum and minimum ranges or amounts were assigned scores proportionately.

[b]Number of servings depends on Recommended Energy Allowance.

From: Kennedy ET, Ohls J, Carlson S, Fleming K. The Healthy Eating Index: design and application. *J Am Diet Assoc.* 1995; 95(10):1103–1108. Reprinted with permission.

of 6- to 11-year-old boys and girls using the Nationwide Food Consumption Survey (NFCS) 1977–1978, the Continuing Survey of Food Intakes by Individuals (CSFII) 1989–1991, and the CSFII 1994, 1996, and 1998 to assess whether the trends in children's food intake changed over time.[30-32] (The CSFII and NHANES have now merged into an integrated survey that acts as the primary source of nationally representative data on dietary intake of foods and nutrients and nutritional status.[33]) Results showed increases in intakes of soft drinks as well as decreases in intakes of total fluid milk due to decreases in whole milk intake. Higher intakes of crackers, popcorn, pretzels, corn chips, and potato chips and higher intakes of non-citrus juices, candy, and fruit drinks were observed. Results also showed lower intakes of yeast breads, rolls, green beans, corn, green peas, lima beans, beef, pork, and eggs.[29] These findings imply that these children were not consuming important nutrients such as vitamins and minerals that can promote growth and development. In addition, this trend of poor quality diet may be one of the reasons for the high incidence of childhood obesity.

Nutrition-Related Concerns During Childhood and Adolescence

Concern has been raised regarding poor dietary habits during childhood and adolescence. Appropriate food selection is essential because children of this age are still growing. Appropriate food selection also can reduce some of the negative consequences of inadequate food intake. Hence, it is important to monitor children's food and nutrient intakes to reduce nutrition-related health conditions, which includes but are not limited to iron deficiency anemia, lead poisoning, dental caries, overweight and obesity, and high blood cholesterol.

Iron Deficiency Anemia

Iron deficiency anemia is a problem for all ages, but especially for children. Many iron-deficient children come from low-income families with poor diets.[34] Cultural traditions and lack of nutrition knowledge about iron requirements are also factors that contribute to iron deficiencies.[35] *Iron deficiency* is defined as absent bone marrow iron stores, an increase in hemoglobin concentration of < 1.0 g/dl after treatment with iron, or other abnormal laboratory values, such as serum *ferritin* concentration.[36] Age- and sex-specific cutoff values for anemia are derived from NHANES III data. For children 1 to 2 years of age, the diagnosis of anemia would be made if the hemoglobin concentrations were < 11.0 g/dl and hematocrit was < 32.9 percent. For children ages 2 to 5 years, a hemoglobin value of 11.1 g/dl or a hematocrit of 33.0 percent signifies iron deficiency anemia.[37]

One of the Healthy People 2010 objectives is to reduce iron deficiency in children ages 1 to 2 years from 9 percent to 5 percent and in children ages 3 to 4 years from 4 percent to 1 percent.[38] A progress report in 2002 showed a decrease to 7 percent in 1 to 2 year olds (see **Table 9.2**).[39] Reaching this goal will require reducing or eliminating disparities in iron deficiency by race and family income level.

The prevalence of iron deficiency is higher in African Americans than in European American children (10 percent versus 8 percent for children ages 1 to 2 years) and is highest in Mexican American children (17 percent of children ages 1 to 2 years).[38] Also, children of families with incomes less than 130 percent of the poverty threshold have higher incidences of iron deficiency than those with a higher income (12 percent versus 7 percent).

Low blood iron levels affect a child's resistance to disease, attention span, behavior, and intellectual performance.[40,41] It is reported that

Successful Community Strategies 🏠🏠🏠

Lead Poisoning Prevention in Hartford, Connecticut[58]

The Hartford Health Department, the Hartford Regional Lead Treatment Center, and the Hartford Lead Safe House established a Lead Poisoning Prevention and Education Program (LPPEP) in 1999. The program was a citywide effort to increase lead poisoning awareness and promote behaviors leading to lead-poisoning prevention among the residents within the city of Hartford, Connecticut. They implemented a multifaceted public health campaign that involved several partnerships. The program was funded by the Centers for Disease Control and Prevention, the U.S. Department of Housing and Urban Development, the Connecticut Department of Public Health, and the U.S. Environmental Protection Agency. The campaign used 10 different strategies to carry out the intervention program, including an educational video that aired on public access television and

was made available to 10 of the city's public libraries; drawings showing the hazards of lead poisoning that were chosen from a poster contest were displayed at the capitol building; and an educational table was displayed in front of a local Hartford hardware store for almost one year to reach patrons and pedestrians with messages about lead poisoning and lead-safe work practices. Also, four educational advertisements highlighting lead poisoning prevention were placed for two consecutive months from April 1 to June 30, 2000 in Connecticut's major newspaper and two smaller, local Hartford newspapers, to reach different segments of the population. One of the ads featured two African American boys encouraging readers to test their children and homes for lead. The ads included phone numbers for both the Hartford Health Department and the Connecticut

Children's Medical Center. From April 2000 through April 2001, the Hartford Health Department posted an educational awareness message in English and in Spanish on 16 Hartford billboards. These messages featured a woman playing with a child; underneath was the phrase, "He got his eyes from grandma, his laugh form Daddy, and his lead poisoning from home." The billboards have continued to be posted throughout the city. In addition, the Hartford Health Department partnered with a local dairy to place lead awareness messages on almost 1 million milk cartons and 300,000 orange juice cartons that were distributed throughout Connecticut, Rhode Island, Westchester County in New York, and western Massachusetts. These ads featured drawings of children, along with the phrase "One good reason to prevent lead poisoning."

excessive consumption of milk could contribute to low iron intake. Milk/soymilk intake should be limited to 3 to 4 cups per day, or no more than 24 ounces; this will permit inclusion of iron-rich foods, such as lean meats, legumes, fish, poultry, and iron-enriched breads and cereals.[36] Larger intakes of milk or soymilk may replace foods that are high in iron.

Cultural and religious practices also may affect children's iron status. For example, it was reported that East Indian mothers living in Great Britain do not feed their children beef if they are Hindu; if they are Moslem, they do not feed children pork or meats that are not "halal." (Permitted, or lawful, foods are called halal.) They often do not replace the nutrients in those items with equivalent foods, consequently causing anemia.[42] In contrast, it was reported that in Spain, preschool children showed better iron status when meat was included in their diets during their eighth month or earlier, compared to those who were given meat later.[43] There are no reports on the effect of kosher meat on iron status.

Iron deficiency anemia is not common in school-age children. The NHANES III data from 1988–1994 and other studies have shown that more than 7 percent of older children were iron deficient, however.[44–46] It was reported that iron deficiency among adolescents was 2.8 to 3.5 percent of 11- to 14-year-old females, 4.1 percent of 11- to 14-year-old males, 6.0 to 7.2 percent of 15- to 19-year-old females, and 0.6 percent of 15- to 19-year-old males.[47,48] Dietary intake of iron ranges from 10.0 to 12.5 milligrams per day in females (ages 14 to 18 years old).[48] The Dietary Reference Intakes (DRIs) are 15 mg per day for girls and 11 mg per day for boys. Donovan et al. reported that 32 percent of male and 83 percent of female adolescents consume less than the DRI for iron.[49,50]

Lead Poisoning

About 4.4 percent of children ages 1 to 5 years have high blood lead levels—higher than 10 mg/dl. Lead poisoning is common among children under age 6 and can cause learning disabilities and behavior problems, slow growth, brain damage, and central nervous system damage. Lead poisoning also can cause iron deficiency, and in turn, iron deficiency can impair the body's ability to prevent lead absorption.[38,51] Satisfactory calcium intake may slow lead's absorption or interfere with its toxicity.

The U.S. Environmental Protection Agency's (EPA's) "Keep It Clean" public health campaigns to prevent lead poisoning have significantly reduced the amount of lead in the environment. Also, the U.S. ban on the use of leaded gasoline, leaded house paint, and lead-soldered food cans have helped to reduce lead poisoning.[52] Other strategies for preventing lead poisoning include providing nutritious foods, screening children for lead poisoning, preventing children from eating non-food items, avoiding water containing lead, and preventing children from putting dirty or old painted objects in their mouths. In addition, food providers must wash their hands before handling foods and require children to also wash their hands before eating.[22,37,53]

The problem of lead exposure is still prevalent in the United States. Nearly 900,000 children younger than 6 years

iron deficiency Absent bone marrow iron stores, an increase in hemoglobin concentration of < 1.0 g/dl after treatment with iron, or other abnormal laboratory values, such as serum ferritin concentration.

ferritin A complex of iron and apoferritin that is a major storage form of iron.

Additionally, the Hartford Health Department partnered with the Connecticut Transit Authority to place educational signs on the interiors of 120 city buses, on the exterior bus tails of 20 additional buses, and on the walls of five of the city's shelters. Plus, a series of 4-foot by 8-foot lead poisoning awareness signs were placed on the sides of Hartford's 13 municipal sanitation trucks. The sign posted messages in English and in Spanish about the hazards of lead poisoning and the importance of having children tested for lead. In addition, the city of Hartford collaborated with the U.S. Postal Service and the U.S. Department of Housing and Urban Development to implement, for the first time in the United States, postmarks aimed at the prevention of lead poisoning. This postmark was applied to almost every stamped, first-class card and letter mailed in Connecticut in October 2001.

The postmark featured an illustration of a house accompanied by the phrase "Let's give every child a lead safe home."

At the end of the campaign, the Hartford Health Department conducted a survey to evaluate its effectiveness. About 45 percent of the respondents said that they took specific steps to learn more about lead poisoning because of the campaigns described above. The survey also showed that:

- About 73.3 percent of the respondents said that they asked their doctor about blood tests for lead poisoning.
- 21.3 percent said that they called a phone number to learn more about lead poisoning.
- 76 percent said that they changed the way they cooked or cleaned.

- 42.7 percent said that they changed the kinds of foods they fed their families.
- 41.3 percent said that they spoke to their landlord.
- 60 percent said that they took other steps to prevent lead poisoning.

Among those reporting that they took specific steps to learn more about how to prevent lead poisoning: About 51 percent specified that they took steps because of the newspaper advertisements. Consequently, the newspaper ads were the most effective campaign strategy in terms of self-reported lead-poisoning prevention behavior.

dental caries Tooth decay.

old still have elevated blood lead levels.[54] Low-income children and African American children are at eight and five times higher risk for lead poisoning, respectively, than other U.S. children.[55] A study conducted in California identified Mexican-born children as being at a higher risk than Hispanic children born in the United States.[56] The Centers for Disease Control and Prevention (CDC) recommends universal lead screening for children living in neighborhoods where the risk of lead exposure is widespread, and the federal Medicaid program requires that all eligible children be screened for elevated blood lead levels. Children who live in housing built before 1950 are at high risk for lead poisoning because of the presence of lead-based paints.[57] Children who live in inner cities are also at risk of lead poisoning because of the lead in dirt. Successful Community Strategies 9-1 presents a successful lead intervention program.

Dental Caries

Dental caries is a widespread problem for all age groups. About one in five children ages 2 to 4 years has decay in their primary or permanent teeth.[59] Foods containing carbohydrates that stick to the surface of the teeth, such as sticky candy like caramel, can interact with the bacteria *Streptococcus mutans* and cause tooth decay.[60] The following suggestions may help reduce dental caries in children:[22,37,61]

- Brush the child's teeth to remove carbohydrates.
- Rinse the child's mouth with water.
- Use fluoridated water.
- Provide crunchy foods such as carrot sticks and apple slices for a snack. These are less likely to promote tooth decay than sticky candies or raisins.

Tooth decay occurs when sugar in liquids is in contact with teeth for a prolonged time. Milk, formula, juice, Kool-Aid, and soft drinks contain sugar.

Overweight and Obesity

There has been a significant increase in the United States in the prevalence of overweight and obesity in children and adolescents. A body mass index (BMI) between the 85th and 95th percentiles for age and sex is considered at risk for overweight, and a BMI at or above the 95th percentile is considered overweight or obese.[62] According to the 2003–2004 NHANES data, about 18.8 percent of children (6 to 11 years old) and 17.4 percent of adolescents 12 to 19 years are overweight. A research study conducted by Krebs and Baker showed that about 15.3 percent of 6- to 11-year-olds and 15.5 percent of 12- to 19-year-olds were at or above the 95th percentile for BMI on standard growth charts developed by the CDC.[62] One of the Healthy People 2010 objectives is to reduce the prevalence of overweight from the baseline of 11 percent to 5 percent. However, **Figure 9-1** shows a progressive and constant trend of overweight in children and adolescents through 2004 when the BMI criterion was applied to data from previous NHANES since the 1960s. The data show an increase of almost 45 percent from estimates of 11 percent obtained from NHANES III data (1988–1994) and a three-fold increase from the 1960s.[63]

Overweight and obesity occur at a higher rate in African American girls than Hispanic and European Americans. For example, the prevalence of overweight in girls ages 12 to 19 years for African Americans was 25.4 percent, Mexican Americans was 14.1 percent and European Americans was 15.4 percent.[64] But for a boy of the same age group, there was a slight difference: for African Americans, 18.5 percent; for Mexican Americans, 18.3 percent; and for European Americans, 19.1 percent. In addition, Hedley et al. reported that 42.8 percent of Mexican American boys ages 6 to 19 years were at risk of overweight compared with 31 percent of African American boys and 29.2 percent of European American boys.[65] Among girls, 40.1 percent of African American girls were at risk of overweight compared to 36.6 percent of Mexican American girls and 27.0 percent of European American girls.[65]

The mechanism of obesity development is not well understood, but it is confirmed that obesity develops when energy intake exceeds energy expenditure. Many factors contribute to obesity in children and adolescents worldwide, including the amount of television viewing, an inactive and sedentary lifestyle, genetic factors, environmental factors, and cultural environment.[66,67] In a small number of cases, childhood obesity is due to medical causes such as hypothyroidism and

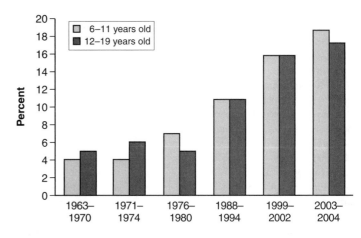

FIGURE 9-1　Prevalence of Overweight Among Children and Adolescents Ages 6–19 Years, for Selected Years 1963–1970 Through 2003–2004

growth hormone deficiency.[68] Other causes may be that low-income families lack safe places for physical activity and lack consistent access to healthful food choices, mainly fruits and vegetables.

The situations that encourage overweight or obesity evolved over a period of years; therefore, no single change will reverse the trend. Multi-component, family-based, community-based, school-based approaches including diet, physical activity, and behavior modification for reducing overweight in children and adolescents may be the best strategy.

Obesity is associated with major health problems in children and is an early risk factor for morbidity and mortality in adults.[69] Studies show that about one-third of overweight preschool children, one-half of overweight school-age children, and three-quarters of overweight teenagers grow up to be obese adults.[70–72]

Medical Problems Related to Childhood Obesity

Obese children and adolescents commonly have problems that affect cardiovascular health (hypercholesterolemia, dyslipidemia, and hypertension),[69] the endocrine system (hyperinsulinism, insulin resistance, impaired glucose tolerance, type 2 diabetes mellitus, and menstrual irregularity),[73] and mental health (depression and low self-esteem).[74–76] Other major problems that can be caused by overweight and obesity include osteoporosis and some cancers (such as ovarian and breast cancer).[77] In addition, some children may develop sleep apnea, and liver and gall bladder diseases.[78]

One health risk of notable concern is the prevalence of diagnosed diabetes coincident with increases in the prevalence of obesity and sedentary lifestyle.[79,80] Diabetes is a group of diseases marked by high levels of blood glucose due to defects in insulin production, insulin action, or both.[81] Type 1 diabetes is usually diagnosed in children and young adults, and was known as juvenile diabetes. Type 1 diabetes develops when the body's immune system destroys pancreatic beta cells, the only cells in the body that make the hormone insulin that regulates blood glucose. People with type 1 diabetes must have insulin administered by injection or a pump to help move glucose from the blood to the cells. Type 1 diabetes accounts for 5 to 10 percent of all diagnosed cases of diabetes.

Another kind of diabetes is called type 2 diabetes. This is the most common form of diabetes, and accounts for about 90 to 95 percent of all diagnosed cases. It usually begins as insulin resistance, a disorder in which the cells do not use insulin properly. As the need for insulin increases, the pancreas gradually loses its ability to produce it. Type 2 diabetes is associated with older age, obesity, a family history of diabetes, a history of gestational diabetes, impaired glucose metabolism, physical inactivity, and certain races/ethnicities. African Americans, Hispanic Americans, American Indians, and some Asian Americans and native Hawaiians are at high risk for type 2 diabetes.[81] Clinically based reports and regional studies show that type 2 diabetes is increasing in children and adolescents.[82–85] Several factors are linked to type 2 diabetes. These children and adolescents are usually between 10 and 19 years old, obese, have a strong family history for type 2 diabetes, and have insulin resistance.

This trend of obesity and its relationship to diabetes is not restricted to only U.S. children. Among Japanese schoolchildren, the incidence of Type 2 diabetes increased from 0.2 to 7.3 per 100,000 children per year between 1976 and 1995.[86] The increase was associated with changing dietary patterns and increasing rates of obesity among these children.[86] Similarly, Sinha et al. reported the prevalence of impaired glucose tolerance in 25 percent of 55 obese children (4 to 10 years of age) and in 21 percent of 112 obese adolescents (11 to 18 years of age).[87] In addition, type 2 diabetes was observed in 4 percent of the 112 obese adolescents.[87]

The prevalence of childhood obesity indicates an urgent need for the development of effective strategies for primary, secondary, and tertiary prevention. Primary prevention may include family and/or school-based programs, regardless of the children's risk status. Secondary prevention may include routine assessments of eating and activity patterns that may include school-based or institution-based programs. Tertiary prevention efforts may include individual, family-based, and multiple-component–based (diet, physical activity, behavior, and parent training) programs.

Dealing with Overweight and Obesity

Overweight and obesity are easier to prevent than to treat. Early intervention and prevention of obesity are valuable. (See Chapter 10 for more information on prevention of obesity in adults.) There is evidence that childhood eating and exercise habits can be modified more easily than adult habits.[88] Prevention of obesity needs to focus on parents' knowledge of nutrition. Parental education should include information about low-fat foods, good physical activities, and monitoring of television viewing. Wolf et al. reported that adolescents spend an average of 22 to 25 hours per week watching television.[89] (More about television viewing later in this chapter.)

Reports from national surveys of parents showed that:[90–92]

- Ninety-five percent believed that physical education should be a part of school curriculum for all students K–12, and that regular, daily physical activity could help children do better academically.
- About 85 percent believed that parents and school officials should work together to decide what students should eat and drink at school and that they would support programs in schools to help fight childhood obesity.

Physical activity is one of the answers to childhood obesity.

Parents and family members play an important role in a successful weight loss or healthy lifestyle program. A 10-year follow-up study involving parents in a weight management program with their obese children showed that parental involvement led to a significant weight loss in obese children compared to obese children without parental involvement.[93]

Similarly, a British pilot study showed that school might be an appropriate setting for the promotion of healthy lifestyles in children. However, interventions require replication in other social settings, including the family setting. The researcher stated that successful efforts should be long-lasting, multifaceted, and sustainable; involve all school-age children; and be behaviorally focused.[94]

One program designed to encourage young children to be physical fit is VERB. The VERB campaign encourages young people ages 9 to 13 years (tweens) to be physically active every day. This is a national, multicultural, social marketing campaign coordinated by the CDC. The campaign uses a combination of paid advertising, marketing strategies, and partnership efforts to reach the distinct audiences of tweens and adult role models. More information about VERB can be obtained from the CDC website (http://www.cdc.gov). Successful Community Strategies 9-2 presents a different successful obesity prevention program.

High Blood Cholesterol

Atherosclerosis is a progressive, complex disease that often begins in childhood and adolescence. It is related to high serum total cholesterol levels, consisting of low-density lipoprotein (LDL), very low-density lipoprotein (VLDL), and high-density lipoprotein (HDL) levels. Children and adolescents with elevated serum cholesterol levels, mainly LDL cholesterol levels, often have family members with high incidence of coronary heart disease.[69]

Most parents do not know their children's cholesterol levels. The children fitting the following criteria are at risk:[96]

- If a parent or grandparent had coronary heart disease when age 55 years or younger.

- If a parent has a blood cholesterol level 240 mg/dl or above. (About 90 percent of children with high cholesterol have a parent who also has high blood cholesterol.)
- If lipid abnormalities are in the family history.
- If a child has a medical condition that predisposes him or her to coronary heart disease, such as severe obesity, diabetes, elevated blood pressure, renal disease, or low thyroid activity.
- If family history is unknown.

Once a lipoprotein analysis is obtained, it should be repeated so that an average LDL cholesterol level can be established. The average LDL cholesterol level determines the steps for risk assessment and treatment. **Table 9.4** lists the acceptable blood cholesterol profile for children as determined by the National Cholesterol Education Program's Expert Panel (NCEPEP) and major health organizations including the American Heart Association (AHA) and the American Academy of Pediatrics (AAP).

It is encouraging to know that some children are making efforts to reduce fat intake. For instance, the results from the Bogalusa Heart Study showed a significant increase in the percentage of energy supplied by protein and carbohydrates and a significant decrease in the percentage of energy received from fat, mainly saturated and monounsaturated fat. The general dietary recommendations of the AHA for those age 2 years or older stress a diet that depends on fruits and vegetables, whole grains, low-fat and non-fat dairy products, beans, fish, and lean meat.[97,98]

Research also shows that children with high blood cholesterol levels can benefit from reducing the amount of fat, saturated fat, and cholesterol in their diets without adversely affecting their normal development. In the Dietary Intervention Study in Children (DISC), children were asked to adopt a low-fat, low-cholesterol diet. The children maintained this diet for 7 years. The dietary modifications did not alter the children's growth, nutritional status, or sexual maturation throughout the 7-year study. In addition, the diet significantly helped decrease the children's blood levels of LDL for up to 3 years after they stopped being on the diet.[99,100]

Successful Community Strategies 🏠🏠🏠

Pathways: An Obesity Prevention Program for American Indian Schoolchildren[95]

Pathways is a culturally appropriate obesity prevention program for third-, fourth-, and fifth-grade American Indian schoolchildren. The purpose of the program was to increase individual attributes such as children's knowledge about physical activity and food selections; their values about health, physical activity, and nutrition; and their sense of personal control over their choices.

An intervention committee composed of universities, American Indian nations, schools, and families (working groups) coordinated the

development of the Pathways intervention program. The committee modified the intervention based on feedback from the review process and from a highly organized process evaluation that included feedback from students, teachers, school administrators, families, and food service workers. Approval for the study was obtained from each academic institution's review board. Similar approval was obtained from each tribe. The content and approach of the Pathways intervention combined constructs from social learning theory and cultural concepts that

included American Indian customs and practices. Therefore, the intervention team drew on the indigenous beliefs and values of each participating American Indian nation to create a program that supported healthier lifestyles and reflected the nations' traditional cultures. The program also equipped children with experience in self-monitoring and goal setting to effect changes in their existing habits.

The Pathways intervention targeted four areas: 1) classroom curriculum, 2) physical education,

TABLE 9.4	Cholesterol Levels in Children and Adolescents Ages 2–19 Years[101]		
Cholesterol	**Acceptable, mg/dl**	**Borderline, mg/dl[a]**	**High, mg/dl[b]**
Total cholesterol	Less than 170	170–199	200 or more
LDL cholesterol	Less than 110	110–129	130 or more

HDL levels should be greater than or equal to 35 mg/dl and triglycerides should be less than or equal to 150 mg/dl.

[a] May require moderate changes to diet

[b] May require changes in diet and possible drug treatment

Dieting Behavior and Abnormal Eating

Dieting and abnormal eating behaviors among adolescents, especially among girls, is very common. Studies indicate that overweight individuals are more likely to report engaging in dieting and other weight-control behaviors than non-overweight individuals.[102,103] For instance, in a cross-sectional study, 17.5 percent of underweight girls (BMI < 15th percentile), 37.9 percent of average weight girls (BMI 15th–85th percentile), 49.3 percent of moderately overweight girls (BMI 85th–95th percentile), and 52.1 percent of very overweight girls (BMI > 95th percentile) reported dieting behaviors.[104] Due to the nature of this study, it is not clear whether dieting led to higher BMI values or whether overweight status led to increased dieting behavior. However, Stice et al. found that baseline dieting behaviors and dietary restraint were associated with the onset of obesity.[102]

Adolescents who diet are more likely to have poor body image and indulge in fasting, vomiting, taking diet pills, and binge eating.[102,105,106]

It is estimated that 0.5–1 percent of the general population suffers from *anorexia nervosa*, 2 percent suffer from *bulimia nervosa*, and 2 percent suffer from *binge eating* disorders.[107] In general, 95 percent of individuals diagnosed with clinical eating disorders are female.

Clinical diagnosis of these disorders is based on the psychological, behavioral, and physiological characteristics described by the *Diagnostic and Statistical Manual of Mental Disorders*, fourth edition (*DSM-IV*), criteria.[108,109] Some of the criteria for anorexia nervosa, bulimia nervosa, and binge eating disorders are presented in **Box 9-1**.

Eating disorders have many causes, and it is likely that several factors contribute to the development of the disorders in any given case. In some cases, sociocultural pressures may explain why eating disorders are high in economically privileged communities and countries; a cultural obsession with weight and thinness in women has been linked with increasing incidences of eating disorders during the past two decades.[109,110]

atherosclerosis A progressive, complex disease that often begins in childhood and adolescence and is related to high serum total cholesterol levels.

anorexia nervosa An eating disorder characterized by extreme weight loss, poor body image, and irrational fears of weight gain and obesity.

bulimia nervosa An eating disorder characterized by recurrent episodes of rapid, uncontrolled eating of large amounts of food in a short period of time. Purging often follows episodes of binge eating.

binge eating This disorder is characterized by consuming large quantities of food in a very short period of time until the individual is uncomfortably full, which normally is not followed by vomiting or the use of laxatives. The individual typically feel out of control during a binge episode, followed by feelings of guilt and shame. People must experience eating binges twice a week on average for over 6 months to qualify for this diagnosis.

3) family education, and 4) school food service. Formative assessment was conducted in each of the participating communities to identify the main risk factors for obesity specific to the study populations; design and evaluate culturally appropriate interventions, based on people's beliefs, perceptions, and behaviors; and engage members of each tribe in the development and implementation of the program.

The data collection methods used to gather information from the participants were in-depth interviews, semistructured interviews, focus groups, and direct observation. Data were collected from school staff members (teachers, food service workers, and administrators), third- to fifth-grade students and their caregivers, and other community members using in-depth interviews, semi-structured interviews, focus groups, and direct observation.

Teacher response to the 12 lessons of the third-grade curriculum showed a trend toward increased satisfaction with the lessons overall, with the students' enjoyment of the lessons, and with the students' attainment of knowledge and skills as the weeks advanced. Classroom observation by Pathways staff members complemented these responses, showing that the children participated actively in and enjoyed the lessons (particularly the story circle and music) and clearly retained some of the primary concepts.

$\mathscr{B}$ox 9-1　**Some Criteria for Eating Disorders**[108,109]

Anorexia nervosa:
- BMI of less than 17.5 kg/m² in adults
- Intense fear of gaining weight
- Disturbance in the way in which body size or weight is perceived
- Amenorrhea if the individual is a postmenarchal female

Bulimia nervosa:
- Recurrent episodes of binge eating
- Recurrent purging behavior
- Excessive exercise or fasting
- Excessive concern about body weight or shape, and absence of anorexia nervosa
- Self-evaluation unduly influenced by body shape and weight

Provisional criteria for binge eating:
- Recurrent episodes of binge eating associated with at least three behavioral and attitudinal characteristics, such as:
  - Eating large amounts when not physically hungry
  - Feeling disgusted or guilty after overeating
  - Eating much more rapidly than normal
- Occurs, on average, at least 2 days a week for 6 months
- The regular use of purging, fasting, and excessive exercise

$\mathscr{B}$ox 9-2　**Primary Causes of Protein-Energy Malnutrition (PEM)**[117]

Biological:
- Maternal malnutrition prior to or during pregnancy and lactation
- Genetic factors

Sociological:
- Poverty
- Limited or selective unavailability of food

Ecological:
- Disasters leading to famine
- Profound social inequalities either at the individual level (discrimination, refugees, prisoners) or at the community or country level
- War

Nutritional factors and dieting behavior may also contribute to the development and course of eating disorders. The onset of bulimia nervosa usually follows a period of dieting to lose weight,[111,112] and a contributory link between dietary restraint and bulimia is strengthened by similar behavior among obese patients who binge eat following diet restriction and among normal subjects following a period of food deprivation.[113,114] Their abnormal eating patterns, as well as the physiological consequences of those patterns, serve to perpetuate the disorder and contribute to its often difficult nature.

Malnutrition in Children

Malnutrition and hunger are responsible for nearly half of the deaths of preschool children throughout the world. Deficiencies in vitamin A, zinc, iron, and protein also result in illness, stunted growth, and limited development, and in the case of vitamin A, possibly permanent blindness.[115,116]

Malnutrition is caused by continual consumption of foods that provide less or more than the nutrients or energy required to support the everyday needs of the human body. Malnutrition includes **undernutrition**, which means the body is not receiving enough nutrients, and overnutrition, which includes excessive consumption of any particular nutrient.[117,118]

Undernutrition is a significant cause of malnutrition in developing countries, and poverty is its main cause. Poor families often do not have the economic, social, or environmental resources to purchase or produce enough food. Poor soil conditions also contribute to a family's inability to grow enough food to prevent malnutrition and its complications. In addition, low wages, underemployment, and food prices beyond the reach of families contribute to undernutrition in the urban poor.

Children, mainly infants and those under 5 years of age are at an increased risk for undernutrition due to the greater need for energy and nutrients during periods of rapid growth and development. Protein-energy malnutrition (PEM) occurs throughout the life cycle, but is more common during infancy/childhood and in the elderly. PEM is classified into two parts: primary and secondary. Primary PEM, presented in **Box 9-2**, refers to a deficit of available food. This may be due to biological, sociological, economic, and ecological conditions. Secondary causes of PEM, presented in **Box 9-3**, may be biological or social. Biological conditions may interfere with food intake or utilization or may increase the need for energy and other nutrients. In most cases, PEM is caused by a combination of both, but the concept of two parts may be useful for targeting interventions.[117]

The Prevalence and Effect of Malnutrition in Children

In the United States, about 13 million children live in families with incomes below the federal poverty level. About 20 percent of children under 6 years old and approximately 17.8 percent of children 6 years or older live in poor families.[119] About 15.6 percent of households with children under 6 years old were food-insecure, and more than 31 percent of these households experienced hunger in 2005.[120,121] In 2005, 15 percent of U.S. households obtained food from food pantries.[120]

The World Health Organization (WHO) Program of Nutrition compiled the most recent estimates about the distribution of PEM worldwide; the report is available online at http://www.worldhunger.org. The database covered 95 percent of the total population of children less than 5 years of age who lived in about 200 countries, as was reported in nationally representative surveys available in 2003. According to the data:

Box 9-3 Secondary Causes of Protein-Energy Malnutrition (PEM)[117]

Biological conditions that may interfere with food intake and utilization:
- Congenital anomalies (e.g., cleft lip)
- Gastrointestinal problems that may cause malabsorption of nutrients (e.g., tropical sprue)
- Genetic factors (e.g., phenylketonuria [PKU])

Biological conditions that may increase the need for energy and other nutrients:
- AIDS
- All infectious diseases accompanied with fever
- Other diseases that increase catabolism (e.g., tuberculosis)

Social causes:
- Lack of education
- Inadequate weaning practices
- Child abuse
- Alcoholism and other drug addictions

- About 182 million children, who represent 32.5 percent of all children under 5 years old, were stunted (low height for age).[122]
- About 150 million children (26.7 percent) were underweight (low weight for age).
- The largest percentage of children diagnosed with PEM was from Asia at 70 percent.
- Africa had 26 percent of children diagnosed with PEM.
- Latin America and the Caribbean showed 4 percent stunted growth.
- About 5 million children died of malnutrition worldwide.[117,122]

Globally, there is an adequate food supply and the technical expertise necessary to address the problems and complications of malnutrition. All that is lacking is the political cooperation to address this devastating situation.[117]

In the United States, federal programs such as the WIC Program, National School Lunch Program, School Breakfast Program, Summer Feeding Program, and Special Milk Program provide a safety net for children. The WIC program is designed to follow children through their fifth birthday. It provides vouchers for milk, eggs, cereal, juice, cheese, and either peanut butter or dried beans. However, the WIC program does not reach all the children in need. Many parents do not understand that WIC is still available after a child is weaned from formula, do not have transportation to get to a WIC grocery site, or are homeless.

Children and Adolescents with Special Healthcare Needs/Childhood Disability

The prevalence of ***childhood disability*** is increasing—about 7 to 18 percent of children and adolescents from birth to 18 years in the United States have a chronic physical, behavioral, developmental, or emotional condition. These conditions limit their activities and/or require

special care.[123-125] The health and health-related needs of children with disabilities are very broad and it is not possible to adequately cover all aspects in this chapter.

There are various causes of developmental disabilities, and special healthcare needs are comprehensive. Children may have physical impairments, developmental delays, or chronic medical conditions that are caused by or associated with the following factors:[126,127]

- Genetic conditions (e.g., diabetes, sickle cell anemia)
- Congenital infections
- Inborn errors of metabolism (e.g., phenylketonuria, lactose intolerance, galactosemia)
- Prematurity
- Neural tube defects
- Maternal substance abuse
- Environmental toxins (e.g., lead, mercury)

Children and adolescents with special healthcare needs are at risk for nutrition-related health problems. It is estimated that up to 40 to 50 percent of children and adolescents with special healthcare needs have nutrition-related risk factors or health problems that require the attention of a registered dietitian, nutritionist, or healthcare professional.[128,129] Some of the nutrition risk factors include, but are not limited to, physical, biochemical, psychological, or environmental in nature. Physical conditions such as a cleft lip or palate or a disease process such as ***galactosemia*** may limit an individual's ability to feed, digest, or absorb food. Drug–nutrient interactions may alter digestion, absorption, or the bioavailability of nutrients from the diet. Also, psychological factors may contribute to an individual's ability to accept and cope with a disability or treatment plan.[129] For example, depression or stress may alter an individual's appetite and motivation to follow a specified diet plan. Environmental factors such as family and social support, finances, and other factors will have a significant impact on the children's access to nutritious foods and support for following certain dietary regimens. One or a combination of these factors may put a child or an adolescent with special needs at nutritional risk.[130] Common nutrition problems for children and adolescents with special healthcare needs may include the following:[128,129,131,132]

- Altered energy and nutrient needs
- Delayed or stunted linear growth
- Underweight
- Overweight or obesity
- Feeding delays or oral-motor dysfunction
- Drug–nutrient interactions
- Appetite disturbances
- Unusual food habits (e.g., rumination, voluntary regurgitation of food, pica, disordered eating)
- Dental and gum disease

It is important to perform comprehensive assessment of the problems. The assessment process should include anthropometric data, biochemical and lab data, clinical findings, medical history, a dietary history or food frequency questionnaire, and feeding skills assessment

undernutrition A health condition caused by a deficiency of one or more nutrients.

childhood disability Children and adolescents who have or are at increased risk for a chronic physical, developmental, behavioral, or emotional condition and who require health and related services.

galactosemia Lack of the enzyme needed to metabolize galactose.

(chewing ability, etc.).[132] The assessment and care plan processes require a multidisciplinary team approach that allows individuals from different disciplines to address the problems that may impact nutrition and other needs. The multidisciplinary team members can include physicians, nurses, dietitians, dentists, community resource personnel, and social workers.[131] The child and caregiver(s) should be the main members of the team who identify problems and set priorities to be addressed in the treatment plan.

After the assessment process is completed and a treatment plan is established, the best strategy for incorporating nutrition goals and objectives outside the home is to collaborate with the school system. In local communities, public schools use the Child and Adult Care Food Program to provide resources to children and adolescents with special needs. Public schools also administer the National School Lunch and National School Breakfast Programs. Federal government regulations allow modified school meals for students with disabilities or chronic medical problems needing special diets at no extra cost. Food substitutions and modified meals required for a medical or special dietary need are provided for individuals identified by the school system as having a disability.[129] The provision of comprehensive nutrition services to 3 to 5 year olds with disability was mandated by Congress in 1986 (Education of the Handicapped Act Amendments PL99-457).[133] In this provision, nutritionists are recognized as the health professionals qualified to provide developmental services to children with special healthcare needs.[133]

The Special Olympics program is a non-governmental program that promotes health, nutrition and physical fitness for disabled children and adolescents. This program provides year-round sports training and athletic competition in a variety of community-based Olympic-type sports for children. The activities include nutrition, physical fitness, and the sharing of gifts, skills, and friendship. To receive the nutrition benefits, the child must have a diet prescription from a physician. The prescription must include the following information:[129,131]

- A statement identifying the disability, and how the disability affects the adolescent's diet
- A statement identifying the major life activity affected by the disability
- A specific list of dietary changes, modifications, or substitutions required for the diet

The goals set by Healthy People 2010 for the nation's disabled children and adolescents were to achieve more physical activity, better nutrition, weight control, and improved access to healthcare and preventive services and mental health services.

The Effect of Television on Children's Eating Habits

It appears that television advertisements influence children's dietary habits. Children watch an average of 3 hours of advertisements per week and 19,000 to 22,000 commercials over a 1-year period.[134] It is reported that children from families with high television use consume an average of 6 percent more of their total daily energy intake from meats; 5 percent more from pizza, salty snacks, and soda; and nearly 5 percent less of their energy intake from fruits, vegetables, and juices than children from families with low television use.[134-138] Research shows that nutrient content of advertised foods exceeded the recommended amounts for fat, saturated fat, and sodium, and failed to provide the recommended amount of fiber and certain vitamins and minerals.[37,139] Children from high television viewing families derived less of their total calories from carbohydrates and consumed twice as much caffeine as children from low television viewing families.[140]

Television is the favorite medium of advertising by the food industry,[141] and it is reported that children are exposed to too much television advertising.[142] Research studies examined food advertising during children's Saturday morning television programming and found that over half (56 percent) of all advertisements were for food. The foods promoted were high in fat or sugar, and many were low in nutritional value. As such, the diet presented on Saturday morning television is in direct contrast to what is recommended for healthful eating for children.[139,142] There is also a growing trend toward food commercialism and marketing in schools. Channel One, the daily news program that broadcasts to millions of students in grades 6–12 in thousands of schools, has 2 minutes out of each daily 12-minute program devoted to paid commercials for products that include candy bars, snack chips, and soft drinks.[142] One of the Healthy People 2010 objectives is to increase the proportion of children who view television 2 or fewer hours per day from 60 percent to 75 percent. A progress report shows little or no change.

Nutrition During Childhood and Adolescence

Adequate nutrition is very important during the school-age years. Although clinical signs of malnutrition are not common in children in North America, there are children who receive diets that are inadequate in quantity or quality. Nutrients most likely to be low or deficient are calcium, iron, zinc, vitamin B_6, and vitamin A.[143,144] Similarly, national survey data show that children continue to consume foods high in sugar and sodium and insufficient amounts of fruits and vegetables.[29] Children living in poor families are more likely to follow diets that are low in calories; vitamins A, C, E, and B_6; folate; iron; zinc; thiamin; and magnesium.[145] Community nutritionists can encourage parents and caregivers to provide adequate foods using the food guide presented in **Table 9.5**.

Growth and Development

The normal events of puberty and the simultaneous growth spurt are the primary influences on nutritional requirements during adolescence. During puberty, height and weight increase, many organ systems enlarge, and body composition is altered due to increased lean body mass

TABLE 9.5	**The Recommended Daily Calorie Intake**		
Age Category		**Not Active**	**Active**
Children 2–3 yrs		1,000	1,400
Females 4–8 yrs		1,200	1,800
Females 9–13 yrs		1,600	2,200
Females 13–18 yrs		1,800	2,400
Females 19–30 yrs		2,000	2,400
Males 4–8 yrs		1,400	2,200
Males 9–13 yrs		1,800	2,600
Males 14–18 yrs		2,200	3,200
Males 19–30 yrs		2,400	3,000

Source: U.S. Department of Agriculture. MyPyramid Sample Menu. Available at: http://www.mypyramid.gov/professionals/index.html. Accessed November 28, 2005.

and changes in the quantity and distribution of fat. The timing of the growth spurt is influenced by genetic as well as environmental factors. Children who weigh more than average for their height tend to mature early and vice versa.[20]

Normally, growth spurts begin between ages 10.5 and 11 for girls, and peak at about 12 years of age. Boys' growth spurts start between 12.5 and 13 and peak at about age 14. This spurt lasts about 2 years.[22] The most rapid linear growth spurt for an average American boy occurs between 12 and 15 years of age. For the average American girl, the spurt occurs about 2 years earlier, between 10 and 13 years of age. The growth spurt during adolescence contributes about 15 percent of final adult height and about 50 percent of adult weight. During adolescence, boys tend to gain more weight than girls, and boys experience greater increases in lean body mass. Girls accumulate more body fat, specifically around the hips and buttocks, upper arms, breasts, and upper back.

Growth charts are tools used for monitoring the growth of a child.[146] These charts, which are pertinent to the school-age child, include weight-for-age, stature-for-age, and BMI-for-age for boys and girls.

Adolescent Eating Behaviors

The eating habits of adolescents are not static; they fluctuate throughout adolescence. Adolescents may use foods to establish individuality and to express their identity. Experimentation may lead to certain eating behaviors such as skipping meals, and the rate of meal skipping may increase as they mature.[137] Breakfast is the most-skipped meal; only 29 percent of adolescent females eat breakfast daily.[138,147] Adequate nutrition, especially eating breakfast, has been associated with improved academic performance and reduced tardiness and absences.[148] Lunch is another meal that about 25 percent of adolescents skip.[138,149,150] Reasons for their changes in eating habits include spending less time with family and more time with their peer group.[138] They eat more meals and snacks away from home, including many fast foods high in fat and calories.[15] The average teenager eats at fast food restaurants twice a week. Fast food visits account for 31 percent of all food eaten away from home and make up 83 percent of their visits to restaurants.[149,151]

The results of the Healthy Eating Index (HEI) showed that in general, children ages 11 through 18 had poorer quality diets compared to younger children (2 to 3 years old). The possible reasons for the poor diet may be that parents are less attentive to the diets of this age group (11 through 18) and that children from low-income families are more likely to have a poorer diet. In addition, studies show that as children become more independent, they make inadequate dietary choices such as consuming more fast foods and salty snacks.[149,151] The average HEI scores for females ages 11 to 18 was 61.5 and for males of the same age was 60.4. As mentioned earlier in the chapter, an HEI score over 80 implies that the person has a good diet; a score between 51 and 80 means the diet needs improvement.

Food and Nutrition Programs for Children and Adolescents

Child nutrition programs contribute significantly to the food and nutrient intake of school-age children. The purpose of these programs is to provide nutritious meals to all children. These programs can also reinforce nutrition education in the classroom. Child nutrition programs include the National School Lunch Program, School Breakfast Program, Summer Food Service Program, and Special Milk Program (see also Chapter 4).

National School Lunch Program

The National School Lunch Program provides nutritious lunches and the opportunity for professionals to practice skills learned in nutrition education classes. This program also offers after-school snacks at sites that meet eligibility requirements.

School food programs for children started in the early 1900s when free, compulsory, and universal education was established.[152] Philanthropic organizations, local school districts, and private individuals made the first efforts to establish free lunches in schools. With increasing federal involvement, primarily in the form of donations from the accumulation of surplus foods, states gradually expanded the number of food programs.[152] In 1946, legislation was passed establishing the National School Lunch Program under the direction of the USDA. Today, federal cash reimbursements and donated foods from the Commodity Supplemental Food Program are provided to schools that serve a lunch meeting specified nutritional requirements (see **Table 9.6**). Modifications in 1971 established the provision that children from families with incomes at or below 130 percent poverty level are eligible for a free lunch, and children in families with incomes between 130 percent and 185 percent below the poverty level are eligible for a reduced price lunch.[153] **Table 9.7** shows the eligibility standards for the federal child nutrition programs.

A small reimbursement is also provided to the school for all lunches, but children from families with incomes above 185 percent of the poverty level pay the established price (see **Table 9.8**). Most of the support that the USDA provides to schools in the National School Lunch Program comes in the form of a cash reimbursement for each meal served.

TABLE 9.6	**Acceptable National School Lunch Program Meals**		
Food Items		**Type A***	**Type B***
Milk, whole		½ pint	2 pints
Protein-rich foods consisting of any of the following or a combination thereof:		2 oz	1 oz
Fresh or processed meat and poultry			
Cheese, cooked or canned fish			
Dry peas, or beans, or soybeans, cooked		½ cup	¼ cup
Peanut butter		4 Tbsp	2 Tbsp
Eggs		1	½
Raw, cooked, or canned vegetables, fruits, or both		¾ cup	½ cup
Bread, muffins, or hot bread made of whole grain cereal or enriched flour		1 portion	1 portion
Butter or fortified margarine		2 tsp	1 tsp

*The Type A lunch was designed to meet one-third to one-half of the minimum daily nutritional requirements of a child 10 to 12 years of age. The Type B pattern was devised to provide a supplementary lunch in schools where adequate facilities for the preparation of a Type A lunch could not be provided.

Source: U.S. Department of Agriculture, Food and Nutrition Services. School Meal Programs Income Eligibility Guidelines. Available at: http://www.fns.usda.gov/cnd. Accessed April 24, 2005.

TABLE 9.7 Annual Income Eligibility Guidelines for the Federal Child Nutrition Programs, July 1, 2005–July 1, 2006

Household Size	Annual Federal Poverty Guidelines	Reduced Price Meals—185%					Free Meals—130%				
		Annual	Monthly	Twice per Year	Every Two Weeks	Weekly	Annual	Monthly	Twice per Month	Every Two Weeks	Weekly
48 CONTIGUOUS STATES, DISTRICT OF COLUMBIA, GUAM, AND TERRITORIES											
1	9,570	17,705	1,476	738	681	341	12,441	1,037	519	479	240
2	12,830	23,736	1,978	989	913	457	16,679	1,390	695	642	321
3	16,090	29,767	2,481	1,241	1,145	573	20,917	1,744	872	805	403
4	19,350	35,798	2,984	1,492	1,377	689	25,155	2,097	1,049	968	484
5	22,610	41,829	3,486	1,743	1,609	815	29,393	2,450	1,225	1,131	566
6	25,870	47,860	3,989	1,995	1,841	921	33,631	2,803	1,402	1,294	647
7	29,130	53,891	4,491	2,246	2,073	1,037	37,869	3,156	1,578	1,457	729
8	32,390	59,922	4,994	2,497	2,305	1,153	42,107	3,509	1,755	1,620	810
For each additional family member, add	3,260	6,031	503	252	232	116	4,238	354	177	163	82
ALASKA											
1	11,950	22,108	1,843	922	851	426	15,535	1,295	648	598	299
2	16,030	29,656	2,472	1,236	1,141	571	20,839	1,737	869	802	401
3	20,110	37,204	3,101	1,551	1,431	716	26,143	2,179	1,090	1,006	503
4	24,190	44,752	3,730	1,865	1,722	861	31,447	2,621	1,311	1,210	605
5	28,270	52,300	4,359	2,180	2,012	1,006	36,751	3,063	1,532	1,414	707
6	32,350	59,848	4,988	2,494	2,302	1,151	42,055	3,505	1,753	1,618	809
7	36,430	67,396	5,617	2,809	2,593	1,297	47,359	3,947	1,974	1,822	911
8	40,510	74,944	6,246	3,123	2,883	1,442	52,663	4,389	2,195	2,026	1,013
For each additional family member, add	4,080	7,548	629	315	291	146	5,304	442	221	204	102
HAWAII											
1	11,010	20,369	1,698	849	784	392	14,313	1,193	597	551	276
2	14,760	27,306	2,276	1,138	1,051	526	19,188	1,599	800	738	369
3	18,510	34,244	2,854	1,427	1,318	659	24,063	2,006	1,003	926	463
4	22,260	41,181	3,432	1,716	1,584	792	28,938	2,412	1,206	1,113	557
5	26,010	48,119	4,010	2,005	1,851	926	33,813	2,818	1,409	1,301	651
6	29,760	55,056	4,588	2,294	2,118	1,059	38,688	3,224	1,612	1,488	744
7	33,510	61,994	5,167	2,584	2,385	1,193	43,563	3,631	1,816	1,676	838
8	37,260	68,931	5,745	2,873	2,652	1,326	48,438	4,037	2,019	1,863	932
For each additional family member, add	3750	6,938	579	290	567	134	4,875	407	204	188	94

Source: U.S. Department of Agriculture, Food and Nutrition Services. School Meal Programs Income Eligibility Guidelines. Available at: http://www.fns.usda.gov/cnd. Accessed April 24, 2005.

TABLE 9.8	**Current Basic Cash Reimbursement Rates (July 1, 2006–June 30, 2007)[a,154]**		
Free lunches:	$2.40	Free snacks:	$0.65
Reduced-price lunches:	$2.00	Reduced-price snacks:	$0.32
Paid lunches:	$0.23	Paid snacks:	$0.06

[a] Higher reimbursement rates are in effect for Alaska and Hawaii, and for some schools with high percentages of low-income children.

In 1994, the Food and Nutrition Service (formerly Food and Consumer Service) launched the School Meals Initiative for Healthy Children. The purpose of this initiative was twofold: 1) to educate children about the importance of making healthy food choices and 2) to provide support for school food service professionals to offer healthy school meals that meet the *Dietary Guidelines for Americans*. The recommendation included that no more than 30 percent of an individual's calories come from fat and less than 10 percent from saturated fat. Regulations also established a standard for school lunches to provide one-third of the Recommended Dietary Allowances for protein, vitamin A, vitamin C, iron, calcium, and calories. School lunches must meet federal nutrition requirements, but local school food authorities make decisions about what specific foods to serve and how they are prepared. The initiative was implemented in schools throughout the United States at the beginning of the 1996–1997 school year.[154]

In fiscal year 2007, more than 30.1 million children received their lunch through the National School Lunch Program each day. Since the modern program began, more than 187 billion lunches have been served.[155] However, not all children participate in the National School Lunch Program or the School Breakfast Program.[156]

School Breakfast Program

The School Breakfast Program began as a pilot project in 1966 and was made permanent in 1975. Eligibility criteria are the same as for the School Lunch Program. There are many reasons the School Breakfast Program was implemented, some of which are the obvious nutrition-related ones. However, studies have shown that children who participated in the School Breakfast Program also have higher standardized achievement test scores than eligible non-participants.[152]

Children often skip breakfast because of busy schedules, long bus rides, and lack of resources.[157] Meal standards and children's access to healthy foods improve the health status and academic performance of students. School breakfasts must provide one-fourth of the RDA for calories, protein, calcium, iron, vitamin A, and vitamin C for the applicable age or grade groups.[158,159]

In fiscal year 2005, an average of 9.7 million children participated in the School Breakfast Program every day. That number grew to 9.77 million in the early months of fiscal year 2006 when millions of the participants received their meals free or at a reduced price.[160]

Special Milk Program

The Special Milk Program, established in 1955 by the USDA, provides reimbursement for milk served to children. It is available to schools and childcare institutions that are not eligible for other federal child nutrition service programs. Children whose families are eligible for free school lunches or breakfasts are also eligible for free milk through this program.[152,161] In fiscal year 2006, 96 million half-pints of milk were served through the Special Milk Program.

In 2005, nearly 5,375 schools and residential childcare institutions participated, along with 1,011 summer camps and 642 non-residential childcare institutions. The Special Milk Program may also provide milk to children in half-day prekindergarten and kindergarten programs where children do not have access to the school meal programs.

Schools or institutions may choose pasteurized fluid types of unflavored or flavored whole milk, low-fat milk, skim milk, and cultured buttermilk that meet state and local standards. All milk should contain vitamins A and D at levels specified by the Food and Drug Administration. The federal reimbursement for each half-pint of milk sold to children in school year 2006–2007 was 14.5 cents.[7] For children who receive free milk, the USDA reimburses schools the net purchase price of the milk.

Because of the expansions made in the National School Lunch Program, there has been a substantial decrease in the Special Milk Program since the 1960s. In fiscal year 2005 the Special Milk Program cost $16.6 million. By comparison, the program cost $101.2 million in 1970, $145.2 million in 1980, and $19.2 million in 1990.[162]

Summer Food Service Program

The Summer Food Service Program was established in 1975 after a pilot program in 1968. The program provides free nutritious meals to low-income children during school vacations. It is offered in areas or at activity programs, such as day camps, where at least half of the children are from households with incomes below 185 percent of the poverty level.

The program provides one to two meals per day except in special conditions when three meals are provided daily. All meals are served free to eligible participants, and the USDA reimburses the sites for the meals served. During the summer of 2007, 1,924,799 children participated in this program.[153]

About 29 million U.S. children depend on free and reduced-price school meals for 9 months of the year, but only about 2.3 million participate in the summer food program (discussed in a later section). Many communities do not offer this important program; therefore, a large number of children do not eat breakfast during summer months; consequently contributing to overall poor eating habits.[163]

Team Nutrition Program

In 1995, the USDA started its School Meals Initiative for Healthy Children, called Team Nutrition, to "improve the health and education of children through better nutrition."[164] The initiative's major objectives are 1) to provide meals that are consistent with the *Dietary Guidelines for Americans* and other current scientific recommendations for children at school, and 2) to improve child health and nutrition by developing creative public and private partnerships through the media, schools, businesses, families, and the community. Partnership with private sectors also enhances the nutrition education efforts. For instance, a subsidiary of the Walt Disney Company used two movie characters to help promote nutrition. Scholastic, Inc., an educational publisher, developed teaching kits for use in schools. And the Cooperative State Research, Education, and Extension Services (CSREES) implemented community nutrition action kits. Training and technical assistance were provided to develop new recipes for use in the updated school meals program by changing the specification for foods offered in school meals and by funding training grants to assist states in developing a sustainable training infrastructure for local school districts.[164] The Healthy School Meals Resource System is an information system for food service professionals available in print form, computer disk, and on the Internet at http://www.fns.usda.gov/cnd/summer/about/ program_data.html.

Team Nutrition uses an extensive nationwide network of public and private organizations to develop and disseminate products, including private sector companies, nonprofit organizations, and advocacy groups. The purpose of the relationships is to leverage resources, expand the reach of messages, and build a broad base of support.

The success of Team Nutrition depends on effective partnerships among federal, state, and local agencies that administer child nutrition programs. Team Nutrition schools are the focal point for this initiative; however, the roles and responsibilities presented in **Table 9.9** are critical at each level.[165]

Head Start Program

The Head Start program is a comprehensive child health development program for children between the ages of 3 and 5 from families that meet the federal poverty guidelines. The Head Start Act of 1965 established this program, which provides all enrolled children with a broad array of services including education, health services (medical, nutritional, dental, and mental health), social services, parent involvement activities, and special services to children with disabilities.[166]

In fiscal year 2006, $6,776,784,000 was spent to support nearly 18,875 centers to provide development and family support services in all 50 states and in the District of Columbia and Puerto Rico. These programs served about 905,850 children ages 3 to 5 years. Twenty-nine percent of Head Start program staff members were parents of current or former Head Start children. Over 1,353,000 parents volunteered in their local Head Start Program in 2004.[166,167]

National Youth Sports Program (NYSP)

The National Youth Sports Program is a federal program designed to assist low-income children ages 10 to 16 in a summer program. The main goal of the program is to motivate low-income children to learn self-respect through a program of sports instruction and competition.

In 1968, representatives of the National Collegiate Athletic Association (NCAA) and the President's Council on Physical Fitness piloted the NYSP concept during the summer at two university athletics facilities. On March 17, 1969, the White House announced that the federal government was committing $3 million to establish a sports program for economically disadvantaged young children. The federal grant has increased significantly since then, and funding appropriations are renewed on a yearly basis. An annual grant is provided to a national, nonprofit organization to operate the NYSP.

The NYSP provides a comprehensive developmental and instructional sports program for about 78,148 low-income children. In fiscal year 2005, more than $17 million was awarded to 206 colleges and universities in 48 states to provide sports instruction and enrichment activities to disadvantaged young people. The program includes supervised sports instruction in at least four sports, using the campus facilities of the colleges and universities. The enrichment part of the program provides the children with information about career and educational opportunities, study habits, drug and alcohol abuse, and nutrition.[167]

In addition, each participant receives a free complete medical examination prior to participation in NYSP. Any physical problems that are identified receive adequate follow-up treatment. Every participant is covered by an accident-medical insurance policy, and liability insur-

TABLE 9.9	The Roles and Responsibilities of Federal, State, and Local Agencies		
FNS and the USDA	**State Agencies**	**School Districts and Other School Food Authorities**	**Schools**
• Establish policies. • Develop materials that meet needs identified by the FNS and its state and local partners. • Disseminate materials in ways that meet state and local needs. • Develop partnerships with other federal agencies and national organizations. • Promote Team Nutrition messages through the national media.	• Make recommendations to FNS regarding Team Nutrition materials and dissemination methods. • Provide training and technical assistance to strengthen current Team Nutrition schools. • Recruit new Team Nutrition schools. • Develop partnerships with other state agencies and organizations. • Promote Team Nutrition messages through the state media.	• Recruit Team Nutrition schools. • Receive Team Nutrition materials from FNS, distribute to schools, and provide training for their use. • Develop partnerships with other school district departments and community organizations. • Coordinate Team Nutrition activities among schools, especially community events. • Provide support as needed by Team Nutrition schools.	• Offer a variety of healthy menu choices. • Provide behavior-based nutrition education in pre-K through grade 12. • Establish policies and provide resources that ensure a school environment supportive of healthy eating and physical activity. • Involve parents and communities in Team Nutrition activities that reinforce team nutrition messages. • Establish partnerships among teachers, food service staff, school administrators, parents, community leaders, and the media.

Source: U.S. Department of Agriculture, Food and Nutrition Service. Team Nutrition Policy Statement. Available at: http://www.fns.usda.gov/tn. Accessed May 24, 2004.

ance is provided for sponsoring institutions. In addition, a minimum of one USDA-approved meal is provided on a daily basis and is funded by the USDA.

Challenges to Implementing Quality School Nutrition Programs

Research shows that students who participate in school meal programs have improved academic performance and healthier eating habits.[168] However, less than 60 percent of students choose the National School Lunch Program (NSLP) or School Breakfast Program (SBP).[169] School meals face a variety of challenges:[169]

- Students' preferences for fast foods, soft drinks, and salty snacks
- Mixed messages sent by school personnel
- School food preparation and serving space limitations
- Inadequate meal periods
- Lack of education standards for school foodservice directors

Studies have shown that school meal programs improve children's academic, behavioral, emotional, and social functioning.[170-172] Children participating in the National School Lunch Program are more likely than non-participants to consume more vegetables, milk and milk products, and meat and meat substitutes, and fewer soft drinks and/or fruit drinks.[173] Consequently, they consume higher amounts of calcium, riboflavin, phosphorus, magnesium, zinc, thiamin, and vitamins B_6 and B_{12} than non-participants. The contribution of school meals to total daily intake of vitamins and minerals ranges from 45 percent for iron (RDA) to 77 percent for calcium (RDA). School lunches provide about 35 percent of total energy intake. Thirty-three percent of the energy is from fat and 12 percent from saturated fatty acids. School lunches contribute one-third of the total sodium intake and 8 percent of total sucrose intake. For some 10-year-old children, about 50 to 60 percent of total daily intake of energy, protein, cholesterol, carbohydrate, and sodium are from school meals.[174]

In many schools, the continued success of child nutrition programs is in trouble. The environment in these schools discourages students from eating meals provided by the NSLP and SBP and encourages food choices and eating habits that are not consistent with the *Dietary Guidelines for Americans*.[175,176]

The sale of foods in snack bars, school stores, and vending machines competes with school meals for students' appetites, time, and money.[176] **Competitive foods** are any foods sold in competition with USDA school meals and are considered as "foods of minimal nutritional value" (FMNV) and "all other foods offered for individual sale."[176] FMNV provide less than 5 percent of the Daily Reference Intake of each of the following eight nutrients per serving: protein, niacin, riboflavin, thiamin, calcium, iron, and vitamins A and C. FMNV include soft drinks, non-fruit water ices, chewing gum, candies, jellies/gums (gum drops, jelly beans, and jellied and fruit-flavored slices), marshmallow candies, fondant (candy, soft mints), licorice, spun candy (cotton candy), and candy-coated popcorn. These foods may not be sold in the food service area during the serving period by law.[176-178]

Many foods that are served in competition with the NSLP and SBP are as a result of school administrators finding loopholes in competitive food regulations. For example:

- Government regulations restrict the sale of FMNV only during actual meal times and only in food service areas where meals are prepared and/or served. They do not prohibit competitive foods

from being sold on school campuses all day in locations other than where school meals are being served.

- The USDA's definition of FMNV does not include many high-fat, high-sodium snack items such as cookies, doughnuts, potato chips, tortilla chips, and cheese puffs.
- Other foods offered for individual sale in food service areas (such as cookies, potato chips, and muffins) are allowed if the income from the sale of such foods benefits the food service, school, or school student organizations. This creates an opportunity for schools to compete with their own NSLP and SBP for revenue, contributing to decreases in student participation in these programs.
- The sale of competitive foods is also not prohibited in elementary schools, a place where most students are not mature enough to make wise food choices.[176]

There is the potential for overconsumption of food when competitive foods are purchased in addition to school meals or in large quantities. This could lead to the risk of overweight or obesity.

To exacerbate these problems, many school districts negotiate exclusive pouring rights and marketing contracts with major beverage companies to promote their beverage and food products. Many of these contracts provide lucrative packages worth millions of dollars and make provisions to increase the percentage of profits schools receive when refreshment stand and vending sales volumes increase. School budgets are continually squeezed, so administrators find pouring rights contracts desirable and often do not consider the nutritional well-being of students.[176] For many schools, competitive foods, especially soft drinks, represent additional income that can be spent for discretionary purposes not necessarily related to food service.

As school populations grow and budgets shrink, schools give higher priority to building classrooms than to expanding food service facilities that are often inadequate for preparing and serving appealing meals to students. In some schools, inadequate cafeteria capacity requires lunch periods to begin as early as 10:00 am and end as late as 1:30 pm. Due to inadequate dining facilities and less time to eat, many students rely on less nutritious foods that are available in vending machines, snack bars, and school stores.[179,180]

Promoting Successful Programs in Schools

Inconsistent funding and severe reduction in funding from year to year, mainly in nutrition education, have decreased the effectiveness of nutrition education for children. An effective way to support nutrition-related action that encourages healthful eating and helps to reduce childhood overweight and obesity is through implementation of a coordinated school health program (CSHP).[157] A CSHP combines health education, disease prevention, health promotion, and access to health and social services in an integrated, comprehensive manner.[181] **Figure 9-2** presents the eight components of a CSHP. Community nutritionists working as CSHP team members can provide leadership and coordination for issues related to many of the components of the school health program.[182]

The CDC provided guidelines that summarize the most effective strategies for promoting

competitive foods Any foods sold in competition with U.S. Department of Agriculture school meals and that are considered as "foods of minimal nutritional value" (FMNV) available at concession stands, vending machines, and fundraisers that are in direct competition with the Child Nutrition Program during meal services anywhere on campus.

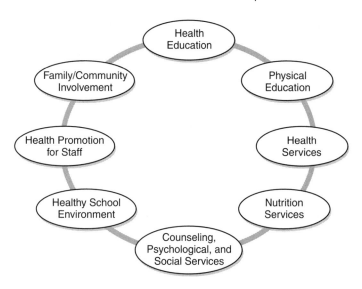

FIGURE 9-2 Eight Components of a Coordinated School Health Program
Source: Centers for Disease Control and Prevention Division of Adolescent and School Health. Available at: www.cdc.gov/healthyyouth/CSHP/index.htm.

healthy eating among school-age children within the CSHP.[182] The guidelines are available at http://www.cdc.gov/HealthyYouth/CSHP.

As **Figure 9-2** shows, nutrition services is one of the eight components of a coordinated CSHP. The other components are discussed in the following sections.

Comprehensive School Health Education

This provides prekindergarten through grade-12 classroom instruction to increase health knowledge, support positive health attitudes, and develop skills necessary for the adoption of a healthful lifestyle. Dietetics professionals can work with school health educators to incorporate health education curricula, nutrition education, and opportunities to practice healthful eating behaviors.

Physical Education

This provides planned and sequential instruction that promotes physical activity designed to develop basic movement skills, sports skills, and physical fitness and to enhance physical, mental, social, and emotional abilities. Dietetics professionals can be advocates for prekindergarten through grade-12 education that promotes lifelong physical activity and focuses on components of health-related fitness.

School Health Services

These are services coordinated by a certified school nurse that provide preventive services, education, emergency care, referral, and management of acute and chronic health conditions. Dietetics profession-

Successful Community Strategies 🏠🏠🏠

The Aptos Middle School (San Francisco, California) Pilot Program[183]

As a pilot project for the San Francisco Unified School District (SFUSD), Aptos Middle School made significant changes in its vending and à la carte food service programs. The purpose of the project was to make more healthful foods and beverages available to students and to establish nutrition standards for competitive foods. About 860 to 900 racially diverse students were enrolled in Aptos Middle School during the 2002–2003 school year. About 36.5 percent of students were eligible for free and reduced-price school meals. The new principal, a new physical education program, and a group of parents, teachers, and volunteers initiated the change in the food service program. The San Francisco superintendent of schools supported this pilot project, which helped to make it successful as a district-wide change.

With strong support from the administration, a nutrition committee composed of parents and teachers was formed to lead the changes. This group met electronically (via e-mail) to share concerns and data and to attain a consensus on appropriate changes for Aptos Middle School. The committee conducted a student survey to discover what foods students wanted the school to provide as à la carte choices. The students' preferences closely matched the parents' ideas of "more fresh foods." The most popular choices were submarine sandwiches, California rolls (sushi), soup, pasta, and smoothies.

The committee collaborated with a creative cafeteria supervisor and investigated products and ingredients that would offer students healthful

versions of the foods they wanted to purchase. This process presented both opportunities and challenges. In several cases, food suppliers and manufacturers were willing to adapt their products to adhere to the nutrition committee's standards (for example, sushi). However, it has not been possible, at least so far, to find smoothie options with appropriate ingredients at an acceptable price.

Changes instituted included:

- All soft drinks were removed from the vending machines located in the physical education department and replaced with bottled water.
- Fruit options for students were expanded

als can assist individuals in these services by developing policies for weight management and obesity programs, and can provide nutrition education programs in conjunction with classroom teachers.

School Nutrition Services

These services integrate nutritious, affordable, and appealing meals; nutrition education; and an environment that promotes healthful eating behaviors. Food service directors, as well as dietetics professionals and parents of school-age children, can advocate for policies to 1) provide more nutritious food offerings, 2) limit or remove competitive food sales and FMNV from school fundraisers, and 3) establish a list of nutritious foods allowed in vending machines, at school parties, and as classroom rewards.

School Counseling, Psychological, and Social Services

These integrate into the school environment activities that focus on the cognitive, emotional, behavioral, and social needs of individuals, groups, and families to prevent and address problems and to facilitate health and learning. Individual and group discussions regarding body image, physical changes, and weight management can also be provided. Dietetics professionals can provide encouragement and support to families who want to practice healthful eating behaviors.

Healthy School Environment

Attention to the school environment means addressing the physical, emotional, and social climates of a school to provide a safe and supportive environment to enhance health and learning. Policies to support healthful eating environments related to vending machines, competitive foods, fundraisers, and classroom rewards and party treats should be developed. Dietetics professionals can help promote healthful eating environments by serving on nutrition-related school committees and advocating for policies that place precedence on nutrition and learning.

School-Site Health Promotion for Staff

This includes assessment of education and fitness activities for school faculty and staff that are designed to maintain and improve students' health and well-being. Faculty and staff should be provided with opportunities to participate in workshops and classes for healthful eating and physical activity. Dietetics professionals can offer nutrition-related workshops and classes to school faculty and staff.

Family and Community Involvement in School Health

Family and community involvement consists of developing partnerships among schools, families, community groups, and individuals to share and maximize resources and expertise in addressing the healthful development of children, adolescents, and families. Dietetics professionals can partner with schools and community organizations to establish nutrition, food preparation, weight management, and exercise programs for students, faculty, staff, and families.[181] Successful Community Strategies 9-3 presents a program created by the Aptos Middle School in San Francisco, California.

---

beyond apples, oranges, and bananas to include such fruits as kiwifruit, grapes, strawberries, and melons; jicama, raw broccoli, spinach, and romaine lettuce were available for salads.

- Soft drinks were removed from the à la carte line in the cafeteria and replaced with water, milk, and 100-percent juice (no more than 12 ounces per serving).
- FMNV and high-fat foods, such as French fries and nachos, were removed from cafeteria meals.
- During the 2002–2003 school year, high-fat/high-sugar foods were also removed from the à la carte line and replaced with fresh, healthier options and more appropriate portion sizes.

- The new food options included turkey sandwiches, sushi, homemade soup, salads, and baked chicken with rice.
- All vending machines, fundraising sales, and any other food sold outside cafeterias had to adhere to the standards by January 2004.

Results showed that students were buying more units of water than they used to buy soft drinks. Since the larger water bottle is sold at a higher price, vending machine revenues in the physical education department increased. Net revenues increased because food costs were lower for the healthier items. The Aptos cafeteria ended the 2002–2003 year with a surplus of $6,000. The administrators and teachers reported better student behavior after lunch, fewer afternoon visits to the counseling office, less litter in the school yard, and more students sitting down to eat. Aptos Middle School also reported higher scores on standardized tests. The "Healthy Food, Healthy Kids" policy at Aptos won an award from the State of California, and the changes made at Aptos were implemented throughout the San Francisco Unified School District (SFUSD) for the school year 2003–2004. The district-wide trend appears to be a move away from à la carte purchases and toward the National School Lunch Program.

Chapter Summary

- The nutrients most likely to be low or deficient in school-age children are calcium, iron, vitamins B_6 and A, and zinc.
- The 1999–2000 Healthy Eating Index (HEI) score showed that children younger than 11 years old had a higher quality diet than older children.
- It is estimated that about 4.4 percent of children ages 1 to 5 years have blood lead levels that are higher than 10 mg/dl.
- PEM is classified into two parts: primary and secondary. Primary PEM refers to a deficit of available food; secondary causes of PEM may be biological or social.
- About 40 to 50 percent of children and adolescents with special healthcare needs have nutrition-related risk factors or health problems that require the attention of a registered dietitian, nutritionist, or healthcare professional. Dietitians are recognized as health professionals qualified to provide developmental services to children with special needs.
- Children from families with high television use consume an average of 6 percent more of their total daily energy intake from meats; 5 percent more from pizza, salty snacks, and soda; and nearly 5 percent less from fruits, vegetables, and juices than children from families with low television use.
- Experimentation and idealism during adolescence may lead to certain eating behaviors such as skipping meals. The rate of meal skipping increases as they mature. Breakfast is the most skipped meal; only 29 percent of adolescent females eat breakfast daily. Lunch is another meal that adolescents tend to skip.
- Eating disorders have many causes, and it is likely that several factors contribute to the development of the disorder in any given case. Nutritional factors and dieting behavior may be contributing factors to the development and course of eating disorders.
- Children from families with incomes at or below 130 percent of the poverty level are eligible for a free lunch, and children in families with incomes between 130 percent and 185 percent below the poverty level are eligible for a reduced price lunch.

Critical Thinking Activities

- In groups of four or five, review the national health objectives in Healthy People 2010 for physical activity and weight control for children and adolescents. Pick an objective from each section, and brainstorm possible community programs a community or public health nutritionist could initiate to reach that objective.
- Visit a high school in the community and evaluate the school lunch meals, including the availability of foods of minimal nutritional value.
- A family with four children (ages 3, 7, 9, and 12) earns $17,000 per year. Using the Annual Income Eligibility Guidelines, determine the different types of food assistance programs from which they are eligible to receive benefits.

Case Study 9-1

Sandra is a single mother with three children: Sara is 2 years old, Alice is 6, and James is 13. To support her family, Sandra has a full-time job with an annual income of $18,000, and lives below the poverty line for a family of four. Recently, Sandra expressed to her friend Lisa that she is concerned about Alice and James's and her own weight gain. She explained that an elderly neighbor, Mary, takes care of the children after school and she likes to bake cookies for the children. Since the children have not made friends in their neighborhood, their main leisure activities are watching television and playing video games. Though time constraints lead Sandra to rely more on take-out and fast food meals, she recently started attending an aerobics class with a friend and is interested in developing healthier eating habits. Since Sara is under 5 years old, Lisa suggested that Sandra enroll her in the Special Supplemental Nutrition Program for Women, Infants, and Children (WIC) and use the opportunity to speak to the WIC nutritionist about her concerns for the other children.

Sandra scheduled an appointment with the WIC nutritionist and nutritional assessments were conducted using such methods as 24-hour recall and anthropometric measurements. The evaluations revealed that Sara receives an inadequate dietary intake of essential nutrients such as calcium and iron. The public health nurse assessments showed that the three children were anemic due to lack of adequate iron intake and the 6- and 13-year-olds were overweight because their BMI was between the 85th and 95th percentiles on the CDC/National Center for Health Statistics growth chart.

Sandra was encouraged to:

- Enroll her children in the after-school program at the YWCA near their neighborhood that includes different types of physical activities. The program also provides after-school transportation assistance.
- Enroll in the WIC Farmers' Market program to obtain more fresh fruits and vegetables.
- Enroll in the Food Stamp Program and School Lunch Program.
- Shop for foods once a week using MyPyramid as a guide and purchase low-fat foods.
- Start weekend activities such as swimming instead of watching television or playing video games.
- Schedule a 3-month follow-up visit to see the WIC nutritionist.

Activities

- Conduct a 24-hour recall on two WIC participants (preferably 4- to 5-year-old children) or on two school-age children to determine nutrient intake.
- Identify what federal and state assistance programs may be needed.
- Provide a list containing foods (vitamins, minerals, and protein) that are high in essential nutrients.
- Determine/calculate the children's daily caloric and nutrient needs.
- Devise a list of foods with high iron content.

References

1. Halterman JS, Kaczorowski JM, Aligne CA, Auinger P, Szilagyi PG. Iron deficiency and cognitive achievement among school-aged children and adolescents in the United States. *Pediatr.* 2001; 107:1381–1386.
2. Liuba P, Pesonen E. Infection and early atherosclerosis: does the evidence support causation? *Acta pædiatr.* 2005; 94(6):643–651.
3. Louey S, Thornburg KL. The prenatal environment and later cardiovascular disease. *Early Hum Dev.* 2005; 81(9):745–751.

4. Borer KT. Physical activity in the prevention and amelioration of osteoporosis in women: interaction of mechanical, hormonal and dietary factors. *Sports Med.* 2005; 35(9):779–830.

5. Chevalley TB, Bonjour JP, Ferrari S, Hans D, Rizzoli R. Skeletal site selectivity in the effects of calcium supplementation on areal bone mineral density gain: a randomized, double-blind, placebo-controlled trial in prepubertal boys. *J Clin Endocrinol Metab.* 2005; 90(6):3342–3349.

6. Grantham-McGregor S. Can the provision of breakfast benefit school performance? *Food Nutr Bull.* 2005; 26(2):S144–S158.

7. Cook JT, Frank DA, Berkowitz C, et al. Food insecurity is associated with adverse health outcomes among human infants and toddlers. *J Nutr.* 2004; 134(6):1432–1438.

8. U.S. Department of Agriculture, U.S. Department of Health and Human Services, Center for Nutrition Policy and Promotion. MyPyramid 2005. Available at: http://www.mypyramid.gov. Accessed March 28, 2008.

9. Gleason P, Suitor C. *Children's Diets in the Mid-1990s: Dietary Intake and Its Relationship with School Meal Participation.* Nutrition Assistance Program Report Series, Report No. CN-01-CD1. Washington, DC: U.S. Department of Agriculture, Food and Nutrition Service; 2001.

10. Gleason P, Suitor C. *Changes in Children's Diets: 1989–1991 to 1994–1996.* Office of Analysis, Nutrition and Evaluation, Report CN-01-CD2. Washington, DC: U.S. Department of Agriculture, Food and Nutrition Service; 2001.

11. Nestle M. Increasing portion sizes in American diets: more calories, more obesity. *J Am Diet Assoc.* 2003; 103:41–47.

12. Smiciklas-Wright HM, Mitchell, DC, Mickle SJ, Goldman JD, Cook A. Foods commonly eaten in the United States, 1989–1991 and 1994–1996: are portion sizes changing? *J Am Diet Assoc.* 2003; 103:39–40.

13. Rampersaud GC, Bailey LB, Kauwell GP. National survey beverage consumption data for children and adolescents indicate the need to encourage a shift toward more nutritive beverages. *J Am Diet Assoc.* 2003; 103:97–100.

14. U.S. Department of Health and Human Services. *The Surgeon General's Call to Action to Prevent and Decrease Overweight and Obesity.* Rockville, MD: Author; 2001.

15. Troiano RP, Flegal KM, Kuczmarski RJ, Campbell SM, Johnson CL. Overweight prevalence and trends for children and adolescents. *Arch Pediatr Adolesc Med.* 1995; 149:1085–1091.

16. American School Food Service Association. Impact of hunger and malnutrition on student achievement. *School Food Serv Res Rev.* 1989; 13:17–21.

17. Parker L. *The Relationship Between Nutrition and Learning.* Washington, DC: National Education Association; 1989.

18. Troccoli K. *Eat to Learn, Learn to Eat: The Link Between Nutrition and Learning in Children.* Washington, DC: National Health/Education Consortium; 1993.

19. U.S. Department of Health and Human Services. *Healthy People 2010 Understanding and Improving Health.* 2nd ed. Washington, DC: Author; 2000.

20. National Center for Health Statistics. Healthy People 2010: Progress Review Focus Area 16. Maternal, Infant, and Child Health. Available at: http://www.cdc.gov/nchs/about/otheract/hpdata2010/focusareas/fa16-mich.htm. Accessed October 14, 2005.

21. Berdanier CD, Feldman EB, Flatt WP, St Jeor S. *Handbook of Nutrition and Food.* New York: CRC Press; 2002.

22. Story M, Holt K, Sofka D, Clark EM. *Bright Futures in Practice: Nutrition Pocket Guide.* Georgetown, VA: National Center for Education in Maternal and Child Health, Georgetown University; 2002.

23. Insel PM, Turner ER, Ross D. *Nutrition 2002 Update.* 5th ed. Sudbury, MA: Jones and Bartlett; 2002.

24. Frank-Spohrer GC. *Community Nutrition: Applying Epidemiology to Contemporary Practice.* Gaithersburg, MD: Aspen; 1996.

25. U.S. Department of Agriculture. MyPyramid Sample Menu. Available at: http://www.mypyramid.gov/professionals/index.html. Accessed November 28, 2005.

26. Kennedy ET, Ohls J, Carlson S, Fleming K. The Healthy Eating Index: design and application. *J Am Diet Assoc.* 1995; 95(10):1103–1108.

27. Basiotis P, Carlson A, Gerrior S, Juan W, Lino M. *The Healthy Eating Index: 1999–2000.* CNPP-12. Washington, DC: U.S. Department of Agriculture, Center for Nutrition Policy and Promotion; 2002. Available at: http://www.cnpp.usda.gov. Accessed March 30, 2008.

28. Basiotis PP, Carlson A, Gerrior SA, Juan WY, Lino M. The Healthy Eating Index, 1999–2000: charting dietary patterns of Americans. *Fam Econ Nutr Rev.* 2004; 16(1):1–11.

29. Wilkinson Enns C, Mickle SJ, Goldman JD. Trends in food and nutrient intakes by children in the United States. *Fam Econ Nutr Rev.* 2002; 14(2):56–68.

30. Wilkinson C, Mickle S, Goldman J. Trends in food and nutrient intakes by adolescents in the United States. *Fam Econ Nutr Rev.* 2003; 15(2):15–27.

31. U.S. Department of Agriculture. *Food Intakes: Individuals in 48 States, Year 1977–78.* Nationwide Food Consumption Survey 1977–78, Rep. I-1; NTIS No. PB91-103523. Hyattsville, MD: Human Nutrition Information Service (USDA); 1983.

32. U.S. Department of Agriculture. *Continuing Survey of Food Intakes by Individuals 1994–96, 1998.* [CD-ROM]. NTIS No. PB2000-500027. Washington, DC: Agricultural Research Service (USDA); 2000.

33. Woteki CE, Briefel RR, Klein CJ, et al. Nutrition monitoring: summary of a statement from an American Society for Nutritional Sciences working group. *J Nutr.* 2002; 132:3782–3783.

34. Bentley ME, Griffiths PL. The burden of anemia among women in India. *Eur J Clin Nutr.* 2003; 57(1):52–60.

35. Thane CW, Bates CJ, Prentice A. Risk factors for low iron intake and poor iron status in a national sample of British young people aged 4–18 years. *Public Health Nutr.* 2003; 6(5):485–496.

36. Centers for Disease Control and Prevention. Recommendation to prevent and control iron deficiency in the United States. *MMWR.* 1998; 47(RR-03):1–36.

37. Brown JE, Sugarman I, Krinke UB, Murtaugh MA, Stang J, Wooldridge NH. *Nutrition Through the Life Cycle.* Belmont, CA: Wadsworth Thomson; 2002.

38. U.S. Department of Health and Human Services. *Healthy People 2010.* Conference ed., two volumes. Washington, DC: Author; 2000.

39. Centers for Disease Control and Prevention, National Center for Health Statistics. *National Center for Health Statistics-at-a-Glance.* Hyattsville, MD: Author; 2002.

40. Kennedy E, Powell R. Changing eating patterns of American children: a view from 1996. *J Amer Coll Nutr.* 1997; 16:524–529.

41. Pollitt E. Iron deficiencies and educational deficiency. *Nutr Rev.* 1997; 55:133–141.

42. Riley E, McGee C. Fetal alcohol spectrum disorders: an overview with emphasis on changes in brain and behavior. *Exp Biol Med.* 2005; 230:357–365.

43. Requejo AM, Navia B, Ortega RM, et al. The age at which meat is first included in the diet affects the incidence of iron deficiency and ferropenic anaemia in a group of pre-school children from Madrid. *Int J Vitam Nutr Res.* 1999; 69:127–131.

44. Hine R. Folic acid: contemporary clinical perspective. *Perspect Appl Nutr.* 1993; 1:3–14.

45. Merkel D, Huerta M, Grotto I, et al. Prevalence of iron deficiency and anemia among strenuously trained adolescents. *J Adolesc Health.* 2005; 37(3):220–223.

46. Morad M, Merrick J. Iron deficiency anemia in adolescence. *Int J Adolesc Med Health.* 2005; 17(2):96–97.

47. Looker A, Dallman PR, Carroll MD, et al. Prevalence of iron deficiency in the United States. *JAMA.* 1998; 277:973–976.

48. Maloni J, Faan D. Reducing the risk for preterm birth: evidence and implications for neonatal nurses. *Ad Neonatal Care.* 2004; 4(3):166–174.

49. Donovan UM, Gibson RS. Iron and zinc status of young women aged 14 to 19 years consuming vegetarian and omnivorous diets. *J Am Coll Nutr.* 1995; 14:463–472.

50. Halterman JS, Kaczorowski JM, Aligne CA, Auinger P, Szilagyi PG. Iron deficiency and cognitive achievement among school-aged children and adolescents in the United States. *Pediatr.* 2001; 107:1381–1386.

51. Goyer RA. Toxic and essential metal interactions. *Ann Rev Nutr.* 1997; 17:37–50.

52. Markowitz M, Rosen JF, Clemente I. Clinician follow-up of children screened for lead poisoning. *Am J Public Health.* 1999; 89:1088.

53. Wardlaw GM, Kessel M. *Perspectives in Nutrition.* 5th ed. New York: McGraw-Hill; 2002.

54. Matte TD. Reducing blood lead levels: benefits and strategies. *JAMA.* 1999; 281:2340–2342.

55. Ryan D, Levy B, Levy BS, Pollack S, Walker B. Protecting children from lead poisoning and building healthy communities. *Am J Public Health.* 1999; 89:822–824.

56. Snyder DC, Mohle-Boetani JC, Palla B, Fenstersheib M. Development of a population-specific risk assessment to predict elevated blood lead levels in Santa Clara County, California. *Pediatr.* 1995; 96:643.

57. Centers for Disease Control and Prevention. Screening Young Children for Lead Poisoning; Guidance for State and Local Public Health Officials. Available at: http://www.cdc.gov/nceh/lead/guide/guide97.htm. Accessed March 28, 2008.

58. McLaughlin TJ, Humphries O, Nguyen T, Maljanian R, McCormack K. Getting the lead out in Hartford, Connecticut: a multifaceted lead-poisoning awareness campaign. *Environ Health Persp.* 2004; 112(1):1–5.

59. Casamassimo P. *Bright Futures in Practice: Oral Health.* Arlington, VA: National Center for Education in Maternal and Child Health; 1996.

60. Mushak P, Crocetti AF. Lead and nutrition. Part 1. Biologic interactions of lead with nutrients. *Nutr Today.* 1996; 31:12–17.

61. Lutz CA, Przytulski KR. *Nutrition and Diet Therapy.* 3rd ed. Philadelphia: Davis; 2001.

62. Krebs NF, Jacobson MS. Prevention of pediatric overweight and obesity. *Pediatr.* 2003; 112(2):424–430.

63. Centers for Disease Control and Prevention, National Center for Health Statistics. Prevalence of Overweight and Obesity Among Adults: United States, 1999–2002. Available at: http://www.cdc.gov/nchs/products/pubs/pubd/hestats/obese/obse99.htm. Accessed November 17, 2005.

64. Hedley AA, Ogden CL, Johnson CL, Carroll MD, Curtin LR, Flegal KM. Prevalence of overweight and obesity among U.S. children, adolescents, and adults, 1999–2002. *JAMA.* 2004; 29(23):2847–2850.

65. Centers for Disease Control and Prevention. Overweight Prevalence. Available at: http://www.cdc.gov/nccdphp/dnpa/obesity/childhood/prevalence.htm. Accessed March 26, 2008.

66. Phillips SM, Bandini LG, Compton DV, Naumova EN, Must A. A longitudinal comparison of body composition by total body water and bioelectrical impedance in adolescent girls. *J Nutr.* 2003; 133:1419–1425.

67. Hill JO, Peters JC. Environmental contributions to the obesity epidemic. *Sci.* 1998; 280:1371–1374.

68. Link K, Moell C, Garwicz S, et al. Growth hormone deficiency predicts cardiovascular risk in young adults treated for acute lymphoblastic leukemia in childhood. *J Clin Endocrinol Metab.* 2004; 89:5003–5012.

69. Freedman DS, Dietz WH, Srinivasan SR, Berenson GS. The relation of overweight to cardiovascular risk factors among children and adolescents: the Bogalusa Heart Study. *Pediatr.* 1999; 103:1175–1182.

70. Saelens BE, Sallis JF, Wilfley DE, Patric K, Cella JA, Vuchta R. Behavioral weight control for overweight adolescents initiated in primary care. *Obes Res.* 2002; 10:22–32.

71. Guo SS, Chumlea WC. Tracking of body mass index in children in relation to overweight in adulthood. *Am J Clin Nutr.* 1999; 70(Suppl):145S–148S.

72. Whitaker RC, Wright JS, Pepe MS, et al. Predicting obesity in young adulthood from childhood and parental obesity. *N Eng J Med.* 1997; 337:869–873.

73. Shinha R, Fisch G, Teague B, et al. Prevalence of impaired glucose tolerance among children and adolescents with marked obesity. *N Engl J Med.* 2002; 346:802–810.

74. Strauss RS. Childhood obesity and self-esteem. *Pediatr.* 2000; 105(1):e15.

75. Davison KK, Birch LL. Weight status, parent reaction, and self-concept in five-year-old girls. *Pediatr.* 2001; 107:46–53.

76. Krebs NF, Jacobson MS. American Academy of Pediatrics Committee on Nutrition. Prevention of pediatric overweight and obesity. *Pediatr.* 2003; 112:424–430.

77. U.S. Department of Health and Human Services, U.S. Department of Agriculture. *Dietary Guidelines for Americans.* 6th ed. Washington, DC: Authors; 2005.

78. Dietz WH. Health consequences of obesity in youth: childhood predictors of adult disease. *Pediatr.* 1998; 101(Suppl 3):518–525.

79. Flegal KM, Carroll MD, Ogden CL, Johnson CL. Prevalence and trends in obesity among U.S. adults, 1999–2000. *JAMA.* 2002; 288:1723–1727.

80. Mokdad AH, Ford ES, Bowman BA, et al. Prevalence of obesity, diabetes, and obesity-related health risk factors. *JAMA.* 2001; 289:76–79.

81. Centers for Disease Control and Prevention. *National Diabetes Fact Sheet: General Information and National Estimates on Diabetes in the United States.* Atlanta, GA: U.S. Department of Health and Human Services; 2005.

82. Aye T, Levitsky LL. Type 2 diabetes: an epidemic disease in childhood. *Pediatr.* 2003; 15(4):411–415.

83. Steinberger JD, Daniels SR; American Heart Association Atherosclerosis, Hypertension, and Obesity in the Young Committee; American Heart Association Diabetes Committee. Obesity, insulin resistance, diabetes, and cardiovascular risk in children. *Circ.* 2003; 107:1448–1456.

84. Sung RY, Tong PC, Yu CW, et al. High prevalence of insulin resistance and metabolic syndrome in overweight/obese preadolescent Hong Kong Chinese children aged 9–12 years. *Diabetes Care.* 2003; 26:250–251.

85. Centers for Disease Control and Prevention. Diabetes project. Available at: http://www.cdc.gov/diabetes/projects/cda2.htm. Accessed March 26, 2008.

86. Kida K, Ito T, Yang SW, Tanpaichitr V. Effects of Western diet on risk factors of chronic diseases in Asia. In: Bendich A, Deckelbaum RJ, eds. *Preventive Nutrition: The Comprehensive Guide for Health Professionals.* 2nd ed. Totowa, NJ: Humana Press; 2001: 435–446.

87. Sinha R, Fisch G, Teague B, et al. Prevalence of impaired glucose tolerance among children and adolescents with marked obesity. *N Engl J Med.* 2002; 346:802–810.

88. Dwyer J, Stone EJ, Yang M. Prevalence of marked overweight and obesity in a multiethnic pediatric population: findings from the Child and Adolescent Trial for Cardiovascular Health (CATCH) Study. *J Am Diet Assoc.* 2000; 100:1149–1156.

89. Wolf M, Cohen KR, Rosenfeld JG. School-based interventions for obesity: current approaches and future prospects. *Psychol Schools.* 1985; 22:187–200.

90. Centers for Disease Control and Prevention. Healthy Schools Healthy Youth! Available at: http://www.cdc.gov/healthyyouth. Accessed November 13, 2005.

91. National Association for Sport & Physical Education. Parents Believe Physical Activity Key to Preventing Childhood Obesity. 2003. Available at: http://www.aahperd.org/aapar. Accessed March 28, 2008.

92. The Center for Health and Healthcare in Schools. Childhood Overweight: What the Research Tells Us. Available at: http://www.healthinschools.org/Health-in-Schools/Health-Services/Schools-and-Childhood-Overweight.aspx. Accessed March 28, 2008.

93. Dietz W, Gortmaker SL. Do we fatten our children at the television set? Obesity and television viewing in children and adolescents. *J Pediatr.* 1985; 75:807–812.

94. Warren JM, Henry CJ, Lightowler HJ, Bradshaw SM, Perwaiz S. Evaluation of a pilot school programme aimed at the prevention of obesity in children. *Health Promotion Int.* 2003; 18(4):287–296.

95. Davis SM, Going D, Nicolette H, et al. Pathways: a culturally appropriate obesity-prevention program for American Indian schoolchildren. *Am J Clin Nutr.* 1999; 69(4):796S–802S.

96. American Academy of Pediatrics. Cholesterol in Childhood. Available at: http://aappolicy.aappublications.org/cgi/content/full/pediatrics;101/1/141. Accessed November 13, 2005.

97. Kavey RE, Daniels SR, Lauer RM, Atkins DL, Hayman LL, Taubert K. American Heart Association guidelines for primary prevention of atherosclerotic cardiovascular disease beginning in childhood. *Circ*. 2003; 107:1562–1566.

98. American Heart Association. Dietary recommendations for children and adolescents. A guide for practitioners: consensus statement from the American Heart Association. *Circ*. 2005; 112:2061–2075.

99. National Heart, Lung, and Blood Institute. New NHLBI-Sponsored Study Shows Programs Can Teach Children to Eat Healthier. Available at: http://www.eurekalert.org/pub_releases/2005-06/nhla-nns060105.php. Accessed November 2005.

100. Obarzanek E, Kimm S, Barton B, et al. Long-term safety and efficacy of cholesterol-lowering diet in children with elevated low-density lipoprotein cholesterol: seven-year results of the Dietary Intervention Study in Children (DISC). *Pediatr*. 2001; 107:256–264.

101. Clearfield M. National Cholesterol Education Program adult treatment panel III guidelines. *J Am Osteopath Assoc*. 2003; 103(1):S1–S5.

102. Stice E, Cameron RP, Killen JD, et al. Naturalistic weight-reduction efforts prospectively predict growth in relative weight and onset of obesity among female adolescents. *J Consult Clin Psychol*. 1999; 67:967–974.

103. Mackey E, La Greca A. Adolescents' eating, exercise and weight control behaviors: does peer crowd affiliation play a role? *J Pediatr Psychol*. 2007; 32(1):13–23.

104. Freedman D, Dietz W, Srinivasan S, Berenson G. The relation of childhood BMI to adult adiposity: the Bogalusa Heart Study. *Pediatr*. 2005; 115(1):22–27.

105. Neumark-Sztainer D, Story M, Falkner NH, Behuring T, Resnick MD. Sociodemographic and personal characteristics of adolescents engaged in weight loss and weight/muscle gain behaviors. Who is doing what? *Prevent Med*. 1999; 28:4–5.

106. Moore D. Body image and eating behavior in adolescents. *J Am Coll Nutr*. 1993; 12:505–510.

107. Polivy J, Herman CP. Dieting and binging. A causal analysis. *Am Psychol*. 1985; 40:193–201.

108. Schweiger U, Fichter M. Eating disorders: clinical presentation, classification and aetiological models. *Bailliere's Clin Psych*. 1997; 3:199–216.

109. Coulston A, Rock C, Monsen E. *Nutrition in the Prevention and Treatment of Disease*. New York: Academic Press; 2001.

110. American Psychiatric Association. *Diagnostic and Statistical Manual of Mental Disorders*. 4th ed. Washington, DC: Author; 1994.

111. Hsu L. Epidemiology of the eating disorders. *Psych Clin N Am*. 1996; 19:681–700.

112. Haiman C, Devlin MJ. Binge eating before the onset of dieting: a distinct subgroup of bulimia nervosa. *Int J Eating Disord*. 1999; 25:151–157.

113. Kirkley BG. Bulimia. Clinical characteristics, development, and etiology. *J Am Diet Assoc*. 1986; 86:472–486.

114. Lilenfeld LR, Kaye WH, Strober M. Genetics and family studies of anorexia nervosa and bulimia nervosa. *Bailliere's Clin Psych*. 1997; 3:177–197.

115. Hamm LA, Holden W. Providing WIC services to homeless families. *J Nutr Edu*. 1999; 31:224–234.

116. American Academy of Pediatrics, Committee on Community Health Services. Health needs of homeless children and families. *Pediatr*. 1996; 98:789–791.

117. Katz SH, Weaver WW. *Encyclopedia of Food and Culture*. New York: Scribner; 2003: 435–437.

118. American Dietetic Association. Position of the American Dietetic Association: dietary guidance for healthy children aged 2 to 11 years. *J Am Diet Assoc*. 1999; 99:93–101.

119. Fass S, Hancy K. Who Are America's Poor Children? Available at: http://www.nccp.org/publications/pub_684.html. Accessed March 29, 2008.

120. Nord M, Andrews M, Carlson S. *Household Food Security in the United States, 2004*. (FANRR42). Washington, DC: U.S. Department of Agriculture; 2005.

121. America's Second Harvest. Hunger Study: Key Findings. Available at: http://www.hungerinamerica.org/key_findings. Accessed August 25, 2006.

122. World Hunger Education Service. World Hunger Facts 2006. Available at: http://www.worldhunger.org/articles/Learn/world%20hunger%20facts%202002.htm. Accessed March 29, 2008.

123. Newacheck PW, Strickland B, Shonkoff JP, et al. An epidemiologic profile of children with special health care needs. *Pediatr*. 1998; 102(1 Pt 1):17–123.

124. Newacheck PW, Halfon N. Prevalence and impact of disabling chronic conditions in childhood. *Am J Public Health*. 1998; 88(4):610–617.

125. McPherson M, Arango P, Fox H, et al. A new definition of children with special health care needs. *Pediatr*. 1998; 102(1 Pt 1):137–140.

126. Newacheck PW. Adolescents with special health needs: prevalence, severity, and access to health services. *Pediatr*. 1989; 84(5):872–881.

127. Stang J, Story M. Guidelines for Adolescent Nutrition Services. Available at: http://www.epi.umn.edu/let/pubs/adol_book.shtm. Accessed December 23, 2005.

128. Hine RJ, Cloud HH, Carithers T, Hickey C, Hinton AW. Early nutrition intervention services for children with special health care needs. *J Am Diet Assoc*. 1989; 89(11):1636–1639.

129. Willis JH. Adolescents with Special Health Needs. In: Stang J, Story M. Guidelines for Adolescent Nutrition Services. Available at: http://www.epi.umn.edu/let/pubs/adol_book.shtm. Accessed March 30, 2008.

130. Stallings V, Zemel B, Davies J, Cronk C, Charney E. Energy expenditure of children and adolescent with severe disabilities: a cerebral palsy model. *Am J Clin Nutr*. 1996; 64(4):627–634.

131. Horsley JW. Children and adolescents with special health care needs. In: Story M, Holt K, Sofka D, eds. *Bright Futures in Practice: Nutrition*. Arlington, VA: National Center for Education in Maternal and Child Health; 2002: 145–152.

132. Baer MT, Harris AB. Pediatric nutrition assessment: identifying children at risk. *J Am Diet Assoc*. 1997; 97(Suppl 2):S107–S115.

133. Boyle M. *Community Nutrition in Action: An Entrepreneurial Approach*. 4th ed. Belmont, CA: Thomson Wadsworth; 2005.

134. Robert Wood Johnson Foundation. *Making the Grade: State and Local Partnerships to Establish School-Based Health Centers*. Washington, DC: The George Washington University; 2000.

135. Coon K, Goldberg J, Rogers B, Tucker K. Relationships between use of television during meals and children's food consumption patterns. *Pediatr*. 2001; 107(1):E1–E9.

136. Marquis M, Filion YP, Dagenais F. Does eating while watching television influence children's food-related behaviors? *Can J Diet Pract Res*. 2005; 66(1):12–18.

137. Grimm GC, Harnack L, Story M. Factors associated with soft drink consumption in school-aged children. *J Am Diet Assoc*. 2004; 104(8):1244–1249.

138. Boynton-Jarrett R, Thomas TN, Peterson KE, Wiecha J, Sobol AM, Gortmaker SL. Impact of television viewing patterns on fruit and vegetable consumption among adolescents. *Pediatr*. 2003; 112(6):1321–1326.

139. Harrison K, Marske AL. Nutritional content of foods advertised during the television programs children watch most. *Am J Public Health*. 2005; 95(9):1568–1574.

140. Gallo AE. Food advertising in the United States. In: Frazao E, ed. *America's Eating Habits: Changes and Consequences*. Washington, DC: U.S. Department of Agriculture; 1999: 173–180.

141. Kotz K, Story M. Food advertisements during children's Saturday morning television programming: Are they consistent with dietary recommendations? *J Am Diet Assoc*. 1994; 94:1296–1300.

142. Consumers Union Education Services. *Captive Kids: Commercial Pressures on Kids at School*. Yonkers, NY: Consumers Union of the United States; 1990.

143. Alaimo K, McDowell MA, Briefel RR, et al. *Dietary Intake of Vitamins, Minerals, and Fiber of Persons Ages 2 Months and Over in the United States:*

Third National Health and Nutrition Examination Survey, Phase I, 1988–91. Hyattsville, MD: National Center for Health Statistics; 1994.

144. Kennedy E, Goldberg J. What are American children eating: implication for public policy. *Nutr Rev.* 1995; 53:111.

145. Cook JT, Martin LS. *Differences in Nutrient Adequacy among Poor and Non-poor Children.* Medford, MA: Tufts University School of Nutrition Center on Hunger; 1995.

146. Centers for Disease Control and Prevention, National Center for Health Statistics. CDC Growth Charts: United States. Available at: http://www.cdc.gov/nchs/about/major/nhanes/growthcharts/charts.htm. Accessed September 1, 2003.

147. Frisch R, McArthur JW. Menstrual cycles: fatness as a determinant of minimum weight for height necessary for their maintenance or onset. *Sci.* 1974; 185:949–951.

148. Meyer A, Sampson AE, Weitzman M, et al. School breakfast program and school performance. *Am J Dis Child.* 1989; 143:1234–1239.

149. American School Health Association, Association for the Advancement of Health Education, Society for Public Health Education. *The National Adolescents Student Health Survey, A Report on the Health of America's Youth.* Oakland, CA: Third Party Publishing Company; 1988.

150. Lin BH, Guthrie J, Blaylock JR. *The Diets of America's Children: Influences of Dining Out, Household Characteristics, and Nutrition Knowledge.* Washington, DC: U.S. Department of Agriculture; 1996: 746.

151. Siega-Ruz A, Carson T, Popkin B. Three squares or mostly snacks—what do teens really eat? A sociodemographic study of meal patterns. *J Adolesc Health.* 1998; 22:29–36.

152. Olver L. The Food Timeline: American Public School Lunch History. Available at: http://www.foodtimeline.org/foodschools.html. Accessed March 28, 2008.

153. U.S. Department of Agriculture, Food and Nutrition Service. Nutrition Assistance Programs. Available at: http://www.fns.usda.gov/fns. Accessed May 24, 2004.

154. U.S. Department of Agriculture, Food and Nutrition Service. Healthy Meals Resource System. Available at: http://schoolmeals.nal.usda.gov. Accessed March 28, 2008.

155. U.S. Department of Agriculture, Food and Nutrition Service. National School Lunch Program. Available at: http://www.fns.usda.gov/cnd/Lunch/AboutLunch/ProgramHistory_5.htm. Accessed October 8, 2006.

156. U.S. Department of Agriculture, Economic Research Service. Child Nutrition Programs: National School Lunch Program. Available at: http://www.ers.usda.gov/Briefing/ChildNutrition/lunch.htm. Accessed April 2, 2005.

157. Briggs M, Safaii D, Beall DL. Position of the American Dietetic Association: nutrition services: an essential component of comprehensive health programs. *J Am Diet Assoc.* 2003; 103:505–514.

158. Aschner JL. New therapies for pulmonary hypertension in neonates and children. *Pediatr Pulmonol.* 2004; 26(Suppl):132–135.

159. National Research Council. *Recommended Dietary Allowances.* 10th ed. Washington, DC: National Academy Press; 1989.

160. U.S. Department of Agriculture, Food and Nutrition Service. School Breakfast Program. Available at: http://www.fns.usda.gov/cnd/breakfast. Accessed March 29, 2008.

161. Mahan LK, Escott-Stump S. *Krause's Food, Nutrition, and Diet Therapy.* 11th ed. Philadelphia, PA: Saunders; 2003.

162. U.S. Department of Agriculture, Food and Nutrition Service. School Lunch Program. Available at: http://www.fns.usda.gov/cnd/lunch. Accessed March 28, 2008.

163. Willis JT. Those lazy, hazy, crazy days of summer. *Nurs Times.* 1997; 93:24–26.

164. U.S. Department of Agriculture. *Team Nutrition: Program Summary.* Washington, DC: Author; 1995.

165. U.S. Department of Agriculture, Food and Nutrition Service. Team Nutrition. Available at: http://www.fns.usda.gov/tn. Accessed May 24, 2004.

166. Administration for Children and Families. Head Start Fact Sheet. Available at: http://www.acf.hhs.gov/programs/ohs/about/fy2006.html. Accessed April 27, 2005.

167. National Youth Sports Program. General Information. Available at: http://www.nyscorp.org/nysp/home.html. Accessed March 29, 2008.

168. Powell CA, Walker SP, Chang SM, Grantham-McGregor SM. Nutrition and education: a randomized trial of the effects of breakfast in rural primary school children. *Am J Clin Nutr.* 1998; 68:873–879.

169. Gross SM, Cinelli B. Coordinated school health program and dietetics professionals: partners in promoting healthful eating. *J Am Diet Assoc.* 2004; 104(5):793–798.

170. Meyers AF, Sampson AE, Weitzman M, Rogers BL, Kayne H. School breakfast program and school performance. *Am J Dis Child.* 1989; 143:1234–1239.

171. Pollitt E. Does breakfast make a difference in school? *J Am Diet Assoc.* 1995; 95:1134–1139.

172. Black S. Nutrition and learning. *Am Sch Board J.* 2000; 187:49–51.

173. U.S. Department of Agriculture, Food and Nutrition Service. *Children's Diets in the Mid-1990s: Dietary Intake and Its Relationship with School Meal Participation.* Washington, DC: Office of Analysis, Nutrition and Evaluation; 2001.

174. Farris RP, Nicklas TA, Webber LS, Berenson GS. Nutrient contribution of the School Lunch Program: implications for Healthy People 2000. *J Sch Health.* 1992; 62:180–184.

175. U.S. Department of Agriculture, U.S. Department of Health and Human Services. *Nutrition and Your Health: Dietary Guidelines for Americans.* 5th ed. Home and Garden Bulletin No. 232. Washington, DC: Authors; 2000.

176. U.S. Department of Agriculture, Food and Nutrition Service. Foods Sold in Competition with USDA Meal Programs. Available at: http://www.fns.usda.gov/cnd/lunch. Accessed March 30, 2008.

177. U.S. Department of Agriculture. National school lunch program and school breakfast program nutrition objectives for school meals (7 CFR 210.220). *Fed Reg.* 1994; 59:3021–3025.

178. Bergman E. Time spent by school children to eat lunch. *J Am Diet Assoc.* 2000; 100:697–698.

179. Conklin MT, Lambert LG, Anderson JB. How long does it take students to eat lunch: a summary of three studies. *J Child Nutr Manage.* 2002; 26:1–6.

180. Marx E, Wolley SF, Northrop D. *Health Is Academic: A Guide to Coordinated School Health Programs.* New York: Teachers College Press; 1998.

181. Nader PR, Sellers DE, Johnson CC, et al. The effect of adult participation in a school-based family intervention to improve children's diet and physical activity: The Child and Adolescent Trial for Cardiovascular Health. *Prev Med.* 1996; 25:455–464.

182. Centers for Disease Control and Prevention. Guidelines for school health programs to promote lifelong healthy eating. *MMWR.* 1996; 45(RR-9):1–41.

183. Centers for Disease Control and Prevention. Success Story: Make More Healthful Foods and Beverages Available. Available at: http://www.cdc.gov/search.do?action = search&queryText = school + lunch + program&x = 14&y = 3. Accessed March 30, 2008.

CHAPTER

10

Adulthood: Special Health Issues

CHAPTER OUTLINE

- Introduction
- Healthy People 2010
- Cardiovascular Disease
- Obesity
- Cancer
- Osteoporosis

LEARNING OBJECTIVES

- Discuss the significance of cardiovascular disease as it relates to morbidity and mortality.
- State the risk factors for cardiovascular disease.
- Discuss different factors that increase or decrease cardiovascular disease.
- Discuss the influence of different types of fat on heart disease.
- List the guidelines for reducing heart disease risk.
- Discuss the prevalence of obesity.
- Discuss the causes of obesity.
- Define obesity and overweight.
- Discuss the medical and social costs of obesity.
- Describe the dietary, behavioral, and physical activity modifications for the management of obesity.
- List major food sources or food components and how they protect the body and reduce the risk of cancer.
- List the ways in which foods are implicated in the development of cancer.
- Discuss the nutrients and other factors important in building bone density.
- Describe normal bone development.

Introduction

A *chronic condition* is an occurrence of a disease that cannot be cured and that extends over a period of time. It has been recognized that chronic illness is an important issue in the health of older adults.[1] The cause of chronic diseases is associated with several factors, not just a single origin. It is often related to factors in lifestyle, genetics, and/or environment, and in some situations is totally unknown.

An important part of public health is risk factor identification, which can lead to risk reduction through specific interventions aimed at reducing morbidity and mortality related to chronic illness. Risk factors can be classified as modifiable or non-modifiable. For instance, modifiable risk factors for stroke include high blood cholesterol, hypertension, cigarette smoking, and obesity. The non-modifiable risk factors are heredity, race, age, and gender.[2,3] Although each chronic disease must be considered individually, the risk factors of dietary practices are significant in several common chronic diseases, including heart disease, stroke, cancer, *obesity*, and *osteoporosis*, all of which will be discussed in this chapter. Diet is a primary intervention in the prevention of nutrition-related chronic health conditions.

The high prevalence of chronic conditions is one of the challenges of health promotion among older adults. It's assumed that the wear and tear that occurs with aging is inevitable and "normal," but that's not necessarily true in all cases because some individuals can age successfully—by slowing the number and rate of aging changes through positive lifestyle choices—and still have chronic conditions like hypertension and osteoporosis. In the United States and other countries, people are living healthy, productive lives through their 70s, 80s, 90s, and beyond. Generally, health deteriorates with aging through an accumulation of chronic disorders and disabilities. According to the Centers for Disease Control and Prevention (CDC), chronic conditions significantly limit daily activity for 39 percent of persons over 65 years of age and account for about 36 percent of persons' healthcare costs.[4]

Community and public health nutritionists are involved in health promotion and disease prevention activities that require taking scientific research information and applying it to the community and to population-based health practices. They are poised to be the primary information resource regarding the relationships among diet, health, and disease prevention.

Healthy People 2010

One of the goals of Healthy People 2010 is to prevent and control chronic diseases such as heart disease, obesity, cancer, and osteoporosis. The Healthy People 2010 progress report on weight status of adults shows that the proportion of adults age 20 years or older who were at a healthy weight (body mass index [BMI] between 18.5 and 25.0) decreased from 42 percent in 1988–1994 to 34 percent in 1999–2000. The decrease was from 45 to 35 percent for females and from 38 to 32 percent for males. The target is 60 percent. Data also show that the age-adjusted proportion of adults age 20 years or older who

> **chronic condition** An occurrence of a disease that cannot be cured and extends over a period of time.
>
> **obesity** A condition characterized by excess body fat. It is defined as a body mass index of 30 kg/m² or greater or a body weight that is 20 percent or more above the healthy body weight standard.
>
> **osteoporosis** Porous bone due to reduction in bone mass.

were obese (i.e., BMI of 30.0 or more) increased from 23 percent in the survey period 1988–1994 to 31 percent in 1999–2000. For males, the increase was from 20 to 28 percent, and for females, from 25 to 33 percent. The 2010 target for adult obesity, based on measured weights and heights, is 15 percent.[5]

As shown in **Table 10.1**, the Healthy People 2010 objectives to reduce the overall cancer and heart disease death rate show little or no change. In regards to the objectives for fruits and vegetables, the age-adjusted average number of daily servings of fruit consumed showed little change, from 1.6 in 1994–1996 to 1.5 in 1999–2000. Two to four servings are recommended. Also, vegetable consumption showed little change: an average of 3.4 daily servings in 1994–1996 compared with 3.3 in 1999–2000. Three to five servings are recommended; at least one-third of the servings should be from dark green or orange vegetables. Data show that in 1999–2000, 11 percent of adults 20 years of age or older ate dark green and orange vegetables while 22 percent consumed fried potatoes. In 1999–2000, the proportion of all grain products consumed that were whole grain was 13 percent for adults. The target for all grain products is that 50 percent should be whole grain. See **Table 10.1** for more information on the 2010 progress report.

These findings are not encouraging in regards to decreasing the incidence of chronic health conditions (obesity, heart disease, cancer, etc.) in older adults. Due to the results of the most recent review of Healthy People 2010 objectives, several strategies have been recommended to advance the progress toward achieving the objectives in relation to promoting healthy weight and food choices. (See **Box 10-1**.)

> ### *Box* 10-1 Recommended Strategies for Achieving Healthy People 2010 Objectives for Weight and Food Choice[5]
>
> - Promote partnerships with community planners to design neighborhoods that encourage and support increased opportunities for physical activity in appropriate and safe locations.
> - Educate the public about the health benefits of being physically active at any size and the possible added benefit of thereby attaining modest weight reduction.
> - Educate the public on how to use the Nutrition Facts Panel on food products and on how to select appropriate portion sizes for healthful diets, including clarification of the difference between "serving size" and "portion size."
> - Urge medical schools to incorporate training on the prevention and treatment of obesity into their curricula. In a parallel effort, work with medical associations and healthcare organizations on developing means for educating healthcare professionals already in practice.
> - Offer incentives for worksites to provide safe, convenient, and affordable venues for employees to engage in physical activity.

TABLE 10.1 **Healthy People 2010 Objectives for Adults**

Healthy People 2010 Objectives Number	Healthy People 2010 Objectives	Baseline (Year)	Progress Review (2002)	2010 Target
3.1	Reduce the overall cancer death rate (age adjusted per 100,000 standard population).	200.8 deaths (1999) 201.0 deaths (2000) 193.3 deaths (2002)	190.1 deaths (2003)	158.6
5.3	Reduce the overall rate of diabetes per 1,000 population.	40 cases (1997) 41 cases (1998–1999) 45 cases (2000)	N/A	25 cases
7.5	Increase the proportion of worksites with 50 or more employees that offer a comprehensive employee health promotion program to their employees.	34%	N/A	75%
12.1	Reduce coronary heart disease deaths (age adjusted per 100,000 standard populations).	204 (1999) 196 (2000)	N/A	166
12.14	Reduce the proportion of adults (age 20 years or over) with high total blood cholesterol levels ($\geq$ 240 mg/dl).	21.0% (1988–1994) 18.3% (2000)	N/A	17%
19.1	Increase the proportion of adults age 20 years or over who are at a healthy weight (BMI 18.5–25).	42% (1988–1994) 34% (1999–2000)	N/A	60%
19.2	Reduce the proportion of adults who are obese.	23% (1988–1994) 31% (1999–2000)	N/A	15%
19.5	Increase the proportion of persons age 2 years or older who consume more than two daily servings of fruit.	28% (1994–1996)	N/A	75%
19.6	Increase the proportion of persons age 2 years or older who consume more than three daily servings of vegetables, with at least one-third being dark green or deep yellow vegetables.	3% (1994–1996)	N/A	50%
19.7	Increase the proportion of persons age 2 years or older who consume at least six daily servings of grain products, with more than three being whole grains.	7% (1994–1996)	N/A	50%
19.8	Increase the proportion of persons age 2 years or older who consume less than 10% of calories from saturated fat.	36% (1994–1996)	N/A	75%
19.9	Increase the proportion of persons age 2 years or older who consume no more than 30% of calories from total fat.	33% (1994–1996)	N/A	75%
19.10	Increase the proportion of persons age 2 years or older who consume 2,400 milligrams or less of sodium daily.	21% (1988–1994)	N/A	65%
19.11	Increase the proportion of persons age 2 years or older who meet dietary recommendations for calcium.	45% (1988–1994)	N/A	75%
19.17	Increase the proportion of physician office visits made by patients with a diagnosis of cardiovascular disease, diabetes, or hyperlipidemia that include counseling or education related to diet and nutrition.	42% (1997) 38% (1998) 36% (1999) 40% (2000)	N/A	75%
19.18	Increase food security among U.S. households and in so doing reduce hunger.	88% (1995) 90% (1999) 89% (2001)	89%	94%
22.2	Increase the proportion of adults who engage regularly, preferably daily, in moderate physical activity for at least 30 minutes per day.	32% (1997)	33% (2003)	50%

Source: National Center for Health Statistics, Department of Health and Human Services. *Healthy People 2010 Progress Review*. Hyattsville, MD: Public Health Service, Healthy People 2010; 2004. Available at: http://www.cdc.gov/nchs/hphome.htm. Accessed April 6, 2008.

Cardiovascular Disease

Cardiovascular disease (CVD) is one of the chronic health conditions affecting millions of people around the world. The cardiovascular system includes the heart, blood vessels, and blood-forming organs. There are common diseases of the heart and blood vessels that can be influenced by diet and behavioral changes through primary and secondary prevention. Cardiovascular diseases are the leading cause of death in the United States and most of the industrialized countries.[6] It kills over 927,448 individuals in the United States each year—more than the next six leading causes of death combined.[7] Men have a greater risk of heart disease and are at risk at an earlier age than women, but this gap closes with age.

One aspect of CVD is *atherosclerosis*. This hardening of the arteries occurs when fibrous plaques, which are composed mainly of cholesterol, build up in the arteries, especially at branch points. The first sign of atherosclerosis is soft fatty streaks visible along the walls of the arteries. This disease process interferes with the pumping of blood through the artery in two ways: 1) the deposits gradually narrow the opening, and 2) the fibrosis makes it increasingly hard for the artery to constrict or dilate in response to the tissues' need for oxygenated blood.

Damaged endothelium

Normal smooth muscle cell

■ Fatty deposits accumulate in muscle cell

Fatty streak

Fibers ⎱ Fibrous
Fats ⎰ plaque

Large plaque obstructing artery

This mold of an artery demonstrates dramatically how plaque build-up can restrict blood flow.

Coronary heart disease (CHD) is the most common form of cardiovascular disease. It usually involves atherosclerosis and *hypertension* and causes one-third of all deaths in both men and women. Despite the dramatic decline in mortality over the past 25 years, it remains the most common cause of death in the United States. Coronary heart disease costs the United States between $50 billion and $100 billion per year in medical treatment and lost wages.[8]

Many long-term studies, including the Framingham Study, the Honolulu Heart Study, and the Chicago Gas and Electric Company Study, have provided unique data concerning the role of genetic and environmental factors that increase the risk for developing atherosclerotic cardiovascular disease (ASCVD).[9-11] The occurrence of CVD in a person cannot be predicted with certainty; however, many attributes and behaviors are believed to interact to produce the illness. These break down into unmodifiable risk factors and modifiable risk factors.

Unmodifiable Risk Factors

Certain risk factors that are not under the control of the individual, such as age, gender, ethnicity, and family history, can be predictive of atherosclerosis and hypertension in some people. Although these factors cannot be controlled, nutritionists, public health professionals, physicians, and other health educators need to increase the awareness of heart disease in people who fall into risky groups.

Family History

A family history of premature CHD in a parent or sibling increases a person's risk for the disease (see **Case Study 10-1**). Premature CHD is defined as occurring in a male under the age of 50 or a female under age 60.[12] Individuals who suffer the highest risk for premature cardiovascular disease have a rare genetic defect that substantially blocks the clearance of chylomicrons and triglycerides from the blood, reduces low-density lipoprotein (LDL) uptake by the liver, limits synthesis of high-density lipoprotein (HDL), or enhances blood clotting.[13] Other medical conditions, such as certain forms of liver and kidney disease, low concentrations of thyroid hormone, and use of certain medications to treat hypertension, can increase LDL and increase the risk for heart disease.[13]

Modifiable Risk Factors

Unlike age, gender, ethnicity, and family history, some risk factors for cardiovascular disease can be modified. The major modifiable risk factors for CVD are hypertension, obesity, cigarette smoking, *hypercholesterolemia*, and diabetes.[14] **Box 10-2** presents strategies treating modifiable dyslipidemia, which is excess levels of blood lipids such as cholesterol, low-density lipoproteins, and triglycerides.

Hypertension

Hypertension is one of the major risk factors for coronary heart disease. There is a direct link between every increase of blood pressure (BP) above normal levels and cardiovascular complications.[18] A decrease in systolic pressure by 2 millimeters of mercury (mm Hg) is estimated to have the potential to reduce annual mortality from stroke by 6 percent and from coronary heart disease by 4 percent.[18]

Approximately 25 percent of U.S. adults have hypertension, a major risk factor for coronary heart disease, stroke, and premature death.[19] It is more common in people of African descent.[20] The cause of hypertension is unknown, except that in about 5 percent of cases, it is secondary to an underlying pathophysiologic correctable condition.

Box 10-2 Successful Strategies for the Treatment of Modifiable Dyslipidemia[15–17]

Research studies from human clinical and epidemiologic trials show that dyslipidemia is one of the most important modifiable risk factors for coronary heart disease. Dyslipidemia is characterized by increased fasting concentrations of total cholesterol (TC), LDL cholesterol (LDL-C), and triglycerides (TG), in addition to decreased concentrations of HDL cholesterol (HDL-C).

The treatment for dyslipidemia has been mostly with pharmacological therapy. But, because of safety concerns about the use of pharmaceutical agents, the demand for alternative nonpharmacological therapies has increased.

The National Cholesterol Education Program (NCEP) Adult Treatment Panel III (ATP III) recommends lifestyle therapies, which include a combination of diet and exercise modifications, in place of drug treatment for individuals who are in the intermediate range of CHD risk. This review examined the effectiveness of cholesterol lowering of the two NCEP-recommended combination therapies:

1. Low-saturated-fat diets combined with exercise
2. Nutritional supplementation (i.e., fish oil, oat bran, or plant sterol supplementation) combined with exercise

Results showed that low-saturated-fat diets combined with exercise:

- Lowered total cholesterol by 7–18%
- Lowered LDL cholesterol by 7–15%
- Lowered triglyceride concentrations by 4–18%
- Increased HDL-C levels by 5–14%

Alternatively, nutritional supplements combined with exercise:

- Decreased total cholesterol by 8–26%
- Decreased LDL-C levels by 8–30%
- Decreased triglyceride concentrations by 12–39%
- Increased HDL-C levels by 2–8%

These findings suggest that community nutritionists should provide nutrition education that uses combination lifestyle therapies because they are more effective strategies for improving cholesterol levels in those diagnosed with dyslipidemia in their community. Also, including a low-saturated-fat diet as part of the combination will increase HDL-C levels.

than 100 mm Hg, and as part of a combination therapy program for high-risk individuals. [21,22] The new guideline for the prevention and management of hypertension is to consider initiating therapy with two agents if blood pressure is more than 20/10 mm Hg above the goal. One of the agents used should be a thiazide-type diuretic. The guideline also states that the most effective therapy prescribed by even the most careful clinician will control hypertension only if individuals are motivated.[21] Magnesium, calcium, fiber, fat, protein, and certain carbohydrates have also been hypothesized to affect blood pressure, although information linking these dietary factors to blood pressure reduction is not consistent.

One objective of Healthy People 2010 is to reduce the proportion of adults with high blood pressure from 28 percent to 18 percent. Research in 1972 showing the importance of blood pressure to health led to the introduction of the first large-scale public outreach and education campaign to reduce high blood pressure by the National Heart, Lung, and Blood Institute (NHLBI).[23] Its promotion of the detection, treatment, and control of high blood pressure has been credited with influencing the dramatic increase in the public's understanding of hypertension and its role in heart attacks and strokes, as well as a related reduction in deaths. The percentage of people who were able to control their high blood pressure through lifestyle changes and through antihypertensive drug therapy increased from about 16 percent in 1971–1972 to about 65 percent in 1988–1994.[24,25] About 90 percent of all adults now have their blood pressure measured at least once every 2 years. Average blood pressure levels have fallen by 10 to 12 mm Hg since the advent of National High Blood Pressure Education Program (NHBPEP).[24]

The Dietary Approaches to Stop Hypertension (DASH) trial, the DASH-Sodium trial, and the Optimal Macro-Nutrient Intake to Prevent Heart Disease (OmniHeart) study evaluated the effects of diets with different macronutrient profiles on established cardiovascular disease risk factors (blood pressure and blood lipids) in the setting of stable weight. The DASH and DASH-Sodium trials showed that a carbohydrate-rich diet that emphasized fruits, vegetables, low-fat dairy products, and reduced saturated fat, total fat, and cholesterol significantly lowered blood pressure and LDL cholesterol. The OmniHeart trial showed that partial replacement of carbohydrates with either protein (about half from plant sources) or unsaturated fat (mostly monounsaturated fat) also reduced blood pressure, LDL cholesterol, and coronary heart disease risk. Results from these trials showed the importance of macronutrients as a determinant of CVD risk.[26] Community nutritionists can use these results to promote heart-healthy diets that provide enough flexibility to increase individuals' ability to consume them.

Community-based programs may be an important strategy for primary prevention of hypertension. The Joint National Committee on Detection, Evaluation and Treatment of High Blood Pressure suggests that communities consider the items presented in **Box 10-3**.

atherosclerosis A common form of arteriosclerosis where plaque forms within the intima of medium and large arteries; a group of diseases characterized by thickening and loss of elasticity of arterial walls.

hypercholesterolemia Elevated cholesterol level in the blood.

hypertension A condition in which blood pressure remains persistently elevated.

low-risk individual An individual without diabetes or cardiovascular disease and with systolic blood pressure less than 160 mm Hg and diastolic blood pressure less than 100 mm Hg.

Data suggest that dietary factors such as salt, alcohol, and body weight are important to regulate blood pressure. Other nonpharmacologic recommendations include increasing potassium intake and aerobic exercise and quitting smoking.[21] These factors are all recommended as part of the first-line therapy for ***low-risk individuals***, defined as those without diabetes or cardiovascular disease and with a systolic blood pressure less than 160 mm Hg and diastolic blood pressure less

TABLE 10.2	Adult Blood Cholesterol and Triglyceride Levels		
Lipids (mg/dL)	**Desirable**	**Borderline**	**High**
Total cholesterol	< 200	200–239	≥ 240
LDL cholesterol	< 100	130–159	≥ 160
Triglycerides	< 150	150–199	≥ 200–499
Body mass index (BMI)	18.5–24.9	25–29.9	≥ 30

Source: National Cholesterol Education Program. *Third Report of the Expert Panel on Detection, Evaluation, and Treatment of High Blood Cholesterol in Adults (Adult Treatment Panel III)*. NIH Publication No. 02-5215. September 2002. Available at: http://www.nhlbi.nih.gov/guidelines/cholesterol/atp3full.pdf. Accessed April 11, 2008.

Other Modifiable Risk Factors

Other major modifiable risk factors include tobacco and cigarette smoking, hypercholesterolemia, and obesity. Smoking stresses the cardiovascular system by depriving the heart of oxygen and raising the blood pressure. It also damages platelets, making blood clot formation more likely. Toxins in tobacco smoke damage the blood vessels, setting the stage for plaque formation. People who smoke cigars and pipes have an increased risk of CHD, but the risk is not as high as the risk for people who smoke cigarettes.

It is reported that the segment of the public who has had their blood cholesterol checked increased from 67.6 percent in 1991 to 73.1 percent in 2003. The recommended frequency for checking blood cholesterol is every 5 years for healthy people.[27] The government's and healthcare practitioners' concern is that mass screenings increase healthcare costs through repetitive testing of known cases.[28]

Disorders of lipoprotein metabolism can lead to alterations in plasma cholesterol and triglyceride levels; these disorders are usually associated with an increased risk of cardiovascular disease. Total blood cholesterol level of over 200 mg/dl, especially when it is at or over 240 mg/dl together with LDL cholesterol over 130 to 159 mg/dl, is associated with CVD. The higher the LDL, the greater the risk of CHD; therefore, the primary target of cholesterol-lowering management is the LDL cholesterol. In contrast, the higher a person's HDL levels, the lower the risk of coronary heart disease. Individuals with high serum cholesterol concentrations are at lower risk if they also show higher levels of HDL cholesterol; conversely, individuals with low HDL cholesterol concentrations (less than 40 mg/dl) are at a higher risk regardless of their total cholesterol concentrations. A high HDL level (60 mg/dl or more) counteracts one other risk factor in totaling a person's risk.[29] **Table 10.2** presents the range of adult blood cholesterol and triglyceride levels.

Although the liver produces cholesterol, diet also influences serum cholesterol levels. Only foods of animal origin contain cholesterol. Limiting foods containing animal products can reduce the risk of cardiovascular diseases. For people with elevated LDL cholesterol, preexisting cardiovascular disease (including a past heart attack or stroke), or diabetes, the recommended diet reduces saturated fat to 7 percent of daily calories and reduces cholesterol to less than 200 milligrams per day. Compared to the diet for healthy people, the diet for high-risk groups provides less lean meat, skinless poultry, fish, and eggs and strictly limits high-fat meats, especially organ meats (liver, brain, and kidney). Dietitians can help plan a person's diet to ensure that saturated fats and cholesterol are reduced without sacrificing the nutritional quality of the diet.[30]

It has been reported that polyunsaturated fatty acids, monounsaturated fatty acids, and, to a lesser extent, soluble fiber lower LDL cholesterol. However, fat from all sources should not exceed 30 percent of the total calories.

Fish oils, rich in omega-3 polyunsaturated fatty acids, improve blood lipids (primarily by lowering triglycerides), prevent blood clots, and reduce the risk of sudden death associated with CHD.[31] For these reasons, the dietary guidelines recommend at least two servings of fish per week. Plant sources of omega-3 fatty acids, such as flaxseed and flaxseed oil, canola oil, soybean oil, and nuts, may also be beneficial.[32]

In comparison to a number of other CVD risk factors, the prevalence of obesity has increased over the past several decades, which has had a negative impact in reducing CVD morbidity and mortality. Some of the increased risk for CHD observed in individuals with diabetes is attributed to the concurrent presence of other risk factors such as hypertension and obesity. Also, the amount and type of fatty acids ingested and the dietary cholesterol level as well as the caloric content and macronutrient composition of the diet can influence the composition, concentration, and metabolism of plasma lipoproteins. **Table 10.3** presents the major dietary components or conditions and their effect on total cholesterol and LDL cholesterol. Lifestyle interventions that combine counseling for dietary management, weight reduction, and increased physical activity are essential in the management of diabetes and CHD.

| TABLE 10.3 | The Major Dietary Components or Conditions and Their Effect on Total Cholesterol and LDL Cholesterol |

Component	Effect
Polyunsaturated Fatty Acids	
Omega-6 fatty acids (corn oil, cottonseed oil, soybean oil, sunflower oil, etc.)	Lower total cholesterol and LDL cholesterol levels.[34]
Omega-3 fatty acids (eicosapentaenoic acid [EPA] and docosahexaenoic acid [DHA] (ocean fish, king mackerel, salmon, sardines, albacore tuna, fish oil capsules, flaxseed, etc.)	Lower blood pressure, total cholesterol, LDL, and triglyceride levels and are antithrombotic (interfere with blood clotting).[35]
	High intake prolongs bleeding time, impairs immune function, and increases the potential intake of environmental toxins. At a high intake level of 30 to 40 ml of cod liver oil per day, a risk of vitamin A and vitamin D toxicity can occur.[36]
Monounsaturated Fatty Acids	
Oleic acid (olive oil, rapeseed, etc.)	Lowers total and LDL cholesterol without lowering HDL.[37]
Cholesterol	
Animal products	Raises total cholesterol and LDL cholesterol levels. Most individuals compensate for different
Meats	exogenous cholesterol levels and show no serum cholesterol change. Other individuals are
Egg yolks	sensitive to changes in cholesterol intake.[38]
Shellfish	
Saturated Fatty Acids	
Lauric acid (coconut, palm kernel oil)	Increases plasma total cholesterol.
Myristic acid (coconut)	Increases plasma total cholesterol (four to six times more hypercholesterolemic than palmitic and lauric acid).
Palmitic acid (palm oil, beef)	Increases plasma total cholesterol.
Stearic acid (cocoa butter, beef)	Neutral—has no effect on blood lipoproteins due to its desaturation to oleic acid shortly after absorption as well as its high incorporation into phosphatidylcholine.[39]
Trans Fatty Acids	
Animal foods	Increase LDL cholesterol to about the same extent as saturated fatty acids and can also reduce
Hydrogenated vegetable oil	HDL cholesterol concentrations.[40]
Margarines (stick margarines have more trans fat than tub margarine, baked goods, etc.)	
Carbohydrates	
Soluble fiber (pectins, gums, mucilages, legumes, oats, fruits, etc.).	Lower serum cholesterol and LDL cholesterol.
High simple sugar (table sugar, candy, fructose, etc.).	Increase plasma triglycerides.[41]
Vegetarianism	
High fiber	Lowers serum cholesterol and LDL cholesterol.
Fruits	
Vegetables	
Complex carbohydrates	
Grains	
The Mediterranean Diet	
High in fruits, vegetables, grains, and legumes	Lowers incidence of coronary heart disease and possibly cancer.[42]
Low in meat	
High monounsaturated to saturated fat ratio	
Moderate consumption of milk and dairy products	
Moderate ethanol consumption	

(continues)

TABLE 10.3	(Continued)

Component	Effect
Protein	
Soy protein	The mechanism is not clear, but the assumption is that soy protein stimulates LDL receptors' activities, which are chronically reduced in hypercholesterolemia.[43]
Animal protein	*Arginine* is high in plant protein and seems to lower blood cholesterol, while *lysine* and *methionine*, amino acids that are higher in animal proteins, seem to raise plasma cholesterol levels.[44]
	Homocysteine, high levels of this amino acid, may contribute to heart disease by promoting atherosclerosis, excessive blood clotting, or blood vessel rigidity.[45]
	Folic acid and vitamins B_6 and B_{12} are all important in the metabolism of homocysteine by reducing its level. Scientists believe that a diet rich in these vitamins helps prevent blood vessel damage from homocysteine.[46]
Moderate Alcohol Intake	
Red or white wine	Has a protective factor.[47]
Beer	In addition to alcohol, wine contains **phytochemicals** that may also protect against cardiovascular disease.[48]
Distilled liquor	These substances may act as antioxidants, reducing LDL oxidation and blood clot formation, and may alter prostaglandin metabolism.
	Wine also contains *resveratrol*, an antifungal compound in grape skins that increases HDL cholesterol and inhibits LDL oxidation.[46]
Regular Aerobic Physical Activity	
	Lowers LDL, raises HDL, lowers blood pressure, speeds weight loss and loss of body fat, improves blood glucose control in people with type 2 diabetes, and reduces emotional stress.[49]
Coffee and Garlic	
	Evidence relating coffee to increases and garlic consumption to decreases in serum total cholesterol, LDL cholesterol levels, or CHD has been inconsistent.[50]

Prevention of cardiovascular disease depends on minimizing a person's risk factors (hypertension, overweight/obesity, sodium intake, irregular exercise, etc.) and moderation in alcohol consumption.[33] Community nutritionists can use such strategies as cessation of tobacco use and cigarette smoking, decreased saturated fat intake, and control of diabetes mellitus for modifying the risk factors for CHD.

The National Cholesterol Education Program
Healthy People 2010 set a goal of reducing total blood cholesterol among adults from an average of 206 mg/dl to 199 mg/dl, as well as reducing the percentage of adults with high blood cholesterol from 21 percent to 17 percent. The Third Report of the National Cholesterol Education Program (NCEP) Expert Panel on Detection, Evaluation, and Treatment of High Blood Cholesterol in Adults provided further evidence of the importance of diet in treating cardiovascular disease.[51] The NCEP recommended several different strategies for identifying and

phytochemicals Non-nutrient compounds found in plant-derived foods that produce biological activity in the body.

overweight A body mass index of 25 to 29.9 kg/m² or a body weight 10 to 19 percent above the healthy body weight standard.

Consuming a variety of fruits and vegetables can reduce the risk of heart disease.

Box **10-4 The NCEP Guidelines for Reducing the Risk of Heart Disease**[51,52]

- Recommend a cholesterol test every 5 years for all adults over age 20.
- Define low HDL as being less than 40 mg/dl compared to an earlier value of 35 mg/dl.
- Intensify the use of nutrition, physical activity, and weight control in the treatment of elevated blood cholesterol.
- Identify metabolic risk factors, collectively known as "metabolic syndrome" risk factors, linked to insulin resistance, which often occur together and dramatically increase the risk of heart attacks.
- Assess diet and lifestyle behaviors, and use behavioral strategies to enhance adherence.
- Treat elevated triglycerides aggressively. **Table 10.2** earlier in the chapter shows triglyceride levels and levels of total and LDL cholesterol considered desirable, borderline high, and high according to the new guidelines.
- Treat high cholesterol more aggressively in people with diabetes.

Since its inception in 1985, the NCEP has made population-wide dietary recommendations. The following are the latest recommendations:

- Choose foods low in saturated fat.
- Choose foods low in total fat.
- Choose foods high in starch and fiber.
- Choose foods low in cholesterol.
- Be more physically active.
- Maintain a healthy weight, and lose weight if you are overweight.

TABLE 10.4	The NCEP Two-Step Approach to Managing Hypercholesterolemia			
Nutrient	**Step 1 Diet**	**Step 2 Diet**	**Therapeutic Lifestyle Changes (TLC)**
Total fat	Less than 30% of total calories	Less than 30% of total calories	25–35% of total calories
Saturated fatty acids*	Less than 8–10% of total calories	Less than 7% of total calories	Less than 7% of total calories
Polyunsaturated fatty acids	Up to 10% of total calories	Up to 10% of total calories	Up to 10% of total calories
Monounsaturated fatty acids	10–15% of total calories	10–15% of total calories	Up to 20% of total calories
Carbohydrates**	50–60% of total calories	50–60% of total calories	50–60% of total calories
Protein	10–29% of total calories	10–20% of total calories	About 15% of total calories
Cholesterol	Less than 300 mg/day	Less than 200 mg/day	Less than 200 mg/day
Fiber	20–35 g/day	20–35 g/day	20–30 g/day
Total calories***	To achieve and maintain desirable weight	To achieve and maintain desirable weight	To balance energy intake and expenditure and to maintain desirable body weight/prevent weight gain

*Trans fatty acids are an LDL-raising fat that should be kept at a low intake.

**Carbohydrate should be derived predominantly from foods rich in complex carbohydrates, including grains (especially whole grains), fruits, and vegetables.

***Daily energy expenditure should include at least moderate physical activity, contributing approximately 200 kcal per day.

Sources: National Institutes of Health. National Heart, Lung, and Blood Institute. National Cholesterol Education Program. *Expert Panel on Detection, Evaluation, and Treatment of High Blood Cholesterol in Adults (Adult Treatment Panel III)*. And National Institutes of Health. National Heart, Lung, and Blood Institute. NIH Publication No. 02-5215. September 2002. Available at: http://www.nhlbi.nih.gov/guidelines/cholesterol/atp3full.pdf. Accessed May 21, 2008.

managing individuals at risk for heart disease. The strategies include either primary prevention for healthy individuals or secondary prevention for those at risk of heart disease. **Box 10-4** and **Table 10.4** present the approaches for reducing the risk of heart disease and managing hypercholesterolemia.

Obesity

Obesity is a persistent disease, and it is one of the most chronic health conditions in the world. It is reported that more than 1 billion adults worldwide are estimated as *overweight* and about 300 million of them are clinically obese.[53] In the United States, more than half of the population is either overweight or obese, and this condition affects all ages, genders, and ethnic groups.[54]

Obesity increases the risk for high blood pressure, high blood cholesterol, type 2 diabetes, insulin resistance, coronary heart disease, and many other physical ailments.[55] Several studies have demonstrated that increases in obesity also increase the number of lives lost to obesity,[56-58] as well as disease burdens of obesity. It is clear that obesity has become a leading public health problem in the United States. The first principle of the 2001 Surgeon General's Call to Action is to "promote the recognition of overweight and obesity as a major public health problem."[59]

Defining Obesity and Overweight

Obesity is caused by the accumulation of excess body fat. Although some methods to measure body fat do exist, they are expensive and unrealistic for general use. Body weight has traditionally been used to measure excess body fat. In recent years, however, the use of the body mass index (BMI) has become the recommended method for screening and monitoring the population's body fat and for defining both overweight and obesity in a clinical setting.[60] BMI is determined by weight in kilograms divided by height in meters squared (BMI = kg/m^2). For adults, a BMI of 25.0 to 29.9 is classified as overweight and a BMI of 30.0 or more is classified as obese. See Chapter 2 for more about BMI calculation.

Although BMI is the most used criterion for obesity, there are limitations to this method. The measure may be incorrect for individuals with large muscle mass (e.g., body builders, weight lifters) or those with low muscle mass (e.g., the elderly). The location of body fat (fat distribution) is also important because fat distributed around the abdomen ("apple" shape or **android obesity**), found mainly in men, is linked to high blood lipids, glucose intolerance and insulin resistance, and high blood pressure. It also increases the risk for heart disease and diabetes mellitus. Fat that is distributed around the hips and thighs ("pear shape" or **gynoid obesity**) is common in women. Excess body fat at both locations has detrimental consequences for both men and women. A waist circumference of larger than 40 inches in men or larger than 35 inches in women is a sign of increased risk of cardiovascular disease.[61]

Excessive body fat in the abdomen is associated with increased risk for morbidity.

Epidemiology of Obesity and Overweight

Obesity and diabetes have reached epidemic proportions in the United States. According to 2005–2006 data from the Centers for Disease Control and Prevention, 33.3 percent of men and 35.3 percent of women are obese (BMI >30 kg/m^2), and those with a BMI of over 40 or higher are at an increased risk of diabetes.[61,62] In 2006, four states had obesity prevalence rates of less than 20 percent; 20 states had rates of about 25 percent; and 2 states (Mississippi and West Virginia) had rates of more than 30 percent.[61,63] The National Center for Health Statistics reported that, in 2003–2004, 66 percent of the U.S. adults were either overweight (BMI >27 kg/m^2) or obese. Obesity is the second leading cause of preventable death in the United States and accounts for at least 112,000 deaths each year. Obesity increases the risk of CVD, hypertension, and diabetes, and accounted for medical care costs above $75 billion in 2003.[61]

The Healthy People 2010 target for adult obesity, based on measured weights and heights, is 15 percent among racial and ethnic groups for whom data were available. The trend towards obesity is high for adult African American females ages 49 to 59 (55 percent of whom were obese in 2003–2004, up from 50 percent in 1999–2000) and for adult Mexican American females (51 percent of whom were obese in 2003–2004, up from 40 percent in 1999–2000). About 39 percent for European American women of the same age are obese. However, among men, the prevalence of obesity did not differ significantly by race or ethnic group.

Medical and Social Costs of Obesity

Overweight and obesity and their associated health problems have substantial economic consequences for the U.S. healthcare system.[63] The increasing prevalence of overweight and obesity is associated with both direct and indirect costs. Direct healthcare costs refer to preventive, diagnostic, and treatment services related to overweight and obesity (for example, physician's office visits, hospital visits, and nursing home care). Indirect costs refer to the value of wages people lost when they were unable to work because of illness or disability, as well as the value of future earnings lost by premature death. In 2003–2004, $431 billion was attributed to the direct and indirect costs of obesity.[64] Most of the cost associated with obesity was due to type 2 diabetes, coronary heart disease, and hypertension. Data show that U.S. medical expenses in 2003 related to obesity was as high as $75 billion. Medicaid and Medicare paid about half of these costs.[65]

At the state level, estimates of Medicare costs due to obesity ranged from $87 million (Wyoming) to $7.7 billion (California), and Medicaid costs due to obesity ranged from $23 million (Wyoming) to $3.5 billion (New York). (The state differences in obesity expenditures were due to differences in the size of each state's population.[65,66]) These state-estimated data are limited to direct medical costs of obesity, not indirect costs (e.g., absenteeism and decreased productivity).[63]

Overweight and obese individuals are at increased risk for many diseases and health conditions, including the following:[63]

- Hypertension
- Dyslipidemia (for example, high total cholesterol or high levels of triglycerides)
- Type 2 diabetes
- Coronary heart disease
- Stroke
- Gallbladder disease
- Osteoarthritis

- Sleep apnea and respiratory problems
- Some cancers (endometrial, breast, prostate, rectum, uterus, cervical, and colon)
- Complications during pregnancy
- Complications during surgical procedures
- Depression

Society's emphasis on body weight may contribute to the emotional suffering of obese people. Emphasis on physical appearance, especially for women, makes overweight people feel unattractive.[67] Obese people regularly encounter prejudice or discrimination in the workplace, at school, and in social situations. Feelings of rejection, shame, or depression are common in obese individuals.[68] One research study suggested that improved self-image may be an avenue to promoting weigh control in women.[69]

Determinants of Obesity

Weight gain occurs due to an imbalance of energy intake and expenditure. Initially, when energy intake exceeds output, fat cells increase in size. When fat cells can no longer expand, they can increase in number. The size of the fat cells can decrease with weight loss, but the number of cells does not decrease. The reasons for the imbalance between energy intake and expenditure vary based on an individual's genes, emotional state, age, gender, psychological makeup, and environmental factors.[70]

Genes

Scientists have identified some genes that cause obesity when they are damaged, but the actual mechanism that predisposes an individual to obesity is not clear. However, it is clear that when both parents are obese (body weight 100 percent above normal), the likelihood that their children will be obese is high (80 percent); however, when neither parent is obese, the chance that their children will be obese is low (less than 10 percent). Conversely, about 25 to 30 percent of obese persons have normal-weight parents.[71] The relationship between genetics and environment is not clear. It is estimated that genes alone account for about 50 to 90 percent of the variation in the amount of body fat stored.[72] However, having an obese relative does not guarantee that an individual will be obese.

Emotions

Some people overeat because of depression, hopelessness, anger, boredom, and many other reasons besides hunger.[68] This doesn't indicate that overweight and obese people have more emotional problems than other people, but that their feelings seem to influence their eating habits, causing them to overeat. In these cases, as with other emotional issues, psychological intervention may be helpful.[73]

Environmental Factors

The most important environmental factor is lifestyle. Individuals' eating habits and activity level may be learned from the people around them. Overeating and sedentary habits (inactivity) are the most important risk factors for obesity. The term *obesogenic environment* is defined as "the sum of influences that the surroundings, opportunities or conditions of life have on promoting obesity in individuals or populations."[74,75] The environment is broader than just the physical environment; it includes costs, laws, policies, social and cultural attitudes, and values.

Gender

Men typically have more muscle mass than women. Individuals with more muscle mass tend to have higher *basal metabolic rate (BMR)*. Other factors that influence BMR include age, genetics, temperature, hormones, growth, and physical activity. Thus, women are more likely than men to gain weight with the same amount of calorie intake. Also, women often gain weight after pregnancy and at menopause. During pregnancy, women store more body fat to be used for lactation. Menopause causes a decrease in estrogen level, causing increased body fat storage. Also, both men and women tend to lose muscle mass and gain more body fat as they age. Their metabolism also slows slightly, which lowers their caloric needs.[76]

Certain Medical Conditions and Medications

Although these situations are less common causes of obesity than overeating and inactivity, community nutritionists should be aware that individuals with the following conditions may gain excess body fat:[77]

- Hypothyroidism
- Cushing syndrome
- Depression
- Prader-Willi syndrome
- Polycystic ovarian syndrome

Also, certain medications (e.g., steroids, antidepressants, birth control pills, etc.) can cause an increase in body fat.

In addition to the causes listed, obesity is associated with other factors such as poverty; portion sizes; types of food consumed (high-fat foods, fast foods, soft drinks, and potato chips, and fewer complex carbohydrates); agricultural and technological innovations, which cause a decrease in food prices; and a sedentary lifestyle.[78,79]

Obesity Prevention and Treatment Intervention

Extensive scientific research in the area of obesity has contributed significantly to the prevention and treatment of overweight and obesity. Obesity is now viewed as a complex disorder with several contributing factors, such as genetic, sociocultural, environmental, and behavioral. Hence, the recommendations for weight management emphasize moderation and a balanced diet, behavior change, and moderate to vigorous physical activity for improving fitness. This section discusses different strategies for weight management.

Lifestyle Modification

The bases of most obesity management programs are diet modification and physical activity. These modifications are inexpensive, and if the lifestyle changes can be maintained, they have

android obesity Excess storage of fat, mainly in the abdominal area.

gynoid obesity Excess storage of fat, mainly in the buttocks and thigh. Also called gynecoid obesity.

obesogenic environments The sum of influences that the surroundings, opportunities, or conditions of life have on promoting obesity in individuals or populations.

basal metabolic rate (BMR) The minimum amount of energy that an awake, fasted resting body needs to maintain itself; often used interchangeably with resting metabolic rate (RMR). BMR measurements are performed in a warm room in the morning before the individual rises, and at least 12 hours after the last food intake and activity.

the potential for long-term effectiveness.[80] In addition to creating changes in diet and physical activity, the lifestyle modification component of obesity interventions usually includes some form of behavioral modification to increase the long-term effectiveness of the program.

In 1994, the National Weight Control Registry, an ongoing observational study, was established to assess factors associated with sustained weight loss.[80] The requirement for this observational study was that participants must have maintained at least 30 pounds of weight loss for at least 1 year. Initial results indicated that more than 3,000 participants (80 percent women, 97 percent European Americans, with a mean age of 45 years) reported an average weight loss of 66 pounds and that the average duration of weight loss was 5.5 years. Approximately 90 percent of the participants reported previous unsuccessful attempts at weight loss. In this report, 89 percent of the participants reported modifying both diet and exercise to achieve their initial weight loss. The most common methods used were restricting certain types of foods (88 percent), limiting quantities (44 percent), and counting calories (44 percent). Overall, 40 percent of the women and 63 percent of the men reported losing weight on their own, while the remainder used a commercial weight loss program to achieve their weight loss. The most common weight loss strategies used for those who modified their dietary intake were 1) eating a low-fat, low-calorie diet; 2) frequent self-monitoring; and 3) engaging in regular physical activity.[81]

Dietary Modification

The interest in dieting is high because the prevalence of overweight and obesity is very high. About 70 percent of U.S. adults are trying to lose or maintain their weight and almost all report modifying their diet in some way to achieve their goals.[82] The common component of dietary modification for weight loss is reduced caloric intake. The recommendation is to encourage a slow rate of weight loss through an energy deficit (energy output minus energy intake). Small changes in reducing calorie intake by 200 to 300 kilocalories each day is more successful in long-term weight control than a drastic diet of only 1,000 to 1,200 total kilocalories per day. An individual can reduce kilocalorie intake by eliminating one can of soda each day, which is about 150 kilocalories; also, eating half a serving of fries instead of a whole serving would save another 100 kilocalories.[61] Making such changes as replacing whole milk with skim milk and including more fruits and vegetables also will reduce the total kilocalorie intake.

Physical Activity Modification

In general, physical activity is used for the management of obesity. However, studies using only physical activity for weight loss show a small reduction in body weight.[83] Weight losses in the range of 0.09 to 0.1 kg/week have been reported when exercise is used alone compared to a no-treatment control group.[84,85]

Although its impact on weight loss may be minimal, physical activity has a critical role in the long-term maintenance of weight loss. One correlation study showed a strong association between self-reported exercise at follow-up and maintenance of a weight loss program.[86]

Behavior Modification

The most effective weight reduction programs use group **behavior modification**. Behavior modification programs are usually conducted on a weekly basis in university or hospital clinics and have produced average reductions of 8 to 10 percent of body weight over 16 to 26 weeks.[87] The main behavioral modification components utilized in the management of obesity include self-monitoring, **stimulus control**, and relapse

prevention strategies. (See **Case Study 10-2**.) Self-monitoring includes the systematic recording of food intake, exercise activities, and/or weight change. The use of stimulus control involves the identification and modification of environmental cues associated with overeating and sedentary activity, and is widely accepted as clinically effective.[85] The available scientific literature on obesity suggests that consistent self-monitoring, particularly of food intake, is associated with improved outcome,[88] even during high-risk periods such as holidays.

When clients decide to participate in a weight loss program, finding a program that meets their needs becomes important. Some clients choose to participate in programs that include spirituality as a central component. Fitzgibbon et al. conducted a faith-based weight loss intervention study that compared a culturally tailored, faith-based weight loss program to a culturally tailored weight loss intervention with no active faith component.[89] The results were not statistically significant, but suggested that the addition of the faith component improved results.[89] Two weight loss programs based on spirituality are the Thin Within Program, which was founded in 1975 and publicizes itself as a spiritually based, 12-week program that teaches participants to listen to their body's natural internal hunger/fullness signals,[90] and the Weight Down Workshop, founded in 1986 by a registered dietitian that takes a similar approach to weight loss.[90] In 2004, it was estimated that nearly 30,000 Weight Down Workshop groups were in existence nationwide, with many offered through churches. Reports indicate that for some women, spirituality was an important aspect of adhering to program principles.[91]

Hearts N' Parks is a national, community-based program that is designed to increase physical activity and reduce the incidence of obesity and other chronic health conditions. It was developed and supported by the National Heart, Lung, and Blood Institute (NHLBI) of the National Institutes of Health (NIH) and the National Recreation and Park Association (NRPA). The purpose of the program, which was created in 1999, is to reduce the growing trend of obesity and the risk of coronary heart disease in the United States. The program encourages all age groups in the United States to aspire for a healthy weight, follow a heart-healthy eating plan, and engage in regular physical activity. The American Dietetic Association (ADA) is also working with Hearts N' Parks communities to provide expertise on heart-healthy nutrition.[92] About 50 Hearts N' Parks sites ("magnet centers") exist in 11 states.

The magnet centers carry out special "FunFit" events in July, including many activities that are tied to local Fourth of July celebrations. For instance, about 40,000 people attended a July 4 event in Athens, Georgia, where a special Hearts N' Parks tent with games, prizes, and health and wellness information were displayed. On July 5, residents of Roswell, New Mexico, measured their body fat and learned how to grill low-fat foods in conjunction with the city's annual Alien Chase. Over 100,000 people attended a July 6 concert and fireworks event in South Bend, Indiana, that featured Hearts N' Parks displays and nutrition and fitness quizzes.

The Hearts N' Parks model supports the Department of Health and Human Services' Steps to a Healthier US initiative, based on President Bush's Healthier US initiative. These initiatives promote healthy lifestyles and behaviors aimed at achieving and maintaining good health for individuals of all ages. They also encourage public–private partnerships to support community-driven programs on healthy lifestyles that contribute directly to the prevention or treatment of one of three main health problems: obesity, diabetes, and asthma.

In 2002, data collected from the magnet centers included information on 68 programs that varied in size and duration. A pre- and posttest were administered and collected by 36 Hearts N' Parks sites during their first year as a magnet center. Programs for adults lasted an average of 12 weeks, attracting mainly seniors and women.

Results showed that adult participants significantly improved their scores in all areas of knowledge, attitude, and behavior. They increased their knowledge of heart-healthy nutrition by 9 percent. Scores increased from 6 to 7 percent in knowledge of overweight/obesity risks, physical activity, causes of high blood pressure, and ways to control cholesterol levels. Results also showed healthier attitudes toward overweight/obesity, heart-healthy eating habits, and physical activity, and improvements on how frequently participants chose nutritious foods, based on self-reports. Adult participants reported adding, on average, 2 hours of moderate physical activity per week (from 8 hours to 10 hours), such as bicycling, walking, and golfing, after participating in the Hearts N' Parks program. In addition, they reduced the time spent in sedentary activities by an average of 8 hours per week, down to 33 hours.

Older adults (60 years or older) showed greater overall improvement than younger adults. Seniors' pretest knowledge scores were lower than younger adults' scores, but posttest knowledge scores were comparable. Seniors also significantly increased time spent weekly in physical activity on average, from slightly fewer than 6 hours to more than 8.5 hours, and significantly lowered the amount of time each week in sedentary tasks by 10 hours.[93]

Public Health Policy for Addressing Global Obesity

In 2006, the Trust for America's Health (TFAH) reported that national and state policies were inadequate for obesity control and reduction. Some important findings from a study it conducted included that:[94]

- The federal government faces organizational issues, including a lack of designated leadership, a bureaucratic tangle of involved agencies, and a need to learn to balance the competing interests of industry and public health.
- Obesity and obesity-related disease rates are increasing throughout the nation. Adult obesity exceeds 20 percent in 41 states and Washington, DC. Alabama ranked as the heaviest state with 28.4 percent obesity; Colorado ranked as the least obese at 16 percent.
- All states were on track to fail the national Healthy People 2010 goal of reducing the proportion of adults who are obese to 15 percent or lower by the year 2010.[95]

Similarly, the Society for Nutrition Education (SNE) designed a public policy position paper (Improved Nutrition and Physical Activity [IMPACT]) to address the obesity epidemic in the United States. SNE supports local communities to promote good nutrition and increased levels of physical activity among their citizens through community interventions, school-based activities, and healthcare delivery programs. In addition, SNE supports establishing grants for training health professionals and health science students to identify those at risk for obesity and to provide health services for prevention and treatment of these conditions. SNE also supports collecting and analyzing data as part of NHANES and other data sources that can monitor and control obesity.[96]

At the international level, a proactive involvement with food, physical activities, and industries is critical to reduce the risks associated with the global obesity epidemic. This requires collective action including the development of international strategies, together with supportive government policies. The World Heart Federation (WHF) is an international organization whose goal is to improve life through prevention and control of heart disease and stroke, with a focus on low- and middle-income countries. It is one of the international nongovernmental organizations (NGOs) for the World Health Organization's (WHO) Global Strategy on Diet, Physical Activity and Health. Through its national members, the WHF supports the development of food labeling programs. The following are two of the nine initiatives of WHF obesity strategies:[97]

- Supporting WHO's strategy on diet, physical activity, and health
- Increasing awareness of the obesity epidemic and the benefits of healthy diets and physical activity among the population and policy makers through active support of the media

Cancer

Cancer, a disease of the body's cells, is one of the most devastating chronic health conditions in the United States and worldwide. It is the second most common fatal disease in the United States. Its development involves damage to cells' DNA; this damage occurs over a long period of time and grows at the expense of the healthy cells. The characteristics common to all types of cancer are uncontrolled growth and the ability to spread to distant sites (to *metastasize*).

Individuals who are alive and without recurrence of cancer 5 years after diagnosis are considered cured. This is termed the *5-year survival rate*. Survival rates vary significantly depending on the site where the cancer occurred. Overall, the survival rate for some types of cancer is about 52 percent for European Americans and 38 percent for African Americans.[98] Regardless of ethnicity, the 5-year survival rate for poor Americans is estimated to be 10 to 15 percent lower than for middle-class and affluent Americans.[99] This chapter discusses cancer prevention and dietary factors implicated in the development of cancer.

Links Between Cancer and Diet

The causes of cancer are complex and often not understood. Certain cancers occur in great numbers in some countries. It has been estimated that 35 percent of the cancer mortality in the U.S. population is attributable to diet and about 80 percent to environmental factors.[100] For example, stomach and esophageal cancers are common where nitrates and nitrites are prevalent in food and water or where cured and pickled foods are popular. Some of the countries where this occurs are the United States, China, Japan, and Iceland.

Studies of migration between cultures demonstrate the strong effect of environmental factors. These studies reveal that the pattern of occurrence of many types of cancer changes when people move to a new country. For example, in Japan there is more stomach cancer and less prostate, colon, and breast cancer than in the United States. In second-generation Japanese immigrants to the United States, however, the rates and types of cancers are similar to those of

behavior modification A process used to gradually and permanently change habitual behaviors.

stimulus control Altering the environment to minimize the stimuli for eating; for example, removing foods from sight and storing them in kitchen cabinets.

metastasize To spread cancer by the movement of cancer cells from one part of the body to another.

5-year survival rate Individuals who are alive and without recurrence of cancer 5 years after diagnosis.

other Americans.[81] Similar outcomes for prostate cancer are reported in Polish men.[100] The changes coincide with differences in environmental exposure, lifestyle, and diet.

Dietary Components and Cancer

It is hard to review the role of dietary components in cancer development without also considering the other factors that might add to the development of cancer. It is estimated that 35 percent of cancers may be related to diet, including 40 percent of those in men and 60 percent of those in women, notwithstanding the fact that women consume a more varied diet and less alcohol than men.[100] Cooking methods also may be linked to cancer, and some nutrients are associated with cancer when they are consumed in large quantities. The nutrients that may cause cancer include fat, calories, calcium, and vitamin D; other factors such as alcohol also may cause cancer. **Table 10.5** presents the dietary components of cancer.

Protective Effects of Certain Food Components Against Cancer

One of the Healthy People 2010 objectives is to reduce both new cases and the current rate of cancer in the United States. This can be accomplished by eating a moderately low-fat diet and by increasing the consumption of fruits, vegetables, and whole grains. These foods contain vitamins, minerals, and other substances that are beneficial to one's health, such as phytochemicals. This section discusses some of the dietary components that can protect people from the risk of cancer.

Fiber

There is strong evidence that fiber has physiologic effects on the gastrointestinal tract that may prevent the occurrence of chronic diseases. Dietary fiber refers to plant materials that are not easily digested by enzymes in the human gut. Water-soluble fibers include pectin, gums, and mucilages. Insoluble fibers include cellulose and other hemicelluloses.

Early studies suggested that fiber intake was related to the low incidence of colorectal cancer in Africans consuming high-fiber diets.[106] In the United States, populations with a higher per capita intake of fiber usually have a lower incidence of colorectal cancer compared with those with a lower intake. However, epidemiologic studies on the relationship between dietary fiber and colorectal cancer are inconclusive. A recent prospective study using the Nurses' Health Study cohort found no association between fiber intake and the risk of colorectal cancer.[107] Two clinical trials have shown that increasing total fiber intake did not influence the risk of recurrent colorectal **adenomas**,[109,110] which are cancers that arise from glandular tissues. Fiber also plays a protective role in preventing breast and ovarian cancer.[108]

The anticarcinogenic effects previously attributed to fiber may be due to the effects of the non-fiber constituents of fruits and vegetables, such as **antioxidants**, vitamins, and minerals. In addition, high-fiber intake is mostly associated with lower caloric intake, which may also decrease the risk of cancer.

Adequate dietary fiber intake is encouraged because of its role in maintaining normal bowel function and its possible role in disease prevention. The recommended amount of dietary fiber ranges from 25 to 30 g/day or 10 to 13 g/1,000 kcal.[111] Mean dietary fiber intake in the United States is about 14 to 15 g/day.[111] Because some of the benefits of high-fiber foods may be due to other components in fiber-rich diets, high-fiber foods, rather than isolated fiber, are recommended. The recommendation is to consume whole fruits and whole grains instead of fruit juices and refined grains.

Certain fibers exist in higher concentrations in specific foods. For example, insoluble fiber such as pectin is found in fruits and vegetables, especially apples, oranges, strawberries, and carrots. Gums are found in oat bran, barley, and legumes. Whole-wheat flour, wheat bran, and vegetables are good sources of celluloses, while hemicellulose is found in wheat bran, whole bran, and whole grains.

Antioxidants

Free radicals are short-lived, highly reactive chemicals often derived from oxygen-containing compounds, which can have detrimental effects on cells, especially cellular DNA and cell membranes. The body has an antioxidant defense system that prevents free radical damage.[61] This includes antioxidant nutrients, which can directly scavenge free

TABLE 10.5	Dietary Components and Cancer[101–104]	
Dietary Components	**Effect**	
Fats		
Animal	Higher incidences of breast, colon, prostate, and pancreatic cancers.	
Linoleic acid (polyunsaturated fat)	A high level promotes cancer rather than initiates it.	
Omega-3 fatty acids	Have a protective effect against the development of cancer.	
Monounsaturated fatty acids	Have a neutral effect.	
Cooking methods	High-temperature cooking of meat, such as frying, broiling, and grilling, produces *carcinogens* such as heterocyclic amines (HCAs), polycyclic aromatic hydrocarbons, and nitrosamines (PAHs) in animals. These substances can damage the DNA and cause mutations, which may result in cancer of the stomach and esophagus.[105]	
	Low-temperature, high-moisture cooking, such as stewing and pot-roasting, does not produce the same level of carcinogens.	
Alcohol	High consumption causes oropharyngeal, laryngeal, esophageal, breast,[106] and colorectal cancer.	

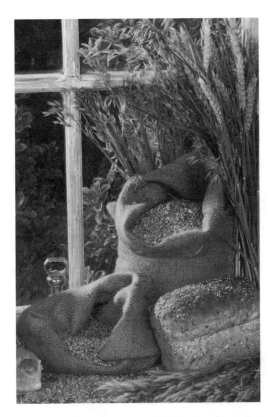

Instead of using white flour, substitute with different types of whole grains in your regular recipes for cookies, muffins, quick breads, and pancakes.

TABLE 10.6	Possible Anticarcinogens in Vegetables and Fruits[13,102,115]
Nutrients/Substances	**Food Sources**
Carotenoids	Carrots, peppers, parsley, greens, spinach
Ascorbate (vitamin C)	Oranges, strawberries, green peppers, tomatoes
Tocopherols (vitamin E)	Wheat germ, safflower oil, sunflower seeds
Selenium	Lean ground beef, crab, turkey, dark meat
Folate	Fortified grain products
Dietary fiber	All plants, fruits, and vegetables
Allium compounds	Onions, garlic
Isoflavones	Soybeans
Flavonoids	Grapefruit, citrus
Protease inhibitors	Seeds, legumes, potatoes, sweet corn
Anthocyanidins	Grapes, cherries, raspberries.
Lignans	Grains, flax seed
Ellagic	Raspberries, spinach, strawberries, blueberries, cranberries
Phytochemical/indoles	Broccoli, brussels sprouts, cabbage, kale

radicals and deactivate them. Alpha-tocopherol (vitamin E), ascorbic acid (vitamin C), beta-carotene (carotenoids, a provitamin A), and flavonoids are antioxidants that have been shown to be active in the prevention of cancer in vitro. Vitamins C and E and green tea can prevent the formation of *carcinogenic* nitrosamines and nitrosamides.[112] A 5-year trial of beta carotene, vitamin E, and selenium showed that consumption of higher levels of these nutrients resulted in the incidence of stomach cancer being reduced by 20 percent and total mortality by 10 percent among residents of Linxian County, China, who have one of the world's highest rates of esophageal and gastric cancer.

The consumption of tomatoes and tomato sauce has been reported to reduce the incidence of prostate and gastrointestinal cancers. Lycopene, found in tomatoes, is the most efficient antioxidant of the carotenoids. A high intake of raw tomatoes, more than seven servings per week, was significantly related to decreased risk for gastrointestinal cancers compared to an intake of less than two servings per week.[113,114] Tomatoes have other components besides lycopene, such as Vitamin C, that may contribute to these findings. Because the cancer-reducing effect may be influenced by other nutrients or a combination of nutrients, eating a variety of whole foods, not individual micronutrients, is the appropriate formula for decreasing the risk of cancer.

Fruits and vegetables are low in calories and good sources of fiber, vitamins, minerals, and other bioactive substances (phytochemicals). (See **Table 10.6**.) Several epidemiologic studies have examined the relationship between fruit and vegetable intake and the occurrence of cancer. Populations with the lowest intake of fruits and vegetables have double the rate of most cancers, such as genitourinary, gastrointestinal,

and pulmonary malignancies as well as stomach, pancreas, oral cavity, esophagus, colorectal, and bladder cancer.[113] Raw vegetables were shown to provide protective effects in 87 percent of studies. Specifically, vegetables from the allium family (e.g., onions, garlic), carrots, green vegetables, cruciferous vegetables (e.g., broccoli, cauliflower), and tomatoes were shown to be protective in 70 to 80 percent of the studies. Total fruits and citrus fruits were shown to be protective in about 65 percent of the studies.[113] The majority of case-control studies indicate that high vs. low consumption of vegetables and fruits reduces the risk of cancer by about half. For example, the risk of stomach cancer decreased by about 60 percent as vegetable intake increased from 100 g/day to 350 g/day and by above 50 percent as fruit intake increased from 50 g/day to 300 g/day.

Physical Activity, Exercise, and Cancer

Several studies, including the Nurses' Health Study, show a direct relationship between physical activity and colon cancer.[102,116] Individuals with high levels of activity throughout their lives were found to have the lowest risk, whereas those who reported high levels of activity

adenomas Cancers that arise from glandular tissues.

antioxidants Vitamins C and E and beta-carotene, which neutralize free radicals and other reactive chemicals and terminate harmful chemical reactions.

linoleic acid An essential omega-6 fatty acid that contains 18 carbon atoms and 2 carbon–carbon double bonds (18:2).

carcinogen An agent that can cause cancer.

carcinogenic Producing cancer; a substance that can produce or enhance the development of cancer.

only in later life were associated with a weaker protective effect of physical activity.[116,117] These studies also reported that mild to moderate physical activity and exercise significantly reduced colon cancer and adenoma risk.[117,118] The American Cancer Society guidelines are consistent with guidelines from the American Heart Association and the American Diabetes Association for the prevention of coronary heart disease and diabetes, as well as for general health promotion, as defined by the Department of Health and Human Services' 2005 *Dietary Guidelines for Americans*. The dietary guidelines are:[119,120]

- Reduce fat intake to less than or equal to 30 percent of calories.
- Increase fiber intake to 20 to 30 g/day, with an upper limit of 35 g/day.
- Include a variety of vegetables and fruits in the daily diet.
- Avoid obesity.
- Consume alcoholic beverages in moderation, if at all.
- Minimize consumption of salt-cured, salt-pickled, or smoked foods, and high-fat meats, particularly those from animal sources.
- Be physically active; achieve and maintain a healthy weight. Be moderately active for 30 minutes or more on most days of the week.

Community and public health nutritionists may find that primary and secondary prevention of all cancers involves a more aggressive approach toward eating behavior. (See **Case Study 10-3**.) Equally, understanding the screening and detection approaches recommended for several major cancers, even if there is no known dietary link, prepares nutritionists with the skills to communicate more effectively with their clients.[121] **Box 10-5** presents a dietary research approach to prevention of cancer, and **Box 10-6** describes a successful strategy for increasing the antioxidant content of pizza crust.

Osteoporosis

Osteoporosis is porous bone due to reduction in bone mass. According to NHANES III, 13 to 18 percent of women, or 4 to 6 million, have osteoporosis, and 37 to 50 percent, or 13 to 17 million, have reduced bone mineral density (BMD). For men, 1 to 2 million have osteoporosis and 28 to 47 percent (8 to 13 million) have reduced BMD. Of women 65 and older, 29.3 percent have osteoporosis.[126–128] Therefore, preventive strategies to retard bone loss and prevent osteoporosis are very important.

Normal Bone Development

Both intrinsic and extrinsic factors determine normal bone mass. Intrinsic factors include genetics, family history, and ethnicity. Extrinsic factors include diet, hormonal milieu, specific illness, and exercise. Each of these factors is discussed in detail in this section.

Genetic factors account for 60 to 80 percent of the variance seen in bone mineral density.[129] Daughters of postmenopausal women with a family history of osteoporosis were found to have a lower than normal BMD,[130,131] and both elderly men and women have an increased risk of osteoporosis when other family members have been affected.[132]

Gender and ethnicity are important factors in the consideration of bone density. Males have a higher bone mass, including peak bone mass, at all ages.[129] Men also have a slower reduction of sex steroids with aging, resulting in less dramatic reduction in BMD. Osteoporosis and fractures are lowest among African Americans compared with other races/ethnicities, and bone mass is higher in African Americans as compared to Hispanics, European Americans, and Asians.[129]

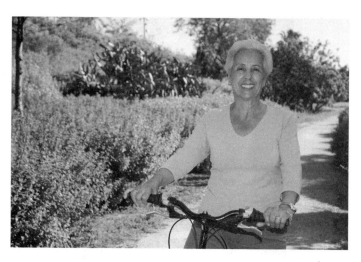

Engaging in leisure time physical activity is the first step toward developing a pattern of regular physical activity.

Box **10-5 Dietary Research Approach Strategy for the Prevention of Cancer**

Dietary Fiber and Colorectal Cancer Risk[122,123]

Le Marchand and colleagues conducted a population-based case-control study among different ethnic groups in Hawaii using personal interviews. (See Chapter 3 for more information on case-control research design.) Between 1987 and 1991, 698 males and 494 females were diagnosed with adenocarcinoma of the colon or rectum, as compared to 1,192 population controls matched by age, sex, and ethnicity. They found a protective association in both sexes with fiber intake from vegetable sources (but not from fruits, except bananas, and cereals). Intakes of carotenoids, light green and yellow-orange vegetables, broccoli, corn, carrots, garlic, and legumes (including soy products) reduced the risk, even after adjustments were made for vegetable fiber. The data supported a protective role of fiber from vegetables against colorectal cancer independent of its water solubility property and the effects of other phytochemicals.

Aligning with these findings, the National Cancer Institute (NCI) designed its Fruits & Veggies—More Matters program to increase per capita fruit and vegetable consumption. The NCI's Five-a-Day program promotes a simple nutrition message that physicians, nurses, community and public health nutritionists, and other healthcare professionals can reinforce to their clients. The basic goal is to promote eating five or more servings of fruits and vegetables every day for better health.

Vigorous physical activity is recommended for improved cardiorespiratory fitness.

Osteoporosis makes the vertebra susceptible to compression fractures from minor trauma. The elderly (especially women) should be concerned about potential fractures if they experience height loss, a limited ability to twist and bend the back, and/or a deformity that develops in the spine.

Box 10-6 Increasing the Antioxidant Content of Pizza Dough[124,125]

Whole grains contain higher levels of fiber and more types of vitamins and minerals, such as folate, vitamin E, and selenium, than refined flour products. These antioxidants have been shown to reduced the risk of some forms of cancer, including prostate and colon cancers. Dr. Liangli Lucy Yu and other nutritionists at the department of nutrition and food science at the University of Maryland conducted a research study to enhance the antioxidant content of pizza dough by incorporating whole wheat flour. The nutritionists increased the antioxidant content by increasing the fermentation process and baking conditions; it is recognized that chemical reactions induced by yeast during the fermentation process release antioxidants that gather in the dough. The researchers extended the time the dough was allowed to rise (48 hours) and baked the dough for a longer period of time (7 to 14 minutes), which increased the antioxidant content of the crust by 60 percent. Also, results showed that the higher the baking temperature (from 400 to 550 degrees Fahrenheit), the more antioxidants accumulated, increasing the antioxidant content in the crust by 82 percent.

Calcium intake seems to increase and maintain bone mass. The recommended daily intake for men and women age 51 years or older is 1,200 mg elemental calcium.[132] Dairy products are the most important sources of dietary calcium, providing approximately 75 percent of the calcium in a typical North American diet.[133] Epidemiologic data suggest that osteoporosis is more prevalent in regions where dairy intake is low and that milk consumption in childhood and adolescence is directly correlated with postmenopausal BMD.[134] (Calcium requirements increase during periods of rapid growth.) It has been reported that calcium alone may not be sufficient for optimal bone accretion. In one study, women consuming more than 1,000 mg of calcium daily exhibited no significant gains in BMD if they did not concomitantly increase their activity patterns.[135] Research evaluating the effects of calcium supplementation on BMD have yielded varying results; controlled supplementation trials in healthy children and adolescents, including twin studies, suggest that calcium supplementation improves bone density.[136,137]

Vitamin D is an important complement to calcium because it facilitates absorption of calcium from the diet. In addition to being absorbed through the intestines, vitamin D is synthesized endogenously in the skin under the influence of ultraviolet sunlight. Risk factors for vitamin D deficiency include inadequate diet, deficient sunlight exposure, low body weight and BMI, the use of anticonvulsants, and malabsorption.[137]

Regular moderate exercise seems to have a beneficial effect on BMD. Studies have suggested that a positive correlation exists between BMD and both body weight and BMI. Low body weight from various conditions has been recognized as an independent risk factor for fractures.[138,139] Several studies have shown that impact (weight-bearing) exercise may have a positive effect on both bone size and mineralization, and a twin study showed that the twin with the longer duration of weight-bearing exercise showed an increased femoral neck BMD.[140,141]

It has been suggested that estrogen helps to preserve bone mass in young women with anorexia nervosa by impairing osteoclast-mediated bone resorption. Oral contraceptive use by these young women in a retrospective cross-sectional study was shown to be associated with a higher BMD.[142] In a small pilot study of women with anorexia nervosa and hypothalamic amenorrhea, estrogen replacement therapy (ERT) increased BMD.[143] Unfortunately, ERT alone has not been shown in other controlled studies to consistently reverse the bone loss in young women with anorexia nervosa, with the possible exception of the most severely underweight patients (less than 70 percent of ideal body weight).[144] Despite the fact that its effects on bone accretion have been disappointing, ERT, combined with psychological support, is a therapy usually used to maintain skeletal health in patients with anorexia.[145] Successful Community Strategies 10-1 presents a successful osteoporosis education program.

Successful Community Strategies 🏠🏠🏠

The University of Nebraska's Osteoporosis Education[146]

A team of healthcare professionals consisting of registered dietitians, faculty, and extension specialists collaborated and designed a community-based health education program. They also formed partnerships and coalitions with individuals, communities, organizations, government agencies, and businesses to educate people about the prevention of osteoporosis.

The program was publicized by placing advertisements in the local newspaper and displaying posters in local businesses. The educational session emphasized prevention, risk factors, diagnosis, and treatment of osteoporosis. The program also had a question and answer session. The participants were able to ask physicians and nutrition professionals questions about osteoporosis. Local health professionals presented the educational session, with local physicians being the primary presenters. Pre- and post data were obtained from the participants using written questionnaires. The following general issues were incorporated into the educational session: knowledge of osteoporosis, the need for an optimal calcium intake and bioavailability; food sources of calcium; parents as role models; issues affecting consumption, such as weight concerns; lactose intolerance; vitamin D inadequacy; dietary factors aiding calcium retention; weight-bearing exercise; prevention and treatment of osteoporosis; bone density scans; and avoidance of smoking and excessive alcohol intake.

Results showed that 82 percent of respondents knew a great deal about osteoporosis after the sessions, as opposed to only 24 percent before the sessions. After the sessions, 86 percent of those who had a bone density scan prior to the sessions indicated that they had a great deal of knowledge about osteoporosis, as compared with only 21 percent before the educational sessions. Also, 55 percent of those who had never had a bone density scan indicated that they had a great deal of knowledge about osteoporosis compared to 27 percent before the sessions.

About 20 percent of the respondents reported "always" taking calcium supplements after the sessions. Thirty-two percent indicated "always" eating a calcium-rich diet prior to the program, whereas 41 percent did following the sessions. Thirty-four percent "always" did weight-bearing exercises at least three times weekly before the sessions, compared to 40 percent after the sessions.

There were requests for additional nutrition and health education sessions due to the success of the educational program. The team approach in presenting the educational sessions and answering/discussing participants' questions contributed to the success of the program.

Chapter Summary

- A low-fat diet accompanied by a high intake of complex carbohydrates may prevent heart disease and cancer.
- In some people, certain risk factors such as age, genetics, gender, and ethnicity can be predictive of atherosclerosis and hypertension.
- Smoking has a significant influence on the risk of acquiring cardiovascular disease.
- A diet containing soybeans may be effective dietary tool to treat hypercholesterolemia.
- The National High Blood Pressure Education Program (NHBPEP) was the first large-scale public outreach and education campaign to reduce high blood pressure. Its promotion of the detection, treatment, and control of high blood pressure has been credited with influencing the dramatic increase in the public's understanding of hypertension and its role in heart attacks and strokes.
- The diet and lifestyle strategies discussed in this chapter to reduce cardiovascular disease risk are appropriate for primary prevention (where a heart attack has not yet taken place, but where there are risk factors).
- There are links between obesity and an increased risk for high blood pressure, high blood cholesterol, type 2 diabetes, insulin resistance, and coronary heart disease.
- BMI is determined by weight in kilograms divided by height in meters squared (BMI = kg/m^2).
- The basis of a weight loss program is diet, behavior, and physical activity modification.
- Cancer is a disease of the body's cells and is one of the most common chronic health issues.
- About 35 percent of the cancer mortality in the U.S. population is due to diet and about 80 percent to environmental factors.
- Many cancers may be related to obesity and excessive caloric intake, as opposed to fat intake.
- Low-temperature, high-moisture cooking methods, such as stewing and pot-roasting, do not produce carcinogens.
- High temperature cooking of meat, for example, frying, broiling, and grilling, may produce carcinogens.
- Excessive alcohol consumption is associated with an increased risk for laryngeal and esophageal cancers.
- Research shows that populations with a higher per capita intake of fiber have a lower incidence of colorectal cancer.
- Fruits and vegetables are good sources of fiber, vitamins, minerals, and other bioactive substances such as phytochemicals. Studies show that populations with the lowest intake of fruits and vegetables have double the rate of most cancers.
- Individuals with high levels of activity throughout their lives were found to have the lowest risk for some cancers.
- Genetic factors account for about 60 to 80 percent of the variance seen in bone mineral density.
- Vitamin D is an important complement to calcium because it facilitates absorption of calcium from the diet.
- Regular moderate exercise seems to have a beneficial effect on bone mineral density.
- Estrogen helps preserve bone mass in young women with anorexia nervosa by impairing osteoclast-mediated bone resorption.

Critical Thinking Activities

Community and public health nutritionists need to be aware of other healthcare professionals (nurses, physicians, health educators) who are also marketing to the same targeted community audience, for example, those needing information about heart disease, obesity, cancer, and osteoporosis prevention. Programs can overlap and negative reactions occur if a competitive/collaborative market analysis is not conducted prior to any prevention or intervention programs in the community.

Activities

- Ask students to identify a nutrition and health education program that the community needs.
- Identify the current providers of heart disease, cancer, osteoporosis, and obesity prevention programs for your community or target audience.
- Determine your strengths and weaknesses in competing with other healthcare professionals who are providing similar education programs.
- Determine how you can collaborate with the current service providers.
- Outline the distinctive characteristic of your program that sets it apart from other healthcare disease prevention programs in your community.

Case Study 10-1

A 28-year-old gold-medal-winning ice skater, Sergei Grinkov, died suddenly of a heart attack as he was ice-skating. After a thorough evaluation, it was established that he died of a protein abnormality in his blood that causes more blood clot formation than normal. Sergei had normal blood lipid levels (total cholesterol 195 mg/dl, HDL of 45 mg/dl, and normal blood triglycerides and LDL). Sergei's major risk factor was that his father died of heart disease at the age of 52.[13]

It is reported that about 25 percent of people living in the United States have this protein abnormality.[13] The only risk factor is a family history of heart-related death under age 60. Therefore, it is important for all adult Americans to ask their physician to evaluate their cardiovascular disease risks.

Chinonye, a community nutritionist, was employed to identify individuals who may have this trait in the community she serves. She wrote a grant proposal and obtained funds from the American Heart Association; she called the program "Know Your Risks for a Heart Attack." She proposed to use the social marketing framework for this program in the community. Social marketing impacts the practice of dietetics by boosting clients' awareness of health issues and helps move clients toward behavioral change. See Chapter 12 for more information on social marketing.

Activities

- Provide a list of different heart disease risk factors.
- Identify other funding agencies that would be interested in funding this program. See http://www.nutrition.jbpub.com/communitynutrition for examples of funding agencies.
- Identify other heart-healthy collaborative agencies and health professionals for the program.
- Provide examples of other ways of making the public aware of the impact of heart disease.

Case Study 10-2

A group of women in the community have been trying to lose weight, but when they feel stressed, they binge. They're having trouble staying on a food plan and exercising regularly, and are becoming discouraged. Cindy, a registered dietitian, listened to their doubts and lack of confidence. She gave them positive feedback, telling them, "I know its frustrating trying to lose weight, but you're doing a good job. You've already lost some weight. I have confidence you can stick to your goals and lose the weight you want to lose." She assured the women that if they worked hard they would lose weight. The group seemed inspired to work harder at their weight loss plan because Cindy listened to their frustration, motivated them by reinforcing their self-esteem, and recognized that they were doing a good job. Cindy did further investigation and found that they were enrolled in a very-low-calorie weight loss program. The program also encouraged minimal physical activity and promised quick weight loss of 6 to 7 pounds per week. Cindy asked the women to keep records of the amount of time and type of physical activities they performed for 1 week. She also provided them the My-Pyramid graphic and asked them to keep a 3-day dietary record.

Activities:

- Create a plan to show the women how to grocery shop using MyPyramid.
- Identify two or three methods of stress management.
- Identify and explain the recommended amount of weight loss per week.
- Explain whether the dietary recommendations and amount of weight loss per week are based on scientifically sound principles.

Case Study 10-3

Chimma, a registered dietitian and a public health nutritionist in an urban-based wellness program, plans to begin a cancer prevention program that includes nutrition education and smoking cessation classes. Her goal is to provide nutrition programs that address some of the Healthy People 2010 objectives. She wants to increase the proportion of persons age 2 years or over who:

- Consume at least two daily servings of fruits from 28 to 75 percent.
- Consume at least three daily servings of vegetables, with at least one-third being dark green or deep yellow vegetables, from 3 to 50 percent.
- Consume at least six daily servings of grain products, with at least three being whole grains, from 7 to 50 percent.
- Consume less than 10 percent of calories from saturated fat from 36 to 75 percent.
- Consume no more than 30 percent of total calories from fat from 33 to 75 percent.
- Participate in at least 30 minutes of daily physical activity.

Chimma attended and completed the Freedom from Smoking course from the American Lung Association and studied hypnosis and behavior modification during her master's degree program in Public Health Nutrition at the University of Minnesota. Chimma's first project will be a needs assessment of the clients attending her program and in the surrounding community in order to determine an ideal time for the classes and the best type of cost-effective nutrition assessment as well as to understand the nutritional knowledge of the community.

Activities

- Divide into groups and indicate how you can publicize classes for smoking cessation using various media methods.
- Provide the clients with a way to change their dietary habits.
- Identify funding sources for the program (see http://www.nutrition.jbpub.com/communitynutrition) for examples.
- Provide the clients different scientific-based methods of reducing stress.
- Identify other healthcare providers with whom the students could collaborate in the community (e.g., American Heart Association to develop a Heart Healthy program).
- Identify different types of screening methods (discussed in Chapter 2) to use in the program.

References

1. Agency for Health Care Research and Quality. Chronic Disease in Adults. Available at: http://www.ahrq.gov/news/focus/chadult.htm. Accessed January 23, 2007.

2. Morrison C, Bare L, Chambless L, Ellis S, Malloy M, Kane J. Prediction of coronary heart disease risk using a genetic risk score: the atherosclerosis risk in communities study. *Am J Epidemiol.* 2007; 166:28–35.

3. American Dietetic Association. The role of dietetics professionals in health promotion and disease prevention. *J Am Diet Assoc.* 2002; 102:1680–1687.

4. Centers for Disease Control and Prevention. Healthy Aging: Preserving Function and Improving Quality of Life Among Older Americans, At a Glance 2008. Available at: http://www.cdc.gov/nccdphp/publications/aag/aging.htm. Accessed April 9, 2008.

5. Department of Health and Human Services. Healthy People 2010. Available at: http://www.healthypeople.gov. Accessed April 9, 2008.

6. Vatten LL, Nilsen TI, Romundstad PR, Drøyvold WB, Holmen J. Adiposity and physical activity as predictors of cardiovascular mortality. *Eur J Cardiovasc Prev Rehabil.* 2006; 13(6):909–915.

7. Thom T, Haase N, Rosamond W, Howard VJ. Heart disease and stroke statistics—2006 update: a report from the American Heart Association statistics committee and stroke statistics subcommittee. *Circulation.* 2006; 113:e85–e151.

8. Centers for Disease Control and Prevention. State-specific trends in high blood cholesterol awareness among persons screened—United States, 1991–1999. *MMWR.* 2001; 50(35):754–758.

9. National Research Council, Food and Nutrition Board. *Diet and Health: Implications for Reducing Chronic Disease Risk.* Washington, DC: National Academy Press; 1989.

10. Keavney B. Genetic epidemiological studies of coronary heart disease. *Int J Epidemiol.* 2002; 31:1730–1738.

11. Simon J, Rosolová H. Family history—and independent risk factors for coronary heart disease, it is time to be practical. *Eur Heart J.* 2002; 23(21):1637–1638.

12. Radomyska B. [Screening programme for hyperlipidemia in children and adolescents. Prophylactic aspects of atherosclerosis]. *Med Wieku Rozwoj.* 2001; 5(1):27–34.

13. Wardlaw G, Kessel M. *Perspectives in Nutrition.* 5th ed. New York: McGraw-Hill; 2002.

14. Hubert H, Eaker E, Garrison R, Castelli W. Life-style correlates of risk factor change in young adults: an eight-year study of coronary heart disease risk factors in the Framingham offspring. *Am J Epidemiol.* 2008; 125(5):812–831.

15. Ferdinand KC. The importance of aggressive lipid management in patients at risk: evidence from recent clinical trials. *Clin Cardiol.* 2004; 27:12–15.

16. Meagher EA. Addressing cardiovascular disease in women: focus on dyslipidemia. *J Am Board Fam Pract.* 2004; 17:424–437.

17. Varady KA, Jones PJ. Combination diet and exercise interventions for the treatment of dyslipidemia: an effective preliminary strategy to lower cholesterol levels? *J Nutr.* 2005; 135:1829–1835.

18. Atilla K, Vassan RS. Prehypertension and risk of cardiovascular disease. *Expert Rev Cardiovasc Ther.* 2006; 4(1):111–117.

19. Wolf-Maier K, Cooper RS, Banegas JR, et al. Hypertension more prevalent in Europe than U.S. and Canada. *JAMA.* 2003; 289:2363–2369.

20. Clark R. Interactive but not direct effects of perceived racism and trait anger predict resting systolic and diastolic blood pressure in black adolescents. *Health Psychol.* 2006; 25(5):580–585.

21. Edward JR. The seventh report of the Joint National Committee on Prevention, Detection, Evaluation, and Treatment of High Blood Pressure. *JAMA.* 2003; 289:2560–2572.

22. Magill MK, Gunning K, Saffel-Shrier S, Gay S. New developments in the management of hypertension. *Am Fam Physician.* 2003; 68:853–858.

23. Burt V, Welton P, Roccella EJ, et al. Prevalence of hypertension in the U.S. adult population. Results from the Third National Health and Nutrition Examination Survey, 1988–1991. *Hypertension.* 1995; 25:305–313.

24. National Center for Health Statistics. *Health, United States with Chartbook on Trends in the Health of Americans.* Hyattsville, MD: Centers for Disease Control and Prevention; 2006. Available at: http://www.cdc.gov/nchs/hus.htm. Accessed January 20, 2007.

25. Jones D, Hall J. Seventh Report of the Joint National Committee on Prevention, Detection, Evaluation, and Treatment of High Blood Pressure and Evidence From New Hypertension Trials. *Hypertension.* 2004; 43(1):1–3.

26. Miller ER, Erlinger TP, Appel LJ. The effects of macronutrients on blood pressure and lipids: an overview of the DASH and OmniHeart trials. *Curr Atheroscler Rep.* 2006; 8(6):460–465.

27. Centers for Disease Control and Prevention, Department of Health and Human Services. Trends in cholesterol screening and awareness of high blood cholesterol—United States, 1991–2003. *MMWR.* 2005; 54(35):865–870.

28. Finkelstein EA, Troped PJ, Will JC, Palombo R. Cost-effectiveness of a cardiovascular disease risk reduction program aimed at financially vulnerable women: the Massachusetts WISEWOMAN project. *J Women's Health Gend Based Med.* 2002; 11(6):519–526.

29. American Heart Association. Cholesterol. Available at: www.americanheart.org/presenter.jhtml?identifier=1516. Accessed January 17, 2007.

30. Allman-Farinelli MA, Gomes K, Favaloro EJ, Petocz P. A diet rich in high-oleic-acid sunflower oil favorably alters low-density lipoprotein cholesterol, triglycerides, and factor VII coagulant activity. *J Am Diet Assoc.* 2005; 105(7):1071–1079.

31. Oh RC, Beresford SA, Lafferty WE. The fish in secondary prevention of heart disease (FISH) survey—primary care physicians and omega3 fatty acid prescribing behaviors. *J Am Board Fam Med.* 2006; 19(5):459–467.

32. Kris-Etherton PM, Harris WS, Appel LJ. Fish consumption, fish oil, omega-3 fatty acids, and cardiovascular disease. *Circ.* 2002; 106:2747–2757.

33. Reeves MJ, Rafferty AP. Healthy lifestyle characteristics among adults in the United States, 2000. *Arch Intern Med.* 2005; 165:854–857.

34. Vijaimohan K, Jainu M, Sabitha KE, Subramaniyam S, Anandhan C, Shyamala Devi CS. Beneficial effects of alpha linolenic acid rich flaxseed oil on growth performance and hepatic cholesterol metabolism in high fat diet fed rats. *Life Sci.* 2006; 79(5):448–454.

35. Denke MA. Dietary fats, fatty acids, and their effects on lipoproteins. *Curr Atheroscler Rep.* 2006; 8(6):466–471.

36. Bourre JM, Galea F. An important source of omega-3 fatty acids, vitamins D and E, carotenoids, iodine and selenium: a new natural multi-enriched egg. *J Nutr Health Aging.* 2006; 10(5):371–376.

37. Appel LJ, Sacks FM, Carey VJ. Effects of protein, monounsaturated fat, and carbohydrate intake on blood pressure and serum lipids: results of the OmniHeart randomized trial. *JAMA.* 2005; 294(19):2455–2464.

38. Herron KL, Vega-Lopez S, Conde K. Pre-menopausal women, classified as hypo- or hyper-responders, do not alter their LDL/HDL ratio following a high dietary cholesterol challenge. *J Am Coll Nutr.* 2002; 21(3):250–258.

39. Haub MD, Wells AM, Campbell WW. Beef and soy-based food supplements differentially affect serum lipoprotein-lipid profiles because of changes in carbohydrate intake and novel nutrient intake ratios in older men who resistive-train. *Metab.* 2005; 54(6):769–774.

40. Pedersen JI, Muller H, Seljeflot I, Kirkhus B. Palm oil versus hydrogenated soybean oil: effects on serum lipids and plasma haemostatic variables. *Asia Pac J Clin Nutr.* 2005; 14(4):348–357.

41. Weggemans R, Zock PL, Ordovas J, Pedro-Botet J, Katan MB. Apoprotein E genotype and the response of serum cholesterol to dietary fat, cholesterol and cafestol. *Atheroscler.* 2001; 154(3):547–555.

42. Nagyova A, Haban P, Klvanova J, Kadrabova J. Effects of dietary extra virgin olive oil on serum lipid resistance to oxidation and fatty acid composition in elderly lipidemic patients. *Bratisl Lék Listy.* 2003; 104(7–8):218–221.

43. Reynolds K, Chin A, Lees KA, Nguyen A, Bujnowski D, He J. A meta-analysis of the effect of soy protein supplementation on serum lipids. *Am J Cardiol.* 2006; 98(5):633–640.

44. Smulyan H. Nitrates, arterial function, wave reflections and coronary heart disease. *Adv Cardiol.* 2007; 44:302–314.

45. Herrmann W. Significance of hyperhomocysteinemia. *Clin Lab.* 2006; 52(7–8):367–374.

46. Clarke R, Lewington S, Sherliker P, Armitage J. Effects of B-vitamins on plasma homocysteine concentrations and on risk of cardiovascular disease and dementia. *Curr Opin Clin Nutr Metab Care.* 2007; 10(1):32–39.

47. Kolovou GD, Salpea KD, Anagnostopoulou KK, Mikhailidis DP. Alcohol use, vascular disease, and lipid-lowering drugs. *J Pharmacol Exp Ther.* 2006; 318(1):1–7.

48. Oak MH, El Bedoui J, Schini-Kerth VB. Antiangiogenic properties of natural polyphenols from red wine and green tea. *J Nutr Biochem.* 2005; 16(1):1–8.

49. Booth FW, Gordon SE, Carlson CJ, Hamilton MT. Waging war on modern chronic diseases: primary prevention through exercise biology. *J Appl Physiol.* 2000; 88:774–787.

50. Tattelman E. Health effects of garlic. *Am Fam Physician.* 2005; 72(1):103–106.

51. National Cholesterol Education Program. Executive summary of the third report of the National Cholesterol Education Program (NCEP) Expert Panel on Detection, Evaluation and Treatment of High Blood Cholesterol in Adults (Adult Treatment Panel II). *JAMA.* 2001; 285:2486–2498.

52. Van Horn L. A summary of the science supporting the new national cholesterol education program dietary recommendations: what dietitians should know. *J Am Diet Assoc.* 2001; 101(10):1148–1154.

53. World Health Organization. Global Strategy on Diet, Physical Activity and Health. Obesity and Overweight. Available at: http://www.who.int/dietphysicalactivity/publications/facts/obesity/en. Accessed January 17, 2007.

54. Ogden CL, Carrol MD, Curtin LR, McDowell MA, Tabak CJ, Flegal KM. Prevalence of overweight and obesity in the United States, 1999–2004. *JAMA.* 2006; 295(13):1549–1555.

55. Department of Health and Human Services. The Surgeon General's Call to Action to Prevent and Decrease Overweight and Obesity. Available at: http://www.surgeongeneral.gov/topics/obesity. Accessed April 9, 2008.

56. Mokdad A, Ford E, Bowman B, et al. Prevalence of obesity, diabetes, and obesity-related health risk factors. *JAMA.* 2003; 289:187.

57. Fontaine KR, Redden DT, Wang C, Westfall AO, Allison DB. Years of life lost due to obesity. *JAMA.* 2003; 289:187–193.

58. Peters A, Barendregt J, Willenkens F, Mackenbach J, Al Mamun A, Bonneux L. Obesity in adulthood and its consequences for life expectancy: a life-table analysis. *Ann Intern Med.* 2003; 138:24–32.

59. Wang G, Dietz WH. Economic burden of obesity in youths aged 6 to 17 years: 1979–1999. *Pediatr.* 2002; 109(5):e81.

60. Moreno L, Blay M, Rodríguez G, Blay V, Mesana M, Olivares J, Jesús F, Sarría A, Bueno M, Zaragoza A. Screening performances of the International Obesity Task Force body mass index cut-off values in adolescents. *J Amer Coll Nutr*. 2006; 25(5):403–408.

61. Insel P, Turner RE, Ross D. *Nutrition*. 3rd ed. Sudbury, MA: Jones and Bartlett; 2007.

62. National Center for Health Statistics. New CDC Study Finds No Increase in Obesity Among Adults, But Levels Still High. Available at: http://www.cdc.gov/nchs/pressroom/07newsreleases/obesity.htm. Accessed April 9, 2008.

63. Mokdad A, Ford ES, Bowman BA, et al. The continuing increase of diabetes in the U.S. *Diabetes Care*. 2001; 24:412.

64. Wang Y, Beydoun M. The obesity epidemic in the United States—gender, age, socioeconomic, racial/ethnic, and geographic characteristics: a systematic review and meta-regression analysis. *Epidemiol Rev*. 2007; 29(1):6–28.

65. Centers for Disease Control and Prevention. Quick Facts: Economic and Health Burden of Chronic Disease. Available at: http://www.cdc.gov/nccdphp/press. Accessed April 9, 2008.

66. Finkelstein EA, Fiebelkorn IC, Wang G. State-level estimates of annual medical expenditures attributable to obesity. *Obesity Res*. 2004; 12(1):18–24.

67. Forrest K, Stuhldreher W. Patterns and correlates of body image dissatisfaction and distortion among college students. *Ame J Health Stud*. 2007; 22(1):18–25.

68. Sjöberg RL, Nilsson KW, Leppert J. Obesity, shame, and depression in school-aged children: a population-based study. *Pediatr*. 2005; 116(3):e389–e392.

69. O'Dea JA, Abraham S. Knowledge, beliefs, attitudes, and behaviors related to weight control, eating disorders, and body image in Australian trainee home economics and physical education teachers. *J Nutr Educ*. 2001; 33(6):332–340.

70. Center for Disease Control and Prevention. Overweight and Obesity: An Overview, Available at: http://www.cdc.gov/nccdphp/dnpa/obesity/contributing_factors.htm. Accessed May 21, 2008.

71. Wright C, Parker L, Lamont D, Craft A. Implications of childhood obesity for adult health: findings from thousand families cohort study. *BMJ*. 2001; 323:1280–1284.

72. Barsh GS, Faroogi S, O'Rahilly S. Genetics of body-weight regulation. *Nature*. 2000; 404:644–651.

73. Wellman N, Friedberg B. Causes and consequences of adult obesity: health, social and economic impacts in the United States. *Asia Pacific J Clin Nutr*. 2002; 11(suppl 8):S705–S709.

74. Swinburn B, Egger G, Raza F. Dissecting obesogenic environments: the development and application of a framework for identifying and prioritizing environmental interventions for obesity. *Prev Med*. 1999; 29:563–570.

75. Swinburn B, Egger G. Preventive strategies against weight gain and obesity. *Obesity Rev*. 2002; 3:289–301.

76. Chang CJ, Wu CH, Yao WJ, Yang YC, Wu JS, Lu FH. Relationships of age, menopause and central obesity on cardiovascular disease risk factors in Chinese women. *Int J Obesity*. 2000; 24:1699–1704.

77. Adler GK, Dipp SL. Cushing Syndrome. WebMed. Available at: http://www.emedicine.com/med/topic485.htm. Accessed January 18, 2007.

78. Finkelstein E, Ruhm CJ, Kosa KM. Economic causes and consequences of obesity. *Ann Rev Public Health*. 2005; 26:239–257.

79. USDA Cooperative State Research, Education, and Extension Service. Obesity and Healthy Weight: Obesity White Paper. Available at: http://www.csrees.usda.gov/nea/food/in_focus/obesity_if_whitepaper.html. Accessed April 11, 2008.

80. McAuley KA, Smith KJ, Taylor RW, McLay RT, Williams SM, Mann JI. Long-term effects of popular dietary approaches on weight loss and features of insulin resistance. *Int J Obesity*. 2006; 30(2):342–349.

81. Appel LJ. Lifestyle modification: is it achievable and durable? The argument for. *J Clin Hypertens*. 2004; 6(10):578–581.

82. Linde JA, Erickson DJ, Jeffery RW, Pronk NP, Boyle RG. The relationship between prevalence and duration of weight loss strategies and weight loss among overweight managed care organization members enrolled in a weight loss trial. *Int J Behav Nutr Phys Act*. 2006; 3:3.

83. Klohe-Lehman DM, Freeland-Graves J, Anderson ER, et al. Nutrition knowledge is associated with greater weight loss in obese and overweight low-income mothers. *J Am Diet Assoc*. 2006; 106(1):65–75.

84. Greenwald A. Current nutritional treatments of obesity. *Adv Psychosom Med*. 2006; 27:24–41.

85. Melin I, Reynisdottir S, Berglund L, Zamfir M, Karlström B. Conservative treatment of obesity in an academic obesity unit. Long-term outcome and drop-out. *Eating Weight Disord*. 2006; 11(1):22–30.

86. Bish CL, Michels Blanck H, Maynard LM, Serdula MK, Thompson NJ, Kettel Khan L. Health-related quality of life and weight loss among overweight and obese U.S. adults, 2001 to 2002. *Obesity*. 2006; 14(11):2042–2053.

87. Suastika K. Update in the management of obesity. *Acta Med Indones*. 2006; 38(4):231–237.

88. Germann JN, Kirschenbaum DS, Rich BH. Child and parental self-monitoring as determinants of success in the treatment of morbid obesity in low-income minority children. *J Pediatr Psychol*. 2007; 32(1):111–121.

89. Fitzgibbon L, Stolley MR, Ganschow P, et.al. Results of a faith-based weight loss intervention for black women. *J Natl Med Assoc*. 2005; 97(10):1393–1402.

90. Thin Within. Frequently Asked Questions. Available at: http://www.thinwithin.org. Accessed May 21, 2008.

91. Reicks M, Mills J, Henry H. Qualitative study of spirituality in a weight loss program: contribution to self-efficacy and locus of control. *J Nutr Educ Behav*. 2004; 36:13–19.

92. National Heart, Lung, and Blood Institute. About Hearts N' Parks. Available at: http://www.nhlbi.nih.gov/health/prof/heart/obesity/hrt_n_pk/hnp_ab.htm. Accessed May 21, 2008.

93. National Institutes of Health, National Heart, Lung, and Blood Institute. Reducing Nationwide Obesity Starts in Neighborhoods. Hearts N' Parks Program Brings Science, Skills to 50 Communities. Available at: http://www.eurekalert.org/pub_releases/2003-07/nhla-rno070303.php. Accessed May 21, 2008.

94. Trust for America's Health. F as in Fat: How Obesity Policies Are Failing in America, 2006. Available at: http://healthyamericans.org/reports/obesity2006. Accessed January 19, 2007.

95. Trust for America's Health. New Report Finds 41 States Have Obesity Levels over 20 Percent; State and Federal Obesity Policies Are Failing. Available at: http://healthyamericans.org/reports/obesity. Accessed May 21, 2008.

96. Orr R, Thompson P, McCullum C, et al. IMPACT Position Paper: SNE. *J Nutr Educ Behav*. 2004; 36(4):169–171.

97. World Heart Federation. A Statement on Obesity from the World Heart Federation. Available at: http://www.world-heart-federation.org/fileadmin/user_upload/documents/whf-obesity-statement.pdf. Accessed May 21, 2008.

98. Reisfield GM, Wallace SK, Munsell MF, Webb FJ, Alvarez ER, Wilson GR. Survival in cancer patients undergoing in-hospital cardiopulmonary resuscitation: a meta-analysis. *Resuscitation*. 2006; 71(2):152–160.

99. Spurlock WR, Cullins, LS. Cancer fatalism and breast cancer screening in African American women. *ABNF J*. 2006; 17(1):38–43.

100. Mahan K, Escott-Stump S. *Food, Nutrition and Diet Therapy*. 10th ed. Philadelphia: W.B. Sanders Company; 2000.

101. Hiom S. Public awareness regarding UV risks and vitamin D—the challenges for UK skin cancer prevention campaigns. *Prog Biophys Mol Biol*. 2006; 92(1):161–166.

102. Kushi LH, Byers T, Doyle C, et al. American Cancer Society guidelines on nutrition and physical activity for cancer prevention: reducing the risk of cancer with healthy food choices and physical activity. *CA Cancer J Clin*. 2006; 56:254–281.

103. Calle EE, Rodriguez C, Walker-Thurmond K, Thun MJ. Overweight, obesity, and mortality from cancer in a prospectively studied cohort of U.S. adults. *New Engl J Med*. 2003; 348 (17):1625–1638.

104. Rodriguez C, Freedland SJ, Deka A, et al. Body mass index, weight change, and risk of prostate cancer in the Cancer Prevention Study II Nutrition Cohort. *Cancer Epidemiol Biomarkers Prev*. 2007; 16:63–69.

105. American Institute of Cancer Research. Foods That Fight Cancer. Available at: http://www.aicr.org/site/PageServer?pagename = dc_foods_home. Accessed May 21, 2008.

106. Navarro Silvera SA, Miller AB, Rohan TE. Risk factors for thyroid cancer: a prospective cohort study. *Int J Cancer*. 2005; 116(3):433–438.

107. Park Y, Hunter DJ, Spiegelman D, Bergkvist L. Dietary fiber intake and risk of colorectal cancer: a pooled analysis of prospective cohort studies. *JAMA*. 2005; 294(22):2849–2857.

108. Shin A, Li H, Shu XO, Yang G, Gao YT, Zheng W. Dietary intake of calcium, fiber and other micronutrients in relation to colorectal cancer risk: results from the Shanghai Women's Health Study. *Int J Cancer*. 2006; 119(12):2938–2942.

109. Schatzkin A, Lanza E, Corie D, et al. Lack of effect of a low-fat, high-fiber diet on the recurrence of colorectal adenomas. *N Engl J Med*. 2000; 342:1149–1155.

110. Alberts D, Martinez ME, Roe DJ, et al. Lack of effect of a high-fiber cereal supplement on the recurrence of colorectal adenomas. *N Engl J Med*. 2000; 342:1156–1162.

111. Position of the American Dietetic Association and Dietitians of Canada: vegetarian diets. *J Am Diet Assoc*. 2003; 103(6):748–765.

112. Adhami VM, Ahmad N, Mukhtar H. Molecular targets for green tea in prostate cancer prevention. *J Nutr*. 2003; 133:2417S–2424S.

113. Kris-Etherton PM, Hecker KD, Bonanome A, et al. Bioactive compounds in foods: their role in the prevention of cardiovascular disease and cancer. *Am J Med*. 2002; 113:71s–88s.

114. Wang S, DeGroff VL, Clinton SK. Tomato and soy polyphenols reduce insulin-like growth factor-I-stimulated rat prostate cancer cell proliferation and apoptotic resistance in vitro via inhibition of intracellular signaling pathways involving tyrosine kinase. *J Nutr*. 2003; 133(7):2367–2376.

115. Kanadaswami C, Lee LT, Hwang JJ, Huang YT. The antitumor activities of flavonoids. *In Vivo*. 2005; 19(5):895–909.

116. World Cancer Research Fund in association with the American Institute for Cancer Research. *Food, Nutrition, and the Prevention of Cancer; A Global Perspective*. Washington, DC: AICR; 1997.

117. Ahmed FE. Effect of diet, life style, and other environmental chemopreventive factors on colorectal cancer development, and assessment of the risks. *J Envir Sci Health C Environ Carcinog Ecotoxicol Rev*. 2004; 22(2):91–147.

118. U.S. Department of Health and Human Services. *Dietary Guidelines for Americans 2005*. Washington, DC: Author; 2005.

119. Department of Health and Human Services. Dietary Guidelines for Americans. Available at: http://www.healthierus.gov/dietaryguidelines. Accessed April 10, 2008.

120. Lichtenstein AH, Appel LJ, Brands M, et al. Diet and lifestyle recommendations revision 2006. A scientific statement from the American Heart Association Nutrition Committee. *Circ*. 2006; 114:82–96.

121. Rashidkhani B, Lindblad P, Wolk A. Fruits, vegetables and risk of renal cell carcinoma: a prospective study of Swedish women. *Int J Cancer*. 2005; 113(3):451–455.

122. Centers for Disease Control and Prevention. 5 a Day. Available at: http://www.cdc.gov/nccdphp/dnpa/5aday/index.htm. Accessed January 12, 2007.

123. Le Marchand L, Hankin JH, Wilkens LR. Dietary fiber and colorectal cancer risk. *Epdemiol*. 1997; 8(6):658–665.

124. USDA Cooperative State Research, Education, and Extension Service. Pizza: The Cancer Fighting Food. Available at: http://www.csrees.usda.gov/newsroom/research/2007/pizza.html. Accessed May 21, 2008

125. Borek C. Dietary antioxidants and human cancer. *Integr Cancer Ther*. 2004; 3(4):333–341.

126. Araujo B, Travison T, Harris S, Holick M, Turner A, McKinlay J. Race/ethnic differences in bone mineral density in men. *Osteo Inter*. 2007; 18(7):943–953.

127. Looker AC, Orwoll ES, Johnston CC Jr. Prevalence of low femoral bone density in older U.S. adults from NHANES III. *J Bone Miner Res*. 1997; 12(11):1761–1768.

128. Centers for Disease Control and Prevention. Hip Fractures Among Older Adults. Available at: http://www.cdc.gov/ncipc/factsheets/adulthipfx.htm. Accessed May 21, 2008.

129. Steelman J, Zeitler P. Osteoporosis in pediatrics. *Pediatr Rev*. 2001; 22:56.

130. Magaña JJ, Gómez R, Cisneros B, et.al. Association of the CT gene (CA) polymorphism with BMD in osteoporotic Mexican women. *Clin Genet*. 2006; 70(5):402–408.

131. Morita A. Genetic factors of osteoporosis and fracture and the application of genetic information to the preventive medicine. *Clin Calcium*. 2005; 15(8):1364–1371.

132. Borges JL, Brandão CM. Low bone mass in children and adolescents. *Arq Bras Endocrinol Metabol*. 2006; 50(4):775–782.

133. Brown JJ, Zacharin MR. Proposals for prevention and management of steroid-induced osteoporosis in children and adolescents. *J Paediatr Child Health*. 2005; 41(11):553–557.

134. Cummings SR. A 55-year-old woman with osteopenia. *JAMA*. 2006; 296(21): 2601–2610.

135. Pongchaiyakul C, Nguyen TV, Kosulwat V, et al. Effects of physical activity and dietary calcium intake on bone mineral density and osteoporosis risk in a rural Thai population. *Osteoporos Int*. 2004; 15(10):807–813.

136. Faibish D, Ott SM, Boskey AL. Mineral changes in osteoporosis: a review. *Clin Orthop Relat Res*. 2006; 443:28–38.

137. Nicklas TA. Calcium intake trends and health consequences from childhood through adulthood. *J Am Coll Nutr*. 2003; 22(5):340–356.

138. Blum M, Harris SS, Must A, et al. Weight and body mass index at menarche are associated with premenopausal bone mass. *Osteoporos Int*. 2001; 12:588.

139. Elgán C, Fridlund B. Bone mineral density in relation to body mass index among young women: a prospective cohort study. *Int J Nurs Stud*. 2006; 43(6):663–672.

140. Rideout CA, McKay HA, Barr SI. Self-reported lifetime physical activity and areal bone mineral density in healthy postmenopausal women: the importance of teenage activity. *Calcif Tissue Int*. 2006; 79(4):214–222.

141. Lewiecki EM, Silverman SL. Redefining osteoporosis treatment: who to treat and how long to treat. *Arq Bras Endocrinol Metab*. 2006; 50(4):694–704.

142. Liu SL, Lebrun CM. Effect of oral contraceptives and hormone replacement therapy on bone mineral density in premenopausal and perimenopausal women: a systematic review. *Br J Sports Med*. 2006; 40:11–24.

143. Golden H, Lanzkowsky N, Schebendach L, Mard J, Palestro J, Shenker C. Hormone replacement therapy (Hrt) and bone mineral density in anorexia nervosa—a 3-year prospective observational study. *J Pediatr Adolesc Gynecol*. 2002; 15(3):135–143.

144. Klibanski A, Biller BM, Schoenfeld DA, et al. The effects of estrogen administration on trabecular bone loss in young women with anorexia nervosa. *J Clin Endocrinol Metab*. 1995; 80:898–904.

145. Robinson E, Bachrach LK, Katzman DK. Use of hormone replacement therapy to reduce the risk of osteopenia in adolescent girls with anorexia nervosa. *J Adolesc Health*. 2001; 26:343–348.

146. Driskell JA, Pohlman DH, Naslund MM. Value of an educational program on osteoporosis. *J Extension*. 2003. Available at: http://www.joe.org/joe/2003october/rb6.shtml. Accessed May 21, 2008.

CHAPTER 11

Promoting Health and Preventing Disease in Older Persons

CHAPTER OUTLINE

- Introduction
- Nutrition, Longevity, and Demographics of Older Persons
- Leading Causes of Death and Disability in Older Persons
- Theories of Aging
- Lifestyle and Socioeconomic Factors That May Influence the Aging Process
- Physiologic Changes That Can Affect Nutritional Status
- Anorexia in the Elderly
- Water Requirements
- Alzheimer's Disease
- Multivitamin/Mineral Supplements
- Nutrition Screening for Older Persons
- Nutrition Assessment
- Nutrition Services That Promote Independent Living
- Home Healthcare Services

LEARNING OBJECTIVES

- Define old age and discuss the demographic shift of the U.S. population.
- Identify the normal physiological changes that can affect nutritional status.
- Discuss the lifestyle and socioeconomic factors that may influence the aging process.
- Describe the Nutrition Screening Initiative.
- List the government nutrition programs for older persons.

Introduction

Aging is a biological, psychological, and social process that most individuals will experience. Although the biological and physical changes that occur during the aging process are unavoidable, the rate and man-

ner at which these changes occur vary among individuals. It is encouraging to know that the older population in the United States is increasing. This is due to advances in modern medicine and technology, which contributed to the increase in longevity of life. Similarly, several

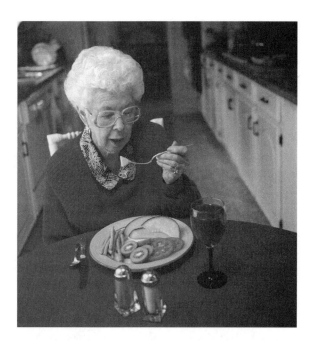

In older persons, appetite is a decisive factor of food intake.

characteristics of older persons influence their health and well-being. Some of the characteristics of aging discussed in this chapter include nutrition, lifestyle, and socioeconomic factors.

Nutrition, Longevity, and Demographics of Older Persons

The average *life expectancy* at birth has increased from 47 years in 1900 to 77.8 years in 2004. In 2004 the life expectancy in the United States was 75.8 years for European American men and 69.5 years for African American men. The same report also showed that the life expectancy for European American women was 80.5 years and for African American women was 76.3 years. Most deaths occurred after age 65.[1] The 65 years and older age group is expected to constitute an increasingly larger share of the U.S. population. In a recent analysis,

foreign-born U.S. residents have a longer life span than native-born persons by 20 percent.[2]

The maximum age to which humans can live (life span) is about 100 to 120 years,[3] but most people do not live this long. The goal to increase life expectancy and the number of years of healthy life is known as *compression of morbidity*. Compression of morbidity can be achieved by slowing the biological changes that accrue over time and delaying the diseases of aging enough to reach the limits of life span before any symptoms emerge.[3-5] **Figure 11-1** presents the life expectancy for people born between 1900 and 2000 at birth and at age 65.

Nutrition plays an important role in *successful aging*. Research suggests that a diet based on rice, fish, vegetable proteins, fruits, vegetables, and some meat contributes to *longevity*.

Adequate food intake is necessary for successful aging. The consequence of inadequate food intake is malnutrition, which can lead to nutrition-related health conditions (osteoporosis, anemia, cancer, etc.), increased disability, decreased resistance to infection, and extended hospital stays among elderly persons.[6,7] Therefore, nutrition is one important component of ensuring that the added years at the end of the lifecycle are healthful and productive. Dietetics professionals are distinctly qualified to provide a wide variety of appropriate, culturally sensitive nutrition programs for older persons. In the United States, nutrition programs (Elderly Nutrition Program, Meals on Wheels, etc.) subsidize meals served to older persons that may help prevent malnutrition. You'll find an overview of some of these programs later in this chapter and in Chapter 4.

As the aged population grows larger, there is an increased awareness that successful aging is not trying to stay young, but rather trying to discover the rewards of a life fully lived to the end.[8] Although many dimensions of successful aging have

life expectancy The average length of life span for a population of individuals.

compression of morbidity The postponement of the onset of chronic disease such that disability occupies a smaller and smaller proportion of the life span.

successful aging Slowing the number and rate of aging changes through positive lifestyle choices or health-related interventions.

longevity A measure of life's duration in years.

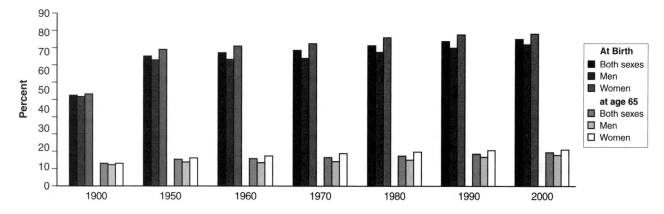

FIGURE 11-1 Life Expectancy at Birth and Age 65: 1900–2000

Source: Centers for Disease Control and Prevention. National Center for Health Statistics, National Vital Statistics System. Final data for 2003. National Vital Statistics Report. Volume 54. Hyattsville, MD.

.n recognized, the four features of successful aging identified by
..sher are outlined below:[9]

- Interactions with others
- Autonomy and sense of purpose
- Personal growth
- Self-acceptance

A positive attitude is the first step toward enhancing quality of life,
whether it is an individual's attitude about his or her own aging or the
attitude toward older persons in the community. It has been reported
that fear and negative attitudes are prevalent among many persons
nearing retirement age, mainly among men.[8] This fear of growing old
may affect an individual's ability to experience an enhanced quality of
life at old age. In addition, many retirement education campaigns focus
on financial security without considering nutrition, fitness, fun, volun-
teerism, community resources, caregiving, or living environments.

Kerschner developed a philosophy of productive aging in the late
1980s, which viewed older adults as representing:[10]

- An opportunity rather than a crisis
- A solution rather than a problem
- An asset rather than a burden
- A resource rather than a drain on resources
- A group that can make social, economic, and cultural contribu-
  tions rather than one that merely constitutes an expanding portion
  of the population

Leading Causes of Death and Disability in Older Persons

Studies show that when older people are asked how they feel about
their health, only 10 percent say their health is fair or poor, whereas
90 percent consider their health to be good, very good, or excellent.[2,11]
Chronic health conditions did not change their perception about how
they felt about their health. In contrast to older adults' perceptions,
public health professionals objectively monitor health by measuring
leading causes of death (mortality) and leading diagnoses of health
conditions (morbidity). Heart disease and cancer are the leading causes
of death for all persons age 65 or older and in all ethnic groups. Other
chronic health conditions, such as cerebrovascular diseases (stroke)
and chronic lower respiratory diseases also affect older persons significantly.[1] **Box 11-1** presents diseases that are common in older persons,
and **Table 11.1** presents the leading causes of death in older persons.

National Goals: Healthy People 2010

The primary goal of the U.S. Department of Health and Human Services'
Healthy People 2010 initiative is to help individuals of all ages increase
life expectancy and improve their
quality of life. Therefore, Healthy
People 2010 includes many objectives related to aging. A few
examples of the objectives set to
promote healthy lifestyles for
older adults include access to
quality healthcare services; reduction of rates of chronic diseases such as arthritis, cancer,
diabetes, kidney disease, and osteoporosis; reduction in hospitalization rates for heart disease

osteopenia Low bone density,
or thinning of the bones, but at a
lower rate than osteoporosis. This
stage of bone loss occurs before
osteoporosis develops.

free radicals Atoms or molecules
that have lost an electron and
vigorously pursue its replacement.
Free radicals can damage normal
cell constituents.

$\mathcal{B}ox$ 11-1 Diseases Common in the Elderly That Impact Their Nutritional Status

- Senile dementia of the Alzheimer's type with cognitive impairment and memory loss
- Arthritis with limited mobility of joints and deformities
- *Osteopenia* with fractures and deformities
- Parkinson's disease with rigidity and tremors
- Dental and oral health problems—problems with chewing
- Gastrointestinal disorders—swallowing difficulties
- Neoplasms with hypercatabolism, anorexia, and cachexia
- Diabetes mellitus with restrictive diet and medication interactions
- Renal insufficiency with restrictive diets and dialysis treatment
- Paralysis that limits mobility

Data from: Berdanier C, Feldman E, Flatt W, Jeor S. *Handbook of Nutrition and Food.* New York: CRC Press; 2002. Reprinted with permission.

---

and stroke; increased immunizations for influenza and pneumococcal
disease; and increased physical activity and fitness for older adults.[12,13]
There has been little progress toward these objectives, however. **Table
10.1** in Chapter 10 provides information on the Healthy People 2010
progress report.

Theories of Aging

Aging is a process that involves the entire body. Individuals age at different rates, but the processes that control the rate at which people age,
and how aging affects the development of chronic diseases, are not well
understood.[14,15] Although the degenerative changes that come with aging are poorly understood, several theories have been proposed to explain the aging process. One theory is that the aging process depends
on genetic, environment, and lifestyle factors.[16] This theory recognizes
that every individual has his or her own unique genetic make-up and
environment, which interact with each other to control the aging process. Another theory of aging is the *free radical* theory. Free radicals
are short-lived, very reactive chemicals often derived from oxygen
compounds that damage cells, especially cellular DNA and cell membranes that may speed up the aging process. However, only the third
theory, the nutritional model, which involves severe caloric restriction,
has been successful in prolonging life in mammalian species.[17]

Genetic, Environment, and Lifestyle Theory

The rates at which changes occur with aging depend on heredity. Genes
determine the competence with which cells are maintained and re-
paired. Fundamental biological processes involved in aging are mostly
determined by genetics.[18] However, environmental factors such as pol-
lution, poor living conditions, and personal lifestyle habits related to
diet, smoking, alcohol abuse, or level of physical activity influence ex-

TABLE 11.1 The Leading Causes of Death in the United States, 2003

Based on Sex	Total Deaths Rank	Total Deaths Percentage of All Deaths	Males Rank	Males Percentage of All Deaths	Females Rank	Females Percentage of All Deaths
Diseases of the heart	1	28.0	1	28.0	1	28.0
Malignant neoplasms	2	22.7	2	24.0	2	21.6
Cerebrovascular diseases	3	6.4	4	5.1	3	7.7
Chronic lower respiratory diseases	4	5.2	5	5.1	4	5.3
Accidents (unintentional injuries)	5	4.5	3	5.9	7	3.1
Diabetes mellitus	6	3.0	6	2.9	6	3.1
Influenza and pneumonia	7	2.7	7	2.4	8	2.9
Alzheimer's disease	8	2.6	10	1.5	5	3.6
Nephritis, nephritic syndrome, and nephrosis	9	1.7	9	1.7	9	1.8
Septicemia	10	1.4	12	1.2	10	1.5
Intentional self-harm (suicide)			8	2.1	17	0.5

Based on Race	Caucasian Rank	%	African American Rank	%	American Indian or Alaska Native Rank	%	Asian or Pacific Islander Rank	%	Hispanic Rank	%
Diseases of the heart	1	28.3	1	26.6	1	20.6	2	25.3	1	23.2
Malignant neoplasms	2	22.9	2	21.5	2	16.4	1	26.2	2	19.7
Cerebrovascular diseases	3	6.4	3	6.5	6	4.2	3	9.0	4	5.5
Chronic lower respiratory diseases	4	5.6	8	2.6	7	3.9	7	3.1	8	2.6
Accidents (unintentional injuries)	5	4.4	5	4.2	3	12.0	4	4.9	3	8.5
Alzheimer's disease	6	2.8	14	1.3	13	0.9	12	1.1	14	1.5
Diabetes mellitus	7	2.8	4	4.4	4	6.0	5	3.6	5	5.1
Influenza and pneumonia	8	2.7	11	2.0	8	3.0	6	3.1	9	2.4
Nephritis, nephritic syndrome, and nephrosis	9	1.6	7	2.7	10	1.9	9	1.6	11	1.8
Intentional self-harm (suicide)	10	1.4	16	0.7	9	2.4	8	1.8	12	1.6
Septicemia	11	1.3	10	2.1	12	1.7	10	1.1	16	1.2
Chronic liver disease and cirrhosis	12	1.1	15	0.9	5	4.3	16	0.8	6	2.8
Assault (homicide)	20	0.4	6	2.9	11	1.8	14	1.0	7	2.7
Human immunodeficiency virus (HIV)	22	0.3	9	2.6	17	0.5	24	0.2	13	1.5
Certain conditions originating in the perinatal period	21	0.4	12	1.6	21	0.5	21	0.5	10	2.2

Source: Heron MP, Smith BL. *Deaths: Leading Causes for 2003*. Hyattsville, MD: National Center for Health Statistics, Centers for Disease Control and Prevention; 2003. Available at: http://www.cdc.gov/nchs/products/pubs/pubd/hestats/leadingdeaths03/leadingdeaths03.htm. Accessed April 11, 2008.

pression of the genetic code by intensifying certain traits. For instance, an individual's height and weight are determined genetically, but diet and other environmental exposures can modify this effect. People with a family history of high levels of LDL cholesterol (i.e., bad cholesterol) and eventually death from cardiovascular disease can deter the effects of their genetic programming by losing weight, consuming diets that are low in saturated fat, performing regular physical activity, and ab-

staining from tobacco use.[19] Individuals with a family history of type 2 diabetes can reduce their risk of developing the disease with a proper diet, physical activity, and maintenance of normal weight.

Free Radicals Theory

Free radicals are unstable oxygen compounds formed normally during metabolism. These can damage cells by initiating reactions that break down cell membranes and modify the normal metabolic processes that protect people from disease.[20] Exposure to oxidizing agents such as environmental pollutants, ozone, smoking, and solar radiation can also damage the cells.[21] Free radicals cause oxidative damage to proteins, lipids, carbohydrates, and DNA and may also indirectly destroy cells by producing toxic products. For instance, spots that appear on the skin with age are caused by the oxidation of lipids, which produces a pigment called lipofuscin, or age pigment.[3,22] The cell damage due to free radicals has been implicated in the development of several chronic diseases, such as cardiovascular disease and cancer, common among older persons.[22-24]

Unstable oxygen compounds can be neutralized when they combine with an antioxidant.[25] The antioxidants prevent them from interfering with normal cell functions. The body can produce antioxidant enzymes (e.g., catalases, glutathione, peroxidase, reductases, and superoxide dismutase).[21] In addition, some antioxidants can be obtained from the diet. Dietary antioxidants include selenium, vitamins E and C, and other phytochemicals, which are plant substances such as beta-carotene, lycopene, flavonoids, lutein, zeaxanthin, resveratrol, and isoflavones that contribute to normal metabolism. For instance, flavonoids found in grapes, apples, broccoli, and onions act as antioxidants. In contrast, it is not effective to consume cellular enzymes designed to break down the damaging compounds, such as superoxide dismutase, because ingested enzymes are broken down during digestion before they can act in the body. Despite this, some health food stores sell superoxide dismutase.[20]

Caloric Restriction Theory

The one nutritional model that has been successful in prolonging life in mice, rats, and other rodents involves severe dietary restriction of energy.[26] The original study in this area demonstrated that dietary restriction in rats increased longevity, but led to diminished sexual maturation and fertility, lower bone strength, and lower bone calcium and phosphorus contents.[27,28] Studies involving less severe dietary restrictions (a 50 to 60 percent lower energy intake than animals allowed to eat as needed) showed increased longevity in rats, mice, and hamsters without developmental abnormalities. Furthermore, the age-related physiologic changes were also delayed. Although the animals in these studies were leaner than the control animals, the results do not point to reduction of body fat as the mechanism by which food restriction extends length of life.[26,29] Research on a moderately reduced energy and protein diet in growing pigs showed a significant increase in intramuscular lipids.[26,29] In obese humans, the accumulation of intramuscular lipids is associated with insulin resistance and the subsequent development of type 2 diabetes mellitus, which is one of the chronic diseases that affects older persons.[30,31]

The most appropriate caloric restriction approach is to add more fruits and vegetables to a diet in order to decrease chronic disease risk and subsequently reduce the aging process. Eating nutrient-dense foods and avoiding obesity enhance prospects for longevity. Therefore, there seems to be a relationship among genetics, environment, nutrition, and lifestyle in the process of aging.

Lifestyle and Socioeconomic Factors That May Influence the Aging Process

A variety of social and economic factors affect aging and can affect the nutritional status of individuals. These factors can interrelate and decrease an individual's ability to socialize, to eat, and the ability to

Box **11-2 Socioeconomic Changes Affecting the Nutritional Status of the Elderly**

Changes with aging include:
- Reduced income with retirement
- Insufficient funds for purchase of food
- Skipping meals
- Increased medical expenses
- Inability to drive to doctor's appointments or to the grocery store
- Inadequate food storage facilities
- Diminished self-esteem
- Social isolation

Data from: Williams SR. *Essentials of Nutrition and Diet Therapy.* 8th ed. Davis, CA: Mosby; 2003.

acquire and enjoy food. The socioeconomic changes affecting the nutritional status of the elderly are presented in **Box 11-2.**

Alcohol Use

Alcohol consumption increases the risk of malnutrition in older persons. Alcohol is high in calories and provides few nutrients. Too much alcohol intake damages the brain, heart, liver, and other organs.[32] It impairs judgment and balance, thereby increasing the frequency of falls. Too much intake also makes it harder to eat and take medications appropriately.[32] Older persons should limit alcohol consumption to no more than one drink (4 to 5 ounces of wine, 12 ounces of beer, or a 1.5 ounce shot of 80-proof liquor) per day for women and two drinks per day for men.[33]

The incidence of alcoholism among the elderly is about 13 percent for men, 2 percent for women, and 6 percent for both sexes.[34] Late-onset alcoholism occurs mainly in women with high socioeconomic status after stressful life events such as the death of a spouse or retirement.[35] It is also important to note that 75 percent of adults 65 years of age or older who misuse alcohol are also taking prescription drugs.[36] Even small amounts of alcohol can react negatively with various medications that many older persons routinely take.

Some of the symptoms of alcoholism in older persons include trembling hands, sleep problems, memory loss, and unsteady gait; these can be easily overlooked simply because they are similar to symptoms of old age.[37] Older adults become intoxicated on a smaller amount of alcohol than younger persons because older persons metabolize alcohol more slowly.[37] In addition to having adverse effects on the liver, drinking large amounts of alcohol increases the risk of hemorrhagic stroke and may exacerbate hypertension in older adults.[20]

Increased Use of Medications and Aging

Persons at highest risk for drug–nutrient interactions (DNI) are those who 1) take many drugs, including alcohol; 2) require long-term drug therapy; or 3) have poor or marginal nutrition status.[38] These and other risk-increasing factors are listed in **Table 11.2.** Older persons are likely to take medications because health problems increase with age.

Almost half of older Americans take multiple medications daily (*poly-pharmacy*).[38,39] The information on DNI is continually updated as new products enter the market or additional, sometimes conflicting, reports appear in the literature.[35]

Twenty-three percent of women and 19 percent of men over 65 years of age take five or more prescription medications a week.[40] Several situations contribute to the increased risk of DNI among the elderly:[41]

- They are more likely to take more medications for longer periods to manage chronic diseases.
- Their medications are more likely to be toxic.
- Their responses to medications vary significantly.
- Their bodies have less capability to handle medications effectively.
- They are more likely to be nutritionally deficient.
- They are more likely to make mistakes in self-care because of illness, mental confusion, or lack of medication information.

The use of over-the-counter and prescription medications can affect nutritional status and contribute to malnutrition. Medications commonly used by older individuals include aspirin, laxatives, diuretics, antacids, anticoagulants (blood thinner), anticonvulsants, heart medications, and pain medications.[41]

Drugs can affect nutritional status by changing food intake patterns. Medications may also interfere with an individual's ability to gather and prepare meals. Drug-induced alterations in mental status, blood pressure, urinary continence, coordination, or gait may affect nutritional status by diminishing interest in food and the ability to carry out activities involved in meal preparation.[38,42] Drugs may have a primary effect on diminishing or increasing appetite or may cause an unwanted side effect; for example, drugs that alter taste perception can also cause gastrointestinal discomfort and decrease food intake. The incidence of nausea and vomiting can be common with many medications and, if severe (e.g., with chemotherapy), may result in weight loss and nutrient deficiencies.[41]

TABLE 11.2	Risk Factors for Drug–Nutrient Interactions[32,35]	
Factors	**Health Conditions**
Restrictive diets	Diabetes and other chronic health conditions
Existing malnutrition	Protein energy malnutrition (PEM)
Drastic changes in eating patterns	Eating disorders
Chronic disease with long-term drug treatment	Cancer, HIV, etc.
Alcohol abuse	Alcoholism
Need for multiple-drug regimens	Heart disease, hypertension, and other chronic health conditions
Extremes in age: young children and the elderly	Underweight and/or frail
Use of a high-potency vitamin or mineral supplement	Quackery and chronic use of medication

Dependent Living

Many older individuals continue to live in a family setting; however, the number and proportion of older U.S. adults living alone have increased significantly in the past three decades, and there is concern that these individuals may have poor dietary quality.[43] Malnutrition can be a problem among older adults regardless of where they live. It is reported that older individuals living independently have reduced intakes of energy and protein.[3,44] Also, older adults who live alone are vulnerable to poverty and social isolation, which affect the quality of food intake and could lead to malnutrition.[43] Alternatively, dependent-living older adults (e.g., those in nursing homes) may have medical conditions that increase nutrient requirements and interfere with food intake and/or nutrient absorption, causing malnutrition. In addition, persons with less education and those who smoke, drink excessive amounts of alcoholic beverages, do not exercise, and have low energy intake are at greater risk for malnutrition. Community nutritionists should consider all of these characteristics when designing programs to improve dietary quality among older persons.[45]

Income Level

Approximately 3.6 million elderly persons live below the poverty level.[2] The rate of poverty is highest among the oldest of the old, minorities, women, persons living alone, and those with disabilities.[3] The poverty rate is higher for the older foreign born than for the older native population.[2] Many older individuals live on a fixed income as they retire from their jobs, which makes it harder for them to afford medication and a nutritious diet. Due to this situation, they often either reduce the amount of food intake or limit the types of foods they consume.

Physiologic Changes That Can Affect Nutritional Status

Aging causes multiple physiologic changes that affect nutrient needs and nutritional status. Individuals age at different rates and many of the decreases in physiologic functions impact the day-to-day lives of many elders. These changes, both physical and mental, can occur rapidly in one organ system and slowly in another. For example, by the age of 70, the kidneys lose about 28 percent of their weight in comparison with values in young adults, the liver loses 25 percent of its weight, and skeletal muscle diminishes by almost half.[41,46,47] **Box 11-3** presents the physiologic changes that are often associated with aging.

Changes in Lean Body Mass

The physiologic changes include a decrease in lean body mass and total body water. Body weight usually decreases after age 60 in men and age 65 in women by an average of 0.5 percent yearly. Many older adults gain body fat and lose about 53 to 60 percent of total body water. Compared to males in their 20s, males in their 70s have about 24 pounds less muscle and 22 pounds more body fat.[35,50,51] The intra-abdominal fat increases the most and is a risk factor for cardiovascular disease and insulin resistance.[52] The reasons for the age-related gains are not clear, but a longitudinal study shows that lack of exercise could be a factor. Results from the Fels Longitudinal Study showed significant age-related decreases in lean body mass and height and increases in total body fat, weight, and body mass index (BMI). However, a shift in body composition was seen in participants who reported high

polypharmacy The use or prescription of two or more different drugs to treat one or more health problems.

Box 11-3 Physiologic Changes Due to Aging[20,35,48,49]

Cardiovascular System
- Reduced blood vessel elasticity and stroke volume output
- Increased blood pressure
- Decreased cardiac output
- Decreased maximal heart rate

Endocrine System
- Reduced levels of estrogen and testosterone
- Decreased secretions of growth hormone
- Reduced glucose tolerance (decreased insulin-like growth factor)
- Decreased ability to convert provitamin D to previtamin D in skin

Gastrointestinal System
- Reduced secretion of saliva and mucus
- Dysphagia or difficulty in swallowing
- Reduced secretion of hydrochloric acid and digestive enzymes
- Slower peristalsis
- Reduced vitamin B_{12} absorption

Musculoskeletal System
- Reduced lean body mass (bone mass, muscle, and water)
- Decreased bone marrow mass and increased bone marrow fat
- Increased fat mass
- Decreased resting metabolic rate
- Missing or poorly fitting teeth
- Reduced work capacity (strength)

Nervous System
- Blunted appetite regulation
- Blunted thirst regulation
- Decreased antibody response
- Decreased brain weight
- Reduced nerve conduction velocity affecting senses of smell, taste, and touch, as well as cognition
- Changed sleep as the wake cycle becomes shorter

Renal System
- Reduced number of nephrons
- Less blood flow
- Slowed glomerular filtration rate
- Decreased renal mass

Respiratory System
- Reduced breathing capacity
- Reduced work capacity (endurance)
- Decreased elasticity in lung tissue

Hepatic System
- Reduced liver volume
- Reduced blood flow

or moderate physical activity levels. For instance, higher levels of physical activity were associated with higher levels of lean body mass in both men and women.[2,53]

Community nutritionists working with older individuals should consider including physical activities (walking, bicycling, swimming, dancing, etc.) when planning programs for older persons. However, they should involve an individual's physician to determine the level of physical activity that is safe.

Aging Bone

Another feature of biologic aging is a decrease in bone density. After age 40, adults tend to lose stature, with a mean height loss of 4.9 cm (1.9 inches) in women and 2.9 cm (1.1 inches) in men. It is important to note that the rate of bone loss is individualized.[35,54,55] Excessive loss of bone density increases the risk of osteoporosis, which is a major cause of morbidity in developed countries. Although hormonal influences account for much of the age-related alteration in bone homeostasis, nutritional factors also play an important role.[56] Several nutrients contribute to bone density, including protein; vitamins C, D, and K; phosphorous; and calcium. Although most North American diets supply an adequate amount of most of these nutrients, calcium intakes are usually below current recommendations. Experts estimate that variations in calcium nutrition in youth may account for a 5 to 10 percent difference in peak adult bone mass, and a 25 to 50 percent difference in hip fracture risk in later life.[57]

Osteoporosis is porous bone due to reduction in bone mass.

Exercises such as walking, running, and dancing, and weight-bearing activities are commonly recommended to increase bone density. Evidence suggests that 20 to 30 minutes of moderate to intense physical activity several times per week produces a favorable skeletal benefit.[57]

The New Jersey Department of Health and Senior Services and Rutgers Cooperative Extension collaborated to provide a community program, Project Healthy Bones, at the state level. They provided education on nutrition, osteoporosis prevention and treatment, home safety, and falls prevention to older persons. More than 1,400 older persons participated in the program. Project Healthy Bones focused on the idea that self-esteem, peer support, and incremental successes were important to change behavior and that having fun should be part of the process. Project Healthy Bones used older adults as peer advocate trainers, who acted as role models and had a better understanding of the beliefs, limitations, and fears of older participants. Analysis of a 3-day dietary assessment showed that, of 57 participants completing 12 to 23 weeks of the program, 39 to 68 percent had increased their calcium intake. The analysis of physical activity levels showed significant progress from exercises in level 1 (introductory) to level 2 (advanced) and an increase in amount of weight lifted. These improvements were evident in participants completing between 12 and 23 weeks of the program and those completing the entire 24-week cycle.[58]

Changes in Taste, Smell, Appetite, and Digestive Juices

Some physiologic changes that occur with age also affect nutritional status. For example, the secretion of certain digestive juices is diminished and gastric acid is reduced, leading to a reduction in the absorption of pH-dependent nutrients such as vitamins C, B_{12}, B_6, and folic acid.[59] The age-related decreased parietal cell secretion of a glycoprotein called intrinsic factor, which binds vitamin B_{12} and permits its efficient absorption, further impairs its bioavailability. In addition, the decrease in gastric acid can lead to bacterial growth, causing the formation of gas.[59,60]

In some individuals, sensory perceptions of taste, smell, hearing, and vision may change. Food consumption is a complex phenomenon that interrelates to the individual's culture, income, health status, and behavioral characteristics. In older persons, appetite is a critical factor in food intake, which is influenced by medication, the presence of physical (e.g., hypertension, chronic infection) or psychological (e.g., depression) disease, and some physiologic sensory functions such as taste and smell. These senses influence appetite and the enjoyment of food and can also influence the amount of food consumed. Because of these reasons, adults need more seasoning of their food.[59]

In older adults, hunger and satiety cues are less than in younger adults. Age has an inverse effect on the variety of foods consumed.[61] The change in palatability of a food once an individual begins to eat it is called *sensory-specific satiety*. This type of satiety is associated with a decreased intake of one food and a switch to another food during an ingestion period. The sensory-specific satiety mechanism promotes more variety and potentially a more well-balanced eating pattern.[62] This mechanism is diminished in older persons compared to younger persons. The reason for the reduced sensory-specific satiety is not clear. The low appetite-regulating mechanism will require older persons to be more aware of their food intake levels and requires them to consume a variety or a combination of foods.

There is a reduction in the ability to taste and smell at about the age of 60, and this reduction becomes more severe in individuals over 70.[63] The reduction of these senses can contribute to impaired nutri-

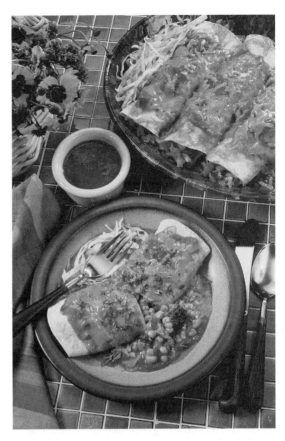

The sensory perceptions of taste and smell diminish with age. Adding adequate spices to foods may motivate an older person to eat.

tional status by decreasing both the appeal and the enjoyment of food. Chemosensory losses that occur with age include the following:[64]

- *Ageusia:* Absence of taste
- *Hypogeusia:* Diminished sensitivity of taste
- *Dysgeusia:* Distortion of normal taste
- *Anosmia:* Absence of smell
- *Hyposmia:* Diminished sensitivity of smell
- *Dysosmia:* Distortion of normal smell

Some research studies show that the reduction in taste acuity is due to a reduction in the number of taste buds on the tongue; other studies suggest that the decrease is the result of changes in sensitivity to specific flavors such as salty and sweet.[65,66] In addition, the ability to distinguish the odors of certain items varies. For instance, the ability to distinguish the odor of breads, vegetables, and coffee reduces significantly with age, but older persons retain the ability to identify green bell peppers and taste sweet foods.[65,66]

Anorexia in the Elderly

Although appetite diminishes with advancing age, severe anorexia that leads to significant weight loss (*anorexia of aging*) is not a normal aspect of aging. The standard for serious weight

sensory-specific satiety The change in palatability of a food once an individual begins to eat it.

anorexia of aging The loss of appetite and wasting associated with old age.

loss used by many nutritionists when monitoring body weight is the loss of 10 pounds or more over a period of 6 months or the loss of 5 percent or more of total body weight over a period of 1 year. Anorexia and weight loss are common in the elderly, especially in individuals suffering from medical or mental illnesses.[67] As mentioned in the previous section, research suggests that many factors contribute to a decline in food consumption with advancing age.[68] With normal aging, men and women may decrease their energy intake as their resting metabolic rate reduces because they are physically less active and their feeding drive (hunger) may decrease and satiety may occur more easily. This physiologic change with aging may be the precursor of pathological anorexia and weight loss that is most commonly due to depression.[12]

Failure to thrive is the term used to designate a weight loss condition recognized in older persons. Previously recognized as a syndrome in infants and children who are neglected, failure to thrive in the developing child is characterized by a failure to grow and develop in both physical and social skills. In older persons, the opposite occurs.[31] This condition is characterized as a failure to maintain as the individual regresses in physical well-being and mental function.[69] Weight loss is the first major symptom of failure to thrive in older adults, and is followed by increasing physical disability, loss of skills for self-care, social withdrawal, diminished mental function, and, finally, death. In most cases, the individuals are living in the community.

In failure to thrive, there is no biologic or physiologic explanation for the weight loss and malnutrition. However, in many incidents, the weight loss is due to a lack of financial resources, social isolation, limited ability to obtain adequate groceries or prepare meals, chronic disease and disability, failing eyesight, or other circumstances that limit food intake.[31,69] Prescription drugs can also have a profound impact on appetite through a variety of mechanisms.[70] If detected early, intervention is both possible and effective.

Water Requirements

Dehydration is a major problem in older adults, especially in the oldest individuals and those who are institutionalized.[71,72] Morley defined dehydration as losing nearly 2 percent of one's initial body weight; this can occur after not drinking any fluids and consuming only dry foods for 24 hours.[72] This happens because the regulation of body water relies on thirst and an individual's response to that thirst. In general, thirst is reduced in older persons, specifically in those with high serum sodium levels (>150 milliequivalents per liter) or a high ratio of blood urea nitrogen to creatinine (>25), which is a good indicator of dehydration."[73]

The symptoms of dehydration among older adults include a swollen tongue, constipation, electrolyte imbalance, nausea and vomiting, hypotension, mental confusion, sunken eyeballs, increased body temperature, decreased urine output, pressure ulcers, and urinary tract infections.[74]

A general guideline of total fluid intake for older adults is 3.7 liters per day for men and 2.7 liters per day for women.[75] A research study reported that more than one in three Americans over the age of 60 may not be consuming enough total water from all sources.[76] Good sources of water include tap and bottled water, milk, juice, carbonated beverages, and soups. Valtin suggested that caffeinated drinks (e.g., coffee and soft drinks) and alcoholic beverages may also count toward daily consumption of fluid.[77] However, because of the diuretic effects of these types of beverages, additional tap or bottled water should be consumed to replace the water that is lost.

Alzheimer's disease (senile dementia of the Alzheimer's type) A disease that results in the relentless and irreversible loss of mental function.

Alzheimer's Disease

Alzheimer's disease (AD) is the most common form of dementia in the United States and Europe. It is estimated that in 2007, there were 4.5 million cases of Alzheimer's disease in the United States.[78] About 5 percent of men and women ages 65 to 74 have AD, and nearly half of those age 85 and older may have the disease. It is important that healthcare professionals understand that the incidence of AD increases with age.

Alzheimer's disease begins with cognitive loss that becomes worse gradually with the extension of cerebral lesions. Other problems occur such as a loss of independence, orientation impairments, loss of sense of self, loss of meaningful relationship with the world, disordered eating behavior, memory loss, behavior and personality changes, reduced ability to think, and weight loss.[79] This weight loss increases the risk of infections, skin ulcers, and falls, and consequently decreases quality of life in individuals with Alzheimer's.[78,80] The disease seems to affect many different cells involving several of the neurotransmitters. Free radical damage is suspected as a mechanism of cell loss in Alzheimer's, but the cause is unknown.[78]

Individuals with Alzheimer's often suffer from a chronically poor diet or from an increased nutrient need. They often suffer from protein malnutrition and other nutritional deficiencies that improve the status of the individual when corrected. Low blood levels of folate and vitamin B_{12} are often found in individuals with Alzheimer's disease.[81] Low folate blood levels may be associated with depressed individuals experiencing a weaker response to antidepressants.[82,83] According to research from the Alzheimer's Disease Cooperative Study, large intakes of vitamin E are associated with slowing the progression of Alzheimer's disease. The study found that individuals with Alzheimer's disease of moderate severity extended the time they were able to care for themselves by consuming 2,000 IU per day of vitamin E compared to those taking a placebo.[82,84]

Vitamin E, thiamine, and vitamin B_{12} have been associated with improved symptoms when blood levels are corrected to normal:[82,84]

- Vitamin E may help by slowing the rate of free radical–induced tissue damage.
- Thiamine may help to produce acetylcholine through its participation in the synthesis of acetyl CoA, a precursor to acetylcholine, the neurotransmitter most closely associated with Alzheimer's symptoms.
- Vitamin B_{12} is required for the generation of methyl groups that are involved in either the synthesis or the conservation of choline, the other component of acetylcholine.
- High doses of acetyl-L-carnitine (1,000 mg with breakfast, 1,000 mg with lunch) have also been reported to slow the progression of Alzheimer's disease.[63]

Alzheimer's disease has three stages, which are presented in **Table 11.3**. During stage one, the individual is encouraged to complete as many tasks as possible, including food preparation and washing dishes. In stage two, the individual needs help keeping track of food intake because they tend to forget. A helper should provide the individual with various stimulating activities such as different types of physical

TABLE 11.3	Major Stages of Alzheimer's Disease[85,87]

Stage	Food-Related Symptoms
1	Purchases and prepares own food; feeds self
	Washes dishes
2	Can feed self, but needs direction and assistance at mealtime
	Needs assistance on food intake
	Needs to be reminded about eating
	Unable to sit still for a long time to eat
	May forget how to prepare food
3	Requires total feeding assistance
	Cannot feed self; may refuse to chew and swallow food
	Is at risk for malnutrition
	May not recognize foods
	Forgets what to do with foods

Alzheimer's disease begins with cognitive loss that gradually becomes worse with the extension of cerebral lesions.

activities. In stage three, the individual may not recognize foods, may forget to eat, or may forget what to do with the food. In this stage, there is loss of muscle mass and body fat due to the lack of food intake.[85] The individual needs help eating and participating in stimulating activities.

Nutrition recommendations for Alzheimer's individuals are difficult because there is limited nutritional data available to healthcare professionals. Additional calories may be needed for increased energy expended by individuals in stages one and two. Foods that are high in antioxidants such as vitamin E, selenium, and vitamin C are recommended; tuna, chicken breasts, cashews, sunflower seed kernels, yellow peppers, papaya, kiwi, oranges, sunflower oil, and enriched grains and cereals are good sources of these nutrients.

Alzheimer's disease is difficult for the caregiver and, in many cases, is perceived as a heavy burden to bear. The caregiver, stressed and often depressed, may become socially isolated. This, in turn, can affect the person with Alzheimer's. It has been reported that the burden Alzheimer's disease imposes on the caregiver caused weight loss in the individual with Alzheimer's disease.[86] The more stressed, depressed, and tired the caregiver becomes, the more the individual with Alzheimer's disease tends to lose weight.

Multivitamin/Mineral Supplements

The use of dietary supplements including vitamins, minerals, and herbal and botanical products is growing. Some older persons use supplements in order to meet their nutrient needs and, in some cases, prolong life. Food contributes more than just its nutrient content; therefore, replacing food with supplements is not an appropriate trade-off.[3] In addition, some nutrients in large amounts can be toxic. Large amounts of one particular nutrient can interact and affect the absorption of other nutrients or interfere with the absorption and metabolism of prescription medications.[88]

The recommendation is to use multivitamin and mineral supplements that do not exceed 100 percent of the Daily Value for any nutrient. This is the safest way to supplement the diet. Supplements con-

taining megadoses or non-nutrient substances may be toxic and should be avoided.[3,75] For example, superoxide dismutase (SOD), an enzyme that protects against oxidative damage, supposedly slows down aging and can be used to treat Alzheimer's. However, it is a protein that is broken down to amino acids in the gastrointestinal tract, so oral supplements will not increase blood or tissue levels of this enzyme. Coenzyme Q is a synthetic version of a compound in the electron transport chain and is marketed to older adults as a way to slow aging by improving the immune system.[3] It has been reported that coenzyme Q does not boost immune function and may be dangerous for people with poor circulation.[3]

Nutrition Screening for Older Persons

To identify malnutrition risk factors among the aging population, the American Academy of Family Physicians, the American Dietetic Association, and the National Council on Aging collaborated and developed the Nutrition Screening Initiative (NSI) checklist. This 5-year project focused on nutrition screening and interventions that help prevent and manage nutrition-related problems before a person becomes ill or a condition worsens. **Figure 11-2** presents the self-administered Determine Your Nutritional Health checklist. A dietitian, physician, nurse, or other healthcare professional can review the resulting score to determine the person's nutritional risk.

The checklist uses the mnemonic "Determine" to communicate basic nutrition information and help users recall the major risk factors and indicators of poor nutritional status. The checklist is not a diagnostic tool, however.

An individual who scored zero to two is considered at good nutritional status, and a recheck in 6 months is recommended. An individual scoring three to five points, which is considered moderate nutritional risk, is encouraged to recheck his or her nutritional status in 3 months, and a self-help approach to improve nutritional status is encouraged.[89] Individuals with a nutrition score of six or more are regarded as being at high nutritional risk and are encouraged to take the checklist to their physician, dietitian, or other health or social service provider.[90]

A practical approach to nutrition screening recommended by the NSI is presented in **Table 11.4**. Level I Screen is a basic nutrition evaluation tool that can be administered in a community setting. It should

DETERMINE YOUR NUTRITIONAL HEALTH

Warning signs of poor nutritional health are often overlooked. Use this checklist to find out if you or someone you know is at nutritional risk.

Read the statements below. Circle the number in the yes column for those that apply to you or someone you know. For each yes answer, score the number in the box. Total your nutritional score.

	Yes
I have an illness or condition that made me change the kind and/or amount of food I eat.	2
I eat fewer than 2 meals per day.	3
I eat few fruits or vegetables, or milk products.	2
I have 3 or more drinks of beer, liquor, or wine almost every day.	2
I have tooth or mouth problems that make it hard for me to eat.	2
I don't always have enough money to buy the food I need.	4
I eat alone most of the time.	1
I take three or more different prescribed or over-the-counter drugs a day.	1
Without wanting to, I have lost or gained 10 pounds in the last 6 months.	2
I am not always physically able to shop, cook, and/or feed myself.	2
TOTAL	

Total your nutrition score. If it's…

0–2	Good! Recheck your nutritional score in 6 months.

3–5   **You are at moderate nutritional risk.**

See what you can do to improve your eating habits and lifestyle. Your office on aging, senior nutrition program, senior citizens center, or health department can help. Recheck your nutritional score in 3 months.

6+   **You are at high nutritional risk.**

Bring this checklist the next time you see your doctor, dietitian, or other qualified healthcare or social service professional. Talk with them about any problems you may have. Ask for help to improve your nutritional health.

Remember: Warning signs suggest risk, but do not represent diagnosis of any condition.

Source: Nutrition Screening Initiative: Determine your nutritional health checklist. The Nutrition Screening Initiative: Development and implementation of the public awareness checklist and screening tools. The Nutrition Screening Initiative is a joint project of the American Academy of Family Physician and American Dietetic Association, funded in part by a grant from Ross Product Division, Abbott Laboratories Inc. Ross Products Division, Abbott Laboratories, Inc., Columbus, Ohio. 1995. Reprinted with permission.

FIGURE 11-2   Determine Your Nutritional Health Checklist

be administered annually or if a major change in status occurs. Level II Screen is administered by a healthcare professional and requires the participation of a physician and dietitian. If problems are identified, the person must be referred to the proper healthcare professional.[89]

Mitchell et al. compared the food group intakes assessed from questions embedded in the NSI Level II Screen with those from a more comprehensive food frequency questionnaire.[91] Results showed that

---

Box 11-4   Determine: Warning Signs of Poor Nutritional Health

- *Disease:* Any disease, illness, or chronic condition (i.e., confusion, feeling sad or depressed, acute infections) that causes you to change the way you eat or makes it hard for you to eat, or puts your nutritional health at risk.
- *Eating poorly:* Eating too little, too much, or the same food day after day, or not eating fruits, vegetables, and milk products daily will cause poor nutritional health.
- *Tooth loss/mouth pain:* It is hard to eat well with missing, loose, or rotten teeth, or dentures that do not fit well or cause mouth sores.
- *Economic hardship:* Having less (or choosing to spend less) than $34.30 (female) to $38.60 (male) weekly for groceries makes it hard to get the foods needed to stay healthy (http://www.cnpp.usda.gov). Income below the poverty guideline.
- *Reduced social contact:* Being with people has a positive effect on morale, well-being, and eating.
- *Multiple medicines:* The more medicines you take, the greater the chance for side effects such as changes in taste, increased or decreased appetite and thirst, constipation, weakness, drowsiness, diarrhea, nausea, and others. Vitamins or minerals taken in large doses can act like drugs and can cause harm.
- *Involuntary weight loss or gain:* Losing or gaining a lot of weight when you are not trying to do so is a warning sign to discuss with your healthcare provider.
- *Needs assistance in self-care:* Older people who have trouble walking, shopping, and buying and cooking food are at risk for malnutrition.
- *Elder years above 80:* As age increases, risk of frailty and health problems also rises.

The dollar amounts used in economic hardship were modified by the author using September 2003, USDA low-cost food plan.

Source: Nutrition Screening Initiative: Determine your nutritional health checklist. The Nutrition Screening Initiative: Development and implementation of the public awareness checklist and screening tools. The Nutrition Screening Initiative is a joint project of the American Academy of Family Physician and American Dietetic Association, funded in part by a grant from Ross Product Division, Abbott Laboratories Inc. Ross Products Division, Abbott Laboratories, Inc., Columbus, Ohio. 1995. Reprinted with permission.

the Level II Screen is a feasible, low-cost tool to screen for determining nutrition risk in older adults. However, the embedded food group questions in the Level II Screen should be interpreted thoughtfully in the overall screening process. **Box 11-4** presents the warning signs of poor nutrition health.

Indicators of poor nutritional status in the elderly may be detected by a physical sign, specific symptoms, or measurable parameter that shows that poor nutritional status is present in the person and is causing some symptoms.[89] Major indicators of poor nutritional status are shown in **Table 11.5**. These can be identified through interview, observation, physical examination, anthropometric measurements, and laboratory tests. Risk factors associated with poor nutritional status include:[88,89,92,93]

- Inappropriate food and nutrient intake
- Poverty, social isolation
- Dependency and disability
- Acute or chronic diseases or conditions
- Chronic medication use
- Functional disability
- Hunger
- Living alone
- Depression
- Dementia
- Poor dentition and oral health, chewing and swallowing problems
- Minority status
- Advanced age

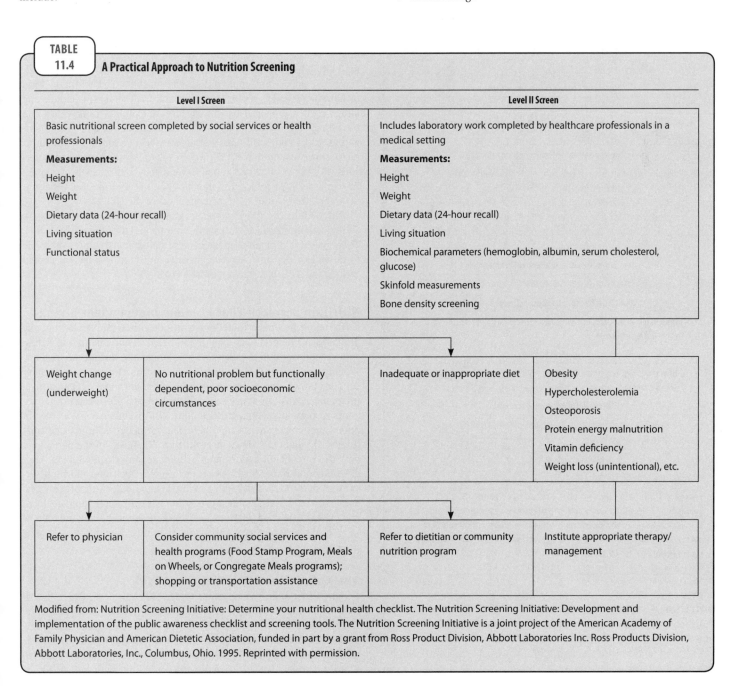

TABLE 11.4 **A Practical Approach to Nutrition Screening**

Level I Screen		Level II Screen	
Basic nutritional screen completed by social services or health professionals		Includes laboratory work completed by healthcare professionals in a medical setting	
Measurements:		**Measurements:**	
Height		Height	
Weight		Weight	
Dietary data (24-hour recall)		Dietary data (24-hour recall)	
Living situation		Living situation	
Functional status		Biochemical parameters (hemoglobin, albumin, serum cholesterol, glucose)	
		Skinfold measurements	
		Bone density screening	
Weight change (underweight)	No nutritional problem but functionally dependent, poor socioeconomic circumstances	Inadequate or inappropriate diet	Obesity Hypercholesterolemia Osteoporosis Protein energy malnutrition Vitamin deficiency Weight loss (unintentional), etc.
Refer to physician	Consider community social services and health programs (Food Stamp Program, Meals on Wheels, or Congregate Meals programs); shopping or transportation assistance	Refer to dietitian or community nutrition program	Institute appropriate therapy/ management

Modified from: Nutrition Screening Initiative: Determine your nutritional health checklist. The Nutrition Screening Initiative: Development and implementation of the public awareness checklist and screening tools. The Nutrition Screening Initiative is a joint project of the American Academy of Family Physician and American Dietetic Association, funded in part by a grant from Ross Product Division, Abbott Laboratories Inc. Ross Products Division, Abbott Laboratories, Inc., Columbus, Ohio. 1995. Reprinted with permission.

TABLE 11.5	Major Indicators of Poor Nutritional Status in Older Americans

Significant Weight Loss Over Time[a]

- 5.0 percent or more of prior body weight in 1 month
- 7.5 percent or more of body weight in 3 months
- 10.0 percent or more of body weight in 6 months or involuntary weight loss

Significant Low or High Weight

- 20 percent or above/below desirable weight for height at a given age (considering loss of height due to vertebral collapse and deformity)

Significant Reduction in Serum Albumin

- Serum albumin of less than 3.5 g/dL

Significant Change in Functional Status

- Change from "independent" to "dependent" in two of the ***activities of daily living*** or one of the nutrition-related ***instrumental activities of daily living***

Significant and Sustained Inappropriate Food Intake

- Failure to consume the recommended minimum from one or more of the food groups suggested in the *Dietary Guidelines for Americans* (e.g., milk and milk products, cereals and grains, fruits, vegetables, meat, legumes, etc.); excessive consumption of fat, saturated fat, and/or alcohol; or a sufficient variety of foods for a period of 3 months or more

Significant Reduction in Mid-Arm Circumference

- To less than 10th percentile (NHANES Standards)

Significant Increase or Decrease in Triceps Skinfolds

- To less than 10th percentile or more than 95th percentile (NHANES Standards)

Significant Obesity

- More than 120 percent of desirable weight, or BMI over 27, or triceps skinfolds above 95th percentile (NHANES Standards)

Other Nutrition-Related Disorders

- Presence of osteoporosis, osteomalacia, folate deficiency, or vitamin B_{12} deficiency

[a]Significant increase in weight requires similar documentation, examination, and interpretation.

Modified from: White JV, Dwyer JT, Wellman N, Posner BM, Ham RJ, Lipschitz DA. Nutrition Screening Initiative: development and implementation of the public awareness checklist and screening tools. *J Am Diet Assoc.* 1991; 91:786–786. Copyright Elsevier (1991). Reprinted with permission by Elsevier.

Nutrition Assessment

Nutrition assessment is the interpretation of information from dietary, laboratory, anthropometric, and clinical evaluations. The information can be used to determine the nutrition status of older persons as influenced by the intake and utilization of nutrients.[94] Older populations can be assessed using surveys, surveillance, screening, or interventions. Information obtained through nutrition assessment can be used to determine baseline data. For example, the data from the National Health and Nutrition Examination Survey (NHANES) of noninstitutionalized older adults using the Healthy Eating Index (HEI) showed that older adults consume poor quality diets.[95] The HEI consists of 10 components and provides an overall picture of the type and quantity of foods people eat, their compliance with specific dietary recommendations, and the variety in their diets. The mean HEI score for 65 years of age and older was 67.6 out of 100, implying that their diets need improvement. The lowest component scores were for milk and fruit intakes. About 20 percent of people 65 years of age or older had good diets, represented by a score of 81 or above. About 14 percent had poor diets, represented by a score of less than 51. The HEI score was significantly lower for poor older persons than for those with high income.[96]

Another study reported that the presence of children in the household was associated with adults 60 years or older consuming more total fat and saturated fat than adults without children. The foods consumed included whole milk; pizza; salty snack foods; beef (in the form of hamburgers); ice cream, ice milk, and milk shakes; calzones and lasagna; cheese dishes; bacon, sausage, and lunch meat; cakes and brownies; pies, donuts, and pastries; chocolate candy and fudge; margarine; and cookies, all representing convenience foods purchased for near-term consumption.[97] Research results also show that older persons with poor dental health had lower dietary intake levels of vitamin A, carotene, folic acid, and vitamin C, and scored low on variety of diet, cholesterol, and sodium components of the HEI.[98]

Older adults are a heterogeneous group, with many different health conditions and broad variations in both mental and functional status. Therefore, it is difficult to make general statements that are applicable to all elderly persons. A comprehensive nutrition assessment should include the ABCDs discussed in **Table 11.6**.

Nutrition Services That Promote Independent Living

Government programs to address nutrition needs and socioeconomic problems for older adults include the USDA's Food Stamp and Extension programs, Adult Day Services food programs, Nutrition Assistance Program for Seniors (NAPS), the Elderly Nutrition Program of the Older Americans Act, and Meals on Wheels and other home-delivered meal programs. Meals on Wheels is designed to provide meals to participants who are homebound due to illness or disability and who cannot attend the congregate meals. The meals are delivered to participants' homes by volunteers. They meet the nutrition needs of the participant and also provide an opportunity for human contact. In addition, nongovernmental home health programs provide food and nutrition services as part of a broader range of nursing and other support services. For instance, home healthcare nutritionists will shop, prepare food, and clean the kitchen afterwards. Home care services allow individuals to receive the necessary support to stay in their homes for as long as possible.

The Elderly Nutrition Program (ENP)

Congress first appropriated funds under Title VII of the Older Americans Act of 1965 to begin the Senior Nutrition Program, also called the Elderly Nutrition Program (ENP), created in 1972. Programs like Meals on Wheels and ENP provide meals to homebound people as well as to those in group settings. Most programs provide meals at least five times per week. The ENP is supported primarily with federal funds,

TABLE 11.6	The ABCDs of Nutritional Assessment for Older Persons[35,99,100]

A: Anthropometric Measurements

- Height (may be difficulty due to poor posture, use knee-to-heel height instead)
- Weight

- Body mass index
- Skinfold measurements (mid-arm muscle circumference, triceps skinfold)

B: Biochemical Parameters

- Serum albumin, hemoglobin
- Serum nutrient levels (vitamins A, D, C; sodium; potassium; iron; calcium; etc.)
- Serum cholesterol and glucose

- Antigen skin tests
- Urine and fecal analysis
- Fecal analysis for nutrients or metabolites that indicate infection or disease

C: Clinical Evaluation

- Mental/cognitive status
- Blood pressure
- Medical history and the physical examination
- Gastrointestinal problems (heartburn, constipation, etc.)
- Hair, skin, fingernails shape, eyes, musculature
- Mouth and teeth, gums

- Dentition status
- Oral status (lesions)
- Breast exam status
- Tongue status
- Vision and hearing status
- Protein energy malnutrition (PEM) status

D: Dietary History/Functional Assessment

Questions about:

- Supplements and medication history
- Polypharmacy
- Poor appetite
- Changes in taste, smell, and digestive juices
- Eating alone
- Adequacy of the diet
- Skipping meals
- Special diets
- Lactose intolerance
- Anorexia
- Food security/food insecurity status

- Abnormal eating habits (anorexia)
- Inadequate bowel movement
- Ability to chew and swallow
- Activities of daily living (ADLs) and/or instrumental activities of daily living (IADLs)
- Social assessment (caregivers, annual income and living conditions, lives alone, housebound)
- Sleep deprivation
- Substance and alcohol abuse
- Lack of transportation and/or cooking and food storage equipment

volunteer time, and in-kind donations. Participant contributions make up the remainder.[101]

The Administration on Aging's Elderly Nutrition Program provides grants to support nutrition services to older people throughout the country. The ENP, authorized under Title III, Grants for State and Community Programs on Aging, and Title VI, Grants for Native Americans under the Older Americans Act, are intended to improve the dietary intake of participants and to offer participants opportunities to form new friendships and to create informal support networks. These meals and other nutrition services are provided in a variety of settings, such as senior centers, schools, and individual homes.[101]

Meals served under the program must provide at least one-third of the daily recommended dietary allowances established by the Food and Nutrition Board of the National Academy of Sciences National Research Council. In practice, the Elderly Nutrition Program's 3.1 million elderly participants are receiving an estimated 40 to 50 percent of most required nutrients.[101]

The ENP also provides a range of related services, including nutrition screening, assessment, education, and counseling, through some of the network's estimated 4,000 nutrition service providers. These services help older participants identify their general and special nutrition needs as they relate to health concerns such as hypertension and diabetes.

The services help older participants learn to shop for, and/or to plan and prepare, meals that are economical and help to manage or improve specific health problems as well as enhance their health and well-being. The congregate meal programs also

activities of daily living (ADL) A person's ability to perform personal care, either independently or with help. It helps to evaluate an older person's ability to care for him- or herself.

instrumental activities of daily living (IADL) A person's ability to perform housekeeping chores and other activities that are required for that person to remain independent.

provide older people with positive social contacts with other seniors at the group meal sites.

Volunteers who deliver meals to older persons who are homebound are encouraged to spend some time with the persons. The volunteers also offer an important opportunity to check on the welfare of the homebound older persons and are encouraged to report any health or other problems that they may observe during their visits. In addition to providing nutrition and nutrition-related services, the Elderly Nutrition Program provides an important link to other needed supportive in-home and community-based services such as homemaker home health aide services, transportation, fitness programs, and even home repair and home modification programs.

Eligibility

The Elderly Nutrition Program services are targeted to older people with the greatest economic or social need, with special attention given to low-income minorities. In addition to focusing on low-income and other older persons at risk of losing their independence, the following individuals may receive services:[101]

- A spouse of any age
- Disabled persons under age 60 who reside in housing facilities occupied primarily by the elderly where congregate meals are served
- Disabled persons who reside at home and accompany older persons to meals
- Nutrition service volunteers

American Indians, Alaskan Natives, and Native Hawaiians tend to have lower life expectancies and higher rates of illnesses at younger ages, so tribal organizations are given the option of setting the age at which older people can participate in the program.[101]

Program Results

Research studies of congregate and home-delivered meals participants showed that the programs improved the dietary intake and nutrition status of their clients.[102,103] Participants had greater diversity in their diets and higher intakes of essential nutrients, and they were less likely to report food insecurity than non-participants.[104] Additional benefits were derived from the activities associated with the congregate meal services: improved diet counseling, exercise, and more opportunities for improved socialization.

But, regardless of these positive results, there are some gaps in the meal programs, such as a lack of weekend or evening meals to those who cannot afford food or cannot cook; a lack of special diets for people with special dietary needs (e.g., people on a low sodium, low-fat, high fiber, or soft diet); and meals that are too high in fat, unappetizing, or lacking in fiber or nutrients (e.g., calcium, selenium, vitamins C and E, or folate).[105] In addition, 41 percent of Title III ENP service providers have waiting lists for home-delivered meals, suggesting a significant unmet need.[106] **Table 11.7** shows the Title III-C (formerly known as Title VII) Meal Pattern.

A 3-year follow-up study to evaluate nutrition status and long-term outcome in the elderly living at home showed that about half of the Meals on Wheels participants were malnourished and that the people with a BMI of 28 or more showed the lowest risk of death within 3 years.[107] The special needs of the homebound elderly need to be given greater priority.[108] Their dietary intake might improve if more than one meal per day were provided, if the meal furnished to the client was pre-

| | TABLE 11.7 | **Title III-C Meal Pattern**[111] |

Food Type	Recommended Portion Size
Meat or meat alternative	3 oz. cooked portion
Vegetables and fruits	Two ½ cup portions*
Enriched white or whole-grain bread or alternate	1 serving (one slice bread or equivalent)
Butter or margarine	1 tsp
Milk	8 oz milk or calcium equivalent
Dessert	1 serving

*A vitamin C–rich fruit or vegetable is served each day; a vitamin A–rich fruit or vegetable is served at least three times per week.

pared with greater percentages of the DRI, and if meals were provided 7 days a week rather than 5.

Other Programs

Low-income individuals who purchase food may also be eligible for hot meals at community "food kitchens" such as Catholic Relief Services and the Salvation Army. These are similar to congregate meals sites, but they serve a broader population. Some food kitchens and emergency food banks also offer groceries or vouchers to purchase food.[109] The Food Stamp Program is another option that provides low-income elderly households with the means to purchase food. Unfortunately, because food stamps carry a "welfare" stigma, some older persons are reluctant to use them.

Although these programs are free, most require determination of eligibility. In some cases, many people who need help buying food cannot meet the eligibility requirements. In 2003, Sharkey found evidence of food insecurity among homebound older women who receive home-delivered meals, regardless of income level.[110] The study also reported that the participants relied on home-delivered meals for long-term food assistance.

Home Healthcare Services

Home healthcare is a satisfactory alternative to care and rehabilitation within a hospital or medical setting. Home healthcare services can also help older individuals avoid institutionalization due to illness or recurrence of a previous illness.[112] Approximately 28 percent of older individuals over 65 years who live independently are unable to perform one or more activities of daily living (ADLs) and 12.9 percent reported difficulties with instrumental activities of daily living (IASLs) without the assistance of another person or the use of physical devices.[112] Homemaker services provide assistance with meal preparation, transportation, bathing, and shopping.

Older persons may need medical nutrition therapy at home involving a variety of health issues, such as heart disease, renal disease, cancer, HIV/AIDS, and/or diabetes, as well as care for one who is on tube feeding such as total parental nutrition (TPN). A community nutritionist can make home visits to assess the elders' health status, monitor their nutritional status, and work closely with the home health agencies (speech, physical, or occupational therapists) to improve the lives of these elderly individuals. Usually, community nutritionists who are

Registered Dietitians (RDs) may receive reimbursement from some insurance companies if a physician or hospital employs the RD or if services are medically supervised or medically necessary.[113]

Activities of Daily Living

An older person's ability to care for him- or herself is typically evaluated using the ADLs and the IADLs. The ADLs listed here are used to evaluate a person's ability to perform personal care, either independently, with some help, or with no help at all:[31,101]

- Bathing oneself
- Dressing oneself
- Feeding oneself
- Using the toilet
- Transferring between bed and chair

The IADLs relate to a person's ability to perform housekeeping chores and other activities required to remain independent:

- Prepare meals
- Perform house-cleaning chores
- Handle money and balance a checkbook
- Shop without help
- Use the telephone
- Leave the house without help

The current practice of elder care is community-based. The goal is to provide services that will enable older persons to remain in their own home or in the home of a family member. Older persons who need help with the ADLs or IADLs may receive help from family members;

An older person's ability to care for him- or herself is typically evaluated using the instrumental activities of daily living (IASLs) such as preparing meals for oneself.

however, increasing numbers of older persons live some distance from their children and others do not have children or other family. To fill this need, services are now being provided by home health agencies, area agencies on aging that receive state and federal funds, and private home care companies.[31]

Successful Community Strategies (below) presents the Senior Farmers' Market Nutrition Program success story. **Box 11-5** presents nutrition programs for promoting health and preventing diseases in older persons.

Successful Community Strategies 🏠🏠🏠🏠

The Seattle Senior Farmers' Market Nutrition Program[114]

The Senior Farmers' Market Nutrition Program is one of the federal food assistance programs for older persons. In the summer and fall of 2001, the Seattle Senior Farmers' Market Nutrition Program supplied a market basket that contained a variety of seasonal local fresh fruits and vegetables to 480 homebound low-income seniors. The purpose of the intervention program was to increase the fresh fruits and vegetables intake of homebound Meals on Wheels participants and compare their intake with other Meals on Wheels homebound seniors who live outside the project service area.

The program was a collaborative effort with five organizations including the University of Washington Health Promotion Research Center. Subjects for both the intervention and control groups were recruited via flyers that were delivered

by Meals on Wheels drivers. Local farmers were contracted to provide the fruits and vegetables in season. The Meals on Wheels drivers volunteered to deliver the market baskets to the participants' homes every 2 weeks. A newsletter that described the produce, provided recipes for less common seasonal foods, and promoted eating fruits and vegetables accompanied each basket. Each basket contained dark green or orange fruits and vegetables. An average of 1.6 servings of vegetables and 0.67 servings of fruit were provided per day over a period of 5 months. The fruits and vegetables supplied 30 percent of the U.S. Recommended Dietary Allowance for vitamin C, 40 percent for vitamin A, and 8 percent for folate daily for 5 months. Both the basket recipients and control respondents were interviewed by telephone before basket deliveries started and

at the end of the intervention. All participants were mailed a serving-size guide with pictures of representative foods. Participants were required to have the guide with them at the time of the telephone survey.

At the end of the intervention period, participants who received the baskets of fruits reported consuming an increase of 1.04 servings of fruits and vegetables per day. At baseline, 22 percent of the basket recipients were consuming 5 or more servings of fruits and vegetables per day, but by the end of the season, 39 percent reported consuming 5 or more servings per day. The conclusion was that home delivery of fruits and vegetables is an effective way to increase fruit and vegetable intake in homebound seniors.

Box 11-5 **Nutrition Programs for Promoting Health and Preventing Diseases in Older Persons**

Older Americans Act—Title III Congregate and Home-Delivered Nutrition Programs

- Serves at least one meal 5 days a week to persons age 60 and older.
- Meals are served at home or in churches, schools, senior centers, or other facilities.
- The government regulates each meal and each is expected to contain at least one-third of the RDAs or DRIs for persons age 60 and older.

Older Americans Act—Title VI Congregate and Home-Delivered Nutrition Programs

- Provides home-delivered and congregate meals to Native American organizations
- Requires that an individual not be physically able to leave the home or be homebound as a result of caring for a disabled spouse

Older Americans Act—Title III Health Promotion and Disease Prevention Program

- Provides health-promotion and disease-prevention services in areas where there are large numbers of economically-in-need older adults

Nutrition Screening Initiative

- Promotes nutritional screening and attention to nutrition in all healthcare and social-service settings that provide for older adults
- Helps identify the need for corrective measures, such as nutrition education or Meals on Wheels

Food Stamp Program

- Provides food stamps to low-income individuals, including the elderly. These can be used instead of cash to purchase food.

- Since October 2002, benefits are issued electronically on a debit card known as the EBT card (Electronic Benefits Transfer card).

Nutrition Program for the Elderly

- Provides grants, cash, and commodity foods to states and tribes to supplement congregate and home-delivered meal programs.
- Increasing socialization was one of the original program goals and continues to be one of the outcomes.

Commodity Supplemental Food Program—Elderly

- Provides food, nutrition education, and health-service referrals to individuals with low incomes, including the elderly.
- Serves target population similar to WIC and persons 60 years of age and older.
- Distribution sites make packages available on a monthly basis.

Child and Adult Care Food Program (Adult Day Care)

- Provides cash reimbursements and food commodities to community daycare centers that serve meals and snacks to children and elderly with special needs.
- Designed to help public and private, nonresidential child and adult daycare programs provide nutritious meals for children up to age 12, the elderly, and certain people with disabilities.
- Sponsors may also receive USDA commodity foods.

Food Distribution Program on Indian Reservations

- Distributes commodity foods to low-income persons, including the elderly, living on or near Indian reservations
- Participants may choose each month whether they will participate in the Food Stamp Program or the Food Distribution Program

Modified from: Grosvenor M, Smolin L. *Nutrition: Science to Life*. Philadelphia: Harcourt College Publisher; 2002. Reprinted with permission by John Wiley and Sons.

Chapter Summary

- The factors that influence aging are interrelated and affect older persons' nutritional status by decreasing their motivation to eat and their ability to acquire and enjoy food.
- Excessive use of over-the-counter and prescription medications can affect nutritional status and contribute to malnutrition.
- According to research from the Alzheimer's Disease Cooperative Study, large intakes of vitamin E are associated with slowing the progression of AD.
- The symptoms of dehydration among older adults include swollen tongue, constipation, electrolyte imbalance, nausea and vomiting, hypertension, mental confusion, sunken eyeballs, increased body temperature, decreased urine output, pressure ulcers, and urinary tract infections.
- The Food Stamp Program is an option that provides low-income elderly households with the means to purchase food. Unfortunately, because food stamps carry a "welfare" stigma, some elders are reluctant to use them.
- Meals on Wheels is designed to provide meals to participants who are homebound due to illness or disability and cannot attend the congregate meals.

Critical Thinking Activities

- Describe your impression of a typical older person and compare it with the demographic information on older adults given in this chapter.
- Watch television for 1 hour and identify both positive and negative ways that older persons are portrayed. What types of merchandise are directed toward older persons? How beneficial are these products to older persons?
- Interview an older person within your family and ask him or her to list any health problems. Are the health problems nutrition related? Ask him or her to include a typical day's activities in the list. Was physical activity listed; if so, how often? Ask the older person to keep a 24-hour dietary recall and determine the nutrient intakes, with specific attention to fluid intake.
- Use the information in the above activity to:
  - Develop screening recommendations for your relative.
  - Find resources in your area that would be able to provide meals and other services.
- Volunteer at a congregate meal or home-delivered nutrition program and provide services such as preparing and serving meals. Participate in fun activities such as playing bingo with the older persons. Prepare and present a 10- to 15-minute demonstration/lecture on how using multiple types of over-the-counter and prescribed medicines affects nutrition.

Case Study 11-1

The Illinois Department of Public Health (IDPH) funded a nutrition education program for persons 60 years and older. The purpose of the education program was to reduce the percentage of obese adults and reduce coronary heart disease deaths. The program's creator, Nikki, was required to recruit and educate at least 300 older adults. She was able to reach the target number of participants by collaborating with the local Illinois Lung and Heart Association.

Activities

- Divide into groups and create a plan to educate congregate meal participants about the health benefits of being physically active at any size and the possibility of attaining weight reduction.
- Educate participants on how to use the Nutrition Facts Panel on food products and on how to select appropriate portion sizes for healthful diets, including clarification of the serving size, using the MyPyramid Food Guide.
- Provide participants with a list of foods that are high in fiber, saturated fat, and cholesterol.
- Identify the types of assessments that could be used to monitor and determine the impact of a nutrition education program.
- Use the Practical Approach to Nutrition Screening tool (Table 11.4) and Determine: Warning Signs of Poor Nutritional Health (Box 11-4) with at least one congregate meal participant, and present the findings.

References

1. Hoyert DL, Heron MP, Murphy SL, Kung H-C. Deaths: final data for 2003. *Natl Vital Stat Rep*. 2006; 54(13):1–104. Available at: http://www.cdc.gov/nchs/products/pubs/pubd/nvsr/nvsr.htm. Accessed May 21, 2008.

2. Administration on Aging, U.S. Department of Health and Human Services. A Profile of Older Americans: 2007. Available at: http://www.aoa.gov/prof/Statistics/profile/2007/profiles2007.asp. Accessed May 21, 2008.

3. Grosvenor MB, Smolin LA. *Nutrition: From Science to Life*. New York: Harcourt College; 2002.

4. Fries JF. The compression of morbidity. *Milbank Quart*. 2005; 83:801–823.

5. Hubert HB, Bloch DA, Oehlert JW, Fries JF. Lifestyle habits and compression of morbidity. *J Gerontol A Biol Sci Med Sci*. 2002; 57(6):M347–M351.

6. Raynaud-Simon A, Lesourd B. [Malnutrition in the elderly. Clinical consequences]. *Presse Med*. 2000; 29(39):2183–2190.

7. Semba RD, Bartali B, Zhou J, Blaum C, Ko CW, Fried LP. Low serum micronutrient concentrations predict frailty among older women living in the community. *J Gerontol A Biol Sci Med Sci*. 2006; 61(6):594–599.

8. Ryff C. Beyond Ponce de Leon and life satisfaction: new directions in quest of successful ageing. *Int J Behav Dev*. 1989; 12(1):35–55.

9. Fisher B. Successful aging, life satisfaction, and generativity in later life. *Int J Aging Human Dev*. 1995; 41(3):239–250.

10. Kerschner H, Pegues J. Productive aging: a quality of life agenda. *J Am Diet Assoc*. 1998; 98(12):1445–1448.

11. U.S. Department of Health and Human Services. *Healthy People 2010. Understanding and Improving Health Objectives for Improving Health*. Vol. 1. Washington, DC: Author; 2000.

12. National Center for Health Statistics, U.S. Department of Health and Human Services. Healthy People 2010. Available at: http://www.healthypeople.gov. Accessed May 21, 2008.

13. Berdanier C, Feldman E, Flatt W, Jeor S. *Handbook of Nutrition and Food*. New York: CRC Press; 2002.

14. Gerberding JL. Healthy Aging: Preserving Function and Improving Quality of Life Among Older Americans, 2008. Available at: http://www.cdc.gov/nccdphp/publications/aag/aging.htm. Accessed April 12, 2008.

15. Ben-Shlomo Y. A life course approach to chronic disease epidemiology: conceptual models, empirical challenges and interdisciplinary perspectives. *Int J Epidemiol*. 2002; 31:285–293.

16. Kennedy ET. Evidence for nutritional benefits in prolonging wellness. *Am J Clin Nutr*. 2006; 83(2):410S–414S.

17. Heilbronn LK, Ravussin E. Calorie restriction and aging: review of the literature and implications for studies in humans. *Am J Clin Nutr*. 2003; 78(3):361–369.

18. Mathers JC. Nutritional modulation of ageing: genomic and epigenetic approaches. *Mech Ageing Dev*. 2006; 127(6):584–589.

19. Abete P, Della Morte D, Mazzella F, et al. Lifestyle and prevention of cardiovascular disease in the elderly: an Italian perspective. *Am J Geriatr Cardiol*. 2006; 15(1):28–34.

20. Wardlaw G, Kessel M. *Perspectives in Nutrition*. 5th ed. New York: McGraw-Hill; 2002.

21. Brown JE. *Nutrition Through the Life Cycle*. 2nd ed. Belmont, CA: Thomson Wadsworth; 2005.

22. Evans PH. Free radicals in brain metabolism and pathology. *Brit Med Bull*. 1993; 49:577–587.

23. Yusuf S, Dagenais G, Pogue J, et al. Vitamin E supplementation and cardiovascular events in high-risk patients. The Heart Outcomes Prevention Evaluation study investigators. *N Eng J Med*. 2000; 342:154–160.

24. de Grey AD. Free radicals in aging: causal complexity and its biomedical implications. *Free Radic Res*. 2006; 40(12):1244–1249.

25. Stadtman ER. Protein oxidation and aging. *Free Radic Res*. 2006; 40(12):1250–1258.

26. Harper JM, Leathers CW, Austad SN. Does caloric restriction extend life in wild mice? *Aging Cell*. 2006; 5(6):441–449.

27. McCay C, Crowel M, Maynard L. The effect of retarded growth upon the length of life and upon ultimate size. *J Nutr*. 1935; 10:63–79.

28. Nnakwe NE. The effect of age and dietary restriction on bone strength, calcium and phosphorus contents of male F344 rats. *J Nutr Health Aging*. 1998; 2(3):149–152.

29. Mattison JA, Roth GS, Lane MA, Ingram DK. Dietary restriction in aging nonhuman primates. *Interdisc Top Gerontol*. 2007; 35:137–158.

30. Kelly DE, Goodpaster BH, Storlien L. Muscle triglyceride and insulin resistance. *Ann Rev Nutr*. 2002; 22:325–346.

31. Williams SR. *Essentials of Nutrition and Diet Therapy*. 8th ed. Davis, CA: Mosby; 2003.

32. National Institute on Alcohol Abuse and Alcoholism. Alcohol and Nutrition. Available at: http://alcoholism.about.com/cs/alerts/l/blnaa22.htm. Accessed September 19, 2004.

33. U.S. Department of Agriculture, Department of Health and Human Services. Nutrition and Your Health: Dietary Guidelines for Americans. Backgrounder 2005 Dietary Guidelines Advisory Committee Report. Available at: http://www.health.gov/DietaryGuidelines/dga2005/Backgrounder.htm. Accessed February 6, 2007.

34. Dawson DA, Grant BF, Li TK. Quantifying the risks associated with exceeding recommended drinking limits. *Alcohol Clin Exp Res*. 2005; 29(5):902–908.

35. Worthington PH. *Practical Aspect of Nutritional Support: An Advanced Practice Guide*. Philadelphia, PA: Saunders; 2004.

36. Stout CM, Popovich DJ. Undiagnosed alcoholism and prescription drug misuse among the elderly. *Caring*. 2001; 20(1):20–23.

37. Rigler S. Alcoholism in the elderly. *Am Fam Physician*. 2000; 661:1710.

38. Michel KE, Higgins C. Nutrient–drug interactions in nutritional support. *J Veter Emerg Crit Care*. 2002; 12(3):163–167.

39. Nnakwe NE. Medication and dietary practices of independent living healthy African-American older persons. *J Nutr Elderly*. 2001; 21(1):39–58.

40. Kaufman DW, Kelly JP, Rosenberg L, Anderson TE, Mitchell AA. Recent patterns of medication use in the ambulatory adult population of the United States: the Slone survey. *JAMA*. 2002; 287(3):337–344.

41. Rodwell WS. *Essentials of Nutrition and Diet Therapy*. 8th ed. St. Louis, MO: Mosby; 2003.

42. Pronsky ZM. *Food Medication Interactions*. 13th ed. Birchrunville, PA: Food-Medication Interactions; 2004.

43. Davis MA, Murphy SP, Neuhaus JM, Gee L, Quiroga SS. Living arrangements affect dietary quality for U.S. adults aged 50 years and older: NHANES III 1988–1994. *J Nutr*. 2000; 130:2256–2264.

44. Jung SL, Frongillo EA. Nutritional and health consequences are associated with food insecurity among U.S. elderly persons. *J Nutr*. 2001; 131:1503–1509.

45. Davis MA, Murphy SP, Neuhaus JM, Gee L, Quiroga SS. Living arrangements affect dietary quality for U.S. adults aged 50 years and older: NHANES III 1988–1994. *J Nutr*. 2000; 130:2256–2264.

46. Beers MH, Berkow R. *The Merck Manual of Geriatrics*. 3rd ed. Whitehouse Station, NY: Merck Research Laboratories; 2000.

47. Roubenoff R, Hughes VA. Sarcopenia: current concepts. *J Gerontol A Biol Sci Med Sci*. 2000; 55:716–724.

48. Saltzman JR, Russell RM. The aging gut: nutritional issues. *Gastroenterol Clin North Am*. 1998; 27(2):309–324.

49. Seals DR, Monahan KD, Bell C, Tanaka H, Jones PP. The aging cardiovascular system: changes in autonomic function at rest and in response to exercise. *Int J Sport Nutri Exerc Metab*. 2001; 11:S189–S195.

50. ASPEN Board of Directors, Clinical Guidelines Task Force. Guidelines for the use of parenteral and enteral nutrition in adult and pediatric patients. *J Parenter Enteral Nutr*. 2002; 26(1 suppl):1SA–138SA.

51. McGee M, Binkley J, Jensen GL. *The Science and Practice of Nutrition Support*. Dubuque, Iowa: Kendall/Hunt; 2001.

52. Harris TB. Waist circumference and sagittal diameter reflect total body fat better than visceral fat in older men and women: the Health, Aging and Body Composition Study. *Ann New York Acad Sci*. 2000; 904:462–473.

53. Guo SS, Zeller C, Chumlea WC, Siervogel RM. Aging, body composition, and lifestyle: the Fels Longitudinal Study. *Am J Clin Nutr*. 1999; 70(3):405–411.

54. van den Beld AW, de Jong FH, Grobbee DE, Pols HA, Lamberts SW. Measures of bioavailable serum testosterone and estradiol and their relationships with muscle strength, bone density, and body composition in elderly men. *J Clin Endocrinol Metab*. 2000; 85(9):3276–3282.

55. Khosla S, Melton LJ 3rd, Atkinson EJ, O'Fallon WM. Relationship of serum sex steroid levels to longitudinal changes in bone density in young versus elderly men. *J Clin Endocrinol Metab*. 2001; 86(8):3555–3561.

56. Sahota O, Hosking DJ. The contribution of nutritional factors to osteopenia in the elderly. *Curr Opin Clin Nutr Metab Care*. 2001; 4(1):15–19.

57. Vicente-Rodriguez G, Ara I, Perez-Gomez J, Dorado C, Calbet J. Muscular development and physical activity as major determinants of femoral bone mass acquisition during growth. *Brit J Sports Med*. 2005; 39:611–616.

58. Klotzbach-Shimomura K. Project Healthy Bones: an osteoporosis prevention program for older adults. *J Extension*. 2001; 39(3): Online. Available at: http://www.joe.org/joe/2001june/iw6.html. Accessed April 12, 2008.

59. Brownie S. Why are elderly individuals at risk of nutritional deficiency? *Int J Nursing Practice*. 2006; 12(2):110–118.

60. National Heart, Lung, and Blood Institute. Diseases and Conditions Index. Pernicious Anemia. Available at: http://www.nhlbi.nih.gov/health/dci/Diseases/prnanmia/prnanmia_all.html. Accessed February 7, 2007.

61. Yukawa H, Takao S. Aging-related changes of food intake in elderly subjects living in an urban community and relation with vital prognosis: results of an 8-year longitudinal study (TMIG-LISA). *Geriatr Gerontol Int*. 2003; 3(suppl 1):S55–S62.

62. Mayo Clinic. Malnutrition and Seniors: When a Relative Doesn't Eat Enough. Available at: http://www.mayoclinic.com/health/senior-health/HA00066. Accessed February 7, 2007.

63. Pribitkin ER, Cowart BJ. Prevalence and causes of severe taste loss in a chemosensory clinic population. *Ann Otol Rhinol Laryngol*. 2003; 112(11):971–978.

64. University of Connecticut. Taste and Smell Center. General Information. Available at: http://www.uchc.edu/uconntasteandsmell/gen.html. Accessed February 7, 2007.

65. Schiffman SS. Intensification of sensory properties of foods for the elderly. *J Nutr*. 2000; 130:927S–930S.

66. Drewnowski A. Sensory control of energy density at different life stages. *Proc Nutr Soc*. 2000; 59: 239–244.

67. Huffman GB. Evaluating and treating unintentional weight loss in the elderly. *Am Fam Physician*. 2002; 65:640–650.

68. Morley JE. Anorexia, body composition, and ageing. *Curr Opin Clin Nutr Metab Care*. 2001; 4(1):9–13.

69. Resnick B. Weight loss and failure to thrive: evaluating and motivating older adults toward recovery. *Ann Long-Term Care Clin Care Aging*. 2001; 9(7):21–31.

70. White R, Ashworth A. How drug therapy can affect, threaten and compromise nutritional status. *J Human Nutr Diet*. 2000; 13(2):119–129.

71. American Dietetic Association. Position of the American Dietetic Association: nutrition, aging and the continuum of care. *J Am Diet Assoc*. 2000; 100:580–595.

72. Armstrong-Esther CA, Browne KD, Armstrong-Esther DC, Sander L. The institutionalized elderly: dry to the bone! *Int J Nurs Stud*. 1996; 33(6):619–628.

73. Bhalla A, Sankaralingam S, Dundas R, Swaminathan R, Wolfe CD, Rudd AG. Influence of raised plasma osmolality on clinical outcome after acute stroke. *Stroke*. 2000; 31:2043–2048.

74. Wingate D, Phillips SF, Lewis SJ. Guidelines for adults on self-medication for the treatment of acute diarrhoea. *Aliment Pharmacol Ther*. 2001; 15(6):773–782.

75. National Institute on Aging, U.S. National Institutes of Health. Alzheimer's Disease Fact Sheet. Available at: http://www.nia.nih.gov/Alzheimers/Publications/adfact.htm. Accessed April 12, 2008.

76. Juan, W-Y, Basiotis PP. More than one in three older Americans may not drink enough water: insight 27 September 2002. *Fam Econ Nutr Rev*. 2004; 16:49–51.

77. Valtin H. "Drink at least eight glasses of water a day." Really? Is there scientific evidence for "8 x 8"? *Am J Physiol Regul Integr Compar Physiol*. 2002; 283(5):R993–R1004.

78. Andorn A, Pappolla MA. Catecholamines inhibit lipid peroxidation in young, aged, and Alzheimer's disease brain. *Free Radic Viol Med*. 2001; 31:315–320.

79. Giannakopoulos P, Gold G, Kövari E, et al. Assessing the cognitive impact of Alzheimer disease pathology and vascular burden in the aging brain: the Geneva experience. *Acta Neuropathol*. 2007; 113(1):1–12.

80. Farias ST, Mungas D, Reed BR, Harvey D, Cahn-Weiner D, Decarli C. MCI is associated with deficits in everyday functioning. *Alzheimer Dis Assoc Disord*. 2006; 20(4):217–223.

81. Otsuka M, Yamaguchi K, Ueki A. Similarities and differences between Alzheimer's disease and vascular dementia from the viewpoint of nutrition. *Ann N Y Acad Sci*. 2002; 977:155–161.

82. Morris MC, Evans DA, Schneider JA, Tangney CC, Bienias JL, Aggarwal NT. Dietary folate and vitamins B-12 and B-6 not associated with incident Alzheimer's disease. *J Alzheimers Dis*. 2006; 9(4):435–443.

83. Abou-Saleh MT, Coppen A. Folic acid and the treatment of depression. *J Psychosomat Res*. 2006; 61(3):285–287.

84. Morris MC, Evans DA, Bienias JL, et al. Dietary intake of antioxidant nutrients and the risk of incident Alzheimer disease in a biracial community study. *JAMA*. 2002; 287(24):3230–3237.

85. Young KW, Greenwood CE, van Reekum R, Binns MA. A randomized, crossover trial of high-carbohydrate foods in nursing home residents with Alzheimer's disease: associations among intervention response. *J Gerontol A Biol Sci Med Sci*. 2005; 60(8):1039–1045.

86. Mittelman MS, Haley WE, Clay OJ, Roth DL. Improving caregiver well-being delays nursing home placement of patients with Alzheimer disease. *Neurol*. 2006; 67(9):1592–1599.

87. Alzheimer's Association. Stages of Alzheimer's. Available at: http://www.alz.org/alzheimers_disease_stages_of_alzheimers.asp. Accessed February 7, 2007.

88. Peng CC, Glassman PA, Trilli LE, Hayes-Hunter J, Good CB. Incidence and severity of potential drug–dietary supplement interactions in primary care patients. *Arch Intern Med*. 2004; 164:630–636.

89. Takahashi R. Nutritional risk in community-dwelling elderly long-term care insurance recipients. *Nippon Ronen Igakkai Zasshi*. 2006; 43(3):375–382.

90. Guigoz Y. The Mini Nutritional Assessment (MNA) review of the literature—what does it tell us? *J Nutr Health Aging*. 2006; 10(6):466–487.

91. Mitchell DC, Smiciklas-Wright H, Friedmann JM, Gordon J. Dietary intake assessed by the nutrition screening initiative level II screen is a sensitive but not a specific indicator of nutrition risk in older adults. *J Am Diet Assoc*. 2002; 102(6):842–844.

92. Shahar D, Shai I, Vardi H, Fraser D. Dietary intake and eating patterns of elderly people in Israel: who is at nutritional risk? *Eur J Clin Nutr*. 2003; 57(1):18–25.

93. Sharkey JR. Variation in nutritional risk among Mexican American and non-Mexican American homebound elders who receive home-delivered meals. *J Nutr Elderly*. 2004; 23(4):1–19.

94. Gibson RS. *Principles of Nutritional Assessment*. 2nd ed. Dunedin, New Zealand: Oxford University Press; 2005.

95. Dixon LB, Winkleby MA, Radimer KL. Dietary intakes and serum nutrients differ between adults from food-insufficient and food-sufficient families: Third National Health and Nutrition Examination Survey, 1988–1994. *J Nutr*. 2001; 131:1232–1246.

96. Lin B-H. Nutrition and Health Characteristics of Low-Income Populations: Healthy Eating Index. Agriculture Information Bulletin 796-1; 2005. United States Department of Agriculture, Economic Research Services. Available at: http://www.ers.usda.gov/publications/aib796/aib796%2D1. Accessed April 13, 2008.

97. Laroche HH, Hofer TP, Davis MM. Adult fat intake associated with the presence of children in households: findings from NHANES III. *J Am Board Fam Med*. 2007; 20(1):9–15.

98. Sahyoun NR, Lin CL, Krall E. Nutritional status of the older adult is associated with dentition status. *J Am Diet Assoc*. 2003; 103(1):61–66.

99. Insel P, Turner E, Ross D. *Nutrition: 2002 Update*. Sudbury, MA: Jones and Bartlett; 2002.

100. Lutz C, Przytulski K. *Nutrition and Diet Therapy*. 3rd ed. Philadelphia: F.A. Davis; 2001.

101. Administration on Aging, U.S. Department of Health and Human Services. The Elderly Nutrition Program. Available at: http://www.aoa.gov/press/fact/alpha/fact_elderly_nutrition.asp. Accessed April 14, 2008.

102. Blecher L. Using forecasting techniques to predict meal demand in Title IIIc congregate lunch programs. *J Am Diet Assoc*. 2004; 104:1281–1283.

103. Millen BE, Ohls JC, Ponza M, McCool AC. The Elderly Nutrition Program: an effective national framework for preventive nutrition interventions. *J Am Diet Assoc*. 2002; 102:234–240.

104. Gollub EA, Weddle D. Improvements in nutritional intake and quality of life among frail homebound older adults receiving home-delivered breakfast and lunch. *J Am Diet Assoc*. 2004; 104:1227–1235.

105. Bartali B, Frongillo E, Bandinelli S, Lauretani F, Semba R, Fried L, Ferrucci L. Low nutrient intake is an essential component of frailty in older persons. *J Gerontol A Biol Sci Med Sci*. 2006; 61:589–593.

106. Administration on Aging, U.S. Department of Health and Human Services. Title III Program Administration and Service Delivery. Available at: http://www.aoa.gov/prof/aoaprog/nutrition/program_eval/er_vol1ch4fh_pf.asp. Accessed April 13, 2008.

107. Fey-Yensan N, English C, Ash S, Wallace C, Museler H. Food safety risk identified in a population of elderly home-delivered meal participants. *J Am Diet Assoc*. 2001; 101:1055–1057.

108. Saletti A, Johansson L, Yifter-Lindgren E, Wissing U, Osterberg K, Cederholm T. Nutritional status and a 3-year follow-up in elderly receiving support at home. *Gerontol*. 2005; 51:192–198.

109. Eppich S, Fernandez CP. Study finds Chapel Hill, NC, soup kitchen serves nutritious meals. *J Am Diet Assoc*. 2004; 104:1284–1286.

110. Sharkey JR. Risk and presence of food insufficiency are associated with low nutrient intakes and multimorbidity among homebound older women who receive home-delivered meals. *J Nutr*. 2003; 133:3485–3491.

111. U.S. Department of Agriculture. Nutrition Services Incentive Program. Available at: http://www.aoa.dhhs.gov/eldfam/Nutrition/Nutrition_services_incentive.asp. Accessed February 7, 2007.

112. Administration on Aging, U.S. Department of Health and Human Services. A Profile of Older Americans: 2007. Available at: http://www.aoa.dhhs.gov/ PROF/Statistics/profile/2007/16.asp. Accessed April 13, 2008.

113. Fox MK, Hamilton W, and Lin B-H. *Effects of Food Assistance and Nutrition Programs on Nutrition and Health.* Vol. 4, Executive Summary of the Literature Review. Washington, DC: Economic Research Service/USDA; 2007.

114. Johnson DB, Beaudoin S, Smith LT, Beresford SA, LoGerfo JP. Increasing fruit and vegetable intake in homebound elders: the Seattle Senior Farmers' Market Nutrition Pilot Program. *Prev Chronic Dis.* 2004; 1(1):A03. Available at: http:// www.pubmedcentral.nih.gov/articlerender.fcgi?artid=544526. Accessed April 13, 2008.

PART III
Delivering Successful
Nutrition Services

CHAPTER 12

Principles of Planning Effective Community Nutrition Programs

LEARNING OBJECTIVES

- Explain the programming processes of planning, implementation, evaluation, and assessment.
- Explain the different types of evaluation.
- Discuss the different data collection methods.
- Discuss the different theories/models that community nutritionists can use to provide effective nutrition programs.

Introduction

The term *program* has a variety of meanings. For our purposes, a program is a collection of activities intended to produce a particular outcome.[1] In community nutrition programs, activities focus directly on nutrition issues or on health problems. The overall purpose is to improve the health of the community or public. *Program planning* is an act of formulating a program for a definite course of action, a process of exploring a situation, deciding on a situation, and designing actions to create the desired outcome.[2] Planning can be more exciting than carrying out the activities related to the program itself. The nutritionist must recognize the importance of continuously critiquing and reevaluating the services that are being provided. The following sections focus on the practicalities of program planning, *program implementation*, and *program evaluation* with high-quality health and well-being as the ultimate goal. Hence, this chapter discusses program planning and

relevant theories of behavior change as they relate to nutrition and health promotion.

The quality of the working relationships among participants is very important to the success of any program. Many *frameworks* have been designed to guide this relationship in health promotion programs. The P-Process has been used mostly for implementing international mass media campaigns, whereas the PRECEDE-PROCEED framework has been used mostly for U.S. worksite programs.[3] This chapter will discuss the P-Process, PRECEDE-PROCEED, and several other frameworks that community nutritionists can utilize to design health promotion programs.

Identifying Issues

In program planning, it is essential to identify issues of interest or concern. Surveys are useful for identifying issues of importance and achiev-

program A collection of activities intended to produce particular results.

program planning The process of exploring a situation, deciding on a more desirable situation, and designing actions to create the desired situation.

program implementation The process of putting a program into action.

program evaluation An ongoing process from the beginning of the planning phase until a program ends.

frameworks Schemes that specify the steps in a process.

ing consensus when it is not practical for people to meet face to face.[4] Community nutritionists can also use data collected from community nutrition assessments, demographic data, maternal and infant mortality rates, and medical records to create a problem list.[5] The problem list compares and ranks perceived needs or those identified by the assessment data. It may reflect a community-wide concern, including ethnic or age groups that are at high nutritional risk. The needs of the groups can be compared and contrasted with the capacity of existing agencies to meet the desired outcome. The problem list can be used to request more funds, plan programs, and evaluate existing programs as well as to determine delivery plans so the community can directly benefit from the program.[6] In addition, community assessment can identify the percentage of low income individuals, the cost of housing in the community, cultural differences, language barriers, housing needs, the location and kinds of local markets, and the quality and prices of the foods they offer. To assess the extent of hunger in the

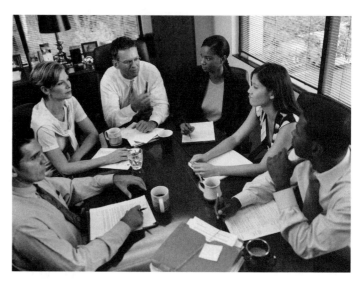

A community needs assessment can be used to generate a list of problems for planning a health and nutrition promotion program.

community, data are needed on local food costs, household resources to obtain and prepare food, and barriers that constrain individuals or families from obtaining adequate food, such as language barriers and cultural differences.[7] **Figure 12-1** presents an assessment instrument that a health promotion program can use to identify a need or concern.

Please take a few minutes to fill out the following survey. Individual information will not be disclosed; only summary results will be tabulated and reported. At no time will individual responses be reported.

1. Listed are various health promotion programs that might be offered by Community X's Fitness and Wellness Program. Please indicate your interest in each of the programs.

Program	Low Interest				High Interest
Nutrition	1	2	3	4	5
Weight loss	1	2	3	4	5
Cancer screening	1	2	3	4	5
Cardiovascular risk reduction	1	2	3	4	5
Hypertension control	1	2	3	4	5
Men's health issues	1	2	3	4	5
Women's health issues	1	2	3	4	5
Parenting skills	1	2	3	4	5
Developing communication skills	1	2	3	4	5
Assertiveness training	1	2	3	4	5
Healthy back	1	2	3	4	5
Stress management skills	1	2	3	4	5
Time management	1	2	3	4	5
HIV and AIDS education	1	2	3	4	5
Drug education	1	2	3	4	5
Home and personal safety	1	2	3	4	5
Exercise and fitness programs	1	2	3	4	5
Smoking cessation	1	2	3	4	5
Other suggestions _____					

FIGURE 12-1 Sample Survey Instruments for Assessing Interests and Readiness for Health Promotion

Source: Anspaugh DJ, Dignan MB, Anspaugh SL. *Developing health promotion programs*. 2 ed. 2006. Long Grove, Illinois: Waveland Press. Reprinted with permission.

Factors That Prompt Program Planning

The nutrition-related health issues that have been identified through a community needs assessment may trigger the decision to develop a nutrition program. For example, the community needs assessment may show that many newly immigrated Hispanic people are not aware of the Special Supplemental Nutrition Program for Women, Infants, and Children (WIC) or that the majority of the children living in a poor neighborhood are not enrolled in the National School Lunch Program.

Additional factors that may prompt program planning include research findings. For example, research shows that the number of women reaching menopause and postmenopause age has increased as well as the incidence of nutrition-related conditions such as heart disease, osteoporosis, and cancer in women. Hence, the Illinois Department of Public Health Office of Women's Health funded education programs to address these health issues. Other factors that may trigger program planning include government policy, such as increasing nutritious foods in schools; the availability of funds to improve an existing program or to create new programs; and federal or state mandates.

At the national level, health problems are changing. Epidemiologic data show high mortality and morbidity rates due to nutrition-related issues (i.e., malnutrition, obesity, heart disease, cancer, and diabetes).[8–10] Hence, the Hearts N' Parks Magnet Centers in 11 states became part of the well-known community-based program that works to reduce some of the nutrition-related health conditions. Hearts N' Parks is an innovative program that aims to reduce the trend of obesity and the risk of coronary heart disease in the United States by encouraging Americans of all ages to aim for a healthy weight, follow a heart-healthy eating plan, and engage in regular physical activity. Hearts N' Parks is supported by the National Heart, Lung, and Blood Institute (NHLBI) of the National Institutes of Health and the National Recreation and

---

2. What classes/programs would you attend if the time of the program was convenient to you?

Program	Would Definitely Attend	Would Probably Attend	Would Not Attend
Nutrition	_____	_____	_____
Weight loss	_____	_____	_____
Cancer screening	_____	_____	_____
Cardiovascular risk reduction	_____	_____	_____
Hypertension control	_____	_____	_____
Men's health issues	_____	_____	_____
Women's health issues	_____	_____	_____
Parenting skills	_____	_____	_____
Developing communication skills	_____	_____	_____
Assertiveness training	_____	_____	_____
Healthy back	_____	_____	_____
Stress management skills	_____	_____	_____
Time management	_____	_____	_____
HIV and AIDS education	_____	_____	_____
Drug education	_____	_____	_____
Home and personal safety	_____	_____	_____
Exercise and fitness programs	_____	_____	_____
Smoking cessation	_____	_____	_____

3. What would be the best time for you to attend these programs?

_____ A. Prior to work   _____ B. Lunch time   _____ C. After work   _____ D. Weekends

4. Would your spouse or significant other take part in the health promotion program?

_____ Yes   _____ No   _____ Maybe

5. Would you participate in an exercise program with males and females (coed)?

_____ Yes   _____ No

6. In what type of exercise programs would you participate?

_____ Aerobics   _____ Swimming   _____ Walking   _____ Jogging

_____ Weight lifting   _____ Tennis   _____ Racquetball   _____ Other (please list)

7. Are you a _____ Female _____ Male?

8. What is your age range?

_____ 20–30   _____ 31–40   _____ 41–50   _____ 51–60   _____ Over 60

9. Are you

_____ Upper management   _____ Middle management   _____ Staff   _____ Production

---

FIGURE 12-1 *(Continued)*.

Park Association (NRPA). Some of the program activities include nutrition and fitness, stress reduction, and family life programs. Typically, the programs for children or adolescents are provided during summer camps or after-school activities for 7 to 11 weeks. The program also serves seniors and women and ends after an average of 12 weeks.

An evaluation of the Hearts N' Parks program showed that children learned to identify nutritious foods and reported being more willing to choose nutritious foods over less nutritious foods. On average, 26 percent of the children increased their heart-healthy eating knowledge, and 15 percent increased their heart-healthy eating intention. Children also increased their interest in various forms of physical activity.[11]

Another national program is the U.S. National Cancer Institute's (NCI's) Fruits and Veggies More Matters Campaign (formerly known as 5-A-Day for Better Health). In 2003, NCI initiated this campaign to motivate African American men to eat 9 servings of fruits and vegetables a day. This campaign was trigged by the high incidence of cancer in the African American population. The campaign used a series of national radio spots that reached more than 17 million listeners a week for 4 months. Currently, the campaign offers an eight-page brochure designed specifically for African American men, and a 9 A Day website (http://www.fruitsandveggiesmatter.gov) that explains the impact of diet on African American men's health. **Figure 12-2** presents additional factors that may prompt program planning.

Analyzing Subjective and Objective Data

Subjective and objective data are very important in program planning. *Subjective data analysis* involves the collection and analysis of data on the various clients' perceived needs. This includes clarification of community values and analysis of the community (external) and agency (internal) environments in which the nutrition program plan will operate.[6,12,13] Community nutritionists can obtain subjective data by studying the mass media, such as reading local newspapers, including those that serve local neighborhoods or ethnic groups; listening to area radio stations, including those that target ethnic groups or special interests; and watching local television coverage.[13,14] The media typically reflect local values, political views, interests, educational levels, and lifestyles. It is possible to identify and determine current critical issues in the community via media coverage of meetings of local, state, national, or international governmental bodies and their opposing views.[6] In addition, perceived problems and needs for nutrition services can be obtained by interviewing professional colleagues (public health physicians, nurses, community health educators, and clinical dietitians) in health agencies to ascertain their perspectives on the community. Also, the use of in-depth narrative interviews is effective in collecting data. An in-depth interview is a nondirective research technique in which the participant is invited to "tell me the story about your health condition, starting with when you first noticed anything

subjective data analysis The collection and analysis of data on various clients that are observable and measurable, such as listening to radio stations, watching local television coverage, and interviewing key informants/community leaders.

objective data analysis The collection and analysis of available demographic and health statistics to prepare a community diagnosis and problem list.

action plan A concise statement of the methods, activities, or intervention strategies to be undertaken.

The Community and Public Needs Assessment Revealed:
- Infant malnutrition and mortality
- An increase in the low-income minority population
- An increased incidence of obesity in school-age children
- An increased rate of measles in the Hispanic and Asian communities
- An increased rate of osteoporosis in older women living in a retirement community
- Research findings about the high incidence of diseases such as heart disease and cancer
- Concerns of well-known community leaders or stakeholders
- Government policy changes related to health
- The availability of resources from the government and/or private organizations for new programs or to expand existing programs

↓

The public or community acknowledges that the health issues need attention or upgrading.

↓

New programs are developed or revised, or existing programs are expanded.

FIGURE 12-2 Factors That May Prompt Program Planning
Data from Boyle M. *Community Nutrition in Action: An Entrepreneurial Approach.* 4 ed. 2005. Belmont, CA: Thomson Wadsworth.

was wrong," and the only prompts used are "tell me more about that" or "what happened next?"[14,15] Informant interviews, which consist of direct conversations with selected members of a community about community members or groups and events, are an effective method of data collection. Holding informant interviews and involving stakeholders are good ways to generate information about community beliefs, norms, and values.

Objective data analysis involves collecting and analyzing data from available demographic and health statistics to prepare the community diagnosis and problem list. For example, vital statistics on births and deaths that are reported to the state health agency can be used in community assessment. All births and deaths are recorded through a local registrar or clerk, usually in the city or county health department. Death certificates provide information on primary and secondary causes of death (mortality). Objective data are collected to determine what is known about the community's population in total as compared with what is known about individuals.[6,13] **Table 12.1** presents examples of subjective and objective data.

A community nutritionist can assess clients' nutritional status and collect observable data using generally accepted parameters, which are described in Chapter 2. For example, researchers at Ohio University used the subjective method of data collection to assess food insecurity. Food insecurity in rural Southeast Ohio was reported to be about two to three times higher than for the rest of the nation. Funding from the University of Ohio and the support of community agencies helped students enrolled in a community nutrition course to conduct a needs assessment and identify factors influencing food insecurity in rural Appalachian Ohio. The students collected data through a review of literature on food insecurity and hunger and interviews with area agencies. They focused the interviews on the agencies' missions/goals and funding sources, and gathered information from annual reports.

Their assessment confirmed the need for additional emergency food resources, and they developed a program, "Halt Hunger on the Hock-

TABLE 12.1	Examples of Subjective and Objective Data[6]	
Subjective Data	**Sources**	
Beliefs	Media (local newspapers, radio stations, television)	
Values	Stakeholders	
Lifestyles	Informants	
Political views	Physicians	
	Nurses	
Objective Data	**Sources**	
Demographic statistics (age, gender, race, ethnicity, income, and educational level)	Birth and death certificates	
	Census Bureau	
Vital and health statistics (births, deaths, infant mortality rate, and marital status)	Medical records	
	Centers for Disease Control and Prevention	
Physical environment (mild climate, inner-city neighborhood, size of neighborhood, public spaces, roads, and older homes)	National surveys (e.g., National Health and Nutrition Examination Survey [NHANES])	

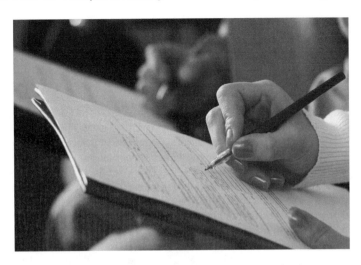

Subjective and objective data are very important in program planning.

ing," to address this need. A food drive was planned as a service-learning project, which improved the community food security status.[16,17]

Writing a Mission Statement

The data collected through subjective and/or objective methods can be used to help write a mission statement. The mission statement is a statement of clear direction for the health program.[3] This statement must be clear, brief, concise, realistic, and inspirational. It is important to choose and rank the most critical issues in order of priority in the mission statement as well as in the subsequent steps of writing the objectives and the *action plan* or activities.[6] When wording the mission statement for nutrition service needs, consider the organization's

philosophy, products, services, markets, values, and concern for the public. It is important to review the mission statement of the organization before writing a mission statement for a specific program. Reviewing the organization's mission statement and matching it with the program's goals will:[18,19]

- Make sure the program is implementing the organization's directive
- Justify the resources, time, and expense the program utilized
- Generate support from supervisors

If the program's goals do not match the organization's mission statement it will be difficult for the nutritionist to justify the use of the organization's resources. He or she will not receive support from supervisors or obtain internal funds and approval for the new program. **Boxes 12-1** and **12-2** present samples of mission statements.

***Box* 12-1 Cornell Cooperative Extension Mission Statement**

The Cornell Cooperative Extension mission statement is to enable people to improve their lives and communities through partnerships that put experience and research knowledge to work.

Source: Cornell University Cooperative Extension Service. Mission Statement. Nutrition. Available at: http://www.cce.cornell.edu. Accessed April 14, 2008. Reprinted with permission.

***Box* 12-2 The Cooperative State Research, Education, and Extension Service**

The Cooperative State Research, Education, and Extension Service (CSREES) mission statement is to advance knowledge for agriculture, the environment, human health and well-being, and communities by supporting research, education, and extension programs in the Land Grant University System and other partner organizations. CSREES doesn't perform actual research, education, and extension but rather helps fund it at the state and local level and provides program leadership in these areas.

Source: Cooperative State Research, Education, and Extension Service. Strategic Plan for 2007–2012. Available at: http://www.crees.usda.gov. Accessed August 27, 2008.

Clarifying Goals

Regardless of the type of data collection method used (subjective or objective), it is import to clarify the program goals because communities often express their goals broadly, which may affect data collection and analysis as well as the program outcome. Goals are general statements about what the program should accomplish (e.g., to improve the health of children, older persons, and pregnant women).[20] For example, the community may want children to grow up healthier. In this case, further exploration is required to identify factors that influence the growth of children in the community (for instance, poor food or a lack of safe places to play and learn).[21]

In the United States, nutritionists can use the national goals and objectives outlined in Healthy People 2010 to plan their programs. The goals are very helpful because they target specific priority needs of the U.S. population identified by a cross-section of practitioners and interested citizens.[21,22] For example, Objective 19-4 is to promote health and reduce chronic diseases associated with diet and weight. To use the Healthy People 2010 objectives, a community might evaluate how well they meet national or state objectives, decide on the significance of the objectives, and then use gaps as starting points for action.

Goals are different from objectives. Goals are broad statements of desired outcome or changes, whereas objectives are specific, measurable actions of the desired outcome to be completed within a specified time frame.[2] For instance, the McLean County Public Health Department identified a high incidence of iron deficiency anemia in their county and aimed to decrease the prevalence of iron deficiency anemia in low-income minority children.

> *Goal:* To reduce iron deficiency anemia in McLean County.
>
> *Objective:* By the end of the nutrition and health promotion program:
>
> - Eighty percent of low-income minority children ages 2 to 5 years will be enrolled in the WIC program.
> - The number of anemic children in McLean County will be reduced by 95 percent.

Developing a Program Plan

It is important to develop a program only after reviewing existing programs and talking to other health professionals such as nurses and other dietitians who have worked with comparable programs or with the target population. Examples of ways to make connections with other professionals are by attending professional conferences, contacting experts in the area, searching the literature, networking via word of mouth, searching the Internet, and becoming a member of an American Dietetic Association practice group. There are six important factors to consider when writing or designing a program plan:[6,23,24]

- The established and emerging scientific evidence from research findings in nutrition and food science that apply to the public's health and/or issues that are relevant to the community that have not been adequately addressed
- The organization's mission and philosophy
- Federal and state legislation either requiring or permitting nutrition services in the community's health and human services system

models physical, symbolic, or mental ways of viewing a real object.

theory A construct that accounts for or organizes events.

- Federal, national, state, local, public, or private sector organizations that provide funds for nutrition services
- Opportunities to contract with other community health and human service agencies to provide nutrition services
- Model nutrition objectives or standards published by expert groups that are pertinent to the community

In addition, community nutritionists can utilize various **models** or **theories** (discussed later in this chapter) to implement a program. The nutritionist can determine which models or theories, if any, provide a good explanation or understanding of the problems that have been selected. For example, there is a model (Stages of Change Model) that can be used to work with people who may not be aware that they are affected by a nutrition-related health condition (such as high blood pressure); other models (Social Learning Theory) can help people acquire skills and motivate them to take preventive action. Depending on the type of health condition, some theories/models may be more useful than others. For many health conditions, especially complex ones, one single theory may not fully address the problems, and it may be necessary to consider and combine multiple theories or parts of a theory.[25]

To continue the previous example, to achieve the goals and objectives related to iron deficiency anemia in low-income minority children, the community nutritionist could develop a program plan that would:[2]

- Evaluate the developmental levels of 95 percent of the low-income minority children by contacting the health department and the neighborhood free clinics that will evaluate the children's developmental levels. WIC program eligibility will be determined for 90 percent of the children observed by the health department and neighborhood free clinics. This will involve WIC program personnel, the health department, and the neighborhood free clinics as the principal change agents.
- Implement an outreach program to identify at-risk infants not identified by the healthcare providers. This activity will involve using key informants, community and public health nurses, community leaders, and clinical dietitians in the community.
- Have as a goal that 85 percent of all the children who are eligible for WIC food supplements will enroll in the program.
- Teach mothers so that 70 percent of the mothers of the children enrolled in WIC will show four different methods of incorporating WIC supplements into their children's diet. The nutritionist will develop the nutrition education components and the marketing plan for the program. The local health department will provide the facilities, teaching rooms, materials, training, equipment, and funds for the program.

Designing Actions

The action plan is a concise statement of the methods, activities, or intervention strategies for a primary, secondary, and/or tertiary prevention program.[20] Interventions must be sufficiently intensive or forceful to achieve the objectives by the target date. Two examples of interventions are nutrition education and social marketing (e.g., public awareness campaigns), which are associated with social planning; these strategies are used in nationwide school and media initiatives in the United States to promote the consumption of fruits and vegetables (e.g., the Fruits & Veggies More Matters program). Social action uses lobbying strategies such as writing letters or making telephone calls to legislators to change a school lunch policy.[21] Community development organizations can use strategies such as community forums and key informants where critical discussion is supported. The following should be considered when designing a program's action plan: [20,21,26]

- Creating a more desirable environment and using communication as a technique
- The resources that are needed and the sources of funding
- The staff needed for the program and their responsibilities
- The theoretical framework that will be appropriate for the program

Another action that must be taken when carrying out a program is keeping accurate records that are designed specifically to support the programming processes and program activities. The nutritionist needs to be responsible for certain tasks:[27]

- Keeping a journal that can assist in tracking the actions and critically reflecting on the outcome.
- Establishing criteria for reviewing the methodologies using statistics. A systematic review is a useful method for summarizing the effectiveness of public health and other population-based interventions.
- Planning nutritional and dietary classes.
- Providing nutritional/dietary guidelines.
- Writing nutrition prescriptions.
- Documenting all activities to save time and prevent conflict.
- Coordinating, controlling, managing, and directing the program.
- Using documentation as a source of data for program evaluation.

Management System

There are two aspects to any management system. The first is the personnel who will manage and organize the program and make sure its goals and objectives will be adequately addressed. The skills and qualification of the staff will influence the quality of the nutrition program. The second aspect is the data system. The nutritionist needs to determine the method the program will use to measure and record data about the participants, their use of the program, and the program outcomes.[12] The use of quantitative methods, qualitative methods, or a combination of data collection methods provides the overall organizational structure needed for an efficient data system.[12,20]

Resources, Budgets, and Feasibility

A feasibility study occurs during a program initiation phase and must be accomplished before significant expenses are carried out. Determining the costs of a program is an essential part of program planning. It is important to calculate the actual cost of a program by determining both the direct costs (personnel salaries, travel reimbursement, equipment, supplies, continuing education for nutrition personnel, printing/postage, and marketing the program) and indirect costs (time lost from work by recipients participating in a program, childcare costs, utilities, building and grounds, and janitorial services). It is also important to plan for situations that may increase the cost of the program, such as an increase in the number of participants or the length of the education program, a need for additional equipment, staff, or space, and so on. Cost analysis, like other components of programming, becomes easier with practice. The community nutritionist who adds the skill of cost analysis to his or her repertoire will be well prepared to carry out a very effective program.[12,20]

Community and public health nutritionists working in nonprofit organizations and government agencies often encounter challenges in obtaining funds for all the components of a program. It is important

The skills and qualifications of the staff will influence the quality of the nutrition program.

that nutritionists link the budget to the program activities. This will reduce unnecessary activities, increase the efficiency of carrying out the program, and reduce costs. Funds may be available to pay personnel salaries, reimburse their travel, buy equipment, and plan a marketing campaign in the present year's budget, but there may not be enough funds to pay for supplies, conduct screening tests, and develop the educational materials.[28] At this stage in the program planning process, the community nutritionist needs to review the budget and other program elements (e.g., travel, marketing campaign) and decide whether outside funding such as cash grants or in-kind funds are available for the program.[12] Once the areas of need are identified, the nutritionist can then prepare and submit grant proposals for funding.

Funding sources include grants and contracts from local, state, or federal agencies; foundations; and private contributions. Grants are a source of initial and ongoing funding. The funding organization generally releases guidelines as to what the organization will fund. The guidelines are frequently released as a request for proposals (RFP). These proposals specify how the nutrition center or program would meet the goals of the granting organization in a given time line. They describe the services and planned client outcomes. See Chapter 13 for more information on grant writing.

Contracts are another source of funding, and can be with the local government, state agencies, or private organizations. Contracts are drawn up for a particular service with project outcomes and a given time line. They provide opportunities for nutrition centers and programs to advance services, practices, and education. For example, the local WIC program may ask for a contract from the local government to perform nutrition screening for admission into the WIC program.

Resources should be sought both within and outside the community. Organizations within the community may serve as resources and can promote community self-reliance. These need to be considered before looking for resources outside the community.[12] For example, students enrolled in a food and nutrition program may collaborate with experienced retired nutritionists and take turns teaching adolescent parents instead of bringing in outside assistance. Possible sources of support both within and outside the community include businesses, social and professional clubs, volunteers, community institutions, and agencies such as churches, schools, and colleges.

The Public Health Service of the U.S. Department of Health and Human Services and the U.S. Department of Agriculture both have been the principal government sources of funding for food and nutrition programs. To take advantage of the funding provided by these agencies, community nutritionists must link their programs to the types of projects/research these agencies fund. Examples of private philanthropic foundations who may provide funding include the W.K. Kellogg Foundation and the Rockefeller Foundation.

Managing Tasks and Time

Program planning needs to be linked with time estimates and task specifications. In the case of a comprehensive nutrition and health program, the time frame necessary for development may be a year or more.[20] For new individual programs, it may require up to 6 months of planning to implement a health promotion effort. To promote success in planning a project, some type of time framework must be established.[20] For example, if students are involved, let the students know when they need to complete their work; if elders need immunizations prior to flu season, note when the immunizations should be finished; or if the project is funded by an agency, state clearly when a final report is expected.[21,29] From these fixed time requirements, the nutritionist and community can work backward to the present; however, if there are no time requirements, working forward from the present is possible.

Time and task management tools can be used during all phases of programming and are helpful when a number of people are working on different aspects of the program. These tools should list goals, objectives, action strategies, and time lines that indicate tasks or activities that must be done, by whom, and when. Creating two time lines—an optimistic time line as well as an alternative one (for if things take longer)—may be a wise choice. All tools can be modified, such as, modifying the language to match the needs of the targeted audience.[21]

Program Implementation

Program implementation is the process of putting a program into action or executing a plan.[21,30] An intervention program's implementation must be based on program goals, objectives, and outcomes. The nutritionist must consider the following:[4]

- The quality of the program implementation
- How to handle unexpected situations
- How to keep the program on track
- The back-up plans for unexpected situations

In the implementation phase of the program planning process, the clients, providers, and administrators must select the best plan to solve the original problem. This stage of the process involves work and activities aimed at achieving the stakeholders' expectations.[31] The person or group who established the goals and objectives may make the implementation efforts or these may be delegated to others. Providing reasons why a particular solution/model was chosen will help the nutritionist get the administration's approval for the plan. It is important to involve clients and administrators throughout the planning process; this helps promote acceptance of the plan.

It is very important to state clearly how the program will be implemented. The implementation of a program may be time limited, such

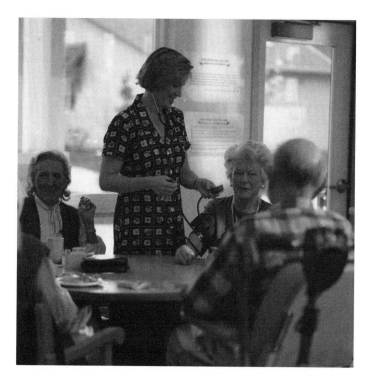

People who do not come to health promotion programs may be the most marginalized or at risk. Hold community forums in settings frequented by seniors; those who attend can help with networking.

as a 10-month program for women's health issues or a 1-year letter-writing campaign to reduce fat intake in school-age children. Tasks, time, and resources must be carefully monitored during implementation to best utilize the program's funds.

Implementation is shaped by the nutritionist's chosen roles, the type of health or nutrition problem selected as the focus for intervention, the community's readiness to take part in problem solving, and the characteristics of the social change process.

Community nutritionists should not be surprised at unexpected situations. There may be glitches in carrying out the program, such as failure to ensure that the promotional materials (handouts, fliers, and illustrations) are culturally appropriate or there were too few public transportation routes to the program site. The need to make changes during the implementation period does not mean that the program was not well planned—changes are inevitable. The nutritionist must anticipate the unexpected, such as reallocation of funds during the program, clients not responding to the invitation to participate in the intervention program, clients not cooperating fully (e.g., not completing a questionnaire for evaluation of the program), or presentation slides not working.[12] Community nutritionists need to continuously consider how things can be improved.

The people who are the hardest to reach are sometimes neglected in the planning phase. These people, who often do not come to events such as community forums, may be the most marginalized or at risk and may be the people whom the program is most intended to benefit. Bracht and Kingsbury argue that it is the practitioner who finds it "hard to hear" rather than the client who is "hard to reach."[32] It is important to make meaningful connections with these people. If the planning phase is not appropriately planned and friendly, people will not be receptive to intervention strategies.

A method of increasing participation (and voice) among seniors was incorporated in one community development project. Hitchcock et al. formed a steering committee with a balance of seniors and practitioners.[21] Community forums were held in settings frequented by seniors. Those who came to community forums were invited to join a networking process whereby they designed questions, practiced interviewing, and then went into the community to interview other seniors. Through this procedure, interviewees suggested additional names of people who had not participated (e.g., house-bound seniors). The interviewers were paid as research assistants from a government grant. Opportunities for empowerment and increased community competence among seniors were obvious in this method, and, amazingly, meaningful information was gained about the seniors' views and goals.

Program Evaluation

Evaluation is defined as the methods used to determine whether a service is needed and likely to be used, whether it is conducted as planned, whether the service actually helps the purpose, and whether objectives are carried out or planned activities are completed.[3] The first item listed also is referred to as *formative evaluation*. This type of evaluation begins with an assessment of the need for a program. The evaluation conducted to assess program outcomes or as a follow-up to the results of the program activities is called *summative evaluation*. An allocation of 10 percent of the program budget is recommended for evaluation.[7]

Evaluation Types

As mentioned earlier, evaluation may be formative, occurring throughout all programming processes, or summative, occurring at an end point. Formative evaluation is ongoing and provides information to those planning and implementing the program during the program implementation. The purpose of this type of evaluation is to strengthen or improve the program being evaluated, to determine the quality of its implementation and permit improvements to the program while activities are in progress.[21,33] Health promotion programs also conduct a formative assessment to:[33,34]

- Understand the perspective in which the intervention will take place and the development of consensus on goals.
- Assess the participants' reactions to the program and improve the health promotion programs.
- Identify specific behaviors of concern and the cause of these behaviors.
- Identify community attitudes that might inhibit or promote program goals.
- Identify resources that are available to the program. Formative assessment is the key to improving the relevance, sustainability, and effectiveness of community-based public health programs.[35]

Summative evaluation on the other hand provides retrospective information about the performance of the program and it is conducted at the completion of the program.[8,33] It assesses changes in behaviors, attitudes, knowledge or health status indicators such as morbidity, mortality, risk behaviors, and others.

Why Program Evaluation and with Whom

Program evaluation is an ongoing process from the beginning of the planning phase until the program ends. The goal of the evaluation must be clear to everyone involved in the program. Program evaluation provides critical information (e.g., the number of participants enrolled, the outcomes, and impact) for funding agencies, top-level decision makers, program accreditation reviewers, and the community at large.[2] Evaluation of an intervention is carried out from the following perspectives:[12,36]

- To see whether the objectives have been achieved
- To determine whether the procedures were carried out according to expectations
- To identify the strengths and weaknesses of the program materials
- To determine the impact of the program
- To test new methods/approaches
- To justify expanding the program, reducing the program, or even closing it

In addition, it shows whether the program is fulfilling its purpose. The major goals of program evaluation are to determine the relevance, progress, efficiency, effectiveness, and impact of program activities. The evaluation aspects include the following:[2,20,37]

- *Evaluation of relevance:* The need for the program
- *Progress:* Tracking of program activities to meet program objectives; assessing whether the program is functioning as planned
- *Efficiency:* The relationship between program outcomes and the resources spent
- *Effectiveness:* The ability to meet program objectives and the results of program efforts
- *Impact:* Long-term changes in the client population
- *Standards:* Determining whether the program staff have the needed credentials; making sure the staff is trained to provide the program

All persons involved in implementing a program need to be a part of the plan for program evaluation. The individuals concerned with evaluation may be divided into four categories:[21,33]

- *The population/community itself:* The community must be invited to participate in the evaluation process, because the actions to be evaluated concern them directly.
- *The change agents (e.g., the community nutritionists, the physician):* They will play an important role in the evaluation process. Moreover, this evaluation will help them improve their performance.
- *The evaluation specialists internal or external to the planning team:* They will provide technical expertise for the evaluation.
- *The sponsors and government representatives:* This will allow them to see the impact of the activities they have promoted and to consider further expansion of the program.

In addition, the results of program evaluation can be used to influence public policy, distribute resources, and persuade politicians and community leaders who have the power to change policies or address a health issue. For example, the high rate of cancer deaths in two rural towns in northeast Colorado prompted community leaders to take action and request an intervention by their local university nutrition department. A research study identified that the rate of cancer incidence was higher (14 percent above the state norm) in these two counties. Citizens, aware that nutrition and eating practices could lower cancer risk, contacted their Colorado State University Cooperative Extension agent for program possibilities. A team was formed to work in these remote small towns to improve nutrition, diet, and health using the

5-A-Day message. The intervention also included fruit and vegetable demonstrations, newspaper articles, pamphlets, discussions, taste testing, and fruit and vegetable puppet shows explaining 5-A-Day and the importance of fruits and vegetables to grades K–6. The nutritionist evaluated the program using 24-hour food recall and pre- and post questionnaires to assess fruit and vegetable consumption.

Results showed that the children had an increased awareness of fruits and vegetables in their diet. The residents of the counties stated that they liked the newspaper articles, pamphlet, and demonstrations and would like the 5-A-Day nutrition and cancer prevention program to continue.[38]

According to the World Health Organization's European Working Group, evaluation of health promotion programs should be participatory. In participatory evaluation, community leaders or participants of the program decide what to evaluate, select the methods and data sources, carry out the evaluation, analyze the data, and present the findings. Participatory evaluation approaches increase the likelihood that results will be directly useful in creating community change.[7] In general, program evaluation consists of three integral parts:[6,21]

- *Responsiveness:* How well the program performed with the problem concerning the program
- *Effectiveness:* How well the desired outcomes were achieved
- *Efficiency:* How much was achieved with the minimum use of resources

The Program Process Evaluation

Program evaluation is often conceptualized in terms of process, structure, impact, and outcomes. *Process* describes all the activities that are conducted to produce change.[2] Process evaluation answers the question, "Was the program implemented as planned?" It centers on program activities instead of outcome. This includes items such as the budget, the program organization, distributing educational materials to all the participants in a timely manner, and accurately anticipating the number of people attending a lunch or after-hours workshop, and if the facilities are accessible.[20,21] Programs are not often implemented exactly as planned. For example, a program activity may be altered based on midterm feedback from the participants. Another example is changing the time the program is offered because working parents could not participate or excuse themselves from work to attend the program. See **Box 12-3** for a program evaluation questionnaire.

Structural evaluation consists of assessing the resources used in providing the nutrition program. Process and structural evaluations provide support for outcome evaluation because the interpretation of program outcomes depends on an understanding of the program as it happens.[2] Structural evaluation also refers to evaluating the settings in which the program is carried out and includes materials, qualifications of the staff, organizational structure, and factors related to program delivery such as the training of personnel and equipment (e.g., blood pressure apparatus, skinfold caliper, bone densitometry).[2,12] This evaluation approach is based on the assumption that, given a proper setting with adequate equipment, good nutrition programming will be achieved.

Outcome evaluation (also known as summative evaluation) is the results of the program. The value of outcome evaluation is that it provides the best information possible about program performance. It evaluates if the program achieved the stated goals and objectives. Outcome evaluation is the most difficult because it involves an assessment of health status indicators and quality of life that were identified in the planning stage. For instance, Rivera et al. studied the nutritional outcome of a large-scale, incentive-based development program on 373 intervention groups in Mexico. Children and pregnant and lactating women in participating households received fortified nutrition supplements, and the families received nutrition education, healthcare, and cash transfers. The outcome measures showed better growth rates in children and lower rates of anemia in low-income, rural infants and children in Mexico.[39] Another example of outcome indicators includes epidemiological statistics such as mortality, morbidity, and disability rates. For instance, a cohort study showed that children who were exposed to methylmercury from traditional seafood diets that include pilot whale meat were significantly associated with deficits in motor, attention, and verbal tests.[40] Additional examples of indicators include safety, behavior, health-related policies, individual and population health status, and use of resources.[41] The satisfaction of stakeholders may or may not be a good indicator of program success (e.g., parents of teens may not be satisfied about after-school physical activities, but the program may help prevent obesity and heart disease).

The terms *outcome* and *impact evaluation* are sometimes used interchangeably, but sometimes are used differently to reflect time differences.[21] Impact evaluation measures the immediate effects of the program on participants' knowledge, attitudes, and behaviors. It assesses changes in the well-being of individuals, households, or communities that can be attributed to the nutrition program. For example, immediate and short-term outcomes are assessed shortly after completion of a program to determine whether the results were as expected (impact). The important impact evaluation question is, "What would have happened to the participant's receiving the intervention if they had not received the program?" For example, upon completion of a Fruit & Veggies More Matters program, the number of participants who consumed fruits and vegetables increased (impact). In the longer term, outcomes are assessed after a certain amount of time has elapsed (e.g., 1 year later) to determine whether changes occurred as anticipated. For example, the number of participants who consumed fruits and vegetables increased and the incidence of high blood pressure and high blood cholesterol decreased (impact) 1 year after the health promotion program. Long-term outcome evaluation is difficult because it requires resources for longitudinal tracking. Also, participants' cooperation and compliance is equally difficult. **Box 12-3** presents an example of program evaluation.

Data Sources and Collection Methods

After the type of evaluation and overall evaluation questions have been decided, the next step is the selection of data sources and data collection methods. Some granting agencies may specify their preferred method or source of data collection. Data sources usually include people and documents. Collection methods include:[6]

- Interviews (face-to-face or telephone)
- Focus groups
- Observations
- Surveys (questionnaire mailings)
- Medical record reviews

Telephone and mail surveys are less expensive than face-to-face interviews and are easier to use for a population-based survey. Not all clients, especially low-income persons, have telephones, however, and this method may produce skewed results.[42] Information about the percentage of the population with telephones is available from the local telephone company. Chart or record reviews are an effective method of collecting data when clinic or program participants are the population of interest or are an appropriate convenience sample.

Box 12-3 Survey Questions for Program Evaluation

Open-Ended

Describe some reasons for attending the program on breastfeeding.

Explain your beliefs about breastfeeding promotion.

Describe your experience with the breastfeeding program

What did you like about the program?

What did you dislike about the program?

Closed-Ended

- Please rate your satisfaction with the breastfeeding program:
  - Very satisfied
  - Somewhat satisfied
  - Unsatisfied
  - Very unsatisfied

Rate the teaching strategies used in the breastfeeding program:

  - Excellent
  - Very Good
  - Good
  - Poor

From: Clark CC. *Health Promotion in Communities: Holistic and Wellness Approaches.* New York: Springer Publishing; 2002. Reproduced with permission of Springer Publishing Company, LLC, New York.

include time lost from work by recipients participating in a program, childcare costs, utilities, building and grounds, and janitorial services.

Benefits are the positive outcomes or consequences of a program. It is easier to determine costs than benefits, which are more complex. For example, if a program benefit is a change in an individual's food purchasing patterns, then that benefit can be valued as the money saved from the new mix of foods purchased. However, intangible costs and benefits, especially benefits, can be measured more directly without using a dollar value.[45] Some examples could include knowledge gained, attitudes changed, skills acquired, reduced healthcare cost, practices adopted, and individual and societal end results. **Figure 12-4** presents potential economic benefits associated with nutrition education on obesity and blood cholesterol.

Program Assessment

Assessment—which includes data-gathering, analyses, and reporting process—of health promotion and disease prevention programs is used to determine program outcomes and measure overall program effectiveness. Most external agencies also require that program directors assess program effectiveness to justify the program's cost.

A wide variety of assessment instruments are used to appraise health promotion programs. Some instruments focus on assessing general health status whereas others focus on more specific health behaviors such as diet. A health risk appraisal can be used to assess current health behaviors, judge the impact of behaviors on health status, and also predict future outcome. An example of a health status assessment is the Duke Health Profile (shown earlier in **Figure 12-3**).[46] It is designed to assess functional health status over a 1-week time period.[47] It has 11 scales: physical health, mental health, social health, general health, perceived health, self-esteem, anxiety, depression, anxiety-depression, pain, and disability.[20]

Nutrition assessment instruments are used in health promotion programs to assess dietary habits and nutrition-related health conditions such as heart disease, obesity, osteoporosis, and diabetes. It is essential to choose a valid and reliable instrument to collect the needed information. In addition to validity and reliability, assessment instruments need to be usable by the intended audiences. A 24-hour recall, food frequency checklist, and 3-day food record are the most widely used nutrition assessment tools and are effective in most cases. These instruments are discussed in Chapter 2.

Nutrition assessment is also used to monitor the progress of national programs. For example, studies show that some modifiable maternal behaviors and experiences before, during, and after pregnancy are associated with undesirable health outcomes for the mother and her infant (e.g., physical abuse, insufficient folic acid consumption, smoking during pregnancy, and improper infant sleep position).[48,49] The Pregnancy Risk Assessment Monitoring System (PRAMS) is an ongoing, state- and population-based surveillance system designed to monitor selected maternal behaviors and experiences that occur before, during, and after pregnancy among women who deliver live-born infants.[50] Between 2000 and 2003, PRAMS mailed a sample of three self-administered surveys to mothers and interviewed non-responders by telephone. The survey data were linked to selected birth certificate data to create annual PRAMS analysis data sets that can be used to produce statewide estimates of perinatal health behaviors and experiences among

Standardized surveys may be used, or they may be created specifically for the program.[43] An example of a questionnaire created for a program is shown in **Figure 12-3**. In the field of nutrition, two commonly used survey methods are the 24-hour recall and the food frequency list. Obtaining accurate 24-hour recall information requires a highly skilled interviewer who uses visual prompts, such as measuring cups or spoons, food models, and different-sized cups and bowls.

Cost-Benefit Analysis

Cost-benefit analysis (CBA) of a nutrition program is the evaluation of the costs of a program in relation to health outcomes. CBA converts program inputs and output into monetary terms and then determines whether there is a net benefit to the program by subtracting costs from benefits.[44] It also evaluates program efficiency.[3] Costs are the value of the resources that must be used to develop, implement, and operate the program being analyzed. Community nutritionists must estimate the tangible and intangible and the direct and indirect costs of the program. The activities in a program that are valued in dollars are referred to as tangible; those that cannot be valued easily in dollars are referred to as intangible. Direct costs are the resources budgeted for or assigned to the program. Direct cost can be directly associated with the project with a high degree of accuracy. Examples of direct costs include personnel salaries, travel reimbursement, equipment, supplies, continuing education for nutrition personnel, printing, and marketing the program. Indirect costs are resources that allow the program to operate, but are not directly attributable to a specific program. Examples

cost-benefit analysis The analytic process whereby the costs and benefits of a program are identified and measured in monetary (dollar) terms.

Date Today: _____ Name: _____ ID Number: _____

Date of Birth: _____ Female _____ Male _____

INSTRUCTIONS: Here are some questions about your health and feelings. Please read each question carefully and check (√) your best answer. You should answer the questions in your own way. There are no right or wrong answers. (Please ignore the small scoring numbers next to each blank.)

	Yes, describes me exactly	Somewhat describes me	No, doesn't describe me at all
1. I like who I am.....................................	12	11	10
2. I am not an easy person to get along with.........	20	21	22
3. I am basically a healthy person....................	32	31	30
4. I give up too easily...............................	40	41	42
5. I have difficulty concentrating	50	51	52
6. I am happy with my family relationships...........	62	61	60
7. I am comfortable being around people............	72	71	70

TODAY would you have any physical trouble or difficulty:

	None	Some	A lot
8. Walking up a flight of stairs	82	81	80
9. Running the length of a football field	92	91	90

During the **PAST WEEK:** How much trouble have you had with:

	None	Some	A lot
10. Sleeping	102	101	100
11. Hurting or aching in any part of your body	112	111	110
12. Getting tired easily	122	121	120
13. Feeling depressed or sad	132	131	130
14. Nervousness	142	141	140

During the **PAST WEEK:** How often did you:

	None	Some	A lot
15. Socialize with other people (talk or visit with friends or relatives)	150	151	152
16. Take part in social, religious, or recreation activities (meetings, church, movies, sports, parties)	160	161	162

During the **PAST WEEK:** How often did you:

	None	1–4 Days	4–7 Days
17. Stay in your home, a nursing home, or hospital because of sickness, injury, or other health problem	172	171	170

FIGURE 12-3 Duke Health Profile

PHYSICAL HEALTH SCORE

Item		Raw Score*
8	=	_____
9	=	_____
10	=	_____
11	=	_____
12	=	_____
Sum	=	_____ × 10 =

MENTAL HEALTH SCORE

Item		Raw Score*
1	=	_____
4	=	_____
5	=	_____
13	=	_____
14	=	_____
Sum	=	_____ × 10 =

SOCIAL HEALTH SCORE

Item		Raw Score*
2	=	_____
6	=	_____
7	=	_____
15	=	_____
16	=	_____
Sum	=	_____ × 10 =

GENERAL HEALTH SCORE

Physical Health score	=	_____
Mental Health score	=	_____
Social Health score	=	_____
Sum	=	_____ ÷ 3 =

PERCEIVED HEALTH SCORE

Item		Raw Score*
3	=	_____ × 50 =

SELF-ESTEEM SCORE

Item		Raw Score*
1	=	_____
2	=	_____
4	=	_____
6	=	_____
7	=	_____
Sum	=	_____ × 10 =

To calculate the scores in this column the raw scores must be revised as follows: If 0, change to 2; if 2, change to 0; if 1, no change.

ANXIETY SCORE

Item		Raw Score*	Revised
2	=	_____	_____
5	=	_____	_____
7	=	_____	_____
10	=	_____	_____
12	=	_____	_____
14	=	_____	_____
	Sum	=	_____ × 8.333 =

DEPRESSION SCORE

Item		Raw Score*	Revised
4	=	_____	_____
5	=	_____	_____
10	=	_____	_____
12	=	_____	_____
13	=	_____	_____
	Sum	=	_____ × 10 =

ANXIETY-DEPRESSION (DUKE-AD) SCORE

Item		Raw Score*	Revised
4	=	_____	_____
5	=	_____	_____
7	=	_____	_____
10	=	_____	_____
12	=	_____	_____
13	=	_____	_____
14	=	_____	_____
	Sum	=	_____ × 7.143 =

PAIN SCORE

Item		Raw Score*	Revised
11	=	_____	_____ × 50 =

DISABILITY SCORE

Item		Raw Score*	Revised
17	=	_____	_____ × 50 =

Raw Score = last digit of the numeral adjacent to the blank checked by the respondent for each item. For example, if the second blank is checked for item 10 (blank numeral = 101), then the raw score is "1," because 1 is the last digit of 101.

Final Score is calculated from the raw scores as shown and entered into the box for each scale. For physical health, mental health, social health, general health, self-esteem, and perceived health, 100 indicates the best health status, and 0 indicates the worst health status. For anxiety, depression, anxiety-depression, pain, and disability, 100 indicates the worst health status and 0 indicates the best health status.

Missing Values: If one or more responses is missing within one of the eleven scales, a score cannot be calculated for that particular scale.

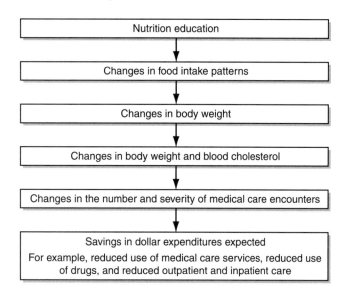

FIGURE 12-4 Potential Economic Benefits Associated with Nutrition Education on Obesity and Blood Cholesterol

Modified from Kaufman M. *Nutrition in promoting the public's health: Strategies, principles, and practice.* 2007. Sudbury, MA: Jones and Bartlett.

women delivering live infants. The data from 19 states measured progress toward achieving HP 2010 objectives for the following eight perinatal indicators:[51]

- *Pregnancy intention:* Results show that in 2003, the prevalence of intended pregnancy among women having a live birth ranged from 48.1 percent in Louisiana to 66.5 percent in Maine.
- *Multivitamin use:* In 2003, the prevalence of multivitamin use at least four times per week during the month before pregnancy ranged from 23.0 percent in Arkansas to 45.2 percent in Maine. During 2000–2003, multivitamin use increased significantly in three states (Illinois, North Carolina, and Utah).
- *Physical abuse:* In 2003, the prevalence of physical abuse by a husband or partner during the 12 months before pregnancy ranged from 2.2 percent in Maine to 7.6 percent in New Mexico; during 2000–2003, significant decreases were recorded in three states (Alaska, Hawaii, and Nebraska).
- *Cigarette smoking during pregnancy:* In 2003, the prevalence of abstinence from cigarette smoking during the last 3 months of pregnancy ranged from 72.5 percent in West Virginia to 96.1 percent in Utah.
- *Cigarette smoking cessation:* In 2003, the prevalence of smoking cessation during pregnancy ranged from 30.2 percent in West Virginia to 65.8 percent in Utah.
- *Drinking alcohol during pregnancy:* In 2003, the prevalence of abstinence from alcohol during the last 3 months of pregnancy ranged from 91.3 percent in Colorado to 98.0 percent in Utah.
- *Breastfeeding initiation:* In 2003, the prevalence of mothers who breastfed their babies in the early postpartum period ranged from 51.2 percent in Louisiana to 90.3 percent in Alaska. During 2000–2003, significant increases were recorded in six states (Arkansas, Illinois, Louisiana, Nebraska, North Carolina, and South Carolina).

- *Infant sleep position:* In 2003, the prevalence of healthy full-term infants who were placed to sleep on their backs ranged from 50.0 percent in Arkansas to 78.7 percent in Washington. During 2000–2003, significant increases were recorded in eight states (Alaska, Colorado, Illinois, Louisiana, Maine, Nebraska, North Carolina, and West Virginia).

Some health promotion program assessments such as PRAMS are continuous. **Figure 12-5** presents five phases of a continuous inquiry and learning process. Each phase comprises two or three concrete steps. Some steps are to be carried out in assessment team meetings and some in meetings with all program participants. The entire process takes about 24 hours to complete over a period of 1 to 4 months, depending on the needs and structure of the program. However, the process is flexible; it allows programs and organizations to carry out the implementation process as needed. The guides for action planning based on assessment results, included in Phase 5 of the process, make the link between the assessment process and program improvement to promote a continuous inquiry cycle.

Reporting Program Success

Results and recommendations from the various program evaluations need to be summarized, analyzed, and interpreted at regular intervals in statistical, graphic, and narrative reports written according to agency requirements and outlines. The program director is often responsible for writing the report. There should be a list of who will receive the report and a strategy for distribution.[3] One aspect of reporting should be weekly, monthly, or quarterly informal feedback to the staff. Quarterly or semiannual written and verbal reports should be reviewed with the staff and administrators, and annual written reports should be sent to the agency board, funding agencies, and the public.

Most agencies publish annual reports that summarize their work during the year and that are disseminated to the community.[52] Nutrition services should be highlighted in these reports and successful programs showcased to the community through media coverage. **Table 12.2** presents an example of a formal report format. See **Box 12-4** for a sample of a program report.

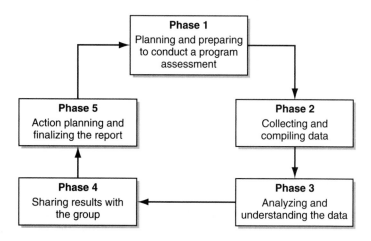

FIGURE 12-5 The Five Phases of the Continuous Assessment

Source: O'Connor C, Zeldin S. Program assessment and improvement through youth-adult partnership: The YALPE Resource Kit. *Journal of Extension.* 2005; 43(5):1–4. Reprinted with permission.

TABLE 12.2 Formal Report Format[12,52-55]

Report Elements	Content
Prefatory section	*Title Page/Front Cover*
	• The title of the report (for some reports, this must be centered, all in caps, and about 1½ inches from the top of the page).
	• The name and title of the person for whom the report is intended.
	• The name, position, and business address of the writer.
	• The date the report is issued.
	• The fiscal year of the report.
	• Begin pagination with the title page.
	• Prefatory parts are paginated with small Roman numerals (i, ii, iii, iv).
	Table of Contents
	• The table of contents provides a map of the structure of the complete report, from the cover page to the appendix.
	Table of Figures
	• List three or more visual aids such as tables and/or figures and their page numbers.
	Abstract/Executive Summary
	• The summary of the entire report.
	• Write the abstract after the report has been written.
Body section	*Background Information*
	• State the objective of the program.
	• Provide background information on the issue or program.
	• Discuss the type of theoretical framework that was used.
	• Describe the equipment (skinfold caliper, blood pressure apparatus, etc.)
	• Provide results/outcomes of the program.
	• Describe how the program was carried out.
	• Use the visual aids to summarize the findings/outcomes.
	• Refer to visual aids within the text before presenting them.
	• Discuss the results.
	• Show how certain outcomes were achieved.
	• Include the strengths and weaknesses of the program.
Terminal section	*Conclusion*
	• Summarize the major findings/outcome of the program.
	Recommendations
	• Recommend specific courses of action (to take or avoid).
	• List the recommendations in order of priority.
	Work Cited
	• List all your sources of information.
	Optional Appendix
	• Contains any other data that would clarify the report.
	• This is supplementary material that would interrupt the flow of the body of the report (such as charts, figures, maps, and pictures).

Box 12-4 **A Sample of a Program Report**

Prefatory Section

Understanding Menopause

By

Dr. Nweze Nnakwe

Program Director
To
Illinois Department of Public Health Office of Women's Health
June 30, 2006

Table of Contents

Table of Figures

Body Section

Background Information

The objective of this program was to increase the knowledge of physiological and emotional changes that may often be experienced during perimenopause and menopause in women 40–60 years old. This program utilized the Health Belief Model. Participants were recruited through a variety of strategies such as distributing flyers throughout McLean County in various businesses and organizations, fitness centers, churches, and newsletters. The program was advertised in newspapers, local TV stations, and radio stations. The local CNN Headline News interviewed the director, which aired for 2 weeks. Gift giveaways such as Boca

coupons were one of the strategies utilized to recruit participants. The nutritionist developed a website and educational materials including a brochure, PowerPoint slides, handouts including nutritional recipes, and posters on how to increase women's knowledge of the physiological and emotional changes that may often be experienced during perimenopause and menopause. The nutritionist conducted 15 workshops and/or seminars to educate women about menopause and health-related issues such as heart disease and osteoporosis, obesity, and stress management. The director initiated a Health Night Fair at an African American church. The program reached the targeted population of 280 for the first year. A 3-month follow-up survey showed that there were some behavior changes such as improved nutrition knowledge, improved level of physical activity, increased number of women beginning hormone replacement therapy, and increase in the use of soy products. The difficulty associated with the program is low attendance at the sessions.

Terminal Section

Conclusion

The targeted population of 280 was reached for the first year. The first quarter of the first year was used to develop the program. Implementation of the program started fully in the second quarter. Eighty-five percent of the participants reported behavior change.

Recommendation

In addition to the first year's strategies, utilizing personal contact with businesses, women's organizations, and churches for the recruitment of participants will be helpful. Continued collaboration with wellness programs and other organizations such as the Heart and Lung Association will be important.

Works Cited and Appendix were not used.

Programming Paradigms, Models, or Theories

Program paradigms are defined as representations of approaches to programming that offer explanations of the processes involved. To provide guidance throughout programming processes, communities and nutritionists together may either create their own model or use an already-tested programming or planning model. Sometimes a model is recommended by a funding agency. Because all models are based on values and assumptions, the nutritionist needs to ensure that the chosen model is either consistent with the nutrition ideas or can be adequately adapted.[21] Community nutritionists can use different models to provide effective nutrition education. The following sections describe different types of models that have been shown to be effective.

program paradigms
Representations of approaches to programming that offer explanations of the processes involved.

Program Planning Using Theories/Models

In the past, program planning, implementation, and evaluation activities were frequently based on the premise that communities were the recipients of programs rather than partners in programming. There is now value in considering other ways of programming that can create opportunities for processes that empower the community (i.e., create opportunities for community control). In this perspective, frameworks refer to schemes that specify the steps in a process.[2] For example, community nutritionists could use a framework that includes listening, critical reflection, participatory dialogue, theme recognition, action, and reflection on action. Regardless of the programming framework the community nutritionist prefers, knowledge of a variety of frameworks is helpful because he or she will be working with people from diverse backgrounds.

When concepts and constructs are related to each other and purposely combined to form a unit, the resulting entity may be labeled a framework, a model, or a theory.[56] Generally, a framework is a planning tool (e.g., the PRECEDE model discussed later in the chapter). It can incorporate theories, models, or parts thereof, and it allows for the organization of a large and unspecified number of potentially predictive or explanatory variables.

Program models are ways of viewing real events, and they can be physical, symbolic, or mental. A program model describes what the nutritionist should do to provide both effective instruction and the support services needed to persist in the learning process long enough to create a behavior change.[57] A physical model is a specific, observable replica of a real structure (e.g., chemical equations, anatomic models, and food models). Symbolic models have a higher level of abstraction than do physical models. For example, signs have symbolic meanings to those who read them. A "No Smoking" sign signifies that the readers should refrain from smoking. Mental models have an even greater level of abstraction than both physical and symbolic models because they convey a mental image, not a real picture. For example, the term *nutrition* has different meanings for different people.[2]

A theory is a construct that accounts for or organizes events. A nutrition theory explains or describes a specific event of nutrition. Theories provide nutritionists with different lenses through which to see situations; each lens provides a different view and understanding. In general, the most effective programs are those that are theory based.[21]

Health Belief Model (HBM)

The Health Belief Model emphasizes perceived threat as a motivating force and perceived benefits (fewer barriers) as a preferred path to action.[58] It asserts that readiness to take action to avoid an illness or condition is possible because people will:[58,59,60]

- Perceive themselves as threatened by the condition, which in turn is determined by a perception of personal vulnerability ("How likely am I to get heart disease and how soon?") and perceived severity of the condition ("How bad would it be to have heart disease?").

- Perceive that the recommended course of action to reduce the threat is feasible and efficacious ("Will I feel better if I change the fats or the diet that I eat?") and that the barriers or costs to it are low ("How hard will it be to make these changes in my diet or fat intake?").

- Believe that they have the ability to successfully perform the recommended behavior ("How confident am I that I can succeed in changing my diet and fat intake?").

Application
Strychar examined the relationship among knowledge, health beliefs, and dietary behaviors of participants using the Health Belief Model.[61,62] A total of 3,432 individuals ages 18 to 74 participated in a screening program conducted in 54 supermarkets in Montreal and Quebec. This program identified participants' risk for cardiovascular disease by measuring total serum cholesterol, blood pressure, height, weight, level of physical activity, and tobacco use. A 10-minute debriefing counseling session interpreted risk factors and recommended follow-up. Seventy percent ($n = 2,420$) also completed a nutrition questionnaire on knowledge, health beliefs, and frequency of consumption of high-fat foods. Respondents increased their knowledge and reduced the frequency of consumption of high-fat foods following the screening program, particularly individuals with higher blood cholesterol levels and high blood pressure. Depending on the relative strength of benefits and

barriers, program strategies could target either the benefits of change or overcoming the barriers.

Knowledge-Attitude-Behavior Model (KABM)

The Knowledge-Attitude-Behavior Model (KABM) stresses that a gain in new knowledge leads to changes in attitude, which, in turn, result in improved dietary behavior or practices.[63] For changes in attitude and behavior to occur, the knowledge provided must be motivational. Research suggests that some types of knowledge are more motivating than others. Rogers refers to "awareness" knowledge as the kind that captures people's attention, increases awareness, and enhances motivation, whereas "how-to" knowledge is the kind people need when they are already motivated.[64] Social psychological research makes a similar distinction, with "anticipated consequences" or expectancies as the kind of knowledge that is likely to enhance motivation to take action (motivational knowledge), whereas "behavioral capabilities" (or knowledge and skills) are needed by people in order to act on their motivations (instrumental knowledge). Also, it is important to consider the acquisition of attitudes. For example, an attitude can be acquired passively by observation (e.g., watching a TV program on how to prepare a low-fat food) or acquired actively by the integration of beliefs about the consequences of an action (e.g., reducing sodium intake to lower blood pressure).[65,66]

General nutrition education interventions have used a stated or implied KABM, which emphasizes dissemination of "how-to" (e.g., how to reduce fat intake) or "skills" information (e.g., shopping with a grocery list). Topics that have been covered include food groups, balanced diets, label reading, high-fat or high-fiber foods, food shopping and preparation skills, managing food budgets, and food sources of nutrients. This kind of instrumental knowledge is essential for those already motivated to eat nutritiously, but for others it is just "information."[60,67] On the other hand, knowledge can be motivating when it is about the potential positive or negative consequences of behavior, particularly if these are of personal relevance or when they tap into other motivators and reinforcers of change.[68] Both motivational and instrumental, or how-to, knowledge are needed for effective nutrition education designed to promote behavioral change.

Application
The KABM is an educational strategy that uses an intervention approach. For example, a list of foods that are good sources of calcium or public announcements of good sources of calcium may be a motivational factor to dietary improvement for individuals who are concerned about the incidence of osteoporosis. However, memorizing a list of foods that are high in calcium does not result in a change in behavior.[69]

Social Learning Theory (SLT)

The Social Learning Theory (SLT) (also called Social Cognitive Theory or Social Influence Theory) emphasizes the interactive nature of the effects of cognitive and other personal factors and environmental events on behavior.[56] The three major constructs/concepts in SLT are behavioral capacity (having the skills necessary for the performance of the desired behavior, such as quitting excessive alcohol drinking), efficacy expectations (beliefs regarding one's ability to successfully carry out a course of action or perform a behavior), and outcome expectations (beliefs that the performance of a behavior will have the desired effects or consequences).[56,70]

The main idea in SLT is that of "reciprocal determinism." This means that behavior is determined by the interaction among three elements: the person, the person's behavior, and the environment.[56,71] The person's actions contribute to creating the environment, and the actions and environment contribute to the person's cognitions or "expectancies." There are three types of expectancies: beliefs about how events are connected, beliefs about the consequences of one's actions (outcome expectations), and beliefs about one's competence to perform the behavior needed to influence the outcomes (efficacy expectations). Incentives also contribute to behavior; incentive or reinforcement is the value of a particular outcome to a person.[56,72]

Application

When problem behaviors are closely tied to social or economic motivations, more comprehensive theories and models, such as the Social Learning Theory may be effective tools for planning nutrition interventions.[73] For instance, if a community nutritionist needs to promote milk-based foods as sources of dietary calcium, SLT would support an educational intervention addressing behavioral capability (knowledge and skills needed to select and prepare milk-based foods), reciprocal determinism (availability of milk-based foods in vending machines and restaurants), expectations (beliefs about osteoporosis as a consequence of avoiding milk-based foods), self-efficacy (confidence in one's ability to use more milk-based foods), observational learning or modeling (seeing peers and other role models drinking milk), and reinforcement (positive or negative feelings that occur when milk drinking is practiced).[74]

In the United States, few children fulfill the current national dietary recommendations to eat five servings of fruits and vegetables per day to promote optimal health and prevent chronic diseases.[75,76] A study examined the effectiveness of a 10-week classroom-based nutrition intervention program that combined child-focused interactive lessons and skill-building activities, repeated food tasting opportunities, and interactive parent-focused lessons on child-feeding strategies to increase children's fruit intake. The change in the children's knowledge, preference, and intake of fruit and parents' use of controlling child-feeding strategies were measured in a pretest/posttest manner. Lessons consisted of 1 hour of instruction provided to children and parents devoted to enhancing knowledge about a fruit, skills necessary to incorporate the fruit into the diet, and techniques to enhance goal-directed behaviors. The sessions included interactive discussions, case studies, brainstorming activities, and games. Topics covered in the classes included exposure (increasing the availability of healthful foods), monitoring (understanding that the children can self-regulate the amount of food they need each day), restriction (learning how to present a variety of foods to children without restricting access to certain foods), rewarding/punishing (understanding that using food as a reward or punishment can be counterproductive), and encouragement (learning how to present food to a child in a less aggressive manner without using verbal prompting).[61] Seventeen parent–child pairs participated in the first class session, which consisted of an orientation and preevaluation session, but were unable to attend any follow-up classes served as the control.

Parents were taken into a separate room, where they were given instruction on child-feeding strategies to enhance fruit acceptance. In the final half-hour of the session, parents rejoined their children in the food laboratory. During this period, parents and children were given the opportunity to sample 10 different fruits (apple, orange, banana, grape, pear, star fruit, mango, papaya, kiwifruit, and cantaloupe). The same 10 fruits were used in each class to give children several opportunities to taste them. Also during this segment of the class, parents were encouraged to practice feeding strategies they had learned earlier. There was a significant increase in knowledge scores and fruit intake by children in the experimental vs. the control group. Fruit preference scores were similar between groups. Additionally, there was a significant decrease in the use of controlling child-feeding strategies by parents in the intervention vs. the control group. This study showed that a nutrition intervention program consisting of extensive food exposure and parent-focused lessons on child-feeding strategies is feasible and can be effective.[77]

Figure 12-6 presents an example of how behavioral models can be used to provide positive nutrition messages for increasing consumption of fruit juice. Each level of the figure adds important concepts addressed by the models discussed in this section.

Theory of Reasoned Action (TRA)

The Theory of Reasoned Action (TRA) is a highly specific theory outlining cognitive and attitudinal determinants of behavior.[56,78] Attitudes and subjective norms determine an individual's intentions, which are

> I realize that fruit juice is a good way to help me get five servings of fruits and vegetables a day, but I have been drinking more soda than juice. I will start buying more juice and less soda the next time I go to the supermarket.
> Stages and processes of change
> **Transtheoretical Model**

> If the vending machines at my office have fruit juice, I would be likely to select it as a beverage.
> Reciprocal determinism
> **Social Cognitive Theory**

> I know that I can drink more fruit juice by making juice part of my weekly shopping list.
> Self-efficacy
> **Social Learning Theory, Transtheoretical and Health Belief Model**

> Vitamin C in fruit juice helps prevent oxidative damage to cells in my skin. If I don't get enough vitamin C, I might have more wrinkles when I get old. Having wrinkles would make me feel ugly. Drinking fruit juice is hard to do because coffee is cheaper.
> Perceived benefits, threats, and barriers
> **Health Belief Model**

> Fruit juice is an excellent source of vitamin C.
> Health information
> **Knowledge-Attitude-Behavior Model**

FIGURE 12-6 How Behavioral Models Can Provide Positive Nutrition Messages

Modified from: Freeland-Graves J, Nitzke S. Position of the American Dietetic Association: Total diet approach to communicating food and nutrition information. *J. Am. Diet. Assoc.* 2002; 102(1):100–108., Reprinted with permission.

foretelling of behavior. Behavior is likely to follow the stated intentions with a shorter the time span between intentions and behavior. The Theory of Reasoned Action is related to the Theory of Planned Behavior (TPB). According to the model, behavior is determined directly by a person's intention to perform the behavior. Intentions are the instructions people give to themselves to behave in certain ways.[79] They are characters that people use for their future behavior. In forming intentions, people tend to consider the outcome of their behavior and the opinion of significant others before committing themselves to a particular action.[80] In other words, attitudes and subjective norms influence an individual's belief that a certain behavior will have a given outcome, and this determines his or her attitudes by evaluating the actual outcome of his or her ability to control the behavior.[81]

Application

Interventions that aim to change dietary behavior provide the possibility for significant public health impact. Theory-based approaches to public health interventions are useful for designing, implementing, and evaluating research. At West Virginia University, Butterfield et al. used TRA to conduct an intervention study targeting high-fat (whole and 2 percent) milk users.[82]

The intervention was composed of systematic combinations of either 1) paid advertising (professionally produced TV, radio, and newspaper ads) played with heavy frequency and strategic placement, 2) public relations (events produced to garner extensive free or "earned" media coverage in local news), or 3) community education (in-store activities such as blind taste testing and school promotions such as poster design contests). Supermarket milk sales data were collected, and randomly selected intervention and comparison community residents were surveyed via telephone to assess milk use. TRA constructs were used in the surveys that were conducted immediately before and after a 6-week mass media campaign. Campaign messages were aimed at changing behavioral rather than normative beliefs.

Results showed significant and predicted changes in intervention participants on intention, attitude, and behavioral beliefs, but not subjective norm outcomes. The message-based intervention that focused upon a specific behavior produced statistically and practically significant public health effects: People reported more switching, and supermarkets showed increased low-fat milk sales. The study also showed that the combination of paid advertising with public relations produced the strongest effects. One of the strongest features of the theory is that it functions as a practical guide for producing behavior change.

Diffusion of Innovation Theory

Diffusion of Innovation Theory examines the process in which an innovative idea or practice achieves acceptance.[56,83] Behavior change in specific cultural groups or populations (e.g., starting physical activity, eating unfamiliar food) may be seen as the adoption of an innovative behavior. Diffusion of Innovation Theory identifies several key components:[56,84,85]

- *Compatibility:* If innovations are consistent with the economic, sociocultural, and philosophical value system of the adopter, then adoption is more likely to happen.
- *Flexibility:* Innovations that can be unraveled and used as separate components will be applicable in a wider variety of user settings.
- *Reversibility:* It is desirable that innovation has the capability of termination in case the adopting individual (or organization) wants

to revert to his or her (or its) previous practices. Innovations that are not capable of termination are less likely to be adopted.

- *Relative advantage:* Adoption is more likely if innovation seems to be more beneficial when compared to previous methods.
- *Complexity:* Complex innovations are more difficult to communicate and understand and are, therefore, less likely to be adopted.
- *Cost efficiency:* Innovation is desirable if its perceived benefits, both tangible and intangible, outweigh its perceived costs.
- *Risk:* The degree of uncertainty introduced by an innovation helps to determine its potential for adoption. Innovations that involve higher risk are less likely to be adopted.

Application

The mass media are an immediate and effective way of introducing new information or trying to influence attitudes, especially during the early stages of reaching audiences susceptible to accepting new ideas.[86] However, at the point of adoption, interpersonal channels are more influential.[87] A communications strategy could consist of using the mass media to introduce the message, provide knowledge, influence attitudes, and reinforce behavior and using interpersonal intervention to teach and encourage the adoption of the behavior.[88] When using the Diffusion of Innovation Theory to promote systemic change within WIC, for example, it is important to talk about the relative benefits of the innovation (e.g., a decrease in iron deficiency anemia in children) rather than mandating use of a new system or process.

Transtheoretical/Stages of Change Model

Another useful model for planning behavioral intervention programs is the Transtheoretical or Stages of Change Model. According to this conceptual model, health behavior change process is gradual, continuous, and dynamic.[89,90] People do not immediately change from old to new behaviors; instead, they progress through a sequence of five discrete states:[56,91]

1. *Precontemplative:* Individuals in this stage have no intention of changing their behavior. They are not aware of the risk, and they deny that adverse outcomes could happen to them or they are aware of the risk, but have made a decision not to change their behavior.
2. *Contemplative:* Individuals in this stage have the intentions to change, but have no specific plans to change soon.
3. *Preparation:* Individuals in this stage have plans to change their behavior and may have taken the first step of changing their behavior.
4. *Action:* Individuals in this stage have started to change their behavior, but the behavior change is fairly recent and may be inconsistent.
5. *Maintenance:* These individuals have maintained consistent behavior change for a long time. The newly acquired behavior has become a part of their lives.

This model suggests that individuals engaging in a new behavior go through the stages of precontemplation, contemplation, preparation, action, and maintenance, but not always in a linear manner; it also may be cyclical because many individuals must make several attempts at behavior change before their goals are realized. The amount of progress people make as a result of intervention tends to be a function of the stage they are in at the start of treatment.[56] **Table 12.3** presents the changes and techniques community nutritionists and participants

TABLE 12.3	**Stages of Change Model**	
Stage of Change	**Characteristics**	**Techniques**
Precontemplation	Not currently considering change: "Ignorance is bliss."	Validate lack of readiness. Clarify that the decision is theirs. Encourage reevaluation of current behavior. Encourage self-exploration, not action. Explain and personalize the risk.
Contemplation	Ambivalent about change: "Sitting on the fence." Not considering change within the next month.	Validate lack of readiness. Clarify that the decision is theirs. Encourage evaluation of pros and cons of behavior change. Identify and promote new, positive outcome expectations.
Preparation	Some experience with change and are trying to change: "Testing the waters." Planning to act within 1 month.	Identify and assist in problem solving regarding obstacles. Help identify social support. Verify that he or she has underlying skills for behavior change. Encourage small initial steps.
Action	Practicing new behavior for 3–6 months.	Focus on restructuring cues and social support. Bolster self-efficacy for dealing with obstacles. Combat feelings of loss and reiterate long-term benefits.
Maintenance	Continued commitment to sustaining new behavior after 6 months to 5 years.	Plan for follow-up support. Reinforce internal rewards. Discuss coping with relapse.
Relapse	Resumption of old behaviors: "Fall from grace."	Evaluate trigger for relapse. Reassess motivation and barriers. Plan stronger coping strategies.

Source: Prochaska JO, DiClemente CC. Stages and processes of self-change of smoking: toward an integrated model of change. *J Consulting Clin Psychol*. 1983; 51:390. Reprinted with permission.

can use to address each stage. The Successful Community Strategies feature in this chapter presents the approach used by Colorado State University at Fort Collins.

Application

The Transtheoretical/Stages of Change Model has direct application to nutrition intervention. Program strategies are more effective when they are designed to match the individual's stage in the change process. For example, individuals in the precontemplation stage would lack awareness or intent to adopt a behavior, such as reducing dietary fat and losing weight. Educational programs for these individuals would put more emphasis on the benefits of making a change. The more practice-oriented "how-to" tips would be diverted to programs and materials targeting individuals in advanced stages, such as action or maintenance.[92] **Box 12-5** outlines interviewing processes that can be used to identify and assist individuals at different stages of change.

Social Marketing Theory (SMT)

Social marketing is the use of marketing concepts and tools to increase the acceptability of social ideas or practices. Social Marketing Theory

Proper display of nutritious foods can motivate consumers to select nutrient-dense foods.

Successful Community Strategies

The Colorado State University Nutrition Education Program[100–106]

Hispanics are projected to be the largest minority group within the United States by the year 2010. Colorado has a large Hispanic population representing about 14 percent of the state's total population. Additionally, there are approximately 21,000 migrant farm laborers who work in agricultural capacities throughout the state. Studies suggest that low-income Hispanics often demonstrate low intakes of vitamins A and C, calcium, iron, and protein and high rates of diabetes, obesity, and infections.

It is very difficult to provide effective nutrition education programs because these individuals are among the poorest in the state, especially when considering the migrant farm worker families. The obstacles to effective nutrition programs involve mainly limited financial resources on the part of both the agencies providing the education and the individuals being served. Other obstacles include lack of transportation, childcare, and time needed for educational endeavors as well as low education levels, low literacy rates, limited opportunities to learn English if English is the second language, culture, health beliefs, and, in some cases, if the nature of the population is especially transient. These factors have severely restricted participation in and success of the nutrition education endeavors. Translation issues, reading level considerations, and complexities of program content have become critical considerations for educators. Community agencies have found these obstacles to be major challenges in providing effective nutrition education programs.

A nutrition education program entitled *La Cocina Saludable* was designed according to the Stages of Change Model and implemented in 10 southern Colorado counties. The objectives of the program were to improve the nutrition-related knowledge, skills, and behaviors that lead to healthy lifestyles

in a low-income Hispanic population. The contents of the program included nutrition information designed to help mothers of preschool children provide for their children's nutritional needs. Materials developed for this program included:

- A free-standing, color photograph, bilingual flip chart
- Corresponding bilingual *La Cocina Saludable Resource Guides*
- A three-dimensional, free-standing, bilingual Food Guide Pyramid
- Coordinating plastic kitchen utensils used as incentives
- Brochures representing the bilingual Food Guide Pyramid
- Food Guide Pyramid magnets

The *Resource Guide* was written in both English and Spanish and included scripted teaching pages corresponding to text background pages. This guide was designed to provide the abuela (Hispanic grandmother) educators, who were minimally trained in nutrition and teaching, with a resource for the nutrition information as well as a script to follow while they taught the classes, thus improving the consistency and accuracy of information presented to participants. The program attempted to overcome barriers by incorporating a flexible program format carried out by abuela educators using the processes described in the Stages of Change Model. The program was evaluated using knowledge, skills, and behavior pretest, posttest, and 6-month follow-up surveys on both the abuela educators and the actual class participants. The materials focused on five units:

- "Make It Healthy" discussed basic nutrition knowledge, including use of the Food Guide Pyramid.

- "Make It Fun" provided tips on making food fun to encourage preschool children to eat healthful foods.
- "Make a Change" explained techniques for lowering fat, lowering salt, lowering sugar, and increasing fiber in diets.
- "Make It Safe" discussed food safety techniques, including cleanliness, the safe cooking of foods, and properly storing foods.
- "Make a Plan" provided tips on choosing healthy foods and on making food resources last longer.

Each of the five units included an experiential and behavioral learning activity designed to reinforce the messages presented in the unit and to use the specific kitchen utensil designated for that unit. The kitchen utensil was then given to the participants as a type of reward for participating and to encourage them to return for the next class meeting.

Results show that the training program was an effective means of disseminating nutrition information and skills to abuela educators, particularly in the areas of healthful eating and the Food Guide Pyramid, where the educators were the most deficient in knowledge and skills. In addition, the results suggested that the five class units led to significant gains in knowledge, skills, and retention of this knowledge. At 6 months, the program participants improved their survey scores after attending the program compared to the control group who didn't attend the program. Additionally, the results suggest that this type of program can be effective in changing selected nutrition-related knowledge, skills, and behaviors leading to healthy lifestyles for low-income Hispanic mothers of preschool children.

Box 12-5 Motivational Interviewing Algorithm

1. Assess and personalize individual's risk status:
   - "Based on your body mass index (BMI), physical exam, family history, and symptoms, I am concerned about the following: _____, _____, and _____."
   - "I want to talk to you about how your weight may be affecting your health."
2. Stages of change evaluation:
   - "How do *you* feel about your weight?"
   - "What concerns do *you* have about health risks?"
   - "Are *you* considering/planning weight loss now?"
   - "Do the pros of changing outweigh the cons?"
3. Educate, risks and advice: weight goal:
   - Educate: Medical Consequences Tip Sheet (longevity and quality of life).
   - Advice: Establish a reasonable goal for weight loss using a clear statement. "A 5–10% weight loss over 6 months for a total loss of _____ to _____ pounds."
4. Assess patient's understanding and concerns:
   - "How do you feel about what I've said?"
   - "On a scale of 1 to 10, with 10 being 100% ready to take action, how ready are you to lose weight?"
5. Facilitate motivation depending on the individual's level of contemplation:

Facilitate Motivation for Precontemplators

- Validate the individual's experience.
- Acknowledge the individual's control of the decision.
- In a simple, direct statement, give your opinion on the medical benefits of weight loss for the individual.
- Explore potential concerns.
- Acknowledge possible feelings of being pressured.
- Validate that they are not ready.
- Restate your position that the decision to lose weight is up to them.
- Encourage reframing of current state of change as the potential beginning of a change rather than a decision to never change.

An answer between 1 and 4 means the individual has very little intention to lose weight.

An answer between 5 and 7 means the individual is ambivalent about taking action to lose weight. The goal is to move the individual from "No" to "I'll think about it."

Facilitate Motivation for Those in Preparation

- Praise the decision to change behavior.
- Prioritize behavior change opportunities.
- Identify and assist in problem solving regarding obstacles.
- Encourage small, initial steps.
- Assist individuals in identifying social supports.

Goal: Provide direction and support.

6. Schedule follow-up:
   - Tell the individual when you would like to see them again.
   - Give the individual a referral to a health specialist (e.g., dietitian, exercise specialist, therapist), if appropriate.

Adapted from: Ockene JK. *Arch Intern Med*. 1997; 157:2334–2341; Simkin-Silverman L, Wing R. *Ob Res*. 1997; 5:603–612; and Taylor S. St. Anthony Family Medicine Residency, Denver, CO., Reprinted with permission.

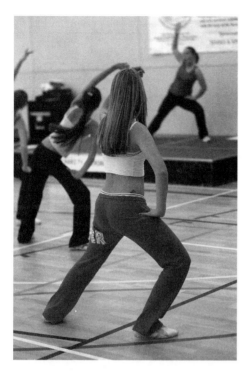

Adopting and maintaining regular aerobic activity is an important part of any health regimen.

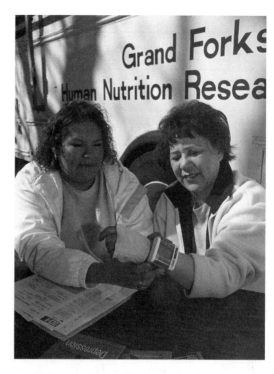

Presenting a positive organizational climate is a significant factor in the success of a program.

(SMT) employs a consumer orientation, audience analysis and segmentation, and aspects of exchange theory in seeking to increase the acceptability of a behavior in a target group.[56,93] An example of a program using SMT is Project LEAN (Low-Fat Eating for America Now), a national campaign whose goal was to reduce dietary fat consumption to 30 percent of total calories through public service advertising, publicity, and point-of purchase programs in restaurants, supermarkets, and school and worksite cafeterias. Project LEAN successfully demonstrated the use of the media, market segmentation, effective spokespersons, and successful partnerships.[94]

Application

Another example of the use of SMT in public health campaigns is Fruits & Veggies More Matters, which was one of the first major health campaigns to follow the principles of SMT. Using data from a variety of research interviews and surveys, designers of this campaign studied the preferences and habits of various audience segments and developed messages that would be perceived as relevant, comprehensible, and actionable by people in those subgroups. By distributing messages based on the needs of consumers in a variety of settings, such as supermarkets, restaurants, and the Internet, the campaign made progress toward the goal of increasing Americans' consumption of fruits and vegetables.[95]

Healthy Communities: The Process

Another program framework model is Healthy Communities: The Process. This is a grass-roots community development process. This model is useful when diverse members of a community come together to work on health issues.[96] The phases of the model are entry, needs assessment, planning, doing, and renewal.[20] **Table 12.4** shows the phases

and the main tasks to be accomplished in each phase. Near the completion of each phase, a pause is recommended so the community group can reflect on several questions: Were the goals accomplished? What is the status of the project? What worked? What didn't and why?[96,97]

This model has been used in grass-roots community development and Healthy Cities/Communities projects. Now that community development is becoming more familiar in healthcare, the model is gaining further acceptance with grantors and with evaluators who use participatory research methods. This model could be used for planning community-based nutrition programs, but the nutritionist may want to change the terminology in the model from "needs" to "issues or interests" to better match a strength-oriented focus.

P-Process

In 1983, the first Population Communication Services project team, which included staff from Johns Hopkins University, developed the framework known as the P-Process.[3] The P-Process provides a communication campaign framework for strategy development, project implementation, technical assistance, institution building, and training.[98] Public health nutritionists can use the P-Process when planning programs for such populations as those with HIV/AIDS, older persons, pregnant women, or the homeless.

The P-Process has been used around the globe for over 15 years and consists of six steps that are followed in sequence to develop and implement effective communication strategies, programs, and activities:[3]

1. *Analysis:* Listen to potential audiences; assess existing programs, policies, resources, strengths, and weaknesses; and analyze communication resources.
2. *Strategic design:* Decide on objectives, identify audience segments, position the concept for the audience, clarify the behavior change

TABLE 12.4	Healthy Communities: The Process

Phase of the Process	Focus of Attention	Major Tasks During This Phase
Entry	The existing situation For example: *Malnutrition in Hispanic infants and children in McLean County.*	• Learn about the environment within which the process will happen. • Introduce yourself into that environment.
Needs assessment	Health needs Public acceptance For example: *Assess feeding methods.* *Determine Hispanic community norms for infant bottle-feeding. Diets are lacking in required nutrients.*	• Gather facts and opinions about community health needs. • Learn what skills and resources already exist. • Have key individuals and the general public accept that health needs are significant. • Gain commitment to action.
Planning	Responding to health needs For example: *Explore WIC program eligibility.* *Investigate the likelihood of qualifying for food stamps.* *Determine the availability of culturally acceptable foods.*	• Explore and choose methods of responding to health needs. • Acquire necessary resources.
Doing	Community action For example: *Locate all county infants, children, and their mothers seen by the Public Health Department for WIC and other programs. Locate or form an outreach program for the community.*	• Implement plans.
Renewal	Evaluation/rejuvenation For example: *75% of the infants and 80% of the children were eligible for WIC food supplements and will be enrolled in the program. Mothers and children who were not qualified due to immigrant status were directed to other food assistance programs, such as food pantries and/ or Catholic Social Services.*	• Evaluate what worked and what didn't. • Determine what has been learned. • Foster self-renewal of those involved. • Re-examine the existing situation.

Modified from: Province of British Columbia, Ministry of Health and Ministry of Responsibility for Seniors. *Health Communities: The Process*. Victoria, British Columbia: Author; 1989. © 1989 by Province of British Columbia, Ministry of Health and Ministry. Reprinted with permission.

model, select channels of communication, plan for interpersonal discussion, draw up an action plan, and design evaluation.

3. *Development, pretesting and revision, and production:* Develop message concepts, pretest with audience members and gatekeepers, revise and produce messages and materials, and retest new and existing materials.

4. *Management, implementation, and monitoring:* Mobilize key organizations, create a positive organizational climate, implement the action plan, and monitor the process of dissemination, transmission, and reception of program outputs.

5. *Impact evaluation:* Measure the impact on audiences, and determine how to improve future projects.

6. *Plan for continuity:* Adjust to changing conditions, and plan for continuity and self-sufficiency.

The P-Process is a well-tested framework that specifies the major steps needed to implement a health communication campaign. It provided the framework for Strategic Communication Planning and Evaluation (SCOPE), which is a CD-ROM–based training tool.

Application

The P-Process is used mainly in developing countries, and is not widely used in the United States. However, funding agencies such as the U.S. Agency for International Development (USAID) may require nutritionists to use the P-Process to carry out their programs. For example, the Mother Care Project intervention program in India was funded by USAID. The intervention program used information, education, and communication (IEC) to increase pregnant women's knowledge about anemia. The purpose of the program was to improve the hematological status between each of the three trimesters of pregnant women in a rural community. Iron supplementation was carried out using ferrous sulfate tablets containing 60 mg of elemental iron. Deworming was provided through administration of 100 mg mebendazole tablets taken twice daily for 3 days. A total of 117 family care volunteers (FCV) were responsible for an average of 200 households each; they were trained to use flash cards to impart knowledge about anemia.

Results showed a significant decrease in the prevalence of anemia by 31, 21.2, and 12 percent, respectively in the first, second, and third trimesters in the intervention groups.[99]

<table>
<tr><td>

TABLE 12.5   **PRECEDE-PROCEED Model**

</td></tr>
</table>

Phase 1. *Social assessment:* A targeted segment of the population in a self-study was asked to identify their needs and desires related to their quality of life.

Program/Application: College students were interviewed and then surveyed about their health interests. Concerns were expressed about unplanned pregnancy and sexually transmitted diseases (STDs).

Phase 2. *Epidemiologic assessment:* Epidemiologic data were used to identify and rank the health goals or problems that might contribute to quality-of-life issues.

Program/Application: Sexually active students reported a lack of condom use. STD and pregnancy rates in national data were similar to those reported by students in the self-study (relates to Healthy People 2010 Objectives 7-3 [health risk behavior information for college and university students] and 23-11 [responsible adolescent sexual behavior]).

Phase 3. *Behavioral and environmental assessment:* Participants were asked to identify and rank health-related behavioral risk factors and environmental risk conditions related to the goals/problems.

Program/Application: Risk factors and conditions included embarrassment, cost, accessibility, partner trust, and partner refusal.

Phase 4. *Educational and ecological assessment:* In relation to the goals/problems, identify factors that have the potential to influence behavior or environment and categorize factors as predisposing (knowledge, attitudes, values, beliefs, perceptions of individuals that can be altered through direct communication), enabling (skills, resources, or barriers controlled largely by societal forces and systems that make possible a change in behavior or environment), or reinforcing (feedback and rewards given to support changes made).

Program/Application: Predisposing factors were relationship skills, sexual health knowledge, and skills in condom use. Enabling factors were readily available condoms at low cost. Feedback and rewards were social support and college credit for involvement in peer education programs.

Phase 5. *Administrative and policy assessment:* Determine capabilities and resources available to develop and implement the program.

Program/Application: Campus health departments were willing to collaborate and to provide funds, teaching time, educational materials, and condoms for 2 years. The college administration agreed to support the program (e.g., physical plant staff assistance).

Phase 6. *Implementation:* Based on resources, select methods, strategies of interventions and implement.

Program/Application: Students, nurses, family and consumer scientists, and faculty developed and implemented peer educational strategies for relationship skill building and sexual health knowledge, including condom use. Faculty arranged credit for students involved. Condom machines ($0.25 per condom) were installed in all washrooms.

Phases 7, 8, and 9. *Process, impact, and outcome evaluation:* Respectively evaluate the implementation of the program, the immediate results, and the long-term results in terms of changes in quality of life for the target population.

Program/Application: Many issues emerged during implementation (for example, the maintenance of condom machines, unplanned pregnancies, iron deficiency anemia, and low-birth-weight babies). Throughout implementation, opportunities to evaluate program activities were provided and activities were adjusted accordingly. At the end of 2 years, students were again interviewed and surveyed. The results were used to determine whether the program should be continued, changed, or stopped.

The depth developed in each phase of the model depends upon resources as well as goals. An advantage is that the model is well recognized by government agencies and grantors.

Modified from: Hitchcock J, Schubert PE, Thomas SA. *Community Health Nursing.* 2nd ed. Clifton Park, NY: Thomson Delmar Learning; 2003. Reprinted with permission.

PRECEDE-PROCEED

The PRECEDE-PROCEED model is another framework that community and public health nutritionists can adopt when planning effective nutrition programs. This model provides a comprehensive guide to planning and implementing health promotion activities in nine phases; the first five involve diagnosis or needs assessment, and the last four involve implementation and evaluation.[98] This framework could be used for planning, implementing, and evaluating many large and small health programs. The long-term use of the model has permitted testing and refinement. It has been modified to ensure more community viewpoints and full participation.[3]

PRECEDE-PROCEED is an acronym for the components of the model. PRECEDE stands for Predisposing, Reinforcing, and Enabling Con-

structs in Educational/Environmental Diagnosis and Evaluation. As its name implies, it represents the process that precedes, or leads up to, an intervention. PROCEED stands for Policy, Regulatory, and Organizational Constructs in Educational and Environmental Development. **Table 12.5** presents the PRECEDE-PROCEED Model.[21]

The Planned Approach to Community Health (PATCH) programs were based on PRECEDE, and the results led to the development of PROCEED. In the model, social, epidemiologic, behavioral, environmental, educational, ecological, policy, and administrative dimensions are assessed and multilevel strategies are designed to improve health status and quality of life.

Chapter Summary

- Community and public health nutritionists use programs to improve the health of communities.
- Factors that may trigger program planning include research findings, a change in existing policy, and availability of resources.
- Formative evaluation provides information to those planning and implementing the program and permits improvements to the program while activities are in progress.
- Summative evaluation provides retrospective information about the performance of the program when the program has been completed.
- To assess the extent of hunger in the community, data are needed on local food costs, household resources to obtain and prepare food, and barriers that constrain individuals or families in obtaining adequate food.
- Funding sources for nutrition programs include grants and contracts from local, state, and federal agencies or foundations and private contributions.
- Data collection methods include interviews, focus groups, observations, and surveys.
- Community nutritionists can plan an effective nutrition education program using one or a combination of models.

Critical Thinking

- Review the general theories of learning summarized in the chapter. Decide which one would most effectively fit the learning needs of a community in which adolescent cigarette smoking is on the rise. Explain the theory you chose.
- Obtain, read, and present at least two research articles that utilized any of the models/theories discussed in this chapter for in-class discussion.

Case Study 12-1

During an initial survey of a community, Ikechi, a public health nutritionist, discovered that migrant and other minority students in the local schools are consuming foods of minimal nutritional value (FMNV) for lunch. In addition, most of the students did not have enough money to purchase nutritious foods. The following barriers to weight management were identified:

- Lack of awareness about the need for and benefits of weight management
- Belief that weight restriction in children can be harmful
- Belief that engaging in a weight management program is expensive and time consuming

Ikechi was asked to develop a nutrition education program using any of the theoretical frameworks discussed in this chapter, such as the Health Belief Model (because of the need to change many of the parents' beliefs about weight management).

Activities

- Divide into groups and perform assessments (on a child and/or an adult) that include body fat measurements using a skinfold caliper, BMI, and diet recall.
- Survey the participants to determine whether the program attendees enjoyed and benefited from the program.
- Use the educational methods and materials presented in the success story of the Colorado State University education program to determine how to provide a more effective program.

References

1. Dignan MB, Carr PA. *Program Planning for Health Education and Promotion.* 2nd ed. Philadelphia: Lea Febiger; 1992.

2. Stanhope M, Lancaster J. *Community and Public Health Nursing.* 5th ed. New York: Mosby; 2000.

3. Valente T. *Evaluating Health Promotion Programs.* New York: Oxford University Press; 2002.

4. Wilson MM, Thomas D, Rubenstein LZ, Chibnall JT, Anderson S, Baxi A. Appetite assessment: simple appetite questionnaire predicts weight loss in community-dwelling adults and nursing home residents. *Am J Clin Nutr.* 2005; 82(5):1074–1081.

5. Shannon J, Shikany JM, Barrett-Connor E, et al. Demographic factors associated with the diet quality of older US men: baseline data from the Osteoporotic Fractures in Men (MrOS) study. *Public Health Nutr.* 2007; 10:1–9.

6. Kaufman M. *Nutrition in Promoting the Public's Health: Strategies, Principles, and Practice.* Sudbury, MA: Jones and Bartlett; 2007.

7. Caravella J. A needs assessment method for Extension educators. *J Extension.* 2006; 44:1–7.

8. Bramley D, Hebert P, Jackson R, Chassin M. Indigenous disparities in disease-specific mortality, a cross-country comparison: New Zealand, Australia, Canada, and the United States. *N Z Med J.* 2004; 117(1207):U1215.

9. Bryce J, Boschi-Pinto C, Shibuya K, Black RE. WHO estimates of the causes of death in children. *Lancet.* 2005; 365(9465):1147–1152.

10. Caulfield LE, Richard SA, Black RE. Undernutrition as an underlying cause of malaria morbidity and mortality in children less than five years old. *Am J Trop Med Hygiene.* 2004; 71(2 Suppl):55–63.

11. National Institutes of Health. Hearts N' Parks Program Continues to Help Participants of All Ages Adopt Hearty-Healthy Behaviors. Available at: http://www.nhlbi.nih.gov/new/press/04-05-27.htm. Accessed May 24, 2007.

12. Boyle M. *Community Nutrition in Action: An Entrepreneurial Approach.* 4th ed. Belmont, CA: Thomson Wadsworth; 2005.

13. Adler NE, Castellazzo GG, Ickovics JR. Relationship of subjective and objective social status with psychological and physiological functioning: preliminary data in healthy white women. *Health Psychol.* 2000; 19(6):586–592.

14. Jensen CJ, Finifter DH, Wilson CE, Koenig BL. Community assessment of senior health using a telephone survey and supplementary methods. *J Appl Gerontol.* 2007; 26(1):17–33.

15. Greenhalgh T, Chowdhury M, Wood GW. Story-based scales: development and validation of questionnaires to measure subjective health status and cultural adherence in British Bangladeshis with diabetes. *Psychol Health Med.* 2006; 11(4):432–448.

16. Dahlberg J, Holben D. Halt hunger on the Hocking—a service-learning project developed in response to a needs assessment of a rural Appalachian Ohio community. *J Am Diet Assoc.* 2004; 104(8):S58.

17. Clark CC. *Health Promotion in Communities: Holistic and Wellness Approaches.* New York: Springer; 2002.

18. McNamara C. Basics of Developing Mission, Vision and Values Statements. Available at: http://www.managementhelp.org/plan_dec/str_plan/stmnts.htm. Accessed May 22, 2008.

19. Cooperative State Research, Education, and Extension Service. About Us. Available at: http://www.csrees.usda.gov/about/background.html. Accessed April 20, 2008.

20. Anspaugh DJ, Dignan MB, Anspaugh SL. *Developing Health Promotion Programs.* 2nd ed. Long Grove, IL: Waveland Press; 2006.

21. Hitchcock J, Schubert PE, Thomas SA. *Community Health Nursing.* 2nd ed. Clifton Park, NY: Thomson Delmar Learning; 2003.

22. U.S. Department of Agriculture, Department of Health and Human Services. *Nutrition and Your Health.* USDA Home and Garden Bulletin No. 232. Washington, DC: Author; 2000.

23. Nelson DE, Kreps GL, Hesse BW, et al. The Health Information National Trends Survey (HINTS): development, design, and dissemination. *J Health Comm.* 2004; 9(5):443–460.

24. Glasgow RE, Lichtenstein E, Marcus AC. Why don't we see more translation of health promotion research to practice? Rethinking the efficacy-to-effectiveness transition. *Am J Public Health.* 2003; 93(8):1261–1267.

25. Kreuter MW, Lezin NA, Green LW. *Community Health Ideas That Work.* 2nd ed. Sudbury, MA: Jones and Bartlett; 2003.

26. Gregory J. Using message strategy to capture audience attention: readers' reactions to health education publications. *J Nonprofit Public Sector Market.* 2006; 15(12):1–23.

27. Briss PA, Brownson RC, Fielding JE, Zaza S. Developing and using the guide to community preventive services: lessons learned about evidence-based public health. *Ann Rev Public Health.* 2004; 25:281–302.

28. Serritzlew S. Linking budgets to activity: a test of the effect of output-purchase budgeting. *Public Budget Finance.* 2006; 26(2):101–120.

29. Russell LB, Suh D-C, Safford MM. Time requirements for diabetes self-management: too much for many? *J Fam Pract.* 2005; 54(1):52–56.

30. Bisset S, Potvin L. Expanding our conceptualization of program implementation: lessons from the genealogy of a school-based nutrition program. Available at: http://her.oxfordjournals.org/cgi/content/full/cyl154v1. Accessed May 22, 2008.

31. Chen H. *Practical Program Implementation: Assessing and Improving Planning, Implementation, and Effectiveness.* London: Sage; 2004.

32. Bracht N. *Health Promotion at the Community Level.* Newbury Park, CA: Sage; 1990.

33. Edelstein S. *Nutrition in Public Health: A Handbook for Developing Programs and Services.* 2nd ed. Sudbury, MA: Jones and Bartlett; 2006.

34. Gittelsohn J, Evans M, Story M, et al. Multisite formative assessment for the Pathways study to prevent obesity in American Indian schoolchildren. *Am J Clin Nutr.* 1999; 69:767S–772S.

35. Merzel C, D'Afflitti J. Reconsidering community-based health promotion: promise, performance, and potential. *Am J Public Health.* 2003; 93:557–574.

36. Health Canada First Nations and Inuit Home and Community Care. *Program Evaluation Guide. The Purpose of Evaluation.* Ottawa, Ontario: Health Canada; 2005.

37. Williams S, Torrens P. *Introduction to Health Services.* New York: Wiley; 1999.

38. Ryan L, Anderson J. The effect of nutrition education on improving fruit and vegetable consumption of youth. *J Extension.* 1995; 33(5):1–5.

39. Rivera JA, Sotres-Alvarez D, Habicht JP, Shamah T, Villalpando S. Impact of the Mexican program for education, health, and nutrition (progress) on rates of growth and anemia in infants and young children. *JAMA.* 2004; 291:2563–2570.

40. Frodi D, Esben BJ, Pal W, White RF, Grandjeance P. Impact of prenatal methylmercury exposure on neurobehavioral function at age 14 years. *Neurotoxicol Teratol.* 2006; 28(3):363–375.

41. Nemcek MA, Sabatier R. State of evaluation: community health workers. *Public Health Nurs.* 2003; 20(4):260–270.

42. Floyd JF, Gallagher P, Stringfellow V, Zaslavsky AM, Thompson JW, Cleary PD. Using telephone interviews to reduce nonresponse bias to mail surveys of health plan members. *Med Care.* 2002; 40(3):190–200.

43. Ariza AJ, Chen EH, Binns HJ, Christoffel KK. Risk factors for overweight in five- to six-year-old Hispanic-American children: a pilot study. *J Urban Health.* 2004; 81(1):150–161.

44. Lambur M, Rajgopal R, Lewis E, Cox RH. Applying Cost Benefit Analysis to Nutrition Education Programs: Focus on the Virginia Expanded Food and Nutrition Education Program. Publication Number 490-403. Available at: http://www.ext.vt.edu/pubs/nutrition/490-403/490-403.html. Accessed May 2, 2007.

45. Rein DB, Constantine RT, Orenstein D, et al. A cost evaluation of the Georgia Stroke and Heart Attack Prevention Program. *Prev Chronic Dis.* 2006; 3(1):A12.

46. Parkerson GR, Broadhead WE, Tse CK. The Duke Health Profile. A 17-item measure of health and dysfunction. *Med Care.* 1990; 28(11):1056–1072.

47. Baró E, Montse F, Vázquez O, et al. Using the Nottingham Health Profile (NHP) among older adult inpatients with varying cognitive function. *Quality Life Res.* 2006; 15(4):575–585.

48. Bell JF, Zimmerman FJ, Mayer JD, Almgren GR, Huebner CE. Associations between residential segregation and smoking during pregnancy among urban African-American women. *J Urban Health.* 2007; 84(3):372–388.

49. Mosley BS, Hobbs CA, Flowers BS, Smith V, Robbins JM. Folic acid and the decline in neural tube defects in Arkansas. *J Arkansas Med Soc.* 2007; 103(10):247–250.

50. Collier SA, Hogue CJ. Modifiable risk factors for low birth weight and their effect on cerebral palsy and mental retardation. *Matern Child Health J.* 2007; 11(1):65–71.

51. Suellentrop K, Morrow B, Williams L, D'Angelo D, Centers for Disease Control and Prevention (CDC). Monitoring progress toward achieving maternal and infant Healthy People 2010 objectives—19 states, Pregnancy Risk Assessment Monitoring System (PRAMS), 2000–2003. *MMWR.* 2006; 6(55):1–11.

52. Hurley PK. A Guide to the Documents: The Formal Report. *University of Hawaii.* Available at: http://emedia.leeward.hawaii.edu/hurley/eng209w/booklet/pages/unit2/frguide.pdf. Accessed May 24, 2007.

53. Boyle M. *Community Nutrition in Action: An Entrepreneurial Approach.* Belmont, CA: Thomson Wadsworth; 2003.

54. Kirmse DW. Formal Technical Report Organization. Gainesville, FL: University of Florida; 2001. Available at: http://pie.che.ufl.edu/guides/reports/formal_report.html. Accessed April 21, 2008.

55. Fischer A, Northey, M. *Formal Reports and Proposals.* Upper Saddle River, NJ: Prentice Hall; 1993.

56. Huff RM, Kline MV. *Promoting Health in Multicultural Populations. A Handbook for Practitioners.* New Delhi, India: Sage; 1999.

57. Comings JP, Soricone L, Santos M. *An Evidence-Based Adult Education Program Model Appropriate for Research.* National Center for the Study of Adult Learning and Literacy (NCSALL) Occasional Paper. Boston: National Center for the Study of Adult Learning and Literacy; 2006.

58. Sapp SG, Weng CY. Examination of the Health-Belief Model to predict the dietary quality and body mass of adults. *Int J Consumer Stud.* 2007; 31(3):189–194.

59. Owen A, Splett PL, Owen GM. *Nutrition in the Community: The Art and Science of Delivering Services.* 4th ed. New York: McGraw-Hill; 1999.

60. Contento IB, Balch GI, Bronner YL, et al. The effectiveness of nutrition education and implications for nutrition education policy, programs, and research: a review of research. *J Nutr Ed.* 1995; 27(6):284–418.

61. Wallace LS. Osteoporosis prevention in college women: application of the Expanded Health Belief Model. *Am J Health Behav.* 2002; 26(3):163–172.

62. Strychar IM, Potvin L, Pineault R, Pineau R, Prévost D. Changes in knowledge and food behaviour following a screening program held in a supermarket. *Can J Public Health.* 1993; 84(6):382–388.

63. Freeland-Graves J, Nitzke S. Position of the American Dietetic Association: total diet approach to communicating food and nutrition information. *J Am Diet Assoc.* 2002; 102(1):100–108.

64. Rogers EM. *Diffusion of Innovations.* 4th ed. New York: Free Press; 1995.

65. Bagozzi RP, Moore DJ, Leone L. Self-control and the self-regulation of dieting decisions: the role of prefactual attitudes. *Basic Appl Soc Psychol.* 2004; 26(273):199–213.

66. Maimanm LA, Becker MH. The Health Belief Model: origins and correlates in psychological theory. In: Becker MH, ed. *The Health Belief Model and Personal Health Behavior.* Thorofare, NJ: Charles Slack; 1974.

67. Dickin KL, Dollahite JS, Habicht J-P. Nutrition behavior change among EFNEP participants is higher at sites that are well managed and whose front-line nutrition educators value the program. *J Nutr.* 2005; 135:2199–2205.

68. Pittet D, Simon A, Hugonnet S, Pessoa-Silva C, Sauvan V, Perneger TV. Hand hygiene among physicians: performance, beliefs, and perceptions. *Ann Intern Med.* 2004; 141:1–8.

69. Monneuse MO, Bellisle F, Koppert G. Eating habits, food and health related attitudes and beliefs reported by French students. *Eur J Clin Nutr.* 1997; 51(1):46–53.

70. Durkin KF, Wolfe KF, Clark GA. College students and binge drinking: an evaluation of social learning theory. *Sociol Spectrum.* 2005; 25(3):255–272.

71. Bodenmann G, Schaer M. Social learning theories. *Sprache Stimme Gehör.* 2006; 30:17–20.

72. Tian PS, Morawska OA. A cognitive model of binge drinking: the influence of alcohol expectancies and drinking refusal self-efficacy. *Addict Behav.* 2004; 29:159–179.

73. Fulkerson JA, French SA, Story M, Nelson H, Hannan PJ. Promotions to increase lower-fat food choices among students in secondary schools: description and outcomes of TACOS (Trying Alternative Cafeteria Options in Schools). *Public Health Nutr.* 2004; 7(5):665–674.

74. Rogers LQ, Matevey C, Hopkins-Price P, Shah P, Dunnington G, Courneya KS. Exploring social cognitive theory constructs for promoting exercise among breast cancer patients. *Cancer Nurs.* 2004; 27(6):462–473.

75. Hansona N, Neumark-Sztainera D, Eisenberga ME, Storya M, Walla M. Associations between parental report of the home food environment and adolescent intakes of fruits, vegetables and dairy foods. *Public Health Nutr.* 2005; 8:77–85.

76. Boynton-Jarrett R, Thomas TN, Peterson KE, Wiecha J, Sobol AM, Gortmaker SL. Impact of television viewing patterns on fruit and vegetable consumption among adolescents. *Pediatr.* 2003; 112(6):1321–1326.

77. Gribble SL, Falciglia G, Davis AM, Couch S. A curriculum based on social learning theory emphasizing fruit exposure and positive parent child-feeding strategies: a pilot study. *J Am Diet Assoc.* 2003; 103(1):100–103.

78. Ajzen I, Fishbein M. *Understanding and Predicting Social Change.* Englewood Cliffs, NJ: Prentice Hall; 1980.

79. Ross L, Kohler CL, Grimley DM, Anderson-Lewis C. The theory of reasoned action and intention to seek cancer information. *Am J Health Behav.* 2007; 31(2):123–134.

80. Carroll LJ, Whyte A. Predicting chronic back pain sufferers' intention to exercise. *Br J Ther Rehab.* 2003; 10(2):53–58.

81. Folta SC, Bell R, Economos C, Landers S, Goldberg JP. Psychosocial factors associated with young elementary school children's intentions to consume legumes: a test of the theory of reasoned action. *Am J Health Promot.* 2006; 21(1):13–15.

82. Booth-Butterfield S, Reger B. The message changes belief and the rest is theory: the 1% or less milk campaign and reasoned action. *Prev Med.* 2004; 39(3):581–588.

83. Britto MT, Pandzik GM, Meeks CS, Kotagal UR. Combining evidence and diffusion of innovation theory to enhance influenza immunization. *Jt Comm J Qual Patient Saf.* 2006; 32(8):426–432.

84. Elder JP, Lytle L, Sallis JF, et al. A description of the social-ecological framework used in the trial of activity for adolescent girls (TAAG). *Health Educ Res.* 2007; 22(2):155–165.

85. Sanson-Fisher RW. Diffusion of innovation theory for clinical change. *Med J Austral.* 2004; 180(6):S55–S56.

86. Valente TW, Fosados R. Diffusion of innovations and network segmentation: the part played by people in promoting health. *Sex Transm Dis.* 2006; 33(7 Suppl):S23–S31.

87. Burgoon JK. Testing the interactivity principle: effects of mediation, propinquity, and verbal and nonverbal modalities in interpersonal interaction. *J Comm.* 2002; 52(3):657.

88. Bandura A. Social cognitive theory of mass communication. *Media Psych.* 2001; 3(3):265.

89. Prochaska JO, DiClemente CC. Stages and processes of self-change of smoking: toward an integrated model of change. *J Consult Clin Psychol.* 1983; 51:390–395.

90. Herzog TA. Are the stages of change for smokers qualitatively distinct? An analysis using an adolescent sample. *Psychol Addict Behav.* 2007; 21(1):120–125.

91. Canales M, Rakowski W. Development of a culturally specific instrument for mammography screening: an example with American Indian women in Vermont. *J Nurs Meas.* 2006; 14(2):99–115.

92. Greene GG, Rossi SR, Rossi JS, Velicer WF, Fava JL, Prochaska JO. Dietary applications of the Stages of Change Model. *J Am Diet Assoc.* 1999; 99:673–678.

93. Dearing JW, Maibach EW, Buller DB. A convergent diffusion and social marketing approach for disseminating proven approaches to physical activity promotion. *Am J Prev Med.* 2006; 31(4):S11–S23.

94. Samuels SE. Project LEAN: a national campaign to reduce dietary fat consumption. *Am J Health Prom.* 1993; 4:435–440.

95. Lefebvre RC, Donner L, Johnson C, Loughrey K, Balch GI, Sutton SM. Use of database marketing and consumer-based health communication in message design: an example from the Office of Cancer Communications' "5 A Day for Better Health" program. In: Maibach E, Parrott R, eds. *Designing Health Messages: Approaches from Communication Theory and Public Health Practice.* Thousand Oaks, CA: Sage; 1995: 217–246.

96. Grier S, Bryant C. Social marketing in public health. *Ann Rev Pub Health.* 2005; 26:319–339.

97. Curran S, Gittelsohn J, Anliker J. Process evaluation of a store-based environmental obesity intervention on two American Indian reservations. *Health Educ Res.* 2005; 20(6):719–729.

98. Green L, Kreuter MW. *Health Promotion Planning: An Education and Environmental Approach.* Mountain View, CA: Mayfield; 1991.

99. Abel R, Rajaratnam J, Kalaimani A, Kirubakaran S. Can iron status be improved in each of the three trimesters? A community-based study. *Eur J Clin Nutr.* 2000; 54:490–493.

100. Taylor T, Serrano E, Anderson J, Kendall P. Knowledge, skills, and behavior improvements on peer educators and low-income Hispanic participants after a stage of change-based bilingual nutrition education program. *J Comm Health.* 2000; 25(3):241–262.

101. U.S. Bureau of the Census. The Official Statistics. Available at: http://www.census.gov/compendia/statab. Accessed May 22, 2008.

102. Colorado Migrant Health Department. *Colorado Migrant Health Program 1996 Report Denver.* Denver: Author; 1996.

103. Diehl AK, Stern MP. Special health problems of Mexican Americans: obesity, gallbladder disease, diabetes mellitus, and cardiovascular disease. *Adv Intern Med.* 1989; 34:79–96.

104. Lopez L, Masse B. Income, body fatness, and fat patterns in Hispanic women from the Hispanic Health and Nutrition Examination Survey. *Health Care Women Int.* 1998; 14:117–128.

105. U.S. Bureau of the Census. *Statistical Abstract of the United States.* Washington, DC: Author; 1990.

106. U.S. Bureau of the Census. *Current Population Survey.* Washington, DC: Author; 1996.

CHAPTER 13

Grantsmanship Skills and Nutrition and Ethics

CHAPTER OUTLINE

- Introduction
- Laying the Foundation for a Grant
- Identifying Funding Sources
- Identifying Possible Collaborators
- Writing the Grant
- Funded Proposals
- What Is Ethics?
- Nutrition and Ethics
- Conflicts of Interest in Research
- Basic Principles of the Protection of Human Subjects
- Business Conflicts
- Ethics in Health Promotion
- Ethical Decision Making
- Code of Ethics for the Profession of Dietetics

LEARNING OBJECTIVES

- Define grant proposal.
- Specify major items in a grant application.
- Identify potential collaborators for a grant proposal.
- Discuss the parts of a grant proposal.
- Discuss the sources for funding community and public health nutrition.
- Define ethics.
- Discuss the possible conflicts of interest in research and business.
- Discuss ethical dilemmas in health promotion.
- Discuss the basic ethical principles.
- Discuss factors to consider in moral decision making.

Introduction

Many community and public health *programs* have experienced reductions in their *budget*. Because of these reductions, they are compelled to become more creative with existing resources and/or obtaining grant funds to develop, expand, or continue their programs. Although many agencies are accomplishing more with less money, several are seeking grant funds to accomplish the organization's goals. For these reasons, grant applications have become very competitive and the number of individuals and organizations seeking funds has increased significantly.[1,2] A *grant* is a fund awarded to individuals or an organization for *research*, educational, and demonstration programs. The grant monies are used to support new innovative programs or expand existing programs to meet community healthcare needs.[2]

Both the grantor and the nutritionist seeking a grant need each other. Community nutritionists can identify community needs and develop creative methods to address them, and foundations, corporations, and other donors have the financial resources necessary to make a program work. The two groups often form productive collaborations, but the grant seeker must take the initiative.

It is important for community nutritionists to acquire grant-writing skills in order to be successful in obtaining money for their research and/or community-related programs. The elements to consider when writing a grant proposal include ethical issues, sources of funds (foundations; federal, state, and local agencies), the length of the proposal, time to write the proposal, and the staff required to carry out the project. Preparing a research study or organizing a community education program and writing a grant proposal are complex endeavors, not only because of the many elements that go into research and/or program design, but also because each element plays an essential role in the success of the program/research.[3]

One of the elements nutritionists encounter in grant writing and in other aspects of dietetics is ethical issues. The American Dietetic Association has provided a set of guidelines for registered dietitians, licensed nutritionists, and registered dietetic technicians entitled the *Code of Ethics for the Profession of Dietetics*. These ethical guidelines are a set of principles that dietitians and nutritionists must apply in every situation coupled with their personal judgments, experience, knowledge, and skills. This chapter discusses the different components of a grant proposal and ethical dilemmas nutritionists encounter in research, business, and health promotion.

Laying the Foundation for a Grant

A *grant proposal* is a written request for money (and occasionally for other resources). Writing a grant proposal compels the nutritionist to create, define, and refine the research idea or community education program.[4] An excellent grant proposal requires very good organization and a strong foundation. To get adequate resources for a program, community nutritionists need to submit a proposal to an agency or foundation that grants funds for health promotion programs. Sometimes nutritionists may need to submit proposals to their own employing agency for funding such as *travel grants* to conferences, *training grants* to learn how to prepare a grant proposal, *demonstration grants* to demonstrate a new approach to delivering community health programs, or *equipment grants* to acquire small tools for a program.[5,6] Also, the nutritionist may submit proposals for *service grants* to support activities and services to the community over and above those outreach programs that are already funded.[7] This could also be accomplished through a *block grant*, which is a sum of money the federal government gives to a state or local government while suggesting a general purpose for the money's use. However, the federal government permits the state or local government to spend the money without meeting specific conditions.

Writing a grant proposal is a systematic, step-by-step process that requires the following:[5]

- Identifying stakeholders
- Generating ideas
- Establishing the need for the grant
- Locating collaborators
- Identifying barriers to overcome (understanding the language of the proposal)
- Locating grant money
- Describing goals
- Finding out how to apply
- Writing a request (i.e., a proposal)

Identifying Funding Sources

The nutritionist or grant-seeking organization should look for funding from an agency that funds a specific type of need in the community. For example, a community service group, such as Kiwanis or the March of Dimes Birth Defects Foundation, may focus on helping pregnant women and children and may be willing to fund a program to improve youth health or prevent folic acid deficiency in a community. Similarly, the American Heart Association may fund a smoking prevention program and the Dairy Council may fund an osteoporosis prevention program. Local, state, and national sources may also have funds available. (See http://nutrition.jbpub.com/communitynutrition for an inventory of U.S., Canadian, and other national funding sources as well as for a sample request for a proposal from the *Federal Register*.)[8]

After locating a potential funding source, it is a good idea to contact the funding agency to discuss whether the nutrition program idea matches the agency's interests and to clarify the agency's requirements (such as questions to be answered, deadlines for submission, and

program A healthcare service designed to meet identified healthcare needs of individuals.

budget Financial plan that shows expenses and income related to a specific service.

grant Money given to an individual or an organization for a need and that does not require repayment. Grants can be given out by foundations, governments, and the like. Grants to individuals can be either scholarships or donations.

research A systematic investigation, including development, testing, and evaluation, designed to develop or contribute to generalizable knowledge.

grant proposal A written request for money (and occasionally for other resources).

travel grant Grant money funding travel and related expenses outside of the state, community, or local area for the purposes of research, both basic and applied, to attend conferences, or to attend a workshop on how to write a grant proposal.

training grant Grant money to learn how to prepare a grant proposal and/or learn new techniques.

demonstration grant A grant given to show a new approach to delivering a community health program or to demonstrate a technique.

equipment grant A grant for small instruments for a start-up fund.

submission format). Guidelines differ among agencies, mainly in the amount of details required; however, the grant writer must answer the following questions in order to be successful:[5]

- What are the objectives/aims, how much will it cost, and what is the time line?
- How is the proposed project related to the grantor's interests?
- What is the maximum amount of money that the applicant can request?
- What has already been accomplished in the research project or program?
- What would be the benefits if this project/program were carried out?
- What are the methods and procedures for the project/program?
- How would the project/program be evaluated?
- Why is the applicant the most qualified to carry out this research project or nutrition program?
- Is collaborative work required?

The search for funding is a step-by-step process. First, the nutritionist/grant seeker must have a clear idea of the project or program needing funding. Second, he or she must search and locate potential grantors. Third, he or she must contact and apply for financial support. Although the grant seeker may modify the program plan later on, it is a good idea to design the project before starting a funding search. The following will help build the proposal:[9,10]

- Start as early as possible.
- Put together a strong, representative grant writing team.
- Identify someone in the community who has grant writing experience.
- Consider all of the people whose skills or knowledge will be needed.
- Involve the major partners early.
- Locate available health data through the Centers for Disease Control and Prevention (CDC) for research information/data (e.g., obesity, heart disease, osteoporosis, mortality and morbidity rates) in your state or community.
- Search for research articles related to the topic.
- Show that the applicant is aware of and plans to work toward local, state, and national standards (if applicable).

Most philanthropic organizations and many corporations are prepared ahead of time for requests for money. They have ready-made grant applications and guidelines describing what kinds of programs they are interested in funding. It is important to not waste these organizations' time if your needs do not match their guidelines. Grantors seldom make exceptions to their grant policies.[9]

After locating the funding source, the next step is to make an initial contact. Potential grantors respond to initial contacts in different ways. Some grantors will fund a project, such as a small grant, directly from a letter of intent. Others will ask for expanded aspects of the letter of intent. The majority of foundations and corporations who regularly fund programs will send out a request for proposal (RFP) grant application form.[11] These forms are usually very clear about what and how much information the foundation needs from applicants. It is important to not exceed the maximum amount of information; give them exactly what they ask for—no more, no less.

Regardless of the form it takes, a typical grant proposal will include the following elements: an introductory overview of the proposal or background information, a statement of need, a project description, and a budget. In addition, grantors may ask for a mission statement (i.e., the rationale and goals of the program), a list of important personnel, and a description of any project partnerships.[9,10]

Identifying Possible Collaborators

Collaboration is a mutual sharing and working together to achieve common goals in such a way that all persons or groups are recognized and growth is enhanced.[12] Many funding agencies look for programs that use a collaborative approach. The proposal has greater potential of being funded if the grant writer seeks partners such as community agencies, local businesses, and individuals who could provide financial backing or an *in-kind* or *matching grant* to support the grant proposal during the planning stage.[13] For example, a service-learning project that can raise matching funds or in-kind donations from a local community member confirms to a grantor that there is community "buy-in." Partnering with another school or community organization on a program can provide additional funding leverage for both partners.

Preparing a grant proposal is very time consuming and labor intensive. Therefore, a professional grant writer may be needed to coordinate the activities and gather materials needed to complete the grant application. Forming a grant writing committee may be beneficial when submitting a grant application for a large sum of money, especially for federal or block grants (such as maternal and child health grants, preventive health and health services grants, and community development grants).[12] The committee may consist of the agency epidemiologist, nurse, nutritionist, accountant, community leaders, statistician, and physician. In addition, the grant seeker can partner with other healthcare professionals, such as the college of nursing, school of public health, or college of dentistry. These professionals also engage in community-based health research and community intervention efforts to reduce morbidity and mortality from diseases and conditions ranging from infant mortality to chronic and genetic diseases.[13-17]

Skills in networking, coordination, and cooperative learning are also necessary in forming a successful partnership.[2,18] You can gain networking experience by attending grant writing workshops and professional develop-

service grant Grant money that supports activities and services to the community over and above those outreach programs already funded. This could also be accomplished through a block grant.

block grant A sum of money the federal government gives to a state or local government, the federal government would suggest a general purpose for the use of the money (e.g., community services or social services) as authorized by legislation, but permits the state or local area to spend the money without meeting specific conditions.

collaboration Mutual sharing and working together to achieve common goals in such a way that all persons or groups are recognized and growth is enhanced.

in-kind Contribution of equipment, supplies, or other tangible resources, as distinguished from a monetary grant. Some organizations may also donate the use of office space or staff time as an in-kind contribution.

matching grant The amount of project costs that the organization, other sponsors, or the institution will contribute toward the project. Support may consist of money, equipment needed for the project, personnel (in-kind), or supplies.

Preparing a grant proposal is very time consuming, and it often requires teamwork to be successful.

ment events as well as associating with colleagues in and outside your local community.

Writing the Grant

Writing a grant is a systematic process. The components of a proposal vary from one grant sponsor to another; therefore, it is very important to read and follow the grantor's instructions very carefully. The components include the items listed in the following sections. However, the sequence of the items may vary according to the needs of the granting agency.

Letter of Intent

The application procedure for writing a research or grant proposal may start with a letter of intent to the funding organization, prior to an invitation to submit a full proposal. The first letter of intent may be sent to indicate to a funding agency the plan to submit a grant proposal. The letter of intent follows many of the same procedures as a proposal, but it is limited to a few pages. Some letters of intent include a limited literature review, but some agencies prefer to receive a more extensive proposal at the beginning. In either case, each step of the proposal must be supported by data. The letter of intent may consist of a one-page summary that may include the following nine items:[19,20]

- Names of the principal and co-investigators, organization/institution/community center, address, telephone and fax numbers, and e-mail address
- Title of the proposed project (brief information about the project)
- Purpose/aim of the project
- Brief description of the project design
- Results of preliminary data
- Time requirements for the project
- Estimated annual and total project budget
- Resume
- Impact or significance of the project to the community

The letter of intent is a good opportunity to describe the positive outcome of a funded grant and the impact this program or research will have on the community if it is funded.

Request for Proposal

After the letter of intent is accepted and the organization asks for submission of a proposal, the detail work of writing the proposal starts. The proposal may begin with the concise one-page summary that was included in the letter of intent.

The grant writer should read the request very carefully and follow the guidelines because the proposal may be disqualified if it is submitted in an improper format.[21] The two major challenges that a grant seeker must address are clarity and consistency within the grant. Assembling a *research grant* or project application is similar to using building blocks. The foundation and structure for the proposal are the specific aims. From the specific aims, the project design and methods are chosen to answer the identified research or program questions and hypotheses. A *hypothesis* is a supposition or question that is raised to explain an event or guide investigation.[22] The community project design and aims are then used to formulate appropriate statistical analyses and evaluation.

Organizing the proposal by the specific aims is one way to promote clarity among hypotheses, variables, instruments, and data analyses. For example, you could use special font styles such as bolding or italics to highlight these variables consistently throughout the sections of the grant; however, make sure that these formatting options are allowed by the funding agency.[18]

The individual sections of a research/project grant are discussed in the following sections. Major components of a proposal grant application include:[19]

- Abstract
- Research or project plan
- References
- Budget
- Curriculum vitae or resume
- Other support (collaboration with business or community organizations)
- Resources (matching funds)
- Institutional review board (IRB) approvals (as needed)
- Appendix
- Dissemination of findings
- Capability

Title

The proposal title should be short, explicit, and informative. It should project the idea of the proposal and inform the grant reviewers as to what they are about to read. Some grantors may limit the number of characters and spaces allowed in the title. It is beneficial to use a catchy project title; it may not be the decisive factor in the grant application, but it may help reviewers remember the proposal better than others reviewed. Some examples of catchy titles might be:

- Nutrition for Fitness
- 21st-Century Nutrition
- Fit for Life
- Fitness Education: In Shape
- Healthy Hearts
- Building Better Bones

Abstract

An abstract is a short summary of the proposed research project/program. It persuades the reviewer to read the proposal, and allows busy reviewers to learn the main ideas without reading the entire proposal.

It is advisable to write the abstract last and use it to summarize the specific aims or objectives, background, significance, research/project design, and method sections. One of the challenging aspects of writing an abstract is adhering to the word limit required by the grantor.[23] An editor can help in reducing unnecessary words and phrases.

It is important to bear in mind that the abstract sets the stage for the remainder of the proposal. It is important to include any changes that were made in the body of the proposal if the abstract was written early in the grant writing process. (This is one reason to write the abstract last.) Attention to detail, especially in the abstract to catch readers' attention, is very important.[18]

Literature Review/Background Information

This section discusses not only what is currently known related to the proposed area of the study, but also, and more importantly, the significance of the research project or program. This section justifies the project, builds the case for the project, and highlights the need for the project.[4] It is vital to convince the reviewers that this project or program is the next logical step based on the state of the science or the community needs. It is also important to show how this program addresses a widespread or significant health concern. Linking the proposed program to national health objectives such as Healthy People 2010 or federal or professional organizational research priorities will strengthen the likelihood of funding for the proposal.[18,24]

In addition, the literature review should focus on the specific aims of the proposal. Critically evaluate existing knowledge and identify gaps in the scientific evidence. Link the **conceptual framework** to the project. A conceptual framework is a way of showing relationships that are known and ones that have not been investigated but may be the focus of the project.[25] The literature reviews found in many journal articles are good examples you can follow when writing your proposal.

Specific Aims

This part of the proposal describes the purpose(s) of the project, what the project intends to accomplish, and the potential value of the research project or program. Although the organization of this section may vary, most nutritionists start with the purpose(s) of the program. The statement of purpose includes the main project variables, their possible interrelationships, and the nature of the population of interest. For example, the purpose of this research project is to assess the relationship among four sets of variables: a) the prevalence of obesity in school children, b) the eating patterns of school children, c) the physiological effects of obesity, and d) the effects of culture on breast-feeding.[11,18] Another example: the aim of this program is to increase the number of fruits and vegetables that men ages 55 years and older consume.

The following example is taken from a grant proposal titled *Perinatal Alcohol Users: Identification and Intervention*. The specific aims of this study were to:[11,18,26]

- Identify alcohol users/abusers at risk for delivering an infant with fetal alcohol syndrome/fetal alcohol effects
- Educate pregnant women's health professionals regarding the identification of and adverse effects of alcohol on the women and their offspring.
- Evaluate the effectiveness of interventions by comparing this group of mothers and infants to those randomly selected as a control group and to those followed in the perinatal, Newborn Division, and Child and Family Health Services Pediatric Tacking databases.

Another example of a grant proposal is the following for a program supported by the Illinois Public Health Department Office of Women's Health titled *Understanding and Managing Menopause*:

- Increase the participants' knowledge of the options available to manage menopause.
- Increase the participants' knowledge of physiological and emotional changes that may often be experienced during peri-menopause and menopause.
- Reinforce health practices that will maintain lifelong good health and vitality.
- Increase the participants' knowledge of the options available to assure well-being and good health and increased assertion to advocate for each woman's individual needs.

After the statement of purpose, the **grantee** can include a description of the problem that the project intends to solve or help solve, for example, "Interventions are needed to increase the identification of women at risk for delivering infants with spina bifida and FAS. Once identified by healthcare practitioners, the participants will be referred to a dietitian who can then enroll and maintain the women in prenatal care."[11]

Research/Program Method

This section must answer the research or program questions. It should contain critical information needed to evaluate the quality of the proposal, independent of any other document. It must be concise, thorough, and specify what the researcher/program coordinator intends to achieve. Although the format for the plan may differ depending on the funding source, most project plans include certain sections: specific aims, background and significance, preliminary results, methods and procedure, and references.[4] The nutritionist must provide a full description of how the objectives will be achieved; how success/outcome will be assessed (for example, an evaluation plan and the number of participants that will be recruited for the program); a description of the participants (or sample/subjects), including who will be involved; the order and time frame of the program activities (time and activity charts, see **Table 13.1**); and the duties and qualifications of the project staff.[27] Citing preliminary results relevant to the project will be a feature unique to the proposal.

Six basic elements comprise the research project design: setting and sample; description of intervention, if applicable; instruments and data collection procedures; data analyses; and

research grant Grant money to support an ongoing research study, develop new hypotheses, or improve existing ideas. Normally there are no, or only very few, conditions associated with the award. The researcher is free to decide on the course of his or her research and to use the funds accordingly, subject only to the general conditions of the sponsor and the policies of the university or organization.

hypothesis A supposition or question that is raised to explain an event or guide investigation.

conceptual framework A visual way of demonstrating relationships that are known and ones that have not been investigated but that may be the focus of the project.

grantee The organization or individual awarded a grant or cooperative agreement by the grantor and who is legally responsible and accountable for the use of the funds provided and for the performance of the grant-supported project or activities.

| TABLE 13.1 | **Grant Activity Chart and Time Line for Nutrition Education Programs** |

Task	January	February	March	April	May	June	July
Develop ideas, needs assessment, proposal goals, objectives, and title. Determine the target audience. Establish need.	X	X					
Plan marketing strategies, review related literature, seek collaborators, and determine methods and procedures.	X	X					
Analyze preliminary data; submit letter of intent; and determine instruments, equipment, and materials.			X	X			
Write proposal and seek second opinion to review the proposal.					X		
Recruit participants and submit proposal.						X	
Write results.						X	
Implement and evaluate.						X	X

formula grant Noncompetitive awards based on a predetermined formula provided to grantees. The amount is established by a formula based on certain criteria (e.g., population, per capita income, poverty, service needs, number of substandard housing units in a community) that are written into the legislation and program regulations. These are directly awarded and administered in a department's program offices. These programs are sometimes referred to as state-administered programs.

time line. These elements are briefly discussed below.[11]

Setting and Sample. The nutritionist must describe the location chosen for the program and the rationale for the selection over other possible locations. Describe the typical client population (older persons, minority groups, infants, etc.). Additionally, if a distant site was selected over a local site, it is important to provide a rationale for that decision. Address how distance will affect data collection, participation, and quality of data collection or the intervention.[11]

Describe the criteria for inclusion and exclusion of participants in the project. It is unethical to exclude any segment of the population

An excellent grant proposal requires good organization and a strong foundation.

that is willing to participate. In addition, the nutritionist has an obligation to convince the reviewer of the adequacy of the site to produce a sufficient number of subjects based on inclusion and exclusion criteria. To address the issue, include in narrative text or table format the number of participants available per month or year for the project at the data collection site who meet the inclusion criteria.[22] In addition to the number of subjects, federal grants such as *formula grants* often require the principal investigator to address the recruitment of special populations, including gender and racial/ethnic groups as well as women and children.[28]

Intervention. The proposal must describe in detail the intervention procedure and administration. Include how the treatment condition differs from the control or comparison group.[11] One example of an intervention is the Brief Intervention Model (BIM), which includes a 10-minute interview with a person in the study. Using the Perinatal Alcohol Users example, following an intervention, the nutritionist and the pregnant women would set a mutual goal for reducing the amount of alcohol the women consume.[11]

Instruments. This part of the proposal describes each of the study or project variables and their measurements. It is essential to describe the population, method of administration, reliability, and validity for each instrument (e.g., bone densitometry, blood pressure apparatus, skinfold caliper) that will be used for the program. If alternate instruments are available, the grantee/nutritionist needs to discuss the rationale for the selection of a particular instrument. Describe any necessary training of project personnel in the use of each instrument. It is helpful to report pilot data or whether any pilot study is planned for the new instruments.[11] Finally, include lists of all instruments needed in an appendix.

Data Collection Procedures. The writer can start describing how potential participants will be identified and recruited into the program in this section of the proposal. This is followed by a clear description of how and when the intervention will be carried out. Also, include an explanation of the control group. It is important to explain the data collection method, and the aspects of how, when, where, and who uses the instruments. Include a description of how the study personnel will be trained in the data collection process.[11] The nutritionist must address any potential problems that may be encountered during the project protocol and should include a plan for how problems will be managed. If the study is complex, the nutritionist should develop a step-by-step procedural checklist that will be used by data collectors to ensure that no procedural item is omitted during the course of the research project.[29]

Data Analysis. This part of the proposal must describe the plans for data management, refinement, and reduction. It is important to describe how the data will be collated, coded, keyed, and verified. This section describes how the data collected will be analyzed to determine the success or outcome of the project. The investigator must provide the name of the statistical test that will be used.[11,29] The principal investigator/nutritionist may want to consider including a statistician on the planning team.

It is important to separate the database of respondents from the results to maintain confidentiality. Also, provide a plan on how to disseminate the findings of the project.[30]

Time Line. This part of the proposal describes the anticipated time frame for project activities, such as the hiring and training of project personnel, identification and recruitment of participants, data collection, data preparation, analysis, marketing the program, and writing the report. It is better to propose an adequate period of time for some aspects of the grant, such as recruitment of participants and hiring personnel. Sometimes, it is better to provide the information in the form of chart or a graph of time relationships or by narrative form.[31]

References

This part of the proposal is the last part of the project plan and consists of references to journal articles, books, and other materials that were quoted in the grant proposal. It is important to provide bibliographic information in a consistent referencing format such as the American Psychological Association (APA) style or any other format the grantor suggested.[32]

Budget

This section of the proposal is very important. The proposed budget and any matching funds must be related to the proposed program activities. It is important for the grant writer to review the grantor's budget criteria meticulously. Grantors typically specify allowable expenses and those that are not fundable.[33] For example, some grants will not allow funding for indirect costs or the salary of the principal investigator, but will allow salaries for consultants and research assistants. Some federal grants do not allow for meals and travel costs related to the presentation of the results, whereas others may. It is essential to link budget items to grant activities (research personnel, consultants, equipment, supplies, travel, computer costs, and other related expenses). The goal is to request exactly what is needed to conduct the project. The funding agencies often require budget justification. Budget justification is a description of the budget items requested and a rationale for why this expense is needed.[11]

Table 13.2 presents a sample budget. This sample budget serves only as a general model and would vary according to the type of research project or program. Also, as already mentioned, some funding agencies do not pay indirect costs.

Curriculum Vitae or Resume

This part of the proposal will highlight the relevant professional accomplishments of the project directors such as their educations, professional experiences, research, publications, honors, and previous grant awards. It is essential to highlight the achievements that are related to the proposed project first because most grantors typically request an abbreviated resume. Check the guidelines; most agencies restrict the resume to two or three pages.[34] The curriculum vitae should include a listing of all publications from the past 3 to 5 years and any additional references specifically related to the topic area of the proposed research/program. Membership in professional organizations or involvement in community service is usually omitted unless it helps to demonstrate the experience or leadership ability to carry out the proposed project.[11]

Dissemination of Findings

Dissemination of findings constitutes the final outcome of a funded research project. This section describes how the community, stakeholders, and other interested individuals will learn about the project and its findings. Disseminating the findings increases the body of knowledge unique to the discipline of nutrition. It is important to describe a possible, effective, and appropriate dissemination plan and indicate who will be responsible for this activity.[11,32] There are many opportunities for disseminating the findings including publication in a related journal, professional meetings, and online presentation. The information that can be presented includes the theory you developed, pilot data, and any instruments that were developed.[35]

The dissemination of findings offers benefits to both the sponsor and the grantee. For example, the community will become aware of the grantor's priorities and commitment. They also become cognizant of the mission and activities of the organization receiving the funds.[11]

Capability

This part of the proposal shows the capacity and dependability of the grantee and his or her organization. The project director (principal investigator) must have the expertise needed to direct all the activities of the grant. The director also must specify the qualifications and abilities of the project staff. He or she must show that the organization has the

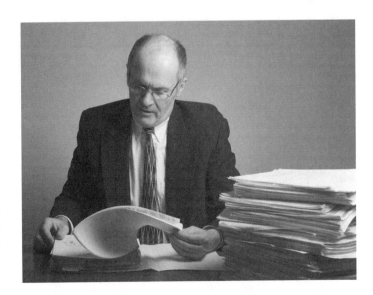

Observe the funder's deadline because late applications are automatically disqualified.

TABLE 13.2 Sample Budget for One Year

Items	Funding Agency/Month	University or Agency/Month	Total/Year
Personnel Salary/Wages			
Principal investigator/senior personnel (director)	$6,000.00	$2,000.00	$96,000.00
One graduate assistant/staff (assists in data collection and processing)	$500.00	-0-	6,000.00
Subtotal	**$6,500.00**	**$2,000.00**	**$102,000.00**
Fringe Benefits			
Life insurance, retirement at 0.33 percent multiplied by salaries	$214.00	$66.00	$2,568.00
Medical insurance, $120 multiplied by the number of months	$120.00	-0-	$1,440.00
Travel (for data collection and for the dissemination of information)			
Mileage (800 @ $0.35)	$280.00	-0-	$280.00
Lodging (5 nights @ $60/night)	$300.00	-0-	$300.00
Per diem (10 days @ $42/day)	$420.00	-0-	$420.00
Equipment	$15,000.00	-0-	$15,000.00
HP computer printer (for preparing flyers, letters)			
Bone density measurement (scanner)			
Supplies	$300.00	-0-	$300.00
Office supplies (pens, paper, etc.)			
Computer printer supplies (ink cartridges)			
Contractual Services			
Telephone	$100.00	-0-	$100.00
Postage	$500.00	-0-	$500.00
Printing	$500.00	-0-	$500.00
Total Direct Costs for the University/Agency	-0-	$2,066.00	$2,066.00
Total Direct Costs for the Funding Agency	$24,234.00	-0-	$125,474.00
Indirect Costs (for program administration) 8% of total direct costs from the funding agency	$1,938.00	$165.00	$2,103.00
Subtotal	**$26,172.00**	**$2,231.00**	**$127,577.00**

capability to support the proposed project and that the project can be carried out on time and within the proposed budget. Also, it is important to include any collaborators' resources and capabilities. The nutritionist must persuade the reviewers that he or she has access to the segment of the population that will be recruited for the project (e.g., older persons, children, pregnant women, postmenopausal women). This can be achieved by providing the number of the targeted audience living in the community (using census data). It is also necessary to include and show that participants are available for the study or project. (Provide a list with the volunteers' signatures, if possible.)[36] Also, describe how you will sustain the program after the funding has ended.[37]

The grantee must include the organization's goal, mission statement, activities, previous achievements, and any unique characteristics that position them for the funding. The nutritionist should also include the facilities, matching funds, equipment, materials, and any other resources that will contribute significantly to the success of the proposed project.

Box 13-1 presents the steps to grant funding success. The Successful Community Strategies feature in this chapter describes a successful proposal that received a Small Grant Program award.

Assembling the Final Product

Once all parts of a grant proposal are written and spell-checked, the whole thing can now be assembled: the cover sheet (containing the name of the principal investigator or project manager, including his or her address, telephone number, and e-mail address), the proposal itself, the budget, and the supplementary materials. Add a cover letter and be sure to note whether the grantor wants multiple copies or if a cover sheet needs to be signed by staff or board members.[16,37] It is important to observe the grantor's deadline because late applications are automatically disqualified.

Box 13-1 Steps to Grant Funding Success

- Start early.
- Ask someone else to read the grant before sending it.
- Work off a preliminary budget; it helps to reduce expansiveness.
- Look for community partnerships.
- Involve a professional grant writer.
- Establish the need for the grant.
- Use national research and statistics to support the application (for example, CDC data).
- Incorporate state and national standards.
- Understand the language for the proposal.
- Don't exceed the page limits, and use 12-point font.
- If the proposal was not funded initially, use the reviewer's comments to revise the proposal.

Reviewing the Grant Proposal

The grantors typically send a letter to the grantee acknowledging the receipt of the proposal and informing him or her of when they plan to announce what proposals will be funded. The grantee can call, e-mail, or send a letter to the grantor if the letter of acknowledgment was not received within 2 to 3 weeks of submission.

Reviewing a grant proposal is a time-consuming activity. The reviews are typically performed by expert committees known as study sections.[38] It may take longer than expected to announce the recipients of the grant because of time constraints, a delay in budget approval by the state or federal government, or availability of the reviewers. Therefore, grant writing requires a great deal of persistence, creativity, and patience.

Funded Proposals

The grant seeker/nutritionist may receive a check with a cover letter if the proposal is funded, or he or she may receive a full-blown **contract** that could stipulate any number of things, such as that the grantee must submit a quarterly and/or final report when the project is completed, that there was a reduction in the amount requested, or that the president of the organization must sign the contract. In all cases, the grantee should write immediately to acknowledge the award. It is important to read the contract first before signing it and note when and what kinds of reports are due.[32]

After receiving the award, check to see whether the grantor has specific reporting forms and guidelines. If the grantor does not ask for a report, send one anyway. Show the grantor how well the money was utilized. If the project generated a newspaper article or other publication, send a copy to the grantor. If it includes a public event, invite the grantor to attend. If you received heartfelt letters of thanks from participants, send samples of the letters to the grantor.[39]

It is important to submit the report on time or send a letter or call to inform the grantor that the report will be late if there are extenuating circumstances that prevent the grantee from submitting the report on time.

If a Proposal Is Rejected

The letter of rejection will probably be a form letter. It is appropriate to contact the grantor and ask for anything that will help when submitting in the future. Perhaps they liked the proposal but did not have enough money or it was not a priority topic at that time.[40] It is important to be cordial when requesting more information. After an objective review of the grantor's guidelines and if the grant seeker believes there is still the potential to receive the award, he or she can apply again in about a year.[32] Many applicants are only successful on their second or third attempt.

What Are Ethics?

Hitchcock et al. defined **ethics** as the study of the nature and justification of **principles** that guide human behaviors and are applied when moral problems arise.[8] Ethical actions involve decisions about which actions, relationships, and policies should be considered right or wrong.[42] The word *ethics* is derived from the Greek *ethos*, "the customary way of acting" or the manner of action that contributes to a person's growth.[43] In the literature, both ethics and morality are, at times, used interchangeably, but distinction can be made between the two. Morality is derived from the Latin *mosmoris*, which means "the customary way of acting," in the sense that "customary" produces proper attributes. Morality can be viewed as the ability to distinguish moral problems from other problems. To be able to differentiate between feelings, facts, and values and reflect on them is a cognitive ability preconditioned by a moral motivation to do good, as it relates to nutrition and health practitioners. Ethics, on the other hand, refers to the methodical analysis of what is right or wrong, good or bad.[43,44]

Nutrition and Ethics

The interests of grant funding agencies, such as food industries and private agencies, can create opportunities for conflicts of interest when conducting grant-related research and reporting findings. A community nutritionist involved in research is prone to conflicts of interest.[45] For example, he or she has an obligation to the funding agency, but also obligations to the profession of dietetics and to the public and the community to provide accurate and complete information that is not misleading.

Ethical codes apply when implementing a community nutrition program just as they do in all other aspects of dietetic practice.[46] The protection of human health involves ensuring adequate nutrition, prevention of malnutrition, and defense against unsafe foods. Healthy people are more able to participate in human affairs and are more able to live productive and meaningful lives if credible scientific knowledge is utilized to adequately improve their lives. Government, private agencies, and healthcare professionals are

contract A written agreement between a grantee and a third party to acquire routine goods and services. The contract could stipulate any number of things, such as that the grantee must submit a quarterly and/or final report when the project is completed, that there was a reduction in the amount requested, or that the president of the organization must sign the contract.

ethics The science or study of moral values; also a code of principles and ideals that guides action.

principles The foundations for rules.

obligated to ensure that human health is improved by providing reliable scientific information.

The ethical questions community and public health nutritionists encounter are similar to those encountered in other disciplines. ***Moral obligation*** is the duty to act in a particular way in response to moral norms. For instance, the community nutritionist must be honest when communicating diet and health information to clients and must ascertain whether scientific findings are sufficient and credible before being translated into dietary advice.[47] The role of community nutritionist requires practices that accept moral responsibility for the growth and development of individuals, families, and communities.

The following is an example of an ethical dilemma encountered by a nutritionist. A community nutritionist was hired to categorize those in the community according to health needs and to decide who should receive first priority for nutrition education and medical nutrition therapy. The categories were as follows:[47,48]

- Those who cannot survive due to lack of food and who are severely malnourished (African American and Hispanic infants, and older persons)
- Those who can be assisted to prevent long-term disability (European American populations at high risk of obesity and individuals experiencing mild hypertension)
- Those who do not have an acute disabling illness or are not at risk of long-term disability (school-age children who are not

obese, women with uncomplicated pregnancies, and elderly individuals with adequate healthcare coverage but who need nutrition education)

This example is connected to the two ethical principles in the American Dietetic Association's *Code of Ethics*, presented later in this chapter: #1, which addresses honesty, integrity, and fairness, and #11, which addresses efforts to avoid bias in any kind of professional evaluation of others. The community nutritionist first selected those who were severely malnourished and then those who were at risk of obesity. Finally, he or she provided nutrition education to the school-age children, women with uncomplicated pregnancies, and elderly individuals.[49]

Conflicts of Interest in Research

Due to a reduction in government funding, increased university overhead expenses, and other reasons, many nutrition scientists obtain research support or funding from non-government sources. These sources can include corporations (e.g., food, drug, biotechnology, and nutrient supplement companies), commodity groups (e.g., walnut or peanut growers, beef or soybean farmers, sugar cane or beet growers, corn growers, etc.), health organizations (e.g., American Heart Association, American Cancer Institute, March of Dimes), and other nonprofit groups (e.g., foundations and research or policy institutes).[50] Dietitians must be cautious about potential conflicts of interest because their research is commonly funded by some of these organizations, along with

Successful Community Strategies 🏠🏠🏠

The UCLA Small Grant: Are Economic Incentives Useful for Improving Dietary Quality Among WIC Participants and Their Families?[41]

The Economic Research Service (ERS) of the U.S. Department of Agriculture created a Small Grant Program in 1998 (titled the Food Assistance and Nutrition Research Program) to stimulate new and innovative food assistance and nutrition issues and to broaden the participation of social science scholars in these issues. These projects focused on the economics of obesity, food insecurity and childhood obesity, food assistance program participation and household well-being, and community influence on food assistance and dietary choices. Several of the projects focused on specific populations, such as people living in the rural South and those living on American Indian reservations.

The grant award selection process included peer review panels composed of experts from the academia, government, and private sectors. In addition to reviewers' comments, the selection process considered coverage of priority research/ program areas, overlap between proposals and

ongoing projects, program needs, and potential benefits from research/program collaborations on particular projects.

To administer the Small Grant Program, the ERS formed partnerships with five academic institutions and research institutes. Partner institutions had the advantage of being closer to the particular regional and state environments that influenced program delivery and outcomes. Each partner institution provided a different emphasis on food and nutrition assistance research.

Dena Herman and colleagues at the University of California Los Angeles received one of the grant awards to investigate whether providing supplemental financial support explicitly for the purchase of fresh fruits and vegetables would result in high uptake of the supplement and whether the individuals would continue to consume more fruits and vegetables after the financial support was removed.

To carry out this project, the researchers/ nutritionists provided vouchers for fresh fruit and vegetable purchases to low-income women participating in the Public Health Foundation Enterprises (PHFE) WIC program in Los Angeles. A total of 602 women who enrolled for postpartum services at three selected WIC program sites (about 200 per site) in Los Angeles were recruited. Sites were assigned to either intervention with vouchers redeemable at a local supermarket; intervention with vouchers redeemable at a nearby year-round farmers' market; or a control site with minimal non-food incentive for participation interviews. Vouchers were issued bimonthly at the level of $10 per week. Interventions were carried out for 6 months, and participants' diets were followed for an additional 6 months following the intervention. Quantitative 24-hour dietary recalls were conducted at four interviews for all participants; in addition, at the intervention sites, two extra interviews spaced 2 months apart were conducted to obtain information on their employer, and the funding agency's interests may conflict with their own.[51] For example, a nutrition scientist may decide to conduct research in osteoporosis (with funding from the dairy council) because the funds are available instead of researching a topic that is more widely needed by the society, such as effective nutrition education methods, but for which funding is limited (funding from local county).

Another aspect of conflict of interest involves the dissemination of the research findings to the public, media, scientific meetings, and interviews with journalists. The interests of the agencies paying for the research may conflict with the actual outcomes of the research and how the results are presented.[52] For instance, the nutrition scientist may be pressured to delay or suppress the outcomes of the research or be pressured to reinterpret the results in a way that's more favorable to the funding source.[50] The ***code of ethics*** of the American Society for Nutritional Sciences (ASNS) states that when members are speaking to the public on a topic where they may be perceived as having a potential conflict of interest, members should reveal those interests to their audience or the person with whom they are speaking. The ASNS code of ethics also states that it is unethical to conduct research if the results determine whether the findings will be published or not.[53]

There may be consequences when nutrition scientists exaggerate the importance of research findings or suppress the outcome of research in favor of the funding agency. The consequences include, but are not to limited to:[50,54–56]

- What is said or not said may add to public confusion on nutrition topics.
- People may be misled about how to select a healthful diet.
- Genuine findings and inferences may be discarded.
- The public's confidence in nutrition science may be undermined.
- Worthwhile treatments/therapy may not be pursued because the original research was discredited.
- Science-based public policy decisions may be affected.

Another possible area of conflict is if nutrition scientists serve on research proposal review boards in their area of expertise and at the same time conduct research on topics related to the proposals being reviewed. A conflict of interest exists if a reviewer's judgment regarding the quality of someone's research proposal is unfairly influenced by his or her own research hypothesis or by the interests of his or her own funding source. Researchers, such as those on review committees, should avoid even the appearance of unfairness in conflicts in the review and evaluation of research and research proposals of other dietitians.[52,57] This is important because such review processes are usually "blind," consequently making

moral obligation Duty to act in a particular way in response to moral norms.

code of ethics A set of statements encompassing rules that apply to people in professional roles.

the fruits and vegetables purchased with the vouchers. Specifically, participants were asked to respond to the question, "What did you buy with your fruit and vegetable coupons last week?" Voucher redemption rates were obtained from scanned data from the supermarket's corporate headquarters. In the farmers' market, vouchers presented for purchase were collected by the farmers' market manager and submitted to the city government's accounting department for tallying; vouchers were then mailed to the study's research staff, who recounted the redeemed vouchers and logged the tallies into an electronic database.

In total, $44,000 worth of vouchers were issued for the supermarket and $44,960 for the farmers' market. Redemption rates were 90.7 percent for the farmers' market and 87.5 percent for the supermarket. Overall, participants reported purchasing 27 and 26 different fruits and 34 and 33 different vegetables in the farmers' market and supermarket outlets, respectively. Five fruits and 5 vegetables accounted for about 70 percent of the items reported for each group with only minor differences in items. The 10 most frequently reported items were oranges, apples, bananas, peaches, grapes, tomatoes, carrots, lettuce, broccoli, and potatoes. A larger number of item purchases were reported for the farmers' market condition, though the total number of types of fruits and vegetables did not differ significantly between the two conditions.

Participants in the intervention conditions increased their consumption of fruits and vegetables with use of the supplement and sustained that increase 6 months after the intervention was completed. At baseline, participants at the farmers' market site reported eating 2.2 servings/1,000 kcal on average, at the supermarket site 2.9 servings/1,000 kcal, and at the control site 2.6 servings/1,000 kcal. Six months post intervention, this same comparison was made and the increase in fruit and vegetable intake reported by the intervention sites was sustained. Both the farmers' market and supermarket sites reported eating 4.0 servings of fruits and vegetables/1,000 kcal on average, while the control site reported eating 3.1 servings/1,000 kcal on average. The difference in consumption between each of the intervention sites and the control site was statistically significant even after adjusting for multiple comparisons. These results were identical when evaluating consumption of fruits and vegetables, excluding beans and potatoes, and of fruits and vegetables, excluding juices. Increases in vegetable consumption were mainly responsible for the overall increases in fruit and vegetable intake. The researchers concluded that the sustained intake of fruits and vegetables may be reflective of the positive cultural habits that the participants have retained as well as the timing of the study at a critical point in the life course. They also attributed the high intake of fruits and vegetables to the large proportion of Latinos included in the study.

potential unfairness hidden. The recommendation is to exempt one-self from the decision making when there is potential for a conflict of interest.

McKnutt suggested the following safeguards to reduce the possibility of conflicts of interest related to sources of research funding:[50,52,58–59]

- What is expected of nutrition scientists when they receive government or non-government funds should be spelled out in a written agreement that is reviewed by a committee of the nutrition scientists' employer/organization. This process decreases the likelihood of investigators doing research that may conflict with the interests of society or the interests of the university.
- Some funding-acceptance policies do not consider it to be a conflict of interest for nutrition scientists to receive funds to do studies if both the researchers and the agency agree before the research starts that results will not be published because the research may be related to a patent application. However, the *Code of Ethics* of the American Society for Nutritional Sciences (ASNS) forbids members to accept money to do research if the grantor has the right to forbid publication of findings if the results are not favorable to the grantor's business or social-marketing objectives. Many other codes, rules, and policies have similar positions. In most contracts between research scientists and grantors, the scientists retain full responsibility for all data and analysis.[53]
- When results are published in a scientific journal, editors and reviewers have an opportunity to assess whether the scientist's relationship with the funding source has influenced the design of a study or interpretation of results. In addition, most nutrition journals publish as part of a research report the source of the investigator's funding, thereby alerting journalists who report scientific findings and other readers to consider whether a study may be influenced by whomever funded it.

Basic Principles of the Protection of Human Subjects

Scientific research has produced substantial social benefits. It has also created some troubling ethical questions. Public attention was particularly drawn to the reported abuses of human subjects in biomedical experiments during the Second World War. During the Nuremberg War Crime Trials, the *Nuremberg Code* was drafted as a set of standards for judging physicians and scientists who had conducted biomedical experiments on concentration camp prisoners. This code became the prototype of many later codes intended to guarantee that research involving human subjects would be carried out in an ethical manner.[60]

Research is defined as a systematic investigation, including research, development, testing, and evaluation, designed to develop or contribute to generalizable knowledge.[61] It also includes activities that meet this definition, whether conducted under a program considered "research" or for other purposes.[62] A ***human subject*** is defined as a living individual about whom an investigator is conducting research to obtain data through intervention or interaction with the individual or to obtain identifiable private information.[62]

The Nuremberg code consists of rules, some general and others more specific, that guide investigators or the reviewers of research in their work. These rules are usually inadequate to cover complex situations; at times they conflict and are often difficult to interpret or apply. Therefore, on July 12, 1974, the National Research Act (Public Law 93-348) was signed into law creating the National Commission for the Protection of Human Subjects of Biomedical and Behavioral Research.

The commission was asked to identify the basic ethical principles that should form the foundation of the conduct of biomedical and behavioral research involving human subjects and to develop guidelines that should be followed to assure that such research is conducted in accordance with those principles.

The Belmont Report is the outgrowth of an intensive 4-day period of discussions that were held in February 1976 at the Smithsonian Institution's Belmont Conference Center, supplemented by the monthly deliberations of the commission that were held over a period of nearly 4 years. The Belmont Report summarized the basic ethical principles identified by the commission in the course of its deliberations. It is a statement of basic ethical principles and guidelines that should assist in resolving the ethical problems that surround conducting research with human subjects. The report is published in the *Federal Register* and reprints are available upon request. The two-volume Appendix (DHEW Publication No. [OS] 78-0013 and No. [OS] 78-0014), containing the lengthy reports of experts and specialists who assisted the commission in fulfilling this part of its charge, is available for purchase from the Superintendent of Documents, U.S. Government Printing Office, Washington, DC 20402.[60] Also, the preliminary papers can be found on the Internet at http://www.irb-irc.com/section6/6.3.03B_BELMONT_App.pdf.

Basic Ethical Principles

The phrase ***basic ethical principles*** refers to those general judgments that serve as a basic justification for the particular ethical prescriptions and evaluations of human actions. Three basic principles, among those generally accepted in the U.S. cultural tradition, are relevant to the ethics of research involving human subjects and are presented in **Box 13-2**: the principles of respect for persons, beneficence, and justice.[60]

Community nutritionists almost always involve human subjects in their work. Sometimes their activities involve limited practice and other times they involve a combination of practice and research. Principally, the term *practice* refers to interventions that are designed exclusively to enhance the well-being of an individual patient or client and that have a reasonable expectation of success.[61] In contrast, the term *research* refers to an activity designed to test a hypothesis, set procedures designed to reach that objective, and permit conclusions to be drawn (e.g., expressed in theories, principles, and statements of relationships).[63] It includes interviewing; surveying, testing, or observing individuals for the purpose of collecting data; and changing the individuals' physical, psychological, and environmental status.

The protection of human subjects is important whether it is for behavioral or biomedical research. The Belmont Report should be used as a guide whenever human beings are involved in any research. Many organizations, universities, and hospitals have an institutional review board (IRB) that is responsible for educating and monitoring research activities for protecting human subjects. Both the participant and the investigator must sign a consent form (see **Figure 13-1**) with accurate and adequate information about the research. Research involving incomplete disclosure is not justified.[60] For instance, an observational study known as the Tuskegee study was a long-term observation of the "natural" course of syphilis in African American men who were recruited into the study without ***informed consent***. The men were observed for several decades but did not receive penicillin, although its effectiveness in the treatment of syphilis was established several years after the initiation of the study.[61] Information about the use of human subjects in research can be found on the National Institutes of Health's website (http://www.nih.gov).

Respect for Persons: Respect for persons incorporates at least two ethical convictions: first, that individuals should be treated as autonomous representatives (individuals with deliberation capacity about personal goals and acting under the direction of such deliberation) and second, that persons with diminished autonomy (children, prisoners, the frail elderly, etc.) are entitled to protection. The principle of respect for persons thus divides into two separate moral requirements: the requirement to acknowledge autonomy and the requirement to protect those with diminished autonomy. In research involving human subjects, participation must be voluntary, and adequate information such as the aim, procedures, risks, and benefits must be disclosed to the participants before they consent for the research. The participants must have the opportunity to ask questions and be informed that they can withdraw from the study at any time.

Beneficence: People are treated in an ethical manner, not only by respecting their decisions and protecting them from harm, but also by making efforts to secure their well-being. Such treatment falls under the principle of beneficence. The term **beneficence** usually includes acts of kindness or charity that go beyond strict obligation. Two general rules have been formulated as complementary expressions of beneficent actions in this sense: 1) do no harm, and 2) maximize possible benefits and minimize possible harms.

Justice: **Justice** is the sense of "fairness in distribution" or "what is deserved." An injustice occurs when some benefit to which a person is entitled is denied without good reason or when some burden is imposed unduly. There are several accepted formulations of just ways to distribute burdens and benefits. Each formulation mentions some relevant property on the basis of which burdens and benefits should be distributed. These formulations are 1) to each person an equal share, 2) to each person according to individual need, 3) to each person according to individual effort, 4) to each person according to societal contribution, and 5) to each person according to merit.

Source: National Institutes of Health. Regulations and Ethical Guidelines. Available at: http://ohsr.od.nih.gov/guidelines/belmont.html#ethical. Accessed February 1, 2006.

Business Conflicts

Many food industries hire Registered Dietitians (RD) or support their research activities. Dietitians who are employed by food industries (such as cereal, dairy, or fast food companies) often encounter moral dilemmas. First, they have obligations to their employer because it is their source of livelihood, and second, they have obligations to the public to do no harm. Society has recognized the field of dietetics as a profession because of its perceived service in public welfare.[52] Dietitians can serve the interests of the public and the employer by looking for acceptable alternatives. For example, a dietitian was hired to educate women 55 years or older about how to prevent osteoporosis. Part of her responsibility was to acquire bone densitometry to measure bone density. A nutrient supplement company provided the Sahara Clinical Bone Sonometer, but asked her to sell their vitamin and mineral supplements to the women and said that the dietitian would receive a commission when she sold these products. This ethical dilemma was stated in the American Dietetic Association *Code of Ethics* Principle #14, which addresses endorsement of products, and Principle #12, which addresses conflicts of interest. In this scenario, the dietitian should not allow financial gain to cloud her professional obligations as stated in the code, should not endorse products, and should not participate in situations leading to conflicts of interest.[59]

The suggestion is to avoid compromising relations as far as it is practical, and when that cannot be done, to disclose the circumstances to all parties that could be affected.[52] When dietitians and other healthcare professionals respect clients as moral agents, they are acting in agreement with the requirements of the moral *principle of autonomy*. Principles are the foundations for rules. The principle of autonomy is the freedom for an individual to choose which actions to take.[2]

Ethics in Health Promotion

The purpose of health promotion is to enable people to increase control over factors that affect their personal health and to prevent the incidence of chronic health conditions. One of the distinctive elements of any profession is the acknowledgment by professionals and the public of the need to keep up-to-date with the latest advances in the field.[64,65] Community dietitians must continue to learn new techniques and the latest evidence-based information and to provide quality services in current and future work settings in order to remain competent with changing public health issues.[66] They also have the responsibility to determine the limits of their competence. A community nutritionist implementing a new program must become competent in that area of practice. For example, he or she may need to learn the latest electronic communication techniques (such as those found on the Internet) as well as legal and ethical issues that may arise when conveying

human subject A living individual about whom an investigator (e.g., professional or student) is conducting research to obtain data through intervention or interaction with the individual or to obtain identifiable private information.

basic ethical principles General judgments that serve as a basic justification for the particular ethical prescriptions and evaluations of human actions.

informed consent When an individual agrees to a treatment plan after receiving sufficient information concerning the proposal, its incumbent risks, and the acceptable alternatives.

beneficence Ethical principle stating that one should do good and prevent or avoid doing harm.

justice Ethical principle that claims that people should be treated equally. It is the standard of fairness that is served when an individual is given what is due, owed, or deserved.

principle of autonomy The freedom of an individual to act as he or she chooses.

(Insert the organization's logo here)

Building Better Bones

Description and Explanation of Procedure: A bone density test is indicated because you have some risk for developing osteoporosis, and you may not already have a diagnosis of osteoporosis. This procedure will be performed using a Hologic Sahara Clinical Bone Sonometer. It is a painless, noninvasive test of the bone mineral density of the heel that takes only a few minutes to perform. The test will be performed by a licensed, trained operator.

Risk: There is little or no discomfort associated with this method of measuring bone density. With this ultrasound machine, there is no radiation involved.

Benefits: I understand that this procedure will provide me with basic information about my bone mineral density.

Confidentiality: I have been assured that information regarding my identity and bone mineral density measurement will be given only to me, my physician, or (organization's name). I understand that any data or answers to questions will remain confidential with regard to my identity.

I have been given an opportunity to ask questions, and all such questions have been answered satisfactorily.

I further understand that I am free to withdraw my consent and terminate my participation at any time.

Signed Consent: I have read the above information and agreed to undergo the procedure to measure my bone mineral density.

_____	_____
Date	Participant's Name (Print)
_____	_____
Date	Participant's Signature
_____	_____
Date	Witness's Signature

Data from: Illinois Department of Public Health, Office of Women's Health. 2007 Grant Application Guideline. Available at: http://www.idph.state.il.us/about/womenshealth/owh.htm. Accessed November 3, 2008.

FIGURE 13-1 Sample Consent Form

---

information using the Internet or electronic mail for nutrition education programs.[49,67]

Benner defined competence as the ability to demonstrate appropriate professional behaviors with desirable outcomes.[64] Dietitians who are competent use up-to-date knowledge and skills, make accurate assessments based on appropriate data, critically evaluate their own practice, communicate effectively with clients and other professionals, and improve performance based on advice from others.[68,69] Therefore, they are uniquely placed to make moral judgments when translating scientific knowledge or information into dietary messages to the public and clients. As promoters of nutrition, it is important to avoid a paternalistic approach, which is a liberty-limiting principle that is often used to overrule people's actions or expressed desires for their own good.[2] Paternalism is justified if the issues that would be prevented are greater than the violation of the moral rule and if the dietitian is willing to allow the violation of the moral rule in all similar circumstances and be able to publicly advocate this kind of violation. For example, a community nutritionist may override a pregnant woman's wish to use illegal drugs and alcohol by referring her to an alcohol and drugs treatment center so that fetal damage can be prevented. Paternalism seems to be limited to those acts that prevent people from committing some serious bodily harm to themselves or others. Additionally, it is morally justified to restrict a person's liberty when not doing so could cause life-threatening physical or mental harm; for example, asking parents to immunize their children against childhood diseases or asking pregnant women to avoid using cocaine.[2]

Similarly, moral sensitivity is a genuine concern for the well-being and dignity of a client that may become a moral burden because they have the right to determine their own plan of life. Moral sensitivity involves a conflict-laden situation and a self-awareness of one's own responsibility in the situation.[70] An example of a moral burden is a community nutritionist not being able to feed animal products to a Hindu pregnant woman who is anemic because of her religious beliefs, which restricts all animal products. Another example is an attempt to feed a client who is suffering from anorexia nervosa who refuses to eat any food.

One ethical conflict is how to achieve the goal of protecting and promoting public health while ensuring individuals' freedom of choice. The principle of beneficence states, "we ought to do good and prevent or avoid doing harm."[71] However, there may be limits on the amount of benefits clients should expect from nutrition education. Surely, nutrition education should not be expected to benefit individuals who continue to put themselves at risk by consuming foods high in fat, calories, and saturated fat and practicing a sedentary lifestyle. The ethical dilemma is how to balance harms and benefits while ensuring freedom of choice. Services that provide the greatest balance of good over bad, or benefit over harm, are in accordance with the ***rule of utility***.[2,72]

Ethical Decision Making

In community nutrition, the main component in *ethical decision making* is focusing on the best interests of the clients while allowing every stakeholder to share in the decision. Ethics is not only about doing what the rules require or making sure that every good goal or value has been carried out. Ethics is about balancing rules, goals, and values to achieve moral justification of decisions. This is the duty of all who participate in making choices.[73]

The skills in making ethical decisions tend to increase over time and with experience for community nutritionists and those in clinical practice. This moral development typically changes as the individual matures.[74] A higher level of ethical consideration is achievable where ethical codes are used only as tools in soul-searching and in culturally sensitive decision-making processes.[75]

Ethical decision making involves several variables. It can be enhanced by an orderly process that considers clients' values, professional obligations, and ethical principles. The following are ways to make ethical decisions:[2,43,76,77]

- *Identify the problem.* The community nutritionist should clarify the issue (for example, values, conflicts, and matters of principles) and gather all the relevant data (facts, norms, principles, rules, and interpretations of the rules).
- *Collect additional information.* The community nutritionist should decide who will be the main decision makers and what the clients or their families want.
- *Identify all the options available to the decision makers.* The community nutritionist should consider all possible courses of action and their outcomes and evaluate the probability that future decisions may have to be made. He or she should realize that all personal judgments contain subjectivity and no one can claim to be totally objective.
- *Understand.* The community nutritionist should understand that all personal judgments have shared dimensions: Human existence is coexistence; consultation of the many opinions in the community is critical; and reflection of the possible consequences of a decision on the community is very important.
- *Think the situation through.* The community nutritionist should consider the basic values and the professional obligations involved, investigate the ethical principles and relevant rules, and realize that every human judgment is fallible.
- *Make the decision.* The decision makers should choose the course of action that reflects their best judgment.
- *Assess the decision and its outcomes.* The community nutritionist should compare the actual outcomes of the situation with the expected outcomes. He or she should determine whether the process of decision making used can be improved for future situations having similar characteristics.

In addition, the American Dietetic Association position paper on ethical issues provides assumptions that may form the basis for ethical deliberation. Community nutritionists may consider using these assumptions when making good moral judgments:[74,77–79]

- *Autonomy:* Respect for the autonomy of the individual is a very strong value in U.S. culture. Adults with decisional capacity should be free to make their own choices about their concerns. There is a limit to freedom, but that limit has to be defined with each situation and should strongly favor the individuals.

- *Nonmaleficence:* "Do no harm." This basic demand has succeeded as a guide to action in clinical medicine. It is the warning to ensure that whatever is done to help the individual does not also hurt the individual (i.e., the balance of "help" and "hurt" must favor helping the individual).
- *Beneficence:* Doing good for clients is the goal of community nutrition. Whatever action is taken should be the right action.
- *Justice:* "Fairness" is the main formula that is used to describe justice in clinical decision making and can be applied in community nutrition. Moral action is the fair action that treats each person equally in similar circumstances.[72]

Code of Ethics for the Profession of Dietetics

The January 1999 *Journal of the American Dietetic Association* stated that the American Dietetic Association and its Commission on Dietetic Registration adopted a voluntary, enforceable code of ethics. This code, entitled the *Code of Ethics for the Profession of Dietetics*, challenged all members, registered dietitians, and registered dietetic technicians to uphold ethical principles. The enforcement process for the *Code of Ethics* establishes a fair system to deal with complaints about members and credentialed practitioners, peers, or the public.[60]

The House of Delegates adopted the first code of ethics in October 1982 and enforcement began in 1985. The code applied only to members of the American Dietetic Association. A second code was adopted by the House of Delegates in October 1987 and applied to all members and Commission on Dietetic Registration credentialed practitioners. A third revision of the code was adopted by the House of Delegates on October 18, 1998, and was enforced on June 1, 1999, for all members and Commission on Dietetic Registration credentialed practitioners.[60]

The Ethics Committee is responsible for reviewing, promoting, and enforcing the code. The committee also educates members, credentialed practitioners, students, and the public about the ethical principles contained in the code. Support of the *Code of Ethics* by members and credentialed practitioners is vital to guiding the profession's actions and to strengthening its credibility. **Boxes 13-3** and **13-4** present the American Dietetic Association's *Code of Ethics* Preamble and Principles.

Public Health Nutrition Code of Ethics

In relation to public health nutrition, the Public Health Leadership Society's publication entitled *Principles of the Ethical Practice of Public Health* established the Public Health Leadership Society, which is founded on ethics.[80] The society created 12 principles that mirrored morality and human rights as a part of their framework. Dietitians employed in a public health setting should utilize both the *Code of Ethics for the Profession of Dietetics* and the *Principles of the Ethical Practice of Public Health* in their practice.

If a member or credentialed practitioner has violated the *Code of Ethics for the Profession of Dietetics*, an appropriate form must be submitted to the Ethics Committee. The complaint must be made within 1 year of the date that the complainant (the person making the complaint)

rule of utility Derived from the principle of beneficence; this includes a moral duty to weigh and balance benefits against harms in order to increase benefits and reduce the occurrence of harms.

ethical decision making Making decisions in an orderly process that considers ethical principles, individual values, and professional obligations.

Box 13-3 *Code of Ethics* Preamble

The American Dietetic Association and its credentialing agency, the Commission on Dietetic Registration, believe it is in the best interest of the profession and the public it serves to have a Code of Ethics in place that provides guidance to dietetics practitioners in their professional practice and conduct. Dietetics practitioners have voluntarily adopted a Code of Ethics to reflect the values and ethical principles guiding the dietetics profession and to outline commitments and obligations of the dietetics practitioner to client, society, self, and the profession.

The Ethics Code applies in its entirety to members of the American Dietetic Association who are Registered Dietitians (RDs) or Dietetic Technicians, Registered (DTRs). Except for sections dealing solely with the credential, the Code applies to all members of the American Dietetic Association who are not RDs or DTRs. Except for aspects solely dealing with membership, the Code applies to all RDs and DTRs who are not members of the American Dietetic Association. All of the aforementioned are referred to in the Code as "dietetics practitioners." By accepting membership in the American Dietetic Association and/or accepting and maintaining Commission on Dietetic Registration credentials, members of the American Dietetic Association and the Commission on Dietetic Registration credentialed dietetics practitioners agree to abide by the Code.

From: American Dietetic Association. Code of ethics for the profession of dietetics. *J Am Diet Assoc.* 1999; 99:109–113. Copyright © 1999. The American Dietetic Association, Chicago, Illinois. Reprinted with permission.

Box 13-4 *Code of Ethics* Principles

1. The dietetics practitioner conducts himself/herself with honesty, integrity, and fairness.
2. The dietetics practitioner practices dietetics based on scientific principles and current information.
3. The dietetics practitioner presents substantiated information and interprets controversial information without personal bias, recognizing that legitimate differences of opinion exist.
4. The dietetics practitioner assumes responsibility and accountability for personal competence in practice, continually striving to increase professional knowledge and skills and to apply them in practice.
5. The dietetics practitioner recognizes and exercises professional judgment within the limits of his/her qualifications and collaborates with others, seeks counsel, or makes referrals as appropriate.
6. The dietetics practitioner provides sufficient information to enable clients and others to make their own informed decisions.
7. The dietetics practitioner protects confidential information and makes full disclosure about any limitations on his/her ability to guarantee full confidentiality.
8. The dietetics practitioner provides professional services with objectivity and with respect for the unique needs and values of individuals.
9. The dietetics practitioner provides professional services in a manner that is sensitive to cultural differences and does not discriminate against others on the basis of race, ethnicity, creed, religion, disability, sex, age, sexual orientation, or national origin.
10. The dietetics practitioner does not engage in sexual harassment in connection with professional practice.
11. The dietetics practitioner provides objective evaluations of performance for employees and coworkers, candidates for employment, students, professional association memberships, awards, or scholarships. The dietetics practitioner makes all reasonable effort to avoid bias in any kind of professional evaluation of others.
12. The dietetics practitioner is alert to situations that might cause a conflict of interest or have the appearance of a conflict. The dietetics practitioner provides full disclosure when a real or potential conflict of interest arises.
13. The dietetics practitioner who wishes to inform the public and colleagues of his/her services does so by using factual information. The dietetics practitioner does not advertise in a false or misleading manner.
14. The dietetics practitioner promotes or endorses products in a manner that is neither false nor misleading.
15. The dietetics practitioner permits the use of his/her name for the purpose of certifying that dietetics services have been rendered only if he/she has provided or supervised the provision of those services.
16. The dietetics practitioner accurately presents professional qualifications and credentials.
    a. The dietetics practitioner uses Commission on Dietetic Registration awarded credentials ("RD" or "Registered

Dietitian"; "DTR" or "Dietetic Technician, Registered"; "CSP" or "Certified Specialist in Pediatric Nutrition"; "CSR" or "Certified Specialist in Renal Nutrition"; and "FADA" or ("Fellow of the American Dietetic Association") only when the credential is current and authorized by the Commission on Dietetic Registration. The dietetics practitioner provides accurate information and complies with all requirements of the Commission on Dietetic Registration program in which he/she is seeking initial or continued credentials from the Commission on Dietetic Registration.

b. The dietetics practitioner is subject to disciplinary action for aiding another person in violating any Commission on Dietetic Registration requirements or aiding another person in representing himself/herself as Commission on Dietetic Registration credentialed when he/she is not.

17. The dietetics practitioner withdraws from professional practice under the following circumstances:
   a. The dietetics practitioner has engaged in any substance abuse that could affect his/her practice;
   b. The dietetics practitioner has been adjudged by a court to be mentally incompetent;
   c. The dietetics practitioner has an emotional or mental disability that affects his/her practice in a manner that could harm the client or others.

18. The dietetics practitioner complies with all applicable laws and regulations concerning the profession and is subject to disciplinary action under the following circumstances:
   a. The dietetics practitioner has been convicted of a crime under the law of the United States, which is a felony or a misdemeanor, an essential element of which is dishonesty, and which is related to the practice of the profession.
   b. The dietetics practitioner has been disciplined by a state, and at least one of the grounds for the discipline is the same or substantially equivalent to these principles.
   c. The dietetics practitioner has committed an act of misfeasance or malfeasance, which is directly related to the practice of the profession as determined by a court of competent jurisdiction, a licensing board, or an agency of a governmental body.

19. The dietetics practitioner supports and promotes high standards of professional practice. The dietetics practitioner accepts the obligation to protect clients, the public, and the profession by upholding the Code of Ethics for the Profession of Dietetics and by reporting alleged violations of the Code through the defined review process of the American Dietetic Association and its credentialing agency, the Commission on Dietetic Registration.

From: American Dietetic Association. Code of ethics for the profession of dietetics. *J Am Diet Assoc* 1999; 99:109–113. Copyright © 1999. The American Dietetic Association, Chicago, Illinois. Reprinted with permission.

first became aware of the alleged violation.[59] The complainant does not have to be a member of the American Dietetic Association or a practitioner credentialed by the Commission on Dietetic Registration. The complaint must provide details on the violation; the basis for the complainant's knowledge of the violation; names, addresses, and telephone numbers of all persons involved or who might have knowledge of the activities; and whether the complaint has been submitted to a court, an administrative body, or a state licensure board. The complaint must also cite the section(s) of the *Code of Ethics for the Profession of Dietetics* allegedly violated. The complaint must be signed and sworn to by the complainant(s).[59,81]

After a hearing on an appeal and citing the provision(s) of the *Code of Ethics for the Profession of Dietetics* that may have been violated, the committee may decide that the dietitian be censured, placed on probation, suspended, or expelled from the American Dietetic Association, or that the credential of the dietitian be suspended or revoked by the Commission on Dietetic Registration of the American Dietetic Association. The decision of the Ethics Committee is sent to the dietitian and the complainant as soon as possible.[59]

Licensure

Many state licensure boards accept the Registered Dietitian (RD) credential from the Commission on Dietetic Registration (CDR). Credentialing is the formal recognition of professional or technical competence.[82,83] Fellow of the American Dietetics Association (FADA), Certified Nutrition Support Dietitian (CNSD), and Board Certified Specialist in Renal Nutrition (CSR) are other certifications that may be required by the state or an employer. Some states have a practice act, which requires that a license be held by the practitioner in order to perform the professional duties allowed in that state by law. Other states have a title act, which specifies that practitioners cannot describe themselves as "dietitians" unless they are licensed in that state. The CDR website (http://www.cdrnet.org) lists various states with state licensure requirements.[84] State licensing boards have the legal authority to enforce the scope of practice in their state, and outline those duties that the practitioner can conduct. Generally, the state board will require that practitioners are certified by a national organization (CDR) in order to meet the requirements for licensure. States often have their own requirements for renewal, and licensees may have to meet the state requirements for continuing education in order to remain licensed.[85] In those states that require certification, it is a violation of state law to practice dietetics without a license.

Chapter Summary

- Writing a grant proposal is a systematic process.
- Grant-seeking organizations or individuals should look for funding from an agency that funds a specific type of need in the community.
- Partnering with another school or community organization on a program can provide additional funding leverage for both partners.
- Many funding agencies look for programs that use a collaborative approach.
- Grant seekers must have a clear idea of the project or program that needs funding.
- Once a funding source that looks promising is located, the next step is to make an initial contact. Potential grantors respond to initial contacts in different ways. Some grantors will fund a project directly from a letter of intent whereas others will ask for expanded aspects of the letter of intent.
- The grant writer should read the request very carefully and follow the guidelines because the proposal may be disqualified due to improper format.
- The research plan is the most critical component of the proposal. It should contain vital information needed to evaluate the quality of the proposal, independent of any other document.
- The grantors usually send a letter to the grant seeker acknowledging the receipt of the proposal and informing him or her of when they plan to announce which proposals will be funded.
- Many applicants are successful only on their second or third attempt.
- A human subject is a living individual about whom an investigator (professional, student, etc.) is conducting research to obtain data through intervention or interaction with the individual or to obtain identifiable private information.
- The phrase *basic ethical principles* refers to those general judgments that serve as a basic justification for the particular ethical prescriptions and evaluations of human actions.
- Respect for persons incorporates at least two ethical convictions: first, that individuals should be treated as autonomous individuals (individuals with deliberation capacity about personal goals and acting under the direction of such deliberation) and second, that persons with diminished autonomy (children, etc.) are entitled to protection.
- Ethical codes apply in implementing a community nutrition program just as they do in all other aspects of dietetic practice.
- Ethical actions refer to decisions about which actions, relationships, and policies should be considered right or wrong.
- A conflict of interest exists if a reviewer's judgment regarding the quality of someone's research proposal is unfairly influenced by their own research hypothesis or by interests of their own funding source.
- In community nutrition, the main component in ethical decision making is focusing on the best interests of the clients while allowing every stakeholder to share in the decision.
- The American Dietetic Association and its Commission on Dietetic Registration adopted a voluntary, enforceable code of ethics. This code, entitled the *Code of Ethics for the Profession of Dietetics*, challenged all members, registered dietitians, and registered dietetic technicians to uphold ethical principles.

Critical Thinking Activities

- Divide into groups and suggest three ways that community nutritionists can utilize the *Code of Ethics for the Profession of Dietetics* when delivering nutrition care services to certain segments of the U.S. population (e.g., older persons, children, minority groups).
- Identify two research studies in the literature relevant to community and public health nutrition, and describe the strengths and limitations of the research.
- Speak with a community member, a community or public health nutritionist, a researcher, and an administrator who have been involved in research. Ask them about their roles and functions in the research and the types of conflicts of interest they have experienced.
- Interview a childcare center staff member and obtain information about how they keep children's records confidential.

Case Study 13-1

Debra Parrish[86] at Keweenaw Bay Ojibwa Community College received funding from the Economic Research Service of the U.S. Department of Agriculture to conduct nutrition screening and other health assessments with the Keweenaw Bay Indian Community, a federally recognized Indian tribe located on the L'Anse Indian Reservation in Baraga County, Michigan. The project developed nutrition surveys for families of children ages 0 to 4 years. Distribution of the surveys proved difficult since tribal operations do not have mailing lists for these children. The goals of the project included:

- Documenting the prevalence of health diseases and obesity among tribal youth
- Reducing the incidence of chronic health diseases
- Creating programs that integrate Ojibwa culture to enhance learning that, in turn, would bring about healthy lifestyle changes

Activities

- Divide into groups and identify funding sources for research in community and public health nutrition for minority groups in the community.
- Identify and write a small grant proposal that may be submitted to the granting agency for funding about a weight loss program for a minority group of children.
- Identify a nutrition problem that has relevance to the community and public health nutrition in your area that could be used to develop a grant proposal.
- Take a human subjects course (if this course is available) or interview the human subjects review chairperson at the college.
- Identify two conflicts of interest that may be expected when conducting research with children.
- Develop nutrition surveys for families of children ages 4 to 6 years.

References

1. Marshall MI, Johnson A, Fulton J. Writing a Successful Grant Proposal. *Purdue Extension, EC-737*. Available at: http://www.ces.purdue.edu/extmedia/. Accessed May 23, 2008.

2. Stanhope M, Lancaster J. *Community and Public Health Nursing.* 5th ed. New York: Mosby; 2000.

3. Bordage G, Dawson B. Experimental study design and grant writing in eight steps and 28 questions. *Med Educ.* 2003; 37:376–385.

4. Inouye SK, Fiellen DA. An evidence-based guide to writing grant proposals for clinical research. *Ann Intern Med.* 2005; 142(4):274–282.

5. Karsh E, Fox AS. *The Only Grant-Writing Book You'll Ever Need.* 2nd ed. New York: Carroll & Graf; 2006.

6. Bartlett JE, Mupinga DM, Higgins C. Grant writing for middle school educators using computer technology. *Clearing House.* 2004; 77(3):122–125.

7. E-Grants Initiative (Grants.gov). Grant Categories. Available at: http://www.grants.gov/aboutgrants/grant_categories.jsp. Accessed May 18, 2007.

8. Hitchcock J, Schubert PE, Thomas SA. *Community Health Nursing.* 2nd ed. Clifton Park, NY: Thomson Delmar Learning; 2003.

9. Colwell JC, Bliss DZ, Engberg S, Moore KN. Preparing a grant proposal—part 5: organization and revision. *J Wound Ostomy Continence Nurs.* 2005; 32(5):291–293.

10. Ryan B. Make your grant proposal successful. *Pharm J.* 2004; 272:475–477.

11. Kenner C, Walden M. *Grant Writing Tips for Nurses and Other Health Professionals.* Washington, DC: American Nurses Association; 2001.

12. Edelstein S. *Nutrition in Public Health: A Handbook for Developing Programs and Services.* 2nd ed. Sudbury, MA: Jones and Bartlett; 2006.

13. Seifer SD. Building and sustaining community–institutional partnerships for prevention research: findings from a national collaborative. *J Urban Health.* 2006; 83(6):989–1003.

14. Fisher EB. The results of the Commit trial. *Am J Public Health.* 1995; 85:159–160.

15. Farquhar JW, Fortmann SP, Flora JA, et al. Effects of communitywide education on cardiovascular disease risk factors: the Stanford Five-City Project. *JAMA.* 1990; 264:359–365.

16. Elder JP, Schmid TL, Dower P, Hedlund S. Community heart health programs: components, rationale, and strategies for effective interventions. *J Public Health Policy.* 1993; 4:463–479.

17. Sullivan M, Kelly JG. *Collaborative Research: University and Community Partnership.* Washington, DC: American Public Health Association; 2001.

18. Rummel N, Spada H. Learning to collaborate: an instructional approach to promoting collaborative problem solving in computer-mediated settings. *J Learn Sci.* 2005; 14(2):201–241.

19. Lofir D, Date AR. Reading and Writing Education Research Grants Program. Available at: www.ed.gov/programs/readingresearch/index.html Accessed May 23, 2008.

20. Philbrick DA. Writing a Successful Grant Application. Available at: www.joe.org/joe/1990summer/tt3.html. Accessed May 23, 2008.

21. Lusk SL. Developing an outstanding grant application. *West J Nurs Res.* 2004; 26(3):367–373.

22. Bliss DZ, Savik K, Whitney JD. Writing a grant proposal—part 2: research methods—part 2. *J Wound Ostomy Continence Nurs.* 2005; 32(4):226–229.

23. Cummings PP, Rivara FP, Frederick P, Koepsell TD, Thomas D. Writing informative abstracts for journal articles. *Arch Pediatr Adolesc Med.* 2004; 158(11):1086–1088.

24. Gray M, Bliss DZ. Preparing a grant proposal—part 2: reviewing the literature. *J Wound Ostomy Continence Nurs.* 2005; 32(2):83–86.

25. Murray CJL, Ezzati M, Lopez AD, Rodgers A, Vander Hoorn S. Comparative quantification of health risks: conceptual framework and methodological issues. *Population Health Metrics.* 2003; 1(1):1–20.

26. Kenner C. *Perinatal Alcohol Users: Identification.* Grant funded by the Centers for Disease Control and Prevention. Atlanta, GA: Ingenta; 1991.

27. Grove LK. Writing winning proposals for research funds. *Tech Comm.* 2004; 51:1–8.

28. Xuehao C. Ridership accuracy and transit formula grants. *Transportation Res Rec.* 2006; 1986:3–10.

29. Hiebert SM. The strong-inference protocol: not just for grant proposals. *Advances Physiol Educ.* 2007; 31(1):93–96.

30. Carlson S, Anderson B. What are data? The many kinds of data and their implications for data re-use. *J Comput Mediated Commun.* 2007; 12(2):635.

31. Burke MA. *Simplified Grant Writing.* Thousand Oaks, CA: Corwin Press; 2002.

32. International Council of Nurses. Guidelines for Writing Grant Proposals. Available at: http://www.icn.ch/guidelines_grants.pdf. Accessed May 23, 2007.

33. Van Zant S. Successful Grant-Writing Strategies. *Leadership.* 2003; 32(4):16.

34. Barrett KE. Preparing your curriculum vitae. *J Pediatr Gastroenterol Nutr.* 2002; 34(4):362–365.

35. Fain JA. *Reading, Understanding, and Applying Nursing Research.* 2nd ed. Philadelphia: F.A. Davis; 2003.

36. Boyle M. *Community Nutrition in Action: An Entrepreneurial Approach.* 4th ed. Belmont, CA: Thomson Wadsworth; 2005.

37. Fredalene B. Securing funds through grant writing. *Exchange Early Child Leaders.* 2006; n168:66–69.

38. Schwartz DA, Mastin JP, Martin M. Improving grant application peer review for the NIEHS. *Environ Health Perspect.* 2006; 114(5):A270.

39. SchoolGrants. Grant Writing Tips. Available at: http://www.schoolgrants.org/tips.htm. Accessed May 21, 2007.

40. Locke L, Spirduso W, Silverman S. *Proposals That Work: A Guide for Planning Dissertations and Grant Proposals.* 4th ed. Thousand Oaks, CA: Sage; 2000.

41. Herman D, Harrison GG, Jenks E, Afifi AA. Are Economic Incentives Useful for Improving Dietary Quality Among WIC Participants and Their Families? Available at: http://www.ers.usda.gov/Briefing/FoodNutritionAssistance/Funding/RIDGEprojectSummary.asp?Summary_ID=28. Accessed May 23, 2007.

42. Monsen ER, Vanderpool HY, Halsted CH, McNutt KW, Sandstead HH. Ethics: responsible scientific conduct. *Am J Clin Nutr.* 1991; 54:1–6.

43. Edelman M. *Health Promotion Throughout the Lifespan.* St. Louis, MO: Mosby; 2002.

44. Lutzen K. Moral sensitivity: a study of subjective aspects of the process of moral decision making in psychiatric nursing (dissertation). Stockholm, Sweden: Karolinska Institute; 1993.

45 Holler H. Resources for ethical dilemmas in dietetics. *J Am Diet Assoc.* 2002; 102(12):1817–1818.

46. Winterfeldt E. Influencing public policy. *Top Clin Nutr.* 2001; 16:8–16.

47. American Dietetic Association. Practice paper of the American Dietetic Association: dietary supplements. *J Am Diet Assoc.* 2005; 105(3):460–470.

48. Fornari A. Promoting professionalism through ethical behaviors in the academic setting. *J Am Diet Assoc.* 2004; 104(3):347–349.

49. Rodriguez JC. Legal, ethical, and professional issues to consider when communicating via the Internet: a suggested response model and policy. *J Am Diet Assoc.* 1999; 99:1428–1432.

50. McNutt K. Conflict of interest. *J Am Diet Assoc.* 1999; 99:29–30.

51. McCaffree J. Characteristics of ethical issues versus poor business practices. *J Am Diet Assoc.* 2003; 103(10):1380–1381.

52. Waymack MH. Ethical conflicts of interest. *J Am Diet Assoc.* 2003; 103(5):555–557.

53. American Society for Nutrition Sciences. *Code of Professional Responsibility for Members of the American Society for Nutritional Sciences.* Bethesda, MD: Author; 1998.

54. Rosenstock L, Lee LJ. Attacks on science: the risks to evidence-based policy. *Am J Public Health.* 2002; 92:14–18.

55. Kassirer J. Financial conflict of interest: an unresolved ethical frontier. *Am J Law Med.* 2000; 27:149–162.

56. Cohen JJ. Trust us to make a difference: ensuring public confidence in the integrity of clinical research. *Acad Med.* 2001; 76:209–214.

57. Rock C. An important issue in nutrition research and communications. *J Am Diet Assoc.* 1999; 99:31–32.

58. Andrews M, Marian M. Ethical framework for the registered dietitian in decisions regarding withholding/withdrawing medically assisted nutrition and hydration. *J Am Diet Assoc.* 2006; 106(2):206–208.

59. American Dietetic Association. Code of ethics for the profession of dietetics. *J Am Diet Assoc.* 1999; 99(1):109–113.

60. National Institutes of Health. Regulations and Ethical Guidelines. Available at: http://ohsr.od.nih.gov/guidelines/belmont.html#ethical. Accessed April 25, 2008.

61. Monsen ER. *Research: Successful Approaches.* 2nd ed. Chicago, IL: American Dietetic Association; 2003.

62. U.S. Department of Education. Information About the Protection of Human Subjects in Research Supported by the Department of Education—Overview. Available at: http://www.ed.gov/policy/fund/guid/humansub/overview.html. Accessed May 18, 2007.

63. Côté-Arsenault D, Morrison-Beedy D. Maintaining your focus in focus groups: avoiding common mistakes. *Res Nurs Health.* 2005; 28:172–179.

64. Benner P. Issues in competency-based testing. *Nurs Outlook.* 1982; 30:303–309.

65. Manore MM, Myers EF. Research and the dietetics profession: making a bigger impact. *J Am Diet Assoc.* 2003; 103(1):108–112.

66. Houle CO. *Continuing Learning in the Professions.* San Francisco, CA: Jossey-Bass; 1981.

67. Gates G. Ethics opinion: dietetics professionals are ethically obligated to maintain personal competence in practice. *J Am Diet Assoc.* 2003; 103(5):633–635.

68. Epstein RM, Hundert EM. Defining and assessing professional competence. *JAMA.* 2002; 287:226–235.

69. Hampl J, Hall R. Dietetic approaches to US hunger and food insecurity. *J Am Diet Assoc.* 2002; 102(7):919–923.

70. Lützén K, Dahlqvist V, Eriksson S, Norberg A. Developing the concept of moral sensitivity in health care practice. *Nurs Ethics.* 2006; 13(2):187–196.

71. Frankena WK. *Ethics.* Englewood Cliffs, NJ: Prentice Hall; 1973.

72. Beauchamp TL, Childress JF. *Principles of Biomedical Ethics.* 5th ed. New York: Oxford Press; 2001.

73. O'Sullivan J, Potter RL, Heller L. Position of the American Dietetic Association: ethical and legal issues in nutrition, hydration, and feeding. *J Am Diet Assoc.* 2002; 102(5):716–726.

74. Neukrug E, Lovell C, Parker R. Employing ethical codes and decision-making models: a developmental process. *Counsel Values.* 1996; 40:103.

75. Curry KR, Jaffe A. *Nutrition Counseling and Communication Skills.* Philadelphia: W.B. Saunders; 1998.

76. Watley LD, May DR. Enhancing moral intensity: the roles of personal and consequential information in ethical decision-making. *J Business Ethics.* 2004; 50(2):105–126.

77. Clayman ML, Roter D, Wissow LS, Lawrence S, Bandeen-Roche K. Autonomy-related behaviors of patient companions and their effect on decision-making activity in geriatric primary care visits. *Social Sci Med.* 2005; 60(7):1583–1591.

78. Elger BS. [Ethics in clinical routine care: example of prognosis information]. *Medizinische Klinik.* 2002; 97(9):533–540.

79. Kennedy W. Beneficence and autonomy in nursing. A moral dilemma. *Brit J Periop Nurs.* 2004; 14(11):500–506.

80. Public Health Leadership Society. *Principles of the Ethical Practice of Public Health.* Vol. 2.2. Chicago, IL: American Public Health Association; 2002.

81. Kieselhorst KJ, Skates J, Pritchett E. American Dietetic Association: standards of practice in nutrition care and updated standards of professional performance. *J Am Diet Assoc.* 2005; 105(4):641–656.

82. American Dietetic Association, Commission on Accreditation for Dietetics Education. *Accreditation Manual for Dietetics Education Programs.* 4th ed. Chicago, IL: Author; 2000.

83. Commission on Dietetic Registration. CDR Certifications and State Licensure. Available at: www.cdrnet.org/certifications/index.htm. Accessed May 23, 2008.

84. Myers EF, Barnhill G, Bryk J. Clinical privileges: missing piece of the puzzle for clinical standards that elevate responsibilities and salaries for registered dietitians? *J Am Diet Assoc.* 2002; 102(1):123–132.

85. Parrish D. Assessing Nutritional Habits of Ojibwa Children. In: Stommes E, ed. *Food Assistance and Nutrition Research Small Grants Program: Executive Summaries of 2004 Research Grants.* Washington, DC: U.S. Department of Agriculture; 2005. Available at: http://www.ers.usda.gov/publications/ccr12/. Accessed May 23, 2008.

CHAPTER

14

Principles of Nutrition Education

LEARNING OBJECTIVES
- Define nutrition education.
- Discuss different educational strategies that may be effective in providing nutrition education throughout the life span.
- List the different components of a nutrition education lesson plan.
- Identify strategies to consider when providing nutrition education to participants with different cultural backgrounds.
- Identify ways to encourage participation in a health promotion program.

Introduction

Nutrition education is an essential major component of health promotion and disease prevention strategies, and most major policy documents require integration of nutrition education into healthcare, worksites, colleges, and elementary and secondary schools. In the food marketplace, nutrition education, or the dissemination of food and nutrition information, has also increased in importance.[1,2] Successful nutrition messages are essentially consumer-oriented. The basic principle of the consumer-oriented communication technique is to understand what consumers know, believe, value, and do relating to food, diet, and

nutrition.[3] This chapter discusses the principles of nutrition education and how community nutritionists can design and implement the nutrition education aspect of an intervention.

Educational Principles

Different types of educational principles can be utilized to guide the selection of nutrition and health information for individuals, families, and the public. The most useful categories of educational principles include those associated with the nature of learning, the events of instruction, and guidelines for effective education.[4]

The Nature of Learning

One way to consider the nature of learning is by examining the *cognitive*, *affective*, and *psychomotor domains* of learning. Each domain has explicit behavioral components that form a hierarchy of steps or levels that build on the previous one.[4,5] Understanding these three learning domains is essential in providing effective nutrition education.

Cognitive domain: This involves knowledge and the development of intellectual skills, including the recall or recognition of specific facts, procedural patterns, and concepts that serve in the development of intellectual abilities and skills.[6,7] It also consists of comprehension, understanding, and application and is divided into a hierarchical classification of behaviors. The clients learn each level of cognition in order of difficulty.[5] For nutrition education to be effective, community nutritionists must first assess the cognitive abilities of their clients so expectations and plans are directed toward the correct level. Teaching above or below the participants'/individuals' level of understanding may lead to frustration and discouragement.[4]

Affective domain: This includes the way individuals deal with things emotionally, for example, feelings, values, appreciation, enthusiasm, motivation, and attitude. It also consists of changes in attitude and the development of values.[4,8] In affective learning, nutritionists consider and try to influence what individuals, families, and communities think, value, and feel about nutrition and health. It is important that dietitians listen carefully to detect clues to feelings that may influence learning because their values and attitudes may be different from those of their clients. As with cognitive learning, affective learning consists of a series of steps.[5] A comparison of the affective and cognitive domains is presented in **Table 14.1**. The domains help the nutritionist determine what he or she should evaluate/identify and how to react/adapt based on client status. It is hard to change well-established characteristics such as values, attitudes, beliefs, and interests. People need support and encouragement from health professionals and those around them to reinforce new behaviors in order to make changes.

Psychomotor domain: This includes the performance of skills that require some level of neuromuscular coordination and use of motor skills. Clients can be taught a variety of psychomotor skills, including preparing foods, measuring blood pressure and blood glucose levels, bathing infants, breastfeeding, and so on.[4] The levels of psychomotor learning, from the simplest to the most intricate level of observable movements, are outlined in **Box 14-1**. Three conditions must be achieved before psychomotor learning occurs:[4,5,8]

- The participants must have the needed ability. For example, the nutritionist may find out that a client participating in the Special Supplemental Nutrition Program for Women, Infants, and Children (WIC) may be capable of following instructions for one or two steps on how to feed her newborn infant. Therefore, the nutritionist needs to adapt the education plan to fit the client's abilities.
- The client must have a sensory image of how to carry out the skill. For instance, when educating a group of obese young adults about the skills for managing their weight, the nutritionist may ask them to picture themselves losing weight.

---

nutrition education Any set of learning experiences designed to facilitate the voluntary adoption of eating and other nutrition-related behaviors conducive to health and well-being.

cognitive domain The domain of learning that involves knowledge and the development of intellectual skills. This includes the recall or recognition of specific facts, procedural patterns, and concepts that serve in the development of intellectual abilities and skills.

affective domain The domain of learning that includes the way individuals deal with things emotionally, such as feelings, values, appreciation, enthusiasm, motivation, and attitude. It also consists of changes in attitudes and the development of values.

psychomotor domain The domain of learning that includes the performance of skills that require some degree of neuromuscular coordination.

TABLE 14.1 Steps in the Cognitive Domain Versus the Affective Domain

Step	Cognitive Domain	Affective Domain
Knowledge	Requires recall of data or information; for example, knows the food safety rules.	Clients receive the information.
Comprehension	Combines recall with understanding; for example, states that milk is a good source of calcium.	Clients respond to what is being taught.
Application	Takes new information and uses it in a different way by applying what was learned; for example, purchasing low-fat milk.	Clients value the information.
Analysis	Breaks down communication into components in order to understand the parts and their relationships; for example, compares the fat content of different types of milk.	Clients make sense of the information.
Synthesis	Builds on the previous four levels by putting the parts back together into a unified whole; for example, plan a low-fat and high-calcium diet.	Clients organize the information.
Evaluation	Judges the value of what has been learned; for example, evaluate/analyze the fat and calcium content of a meal.	Clients adopt behaviors consistent with the new value system.

Modified from: Stanhope M, Lancaster J. *Community and Public Health Nursing.* 5th ed. New York: Mosby; 2000; and Dembo MH. *Applying Educational Psychology.* 5th ed. New York: Longman; 1994. Reprinted with permission.

Box 14-1 Levels of Psychomotor Learning

- *Imitation:* Observing and patterning behavior after someone else. Performance may be of low quality. Example: Peeling a carrot.
- *Manipulation:* Being able to perform certain actions by following instructions and practicing. Example: Preparing foods.
- *Precision:* Refining, becoming more exact. Few errors are apparent. Example: Measuring blood glucose levels using a hand-size meter.
- *Articulation:* Coordinating a series of actions and achieving harmony and internal consistency. Example: Planning and preparing a well-balanced meal.
- *Naturalization:* Having a high level of performance becomes natural; clients do not need to think much about it. Example: Eating three nutritious meals a day.

From: Clark D. Performance, Learning, Leadership, and Knowledge. Available at: http://www.nwlink.com/~donclark. Accessed April 28, 2008. Reprinted with permission.

- The client must have opportunities to practice these new skills. It is important to provide practice sessions during the program because many clients may not have the facilities, motivation, or time to practice what they have learned. For example, a new mother needs to practice breastfeeding until she has learned how to feed her baby.

For a community nutritionist to facilitate skill learning, he or she needs to demonstrate the skills to clients, either in person, electronically, or by using visual aids such as posters, pictures, or food models.[4,9] After the demonstration, the nutritionist needs to allow the clients to practice and correct any errors in carrying out the skill.

The following six principles can help the nutritionist carry out effective nutrition education programs:[4,10]

- *Message:* Send a clear message to the learner. Assess the learner's readiness at various stages of the learning process and be cognizant of factors that may affect the learning process (e.g., emotional, physical, or environmental stressors).
- *Format:* Select the most appropriate learning format (e.g., lecture, small group, storytelling methods).
- *Environment:* Create the best possible learning environment (room, furniture, visual aids, flyers, and other materials).
- *Experience:* Organize positive and meaningful learning experiences (create a pleasant atmosphere, present materials in a well-organized and logical manner).
- *Participation:* Engage the learner in participatory learning (use role play, storytelling, hands-on training, case studies, and critical thinking activities).
- *Evaluation:* Evaluate and give objective feedback to the learner

(use quizzes, demonstrations of skills gained). The nutritionist can use the feedback from the learners to improve the education program.

Applying Educational Principles to Program Design and Interventions

Nutrition education has many definitions. For the purpose of this discussion, nutrition education is a learning experience designed to increase the acceptance of eating and other nutrition-related behaviors contributing to health and well-being.[11] This definition and others suggest that behavioral change is the ultimate criterion for effective nutrition education. The term ***behavior*** does not mean measuring nutrient intake by dietary recalls, records, or food frequency questionnaires. It means the effects of nutrition education (such as the intake of specific foods) or actual behaviors (such as eating five fruits and vegetables per day, having fruits available and visible at home, reducing salting of foods, taking the skin off of chicken, having one's bone density or serum cholesterol checked, quitting smoking, exercising five times a week, limiting alcohol intake, or reading a food label).[11,12,13]

Research studies show that nutrition education works.[12,14,15] It is a significant factor in improving dietary practices when behavioral change is set as the goal and the educational strategies used are designed with that intention.[15] It is also important to note that interventions often do not achieve across-the-board success. Generally, nutrition education works on one criterion but not necessarily on another, with one gender but not with the other, or with one ethnic group but not another. Everyone has a different mixture of backgrounds, cultures, health risks, health beliefs, motivators, learning styles, environment, goals, and expectations.[16] Research studies show that the more effective education programs are behaviorally focused and are based on appropriate theories and prior research.[12,17] Behaviorally focused nutrition education encourages the adoption of food and nutrition-related behaviors that are conducive to health and well-being. The behaviors addressed are identified based on the needs, perceptions, motivations, and desires of the target audience as well as from research-based nutrition and health goals.[18]

Studies also show that effective nutrition programs use a combination of modern models of individual, social, and environmental change.[11,19,20] Additionally, effective programs integrate good instructional design and learning principles and use the mass media (television, radio, newspapers, Internet, etc.) to facilitate a high degree of individualization.[16] Educational research intervention studies show that the degree of the intervention's effect on knowledge and behavior could be predicted based on a quality rating of the intervention's application of the six principles of education: consonance, relevance, individualization, feedback, reinforcement, and facilitation.[16,21] **Table 14.2** summarizes how to utilize these principles for effective nutrition education.

Communication models and expectancy-value theories, such as the Health Belief Model or Theory of Reasoned Action (discussed in Chapter 12), have been used to increase awareness and motivation, whether in direct interpersonal interventions or indirect interventions through media.[11] Lately, the most commonly used planning and implementation tool is social marketing.[4] In social marketing, commercial marketing techniques and principles are used to plan, implement, and

behavior The effects of nutrition education (such as the intake of specific foods) or actual behaviors (such as eating five fruits and vegetables per day).

	TABLE 14.2	Application of Educational Principles to Program Design	

Criteria	Description	Example
Consonance	The degree of fit between a program and its objectives, or the degree to which communication is directed toward accomplishing the intended outcome.	An intervention to improve proper breast pump usage; teaching the benefits of using breast pumps without showing how to use them would be insufficient.
Relevance	The degree to which an intervention is geared toward individuals, including the appropriate reading level and visual acuity.	Programs should be tailored to the individual's knowledge, beliefs, circumstances, and prior experiences as determined by pretests, baseline questionnaires, or interviews.
Individualization	Allows individuals to have personal questions answered or instructions paced according to their individual learning progress.	Because individuals learn in different ways and at different rates, a program is more likely to be effective if the education is tailored to individual needs.
Feedback	Helps individuals learn by providing a measuring stick to determine how much progress they are making, if any.	Feedback can be based on achieving learning objectives (such as increased knowledge about a given subject) or outcomes (such as increased adherence to a glucose monitoring regimen).
Reinforcement	Components of the program (other than feedback) designed to reward the desired behavior.	Praise and congratulations are very effective in rewarding changed behavior.
Facilitation	Measures taken to accomplish desired actions or eliminate obstacles.	A blood glucose monitoring hand-size meter facilitates clients' ability to adhere to a prescribed diet.

From: Patterson R. *Changing Patient Behavior: Improving Outcomes in Health and Disease Management*. 1st ed. San Francisco: Jossey-Bass/AHA Press; 2001. Reprinted with permission by John Wiley & Sons, Inc.

evaluate programs designed to change health or social behaviors. The process, also termed consumer-based health communications (CHC), transforms scientific recommendations into message strategies that are relevant to the consumer.[22]

Developing a Nutrition Education Plan

To plan means to develop a method for achieving a particular outcome. People learn or receive new information in different ways; therefore, having a basic understanding of differences in learning styles and planning programs that address these differences can contribute to successful outcomes or behavior change.[23] Dialogue is one of the educational methods or styles that Vella has used in the community under diverse circumstances.[24] This approach is based on the principle that adults have had sufficient life experiences to maintain a dialogue with any teacher about various subjects and can relate the topics to life experiences. The core concept of the dialogue approach is helping teachers become co-learners and learners become co-teachers, and providing opportunities for participants to apply what they have learned. This approach encourages learners to use interaction to achieve the program objectives.

Joye Norris, the author of *From Telling to Teaching*, introduced the concept of learning through dialogue to paraprofessional educators and learners in the Expanded Food and Nutrition Education Program (EFNEP) in Massachusetts.[25] EFNE audiences are typically diverse, including pregnant women, families with children, youth, the homeless, people in shelters and institutions, and people from different cultures.

For the Massachusetts EFNEP program, Norris worked with the paraprofessionals and learners to determine the lesson topics after several meetings and discussions.[25] Their first step after determining the topics was to incorporate a unique element of the curriculum into the topic's names to reinforce each lesson; for example, "Moving to the Mambo" for the movement lesson (physical activity or exercise),

Nutrition education involves teaching people how to read food labels.

"Foods a Go-Go" for eating on the run, "Whole Grain Twist," "5-A-Day Salsa," "Low-Fat Limbo," "Kitchen Calypso," and "Food Safety 4-Step." The titles gave the lessons energy and a sense of the cultural diversity that characterizes the audience. In addition, music that was consistent with the title of each lesson was used to reinforce the elements in the curriculum. The next step was to develop the nutrition education materials; for instance, seven festive color logos, one for each lesson; posters; sorting cards; food safety bingo; food labels; stickers; and three-dimensional models and other educational materials that reinforced the learning objectives were developed. The lesson began with participants sharing their activities in pairs. The participants were given charts (a small one for personal use, and a large one for the group) on which they could monitor their progress.

The following are the five learning principles that Norris used to conduct successful nutrition education programs: [25]

- *Respect:* Respect the learners as decision makers of their own learning. It is also important to respect their characteristics (who they are, where they've been, and what they know).
- *Inclusion:* The learner must be actively involved in the organization and implementation of the activities. Learners are highly motivated and involved when they are working in small groups or teams. Therefore, it is important to make them feel a part of the group and equal to others in the group.
- *Engagement:* Each learner must do more than just listen. They must be involved in what they are learning.
- *Relevancy:* Determine why the information is important to the learner, and how it has personal meaning to them.
- *Safety:* Create an environment that makes the learner feel free to participate in the activities without fear.

Another way a nutritionist can provide an effective nutrition education program to the community is to use an appropriate theoretical model. For example, when providing educational programs to communities, the nutritionist may decide to use the PRECEDE-PROCEED model to organize the teaching program. However, when delivering education to individuals or families, the nutritionist may choose to use the Health Belief Model to identify the specific beliefs, behaviors, or cultural factors that need to be modified to change behaviors.[4] See Chapter 12, it provides detailed information on these models and how they can be used to provide a nutrition education program.

The focus of community nutrition education should be on health promotion for population aggregates. Such education may happen at the local, state, national, or international level. People of all ages and socioeconomic and sociocultural backgrounds should be included. Education can occur in schools, clinics, prisons, worksites, shelters, and community forums. Education programs may be directed toward a specific population, such as diabetic pregnant women, or toward a specific community, such as a town in Mexico with a high incidence of anemia where people want to learn about reducing iron deficiency anemia. Either way, the education plan must address the needs of the specific population. **Table 14.3** presents the skills and strategies community nutritionists can utilize to develop successful nutrition education for communities and individuals.

Examples of behaviors to be addressed by an education program include those related to food, such as adding less salt to food, eating lower fat foods, or adding two vegetables and two glasses of milk a day; those related to other nutritional concerns, such as breastfeeding; or those related to the environment that impact dietary practices, such as using impure water or buying minimally packaged foods.[11,26] Studies show that variations or combinations of several theories, such as

TABLE 14.3	Skills That Help Provide Successful Nutrition Education for Communities and Individuals			
Community Nutritionist/Manager Skills	**Marketing/Promotional Skills**	**Educator/Motivator Skills**	**Evaluator Skills**	**Counselor Skills**
Develop needs assessments	Develop marketing strategies	Develop educational programs	Design program evaluation tools	Advise clients
Develop mission statement, goals, and objectives	Develop marketing programs/plans	Develop assessment programs	Design staff evaluation	Consult with clients
Develop and administer budgets	Develop format/design	Develop lesson plans	Analyze data	Interpret assessment results to clients
Hire and train staff	Select promotional materials (videotapes, CDs/DVDs, handouts, instructional materials, etc.)	Develop evaluations	Interpret results to supervisor/community	Persuade clients to change
Supervise staff		Form a wellness committee	Serve as a role model for staff/clients	
Evaluate staff		Motivate clients		
Communicate with staff	Teach educational programs	Provide support to clients		
Motivate staff		Support behavioral change		
Purchase equipment		Consult with clients		
Develop schedules		Understand the adult learner		
Understand departmental/organizational culture				
Analyze facilities' needs				
Maintain facilities				
Understand legal and ethical regulations for health, nutrition, fitness/wellness programs				
Communicate with higher authorities/supervisor				

From: Anspaugh DJ, Dignan MB, Anspaugh SL. *Developing Health Promotion Programs.* Long Grove, IL: Waveland Press; 2000; p. 10. Reprinted with permission.

the Social Learning Theory and social marketing, have been effective in producing behavioral change.[27,28] **Box 14-2** presents effective research-based educational strategies.[29-31] However, a program can still be suc-

cessful if cognitive and affective domains were addressed. A short-term nutrition program can't expect behavior change outcomes but may create awareness of the nutrition issue.

Box **14-2 Effective Theoretical Research-Based Educational Strategies**

Program Title: Dietary Fat and Heart Disease Intervention Strategy[31]

Objective: To recognize the fat content of commonly consumed food items

Theory Used: Health Belief Model

Activities

- Display food models (interactive) such as food packages, fat-filled test tubes, syringes filled with shortening, whole and nonfat milk, French fries, baked potatoes, croissants, and potato chips.
- Include foods that are popular with the target audience in the food models.
- Create a table tent for each food item in the display by printing the food's name, serving size, and fat content in teaspoons (5 grams fat = 1 tsp) on a 3 × 5" index card folded in half width-wise.
- To make fat-filled plastic test tubes, fill 12 or more test tubes with different amounts of fat in each (i.e., from ¼ to 3 tsp in ¼ tsp increments).
- Fill plastic test tubes by placing the tubes upright in a test tube rack and pouring melted shortening into the tubes through a funnel.
- Set up the display by grouping similar food types together (e.g., place fast foods in one area, dairy products in another area, etc.). Beside each item, place its table tent and a test tube filled with the amount of fat found in one serving. Combine test tubes until the correct amount of fat is displayed.
- Give each visitor a paper plate and a fat-filled syringe. Ask the participant to plan a meal or snack using the foods displayed. Then have the participant squeeze the amount of fat in the meal or snack from the syringe onto the plate. (The syringes can be refilled with shortening and used again. Keep paper towels and spatulas (for mixing, spreading, or lifting) available.

Program Title: Using Food Calendars to Self-Monitor: Got 5? Nutrition for Kids Program (5 A Day Intervention)[29]

Objective: To help establish enhanced lifestyle practices

Theory Use: Transtheoretical Model/Stages of Change Model

Activities

- Provide each child with a guide containing colored pictures and the names of the top 20 fruits and a similar guide for the top 20 vegetables.
- Provide a total of four 2-week calendars. Use colored fruit and/or vegetable calendars.
- Ask students to write down the names of all the fruits and/or vegetables they consumed for four consecutive 2-week color fruit and/or vegetable calendars.

- Review serving sizes during the first lesson.
- Ask students to complete a tally sheet (provided) for each calendar to assist them in self-evaluation.
- Ask parents to sign each calendar once completed.
- Provide incentives for completing each calendar, such as a jump rope for the first calendar, a Beanie baby for the second, a hula-hoop for the third, and a $5 book fair gift certificate for the fourth.

Program Title: Feed Your Mind: An Interactive Nutrition Evaluation for Teenagers (*Jeopardy*-Like Interactive Activity)[30]

Objectives: To detect knowledge and behavior changes that occurred after the nutrition intervention.

Theory: Social Learning Theory and Knowledge-Attitude Behavior Model

Activities

- Provide six examples of nutrition topics, such as calcium; food label reading; fat, weight, and exercise; fast foods; and My Pyramid.
- Use colorful, eye-catching graphics displayed on exhibit boards at the front of a classroom.
- Set game card values at 20, 40, 60, 80, and 100.
- Group game cards into categories to reflect the objectives (Funny Bones, Label Lingo, Skinny on Fat, Movin' and Munchin', Think Fast, and Grab Bag).
- List one nutrition question for 27 of the 30 game cards. List "Go To" on the remaining game cards, which will direct them to the nutrition questionnaire with "yes/no," multiple choice questions.
- Divide participants into teams of four to six players and distribute questionnaires.
- Read aloud 15 questions in section 1 while participants individually mark their responses on the questionnaire (provided).
- Teams will take turns answering game questions after section 1.
- When a "Go To" card is selected, the educator will read the question aloud and direct participants to answer questions individually.
- The game ends when all game card questions are answered.
- The team with the most points wins a nonperishable food item such as juice box.

Source: Byrd-Bredbenner CF, M. *Dietary fat and heart disease intervention strategies. J of Nutrition Education.* 2000; 32 (1):60A. Copyright © 2000 by Elsevier. Data from Kuczmarski MF, Aljadix L. *Using food Calendars to Self-Monitor: Got 5? Nutrition for kids program. J of Nutrition Education.* 2003; 35:269-270. Copyright © 2003 by Elsevier. Data from Struempler BJ, Cobrin S. *Feed your mind: An interactive nutrition evaluation for teenagers. J of Nutrition Education.* 2002; 34(1):59. Copyright © 2000 by Elsevier.

Identify Educational Needs

Community nutritionists learn about the needs of their clients by performing a systematic and thorough client needs assessment. Needs assessments should be part of the education plan because they help the nutritionist develop a level of awareness and anticipate how the target audience will receive the program activities. In addition, the nutritionist needs to create environmental realms that can create a positive and supportive atmosphere and maximize the learning process. **Box 14-3** provides the environmental realms that can be considered. The steps for needs assessments are listed in **Box 14-4** and Chapter 2. Once the needs have been identified, they should then be prioritized to address the most critical educational needs first.[32]

For a nutrition education program to be effective, the nutritionist must establish a comprehensive time table.[33] This can be accomplished by creating a task development time line like the one presented in **Table 14.4**. The task development time line identifies the tasks needed to complete the project and the month or time period in which those tasks will be accomplished.[34] This time line may be modified according to the activities of other programs.

Education Across the Life Span

Nutrition education that has personal meaning for a particular population group is essential. Educational strategies with individuals and groups are more likely to be effective if they address the specific nutrition concerns. It is also important to examine the different intervention strategies that may be effective in providing nutrition education throughout the life span.

Adult Learners

Adult learning is defined as adults gaining knowledge and expertise.[35] Many older adults are interested in measures they perceive will help them remain healthy or that will manage chronic conditions they may be experiencing. This interest motivates them to implement more health-promoting behaviors.[36] Many older people are enthusiastic readers and are familiar with the current nutrition issues in the media. Health-conscious older persons accept nutrition education offered through the radio, television, local newspapers, magazines, journals, the Internet, or the American Dietetic Association and Cooperative Extension Services hotlines that they can call for answers to their nutrition questions. In addition, adult education programs such as peer or shared learning groups and Cooperative Extension Programs provide nutrition education to older adults.[37]

Educational interventions exist in which a major goal is improving the knowledge of older adults. The nutrition intervention strategies that have been

adult learning Adults gaining knowledge and expertise.

Box 14-3 Environmental Realms

Physical Realm

This realm includes setting up the program and positioning the presenter and the clients in a physical relationship to one another. It also includes lighting and temperature of the room, volume of amplification equipment, furniture, and bathroom facilities. The more subtle effects of environment are those that create a stimulating setting, allow for few external distractions, and assist the learner in concentration and attention.

Interpersonal Realm

This realm consists of human relationships and should be therapeutic, supportive, and conducive to producing quality educational interactions. The interpersonal dynamic should be one in which learners experience a clear sense that the educator cares about their progress and needs. Learners can also contribute to the interpersonal environment by showing interest in the subject and remaining responsible for both peer and group interactions.

Organizational Realm

This realm entails the administrative aspects of the educational program. Beginning with scheduling, announcements, and other preparations, this is the realm that makes the components of the program merge into an effective learning session. Arrangements for parking, delivery of audio-visual materials, ensuring readability of printed or projected materials, and responsiveness to ongoing learner needs and requests are a few examples of the organizational aspects of environment.

From: Stanhope M, Lancaster J. *Community and Public Health Nursing.* 5th ed. New York: Mosby; 2000. Reprinted with permission from Elsevier.

Box 14-4 Steps of a Needs Assessment

1. Identify what the clients want to know.
2. Establish how the clients want to learn, what they think, and what they feel.
3. Identify what will improve the clients' ability and motivation to learn.
4. Collect data from the family, community, and other sources to assess learning needs, willingness to learn, and situational and psychosocial factors that would influence learning. Do presession surveys.
5. Provide a data-based context for the program.
6. Analyze assessment data to identify cognitive, affective, and psychomotor learning needs. Encourage clients' participation in the process. Provide on-the-spot assessments.
7. Help the clients prioritize learning needs.

From: Volker DL. Patient education: needs assessment and resource identification. *Oncol Nurs Forum.* 1991; 18(1):119. Copyright ©1991 by Oncology Nursing Society. Reprinted with permission.

TABLE 14.4 A Task Development Time Line for a Comprehensive Health Promotion Program

Task	Jan	Feb	Mar	Apr	May	Jun	Jul	Aug	Sep	Oct	Nov	Dec
Determine financial commitment	X											
Interview/survey client groups	X											
Conduct needs assessment	X											
Determine target audience	X											
Determine program identifier	X											
Form employee committee	X	X										
Development mission statement		X										
Develop goals and objectives		X										
Determine programs		X										
Determine format		X										
Determine staff needs			X									
Determine equipment needs			X									
Train staff			X	X								
Determine nutrition messages				X	X							
Determine partnerships			X	X								
Develop lesson plan Program I Program II Program III					X	X	X					
Develop program marketing Comprehensive program Individual components								X	X	X	X	X
Plan program evaluation				X								X
Implement program Program I Program II Program III									X	X	X	
Evaluate program Program I Program II Program III											X	X

From: Anspaugh DJ, Dignan MB, Anspaugh SL. *Developing Health Promotion Programs*. Long Grove, IL: Waveland Press; 2000. Reprinted with permission.

effective in increasing nutrition knowledge for improved nutritional adequacy in this population include:[11,38–40]

- *Personalized approaches* such as self-assessment of nutritional status or behaviors and comparison of these with recommendations. Cholesterol and bone density screenings and dietary intake assessments are effective starting points for nutrition education.
- *Behavioral approaches* include individual self-assessments followed by behavioral self-management techniques, such as goal setting, problem solving, and social support.
- *Attention to motivators and reinforcements* include an interest in maintaining health, providing opportunities for social interaction and social support, enhancing self-efficacy, and recognizing the need for good taste and ease of food preparation.

The following are some tips to consider when providing nutrition education to older adults:[41,42]

- Use previous experiences as learning resources. Collaborate with the adult learner by sharing life experiences and knowledge. Use direct experience such as family health history and past experiences. It also is important to note that adults tend to learn in stages. See **Figure 14-1** for the adult learning stages.
- Modify the presentation of learning resources to the learner's level of experience. Consider the impact of chronic conditions/disease, and emotional and cultural factors on the client's ability to communicate or learn the materials.
- Provide feedback about the client's achievement of objectives at periodic intervals. This will help maintain the client's attention span.

Application/Personalized Approach
Hands-on learning experience
Small group experience
Participating in a dialogue about nutrition
Collaborative learning
Behavior change
Having fruits and vegetables available and visible

Direct Experience/ Attention to Motivators
Family health history
Past experiences
Culture
Health beliefs
Chronic health condition

Generalization About Nutrition Knowledge
Knows how to cook
Uses vitamin and mineral supplements

Reflection on Experiences/ Behavioral Approach
Lifestyle
Exercise and eating habits
Health screening and nutrition activities

FIGURE 14-1   The Adult Learning Stages

- Guide the adult learner to reflect on the learning experiences that lead to lifestyle change, such as an increase in physical activities and improved eating habits.
- Connect the adult learner's previous health experiences (such as hypertension, diabetes, or heart disease) to the nutrition education.
- Arrange for a comfortable physical environment conducive to interaction with and among adult learners. Provide hands-on learning experiences using small group experiences and collaborative learning.

Child Learners

Nutrition education for young children is an area of high priority because of the severe consequences hunger and malnutrition can have on this group. Anemia, obesity, dental caries, and growth retardation are nutritional concerns for preschool-age children.[11,43,44] Children are not born with the natural ability to choose nutritious foods, but they are born with a preference for sweet tastes.[45] They also show negative reactions to bitter and sour tastes and a neutral response to salty tastes. It has also been found that preference for a food is a major determinant of food intake in young children.[46] Involving children in meal planning and preparation will increase their food acceptance and intake. Successful nutrition education programs for children have used the following intervention strategies:[11,47–50]

- *Involving parents/families* as the main recipients of the program or in combination with a program offered to preschool and school-age children. Children have shorter attention spans than adults. They tend to learn more through adult active participation.
- *Using a behaviorally focused approach* that targets children's behaviors using a social modeling of peer and adult role models eating nutritious meals and snacks. Adults should offer food to children in a positive social environment and not as rewards.
- *Using developmentally appropriate learning experiences and materials* for children ages 4 to 7 so they understand concepts such as having energy and a strong heart, eating low-fat foods, and keeping germs out of the body.

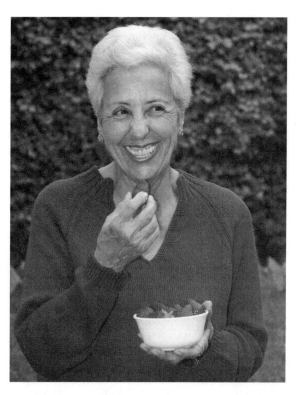

Guide the adult learner to reflect on experiences that lead to lifestyle changes, such as eating habits.

- *Presenting food-based activities* such as tasting parties, food preparation, vegetable and fruit gardens, engaging the five senses with food, eating nutritious meals and snacks, and interactive activities (games, songs, role playing, stories, puppets, and puzzles).
- *Incorporating a self-evaluation or self-assessment and feedback component* is effective in interventions for older children with personalized computer-assisted feedback.
- *Using abstract thinking* as a learning tool for adolescents. Like adults, adolescents are able to reason deductively. Using peer groups is a significant method of enhancing adolescents' learning.

These are additional tips to consider when providing nutrition education to children:[49,50]

- Create a positive attitude toward food.
- Build children's self-esteem by serving cultural and ethnic foods.
- Introduce a variety of unfamiliar nutritious foods.
- Have children participate in mealtime activities, such as setting the table, preparing food, serving food, and cleaning up.

Table 14.5 presents motivating factors for nutrition learning and how adults and children learn.

Pregnant and Lactating Women

The goal of nutrition education for pregnant women, as well as lactating women, is relatively clear: appropriate maternal weight gain, nutritional adequacy of the maternal diet, and positive infant outcomes, such as satisfactory birth weight. (See Chapter 8 for more information

	Motivating Factors and How Adults and Children Learn			
TABLE 14.5	**How Adults Learn**	**Adult Motivators**	**How Children Learn**	**Child Motivators**
	Reading	Health condition	Role models	Parents
	Media (television, radio, magazines, and the Internet)	Health consciousness	Role play/observation	Teachers
	Social interaction	Family history	Stories and songs/music	Peers
	Stories	Health beliefs	Demonstration	Parents
	Hands-on experience	Friends	Hands-on experience	Media (television and magazines)
	Demonstration and dialogue	Relatives/family	Media (videotape, television, and the Internet)	Food tasting
	Observation and reflection		Peers	Curiosity
	Small group discussions		Games and fieldtrips	
	Focus groups and role play			

on pregnant and lactating women.) The methods and timing of interventions are very important. The following are some effective intervention strategies:[11,51,52]

- *Nutrition counseling and classes that focus on pregnant women's specific behaviors* using individualized assessment. The followup sessions should reinforce and maintain behavior.
- *Prenatal exposure to information about the benefits of breastfeeding* with respect to health benefits using group classes and peer breastfeeding classes. Peer education involves inspiring a group of pregnant and lactating women to express health and nutritional messages to each other. The group becomes active participants in the educational process instead of passive recipients.
- *Incentives for participation* are very successful for the Special Supplemental Nutrition Program for Women, Infants, and Children (WIC) population. For example, grocery store discount coupons can motivate participation.

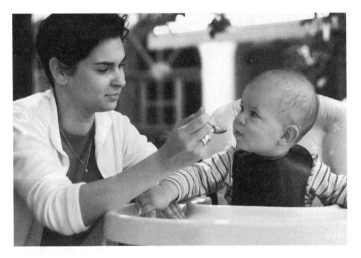

Preference for a food is a major determinant of food intake in young children. It is important to create a positive attitude toward food.

Additional tips for providing an effective nutrition intervention include:[4,11,49]

- Using pamphlets to address the benefits of breastfeeding for mothers and infants
- Asking open-ended questions
- Facilitating cooperative learning skills and group processes
- Being friendly
- Sending clear messages to clients
- Engaging the learner in participatory learning
- Organizing positive and meaningful learning experiences

Education and Culture

How a person interprets messages is based on his or her cultural framework; interpretation of visual elements varies considerably by ethnic group. What may be attractive, appealing, or acceptable to one ethnic group or subgroup may not be so to others.[11] When designing nutrition education materials, it is important to use cultural images that people of the target ethnic group view as positive. It is also important to use those images/symbols within a framework that the target audience feels is appropriate. For example, one educational program created an initial version of a booklet for American Indians on reducing dietary fat that portrayed an eagle on the cover. Although the contents of the booklet were understood and accepted by the target audience, the use of the eagle, a sacred and positive image for this group, was considered inappropriate for the cover of a nutrition education booklet. The cover was redesigned and retested.[11]

Equally important is geography because it influences dietary choices. With regard to dietary practices, the accessibility, affordability, and acceptability of available foods play a more important role than ethnicity in the use of those foods.[53] For example, when a sample poster developed for a Nigerian group with pictures of romaine lettuce, bananas, Brussels sprouts, beets, bean sprouts, seaweed, and peas was used in an area where some of these foods, such as Brussels sprouts, bean sprouts, and seaweed, were not readily available, the group showed poor recognition and acceptance of these items. But these foods were acceptable to another group that had access to them. See Chapter 16 for more information on the influence of culture on the acceptability of foods. The following are additional strategies for nutrition education interventions that may be used for a multicultural group:[11,54,55]

- Review revised materials for illustration/content issues.
- Modify materials based on input from working groups.
- Be knowledgeable about appropriate reading levels (literacy).
- Have an understanding of the cultural appropriateness of vocabulary.
- Limit the number of messages in each educational piece.
- Put people into partnerships—pair up, discuss, and share ideas to engage the participants.
- Use the Health Belief Model when organizing messages.
- Make note of visual appropriateness (with particular attention to cultural preferences/taboos).
- Incorporate an interactive style.
- Use quality visuals.
- Use bilingual interpreters.

Developing a Lesson Plan

An effective nutrition education program requires thorough planning. The nutrition education *lesson plan* needs to describe the desires of the target population. It is the blueprint for organizing a class.[56] A well-designed lesson plan ensures a clear focus and articulates specific learning outcomes. The nutrition messages of a particular educational program may be designed to change the learners' behavior. For example, the nutritionist plans to use MyPyramid chart to demonstrate how to achieve the Fruits and Veggies—More Matters message to "Eat Five to Stay Alive." The chart will portray different types of fruits and vegetables. Fruits and Veggies—More Matters is a national media program designed to encourage the U.S. population to eat five or more servings of fruits and vegetables daily. The program is a joint venture of the National Cancer Institute (NCI) and the Produce for Better Health Foundation.[57]

Lesson plans encourage advanced planning and organization. They help the educator prepare and have instructional materials ready. They also help the nutrition educator think carefully about matching methods and outcomes and think about how to present new information in interesting ways while meeting the needs of different learning styles. See **Table 14.3** for methods that can be used to plan a successful nutrition education program.

The written format of the planned activities should be as individualized as the target audience, but all activity plans should include these basic features: [58]

- Subject/lesson title or concept to be presented
- Specific objectives
- Format
- Materials list
- Procedure/step-by-step learning activities
- Target audience
- Duration
- Evaluation and suggestions for improvement

Components of a Lesson Plan

Each individual lesson should be planned in advance, contain enough information so another person can use it, and follow a format that is consistent. Activities can then be modified to address the needs of a particular segment of the population. Lesson plans usually include the following:[58]

- *Title of the lesson:* The title captures the audience's attention. It is very important because it can make the difference between attendance and non-attendance of the health promotion program. The title is the main concept/component of the marketing plan and should be 10 words or less; for example, "Building Better Bones."
- *Target audience:* It is important to identify the clientele at the beginning of the lesson plan. The target audience determines the communication formats that will be used. Knowing the target audience helps determine the type of promotional strategy to use. For example, if the target audience is of low literacy, then the nutritionist will use an alternative method (i.e., videotapes, demonstration) to ensure that the message is understood.
- *Duration:* Determine the time period that will be most acceptable to the target audience to get the greatest number of participants. Determine how long the program will take, including break time. Some nutrition education programs may take from one to three class periods.
- *Program goal:* The lesson plan should contain a general statement(s) about the desired outcome of the health promotion program; for example, plan a nutritious diet that can reduce the risk of cancer. Each goal should be linked to the objective of the program.
- *Objective:* This establishes the content to be addressed in the lesson and identifies the behavior to be practiced that will yield a successful outcome. It indicates observable clients' behavior and serves as the basis for evaluation of the lesson; for example, the clients will be able to increase the number of fruits and vegetables eaten from two a day to five a day.
- *Procedure:* It is important to determine how the program activities will be carried out in the lesson plan. Include how the activities will be introduced and any background information. List each step sequentially. Include a clear outline of the sequence of activities to be used in a class session. Also include the conclusion/closure of the program.
- *Learning experiences or activities:* It is essential to determine the instructional strategies in the lesson plan. Strategies are methods that can help participants personalize information. They encourage interaction among participants and help them assess their personal feelings about the health promotion information. Examples of strategies include discussion groups, overhead transparencies, participant worksheets and the instructor's answer key, puzzles, games, PowerPoint slides, video clips and discussion, and small group exercises. These activities can give the clients the content and concepts of the program. Outline the different activities/events and tasks that must be accomplished during the learning experience.
- *Method of evaluation:* This helps the instructor see if the participants have achieved the objective. List the strategies for evaluating the effectiveness of the educational program, the amount or level of knowledge acquired, the attitude affected, or the behavioral changes made due to the educational program. Determine how the program outcomes will be evaluated, such as using a questionnaire that asks the participants to write down what they liked or disliked about the program and whether

> **lesson plan** The blueprint for organizing a class. A well-designed lesson plan ensures a clear focus and articulates specific learning outcomes.

it helped them. Another strategy could be to administer a pre- and posttest.

- *Materials needed:* It is important to list all the materials needed for the educational program in the lesson plan. The materials are the tools needed for accomplishing the program's goals and objectives, such as videotapes, foods (e.g., different sizes, colors, and shapes of fruits and vegetables), disposable plates and napkins, an overhead projector, computer, handouts, food models, and so on.

The following section presents a sample lesson plan on bone health.

Lesson Plan Sample

Title: Bone Health

Target Audience: Women 55 years and older

Program Goals: The participants will learn the content of MyPyramid to reduce the risk of osteoporosis.

Objectives: The participants will be able to:

- Identify the main food groups and list foods that are high in calcium and fat.
- Distinguish between a fruit and a vegetable.
- Learn how to select a low-fat, high-calcium diet.

Materials/Equipment:

- Food models
- Paper plates
- Packages from a variety of healthy and "junk" foods
- MyPyramid diagram
- Projector
- Menu (restaurant)
- Table

Duration: One hour (with one 15-minute) break

Procedure:

- Display MyPyramid chart on the overhead projector.
- Exhibit food groups according to similarity using food models; for example, place the dairy products on one area of the table.
- Introduce the activities enthusiastically and encourage participation at the beginning of the session.
- Summarize the session by either summarizing the discussion points or encouraging the participants to try the new strategies from the educational program.

Learning Activities:

- Give each participant a paper plate.
- Allow participants to select a total of five fruits and vegetables for their plate.
- Conduct a discussion about the differences of the foods they have selected.
- Ask the participants to brainstorm all of the foods they can think of that are made with milk.
- Ask the participants to analyze the menu from a popular restaurant and see if the menu contains food from each group.

Evaluation Method:

- Ask the participants to list three high-calcium foods.
- Ask the participants to list two low-fat foods.
- Ask the participants to list the MyPyramid food groups.

Specify the Nutrition Messages

In a lesson plan, it is important to identify nutrition issues and what motivates the audience. The message should go beyond demographics such as race/ethnicity, age, gender, education level, and income level.[58] It is important that the nutrition educator specifies the actions or behavioral change(s) that he or she wants the target audience to adopt. It is also important to use straightforward language that is relevant and compelling to the audience; for example, take a brisk 10-minute walk on your lunch break to encourage physical activity. See **Table 14.6** for communication guidelines for educational interaction. More information on nutrition messages is provided later in this chapter.

Choose a Program Identifier

Choosing a **program identifier** that expresses the main idea of the program is important. A program identifier is a logo, slogan, motto, or tagline that communicates the main concept of the education program.[58] Typically, these make claims about providing an important benefit or solution or about being most suitable for the target audience. The idea behind the concept is to create a memorable phrase that sums up the educational program or reinforces the target audience's memory of the issue. These can be used in promotional materials such as brochures, flyers, and posters. It is important to share the initial logo and promotional materials' concepts with members of the target audience or colleagues for their input.

Develop a Marketing Plan

An effective marketing program is crucial for the nutrition education program to be successful. The main purpose of the marketing plan is to attract the attention of the target audience. Consequently, it is important that the community nutritionist knows the target audience, keeps the message simple and to the point, and avoids clutter. Cluttered media, mainly too many words and pictures, can overpower the program's messages.[33] See Chapter 15 for further details.

Form Partnerships

When developing the marketing plan, it is beneficial to form partnerships with entities such as local businesses, healthcare organizations, and government agencies. For example, local businesses may donate giveaway materials for prizes (e.g., T-shirts, cookbooks, gym bags, gift certificates, restaurant certificates, movie certificates) that can be used as incentives to stimulate interest in the program.[33] The community nutritionist also can form partnerships with other health promotion organizations, such as the American Heart Association or American Cancer Institute, during their health promotion kick-off events. This is a good way to initiate the program and reduce the program's cost. Events can include ribbon cuttings, local celebrity events, drawings, food tasting, or other activities.

Establish Educational Goals and Objectives

Once the clients' needs are determined, the goals and objectives to guide the educational program should be established and stated. *Objectives* are written statements of intended outcomes. They are specific, short-term measures that should be accomplished in steps toward achieving the long-term goal. Objectives are stated in terms of expected outcomes—an end result that must be achieved or an expected change in behavior. The expected outcomes need to be defined in measurable terms;[4] for example, participants are expected to identify high-fat foods from a list provided.

TABLE 14.6	**Communication Guidelines for Educational Interactions**

Communication Method	Action
Begin strong.	People remember the first point.
Use a clear, direct, and succinct style.	This helps the learner remain focused.
Use the active voice.	For example, the educator could say, "We will discuss relaxation techniques" instead of "Relaxation techniques will be discussed."
Accentuate the positive.	For example, the educator could say, "The majority of individuals are able to lose weight with a well-balanced diet and exercise" instead of "A few people have not been able to lose weight with a well-balanced diet and exercise."
Use vivid communication, not statistics or jargon.	Specific case histories are often more meaningful than general, nonspecific terms or dry statistics.
Refer to trustworthy sources.	For example, "the surgeon general" is a more credible source than "some people."
Base strategies on a knowledge of the audience.	Be aware of the perceptions and perspectives of the audience.
Make points explicitly.	Be direct and give clear instructions.
End strong.	The last point made is likely to be remembered.

Source: Stanhope M, Lancaster J. *Community and Public Health Nursing*. 5th ed. New York: Mosby; 2000. Reprinted with permission.

Determine Which Methods to Use

The educational methods chosen for the program need to accomplish the program's goals and objectives. Choose methods that match the clients' strengths and needs. Use the strategies previously listed for adults and children that match the target audience. The lesson plan may require cooking demonstrations, small group sessions, mass media techniques (radio, posters, etc.), case studies, and lectures. You will need to select the appropriate teaching tools, such as audio-visual aids, videotapes, handouts, health assessment equipment, and PowerPoint presentations.[4]

Implement the Program

After the educational methods have been established, they need to be implemented. Implementation entails the following:[4,59]

- Control the starting and stopping of each method and strategy at the most appropriate time and manner (e.g., arrive early, start with greeting the clients first to capture their attention, use warm-ups or icebreakers to get people involved).
- Coordinate and control the environmental factors, the flow of the presentation, and other contributory facets of the program to set the stage for a positive learning environment (e.g., noise, arrange for a babysitter, set a break time).
- Keep the materials logically related to the overall program goals.
- Listen before starting to teach. Encourage participation and acknowledge different viewpoints.
- Edit information. Provide important information first.

Evaluate the Educational Process

Evaluating a nutrition education program is as important in the educational process as it is in the nutrition practice, and it must be included in the lesson plan. Educational evaluation includes:[4]

- Educator evaluation
- Process evaluation
- Product evaluation

Educator evaluation allows for modifications in the teaching process and enables the nutritionists to adequately address the learners' needs.[10,60] The evaluation may occur throughout (formative evaluation) or at the end of the program (summative evaluation). Ongoing evaluation allows the teacher to correct misinformation, misinterpretation, or confusion. The educator may receive feedback verbally or nonverbally. *Process evaluation* examines the components of the education program[61] to determine whether goals and objectives were being addressed throughout the program. The *product evaluation* evaluates the outcome of the educational process.[61] The process can be measured qualitatively and quantitatively.[62] For example, a qualitative assessment answers the question, "How well does the learner appear to understand the content?" A quantitative assessment answers the question, "How much of the content does the learner retain?"[62]

Different approaches can be used to evaluate nutrition and behavioral changes. These include questionnaires, surveys, skills demonstrations, testing, subjective client feedback, and direct observation of improvements in client mastery of materials.

Gather, Organize, and Structure Knowledge

The nutrition educator serves as the facilitator of the education process. Therefore, selecting plans appropriate for the

program identifier A statement or motto that succinctly defines or represents the aim of the program.

objectives Written statements of intended outcomes. The expected outcomes need to be defined in measurable terms.

target audience that support the stated objectives is very important (see **Table 14.6**). Despite the educator's level of knowledge or the quality of the interpersonal relationship that the educator has developed with the learner, good organization of the material is important for learning to happen. Materials need to be presented in a logical and integrated manner, from simple introductory concepts to more complex ideas. As part of the lesson plan, the educator needs to locate, evaluate, and validate the sources of the health and nutrition information that is being communicated to the clients. It is also essential to make the concepts/ideas clear to the participants. The speed of the presentation should match the ability of the learner and leave enough pauses for the learner to absorb the information.[4] The following questions can help the nutrition educator structure the educational concept:[58]

- *What* are the contents/concepts to be addressed in the lesson? Define the objective of the activities; for example, 5-year-old children can name at least two foods that are good for teeth. Make sure the material is culturally sensitive.
- *Where* is the location of the activity? Make sure it is accessible to the target audience.
- *When* will the program start and how often will it take place? Establish the length of the activity.
- *Who* is the segment of the population/target audience participating in the activities? What is the audience's profile (age, gender, race/ethnicity, socioeconomic status, education, and religion)?
- *How* will the activities be carried out effectively? For adult learners, case studies, small group work, computer interactive activities, panel presentations, and demonstrations are very effective;[63] for children, games, demonstration, role playing, and fieldtrips are effective methods; and for large-group presentations, lectures, demonstrations, groups, and panel presentations are effective.[64] It is also essential to use visual aids such as flipcharts, transparencies, handouts, or slides.

Figure 14-2, Dale's Cone of Experience, presents some active learning experiences that can be utilized to carry out educational activities.

Enhancing and Achieving Program Participation

It is reported that effective programs to promote improved dietary practices among low-income families depend on the motivation and performance of the educator. Motivating clients to participate is essential to the progress and success of nutrition and health promotion programs.[65] Hence, the activities of the program require a variety of appealing strategies and an awareness of the practical and psychosocial concerns of potential participants. *Participation*, as it pertains to this discussion, is when clients join others in health promotion activities. One of the strategies for encouraging participation is including health risk assessments, such as screening for blood pressure and other preventive health screenings, as a tool to attract potential participants into health promotion activities. Also, matching clients with partners may increase participation.

For example, Meana and Stewart investigated potential factors affecting decisions to engage in a cardiac rehabilitation program (CRP).[66] One hundred and twenty-nine attendees and 61 nonattendees completed the study. Results showed that physician recommendation was the most important factor influencing both

participation When clients join others in health promotion activities.

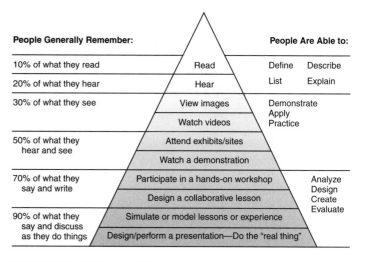

FIGURE 14-2 Dale's Cone of Experience

Adapted from: Edgar Dale's *Cone of Experience, Audio-Visual Methods in Teaching*, 3rd ed. (New York: Holt, Rinehart, and Winston, 1969). Reprinted with permission from Raymond S. Pastore, Bloomsburg University, Bloomsburg, PA 17815-1301.

women's and men's decisions to participate in CRP, followed by encouragement from family members. For women who attended the CRP, encouragement from their adult children was significantly more influential than it was for men. Attention to health promotion was also a significantly more powerful motivator for women.

In addition, more clients will participate in health-promoting activities or programs if they are accessible, affordable, and convenient. Other practical strategies that community nutritionists may use to encourage clients to join health promotion programs include:[32,67]

- Adapting the program literature or educational materials to the demographic characteristics of the target audience
- Considering the educational level of the participants
- Finding convenient class times and locations (e.g., grocery stores, worksites)
- Distributing promotional materials (e.g., newsletters, flyers, radio, e-mail, TV)
- Providing incentives (e.g., T-shirts, magnets, gym bags, headbands, cookbooks, restaurant certificates)

General Ideas for Designing Messages

Health and nutrition messages must be consumer oriented. The community will choose to work with the nutritionist based on the benefits to be gained. Few people will attend a workshop or planning session just out of curiosity.

Many organizations such as the American Dietetic Association, the U.S. Department of Agriculture, the U.S. Department of Health and Human Services, and others have combined efforts to develop positive nutrition messages. In 1998 and 1999, the International Food Information Council (IFIC) conducted focus group research with consumers to determine the barriers that consumers experience in adopting healthy diets. IFIC developed tips for communicating nutrition messages that resonate with consumers.[68] These tips are presented in **Table 14.7**. Community nutritionists can incorporate these messages into different nutrition and education promotion programs. The Successful Community Strategies showcases a successful social marketing message.

Nutrition messages may be designed to change the learners' behavior, such as the USDA's MyPyramid/Steps to a Healthier You initiative.

TABLE 14.7	**Tips for Communicating Nutrition Messages**

Theme	Consumer-Tested Messages/Tips
Be positive.	Split an order of fries with a friend.
	Enjoy a single-scoop ice cream cone instead of a double.
Keep it short and simple.	Open a cookbook and try a new recipe each week.
	Stash packets of instant oatmeal and some juice boxes in your desk.
Make it specific and manageable.	Take a brisk 10-minute walk on your lunch break.
Provide a payoff.	Substitute a glass of milk for a can of soda. You'll build your bone density.
Create a "just for me" message.	Love the taste of whole milk? Balance it with lower-fat foods such as reduced-fat cheese, low-fat sour cream, or fat-free salad dressing.
Talk food and fun.	Try fun snacks, such as fresh fruit kabobs dipped in your favorite fruity yogurt or baked tortilla chips with zesty black bean dip.

Source: International Food Information Council. IFIC Tools for Effective Communications. Available at: http://ific.org/tools. Accessed April 30, 2008. Reprinted with permission.

Designing Nutrition and Health Messages

One role of the community nutritionist is to clarify mixed messages that consumers receive from various sources (family, friends, professional colleagues, the media, the Internet, etc.) and tailor the health messages according to the client's specific needs and health situations. One of the positive aspects of being a nutrition and health educator is that the majority of the U.S. population is interested in nutrition and health messages. For example, research shows that four out of every five persons surveyed agreed that there is a relationship between diet and health,[69,70] 57 percent became more aware of the benefits of a healthy diet in the previous year,[71] and more than half of consumers reported searching for diet and nutrition information in the last month.[72] In addition, 41 percent felt that they were doing all they could to eat healthfully.[73]

The task of educating consumers without overwhelming them is challenging. It means presenting the information in ways consumers want to hear it. For example, positive messages can help prevent the confusion that occurs due to conflicting information. It is reported that the news media disseminate more positive messages than negative ones about food.[40] This positive approach enables consumers to achieve the principles of a healthy diet and physical activity as part of their overall lifestyle. For example, take a 10-minute brisk walk on your lunch break. It will help you feel better, and you will become more energetic.

It is the responsibility of the educator to provide information that is understandable. Medical jargon and technical terms may hinder the clarity of the intended message.[74] For example, when helping clients understand diet control for hypercholesterolemia, the dietitian might use the phrase "high blood cholesterol" rather than the "hypercholesterolemia."

Successful Community Strategies

Social Marketing Nutrition Education Campaign[69]

The 5-A-Day for Better Health program advocated, through media and other channels, that individuals consume five servings of fruits and vegetables each day. The amount of information disseminated by the program was impressive. Within 1 month, there were 1,800 media messages. Within 1 year, all governors had signed proclamations of support, 225 newspapers had carried stories, and 1 million brochures had been distributed about the program. Results showed that the campaign and its principal message had substantial penetration during the 2 years of the campaign; the percentage of Americans who knew that five or more was the number of servings of fruits and vegetables to eat each day for good health increased from a baseline of 8 percent to 29 percent, and the percentage who believed that eating fruits and vegetables would likely help prevent cancer rose from 45 to 64 percent. On the other hand, 13 percent (up from 8 percent) reported that it would be very hard to eat five or more servings of fruits and vegetables per day.

Successful Community Strategies

The Partners for Life Nutrition Education Program for Pregnant Women[75]

The Freedom from Hunger Foundation (FHF) joined the Mississippi Cooperative Extension Service and the State Department of Health to establish the Partners for Life Program (PFLP). The purpose of this joint venture was to address the maternal nutrition problems in the Delta region. Leflore County, a county representative of the Delta region, was selected as the pilot site for a formative evaluation of a nutrition education program for high-risk pregnant women prior to implementation of the PFLP in the other five Delta counties. The investigators and program planner's goal was to collect data that would answer the following questions:

- Could the Expanded Food and Nutrition Education Program (EFNEP) curriculum be adapted to meet the nutritional needs of pregnant women?
- Could peer educators be trained to deliver an effective intervention?
- Could pregnant women be successfully recruited to participate in the program?
- Would the adapted curriculum produce sufficient data in a pilot study to determine its potential for changing dietary knowledge and behavior in pregnancy?
- What are the reactions of pregnant women regarding participation in the program and usability of the nutrition program?

To accomplish this goal an advisory committee consisting of physicians, nurses, nutritionists, health educators, and other health professionals with a maternal and child health viewpoint was formed. The advisory committee provided guidance to the PFLP staff about the development and adaptation of the EFNEP nutrition education program. The investigators adapted EFNEP's methodology for pregnant clients in the local WIC program receiving maternity care at the county health department. The nutrition education lessons were delivered in a sequence of eight consecutive weekly sessions of 60 minutes each. The main teaching format was discussion and observational learning in the clients' homes.

This approach created an interactive education/teaching style. The content areas of the lesson were:

- Maternal and infant nutrition
- Health problems and solutions
- Eating healthy and healthy baby
- How to make decisions
- Saving for mother and baby
- Food, friends, and fun
- Caring for the baby
- Preparation for delivery

Results of the formative evaluation showed both positive and negative outcomes. Positive outcomes were 1) the recruitment and training of the peer educators to provide the intervention had a positive outcome, 2) the recruitment of the targeted population for the pilot study was successful, 3) the successful completion of the project questionnaires and measuring forms, and 4) the improvement in nutrition knowledge and dietary behavior was statistically significant. Two negative outcomes in this formative study were 1) the program experienced problems retaining participants it recruited and 2) deviation of the time frame for intervention delivery. Participants identified program length as the main reason for their dissatisfaction. The authors recommended that nutrition educators and planners can use the results from this formative evaluation to make changes in problem areas (participant retention and length of the program) prior to implementation of a full-scale impact evaluation.

Chapter Summary

- Nutrition education is any set of learning experiences designed to facilitate the voluntary adoption of eating and other nutrition-related behaviors conducive to health and well-being.
- It is important to note that interventions often do not achieve across-the-board success. Generally, nutrition education works on one criterion, but not necessarily on another, or with one gender, but not with the other.
- One way to consider the nature of learning is by examining the cognitive, affective, and psychomotor domains of learning. Each domain has explicit behavioral components that form a hierarchy of steps or levels that build on the previous one.
- The nutrition intervention strategies that have been effective in increasing nutrition knowledge for improved nutritional adequacy in older populations include personalized approaches, behavioral approaches, attention to motivators, and reinforcements.
- The goal of nutrition education for pregnant women, as well as lactating women, is relatively clear: appropriate maternal weight gain, nutritional adequacy of the maternal diet, and positive infant outcomes, such as satisfactory birth weight.
- A lesson plan needs to describe the desires of the target population. It is the blueprint for organizing a class. A well-designed lesson plan ensures a clear focus and specific learning outcomes.
- The program identifier conveys the key theme of the program.
- In developing the marketing plan, it is beneficial to form partnerships with local businesses, healthcare organizations, government agencies, and the like.
- Objectives are written statements of intended outcomes in measurable terms.
- The nutrition educator serves as the facilitator of the education process.

Critical Thinking Activities

- Develop a lesson plan including writing at least two measurable objectives for a nutrition education program on fitness and exercise for high school students.
- Provide two examples of incentives that can motivate high school students to participate in a health promotion program.
- Identify at least four skills essential to a successful nutrition education program and why they are essential.

Case Study 14-1

Elon, a community nutritionist, used different methods of delivering nutrition education to three different geographical areas in Chicago. In one area, she used mass media techniques, including radio announcements, posters, and leaflets. In the second area, she used lectures to deliver nutrition education involving six, 1-hour sessions over 1 month at different sites, and for the third area, she used demonstrations to deliver the nutrition education involving six 1-hour sessions for 3 weeks. The educational sessions were kept didactic, purposely with minimum interaction. The second and third areas served as control groups. The control groups were able to receive the radio spots, but it did not receive leaflets or posters. The face-to-face education groups also may have been exposed to radio broadcasts.

Elon compared the impact of the program on a sample of mothers of children less than 5 years of age in the control areas, face-to-face education, and the mass media group. She collected data about their dietary intake habits and frequency of food intake immediately after the educational programs, 3 months later, and 12 months later. Elon found that nutrition concepts were learned equally among the 3 groups. However, the control groups, which received radio spots, gained more nutrition knowledge than the other groups.

Activities

- Develop a lesson plan to incorporate Elon's activities. Include all the components of a lesson plan presented in this chapter.
- Identify the clients' nutrition education needs and develop a nutrition message for the program. Explain how the nutritional needs were determined.
- Plan a nutrition education program using the theoretical framework presented in Box 14-2. Also, identify two levels of psychomotor skills the clients may possess.
- Identify four strategies that can motivate participation.
- Identify two organizations that can be partners for the program. Include their roles.

References

1. Cowburn G, Stockley L. Consumer understanding and use of nutrition labeling: a systematic review. *Public Health Nutr.* 2005; 8(1):21–28.
2. U.S. Department of Health and Human Services. *Healthy People 2000, National Health Promotion and Disease Objectives*. DHHS Publication No. (PHS) 91-50212. Washington, DC: Author; 1991.
3. Harrison K, Marske AL. Nutritional content of foods advertised during the television programs children watch most. *Am J Public Health.* 2005; 95(9):1568–1574.
4. Stanhope M, Lancaster J. *Community and Public Health Nursing.* 5th ed. New York: Mosby; 2000.
5. Dembo MH. *Applying Educational Psychology.* 5th ed. New York: Longman; 1994.
6. Huitt W. *Bloom et al.'s Taxonomy of the Cognitive Domain. Educational Psychology Interactive.* Valdosta, GA: Valdosta State University; 2004.
7. Computer Strategies. Technology Staff Development: A Different Angle. Dale's Cone of Development. Available at: www.compstrategies.com/staffdevelopment/staffdev/sld004.htm. Accessed May 24, 2008.
8. Denehy J. Health education: an important role for school nurses. *J School Nurs.* 2001; 17(5):233–238.
9. Williams DP, LeBlanc H, Christensen NK. Diabetes stepping up to the plate: an education curriculum focused on food portioning skills. *J Extension.* 2004; 42(3):Online.
10. Knowles M. *The Adult Learner: A Neglected Species.* 5th ed. Houston: Gulf; 1998.
11. Contento IB, Balch GI, Bronner YL, Lytle LA, Maloney S, Olson C, Swadener SS, White S, Randell JS. The effectiveness of nutrition education and implications for nutrition education policy, programs, and research: a review of research. *J Nutr Educ.* 1995; 27(6):284–418.
12. Sims LS. Nutrition education research: reaching toward the leading edge. *J Am Diet Assoc.* 1987; 87(Suppl):S10–18.
13. Steptoe A, Perkins-Porras L, Rink E, Hilton S, Cappuccio FP. Psychological and social predictors of changes in fruit and vegetable consumption over 12 months following behavioral and nutrition education counseling. *Health Psychol.* 2004; 23(6):574–581.
14. Lanerolle P, Atukorala S. Nutrition education improves serum retinol concentration among adolescent school girls. *Asia Pacific J Clin Nutr.* 2006; 15(1):43–49.

15. Assema P, Steenbakkers M, Rademaker C, Brug J. The impact of a nutrition education intervention on main meal quality and fruit intake in people with financial problems. *J Human Nutr Diet.* 2005; 18:205–212.

16. Patterson R. *Changing Patient Behavior: Improving Outcomes in Health and Disease Management.* 1st ed. San Francisco: Jossey-Bass/AHA Press; 2001.

17. Stewart L, Houghton J, Hughes AR, Pearson D, Reilly JJ. Dietetic management of pediatric overweight: development and description of a practical and evidence-based behavioral approach. *J Am Diet Assoc.* 2005; 105(11):1810–1815.

18. Shafer L, Gillespie A, Wilkins JL, Borra ST. Nutrition education for the public—position of ADA. *J Am Diet Assoc.* 1996; 96:1183–1187.

19. Gaglianone CP, Taddei JAAC, Colugnati FAB, et al. Nutrition education in public elementary schools of São Paulo, Brazil: the Reducing Risks of Illness and Death in Adulthood project. *Rev Nutr.* 2006; 19(3):1–11.

20. Williamson D, Copeland A, Anton S, et al. Wise Mind Project: a school-based environmental approach for preventing weight gain in children. *Obesity.* 2007; 15:906–917.

21. Mullen PD, Green LW, Persinger GS. Clinical trials of patient education for chronic condition: a comparative meta-analysis of intervention types. *Prev Med.* 1985; 14:753–781.

22. Sutton SM, Balch GI, Lefebvre RC. Strategic questions for consumer-based health communications. *Public Health Rep.* 1995; 110(6):725–733.

23. McKenzie JF, Neiger BL, Smeltzer JL. *Planning, Implementing, and Evaluating Health Promotion Programs. A Primer.* 4th ed. San Francisco: Benjamin Cummings; 2005.

24. Vella J. *Learning to Listen Learning to Teach. The Power of Dialogue in Educating Adults.* San Francisco: Jossey-Bass; 2002.

25. Norris J. *From Telling to Teaching.* North Myrtle Beach, SC: Learning By Dialogue; 2007.

26. Kim KH, Linnan L, Campbell MK, Brooks C, Koenig HG, Wiesen C. The WORD (wholeness, oneness, righteousness, deliverance): a faith-based weight-loss program utilizing a community-based participatory research approach. *Health Educ Behav.* 2006;Dec 15:1–17.

27. Lefebvre RC, Flora JA. Social marketing and public health intervention. *Health Educ Q.* 1988; 15:299–315.

28. Minkler M. Improving health through community organization. In: Glanz K, Rimer BK, Lewis FM, eds. *Health Behavior and Health Education: Theory, Research, and Practice.* San Francisco: Jossey-Bass; 1990:257–287.

29. Kuczmarski MF, Aljadir L. Using food calendars to self-monitor: got 5? Nutrition for kids program. *J Nutr Educ.* 2003; 35:269–270.

30. Struempler BJ, Cobrin S. Feed your mind: an interactive nutrition evaluation for teenagers. *J Nutr Educ.* 2002; 34(1):59–60.

31. Byrd-Brenner C, Finckenor M. Dietary fat and heart disease intervention strategies. *J Nutr Educ.* 2000; 32(1):60–61.

32. Volker DL. Patient education: needs assessment and resource identification. *Oncol Nurs Forum.* 1991; 18(1):119–123.

33. Anspaugh DJ, Dignan MB, Anspaugh SL. *Developing Health Promotion Programs.* 2nd ed. Long Grove, IL: Waveland Press; 2006.

34. Anspaugh DJ, Dignan MB, Anspaugh SL. *Developing Health Promotion Programs.* Boston: McGraw-Hill Higher Education; 2000.

35. Knowles MS, Holton III EF, Swanson RA. *The Adult Learner: The Definitive Classic in Adult Education and Human Resource Development.* 5th ed. Houston: Gulf; 1998.

36. Radimer K, Bindewald B, Hughes J, Ervin B, Swanson C, Picciano MF. Dietary supplement use by US adults: data from the National Health and Nutrition Examination Survey, 1999–2000. *Am J Epidemiol.* 2004; 160(4):339–349.

37. Dutta-Bergman MJ. Primary sources of health information: comparisons in the domain of health attitudes, health cognitions, and health behaviors. *Health Comm.* 2004; 16(3):273–288.

38. Clark PG, Rossi JS, Greaney ML, et al. Intervening on exercise and nutrition in older adults: the Rhode Island SENIOR project. *J Aging Health.* 2005; 17(6):753–778.

39. Patacca D, Rosenbloom CA, Kicklighter JR, Ball M. Using a focus group approach to determine older adults' opinions and attitudes toward a nutrition education program. *J Nutr Elder.* 2004; 23(3):55–72.

40. International Food Information Council. In The News: A Snapshot of Food and Nutrition Reporting. Available at: ific.org/foodinsight/1998/jf/newsfi198.cfm. Accessed May 24, 2008.

41. Toner HM, Morris JD. A social-psychological perspective of dietary quality in later adulthood. *J Nutr Elderly.* 1992; 11:35–53.

42. International Food Information Council. Sharpen Your Skills. Available at: ific. org/tools/skills.cfm. Accessed May 24, 2008.

43. Ghoneim EH, Hassan MH, Amine EK. An intervention programme for improving the nutritional status of children aged 2–5 years in Alexandria. *East Med Health J.* 2004; 10(6):828–843.

44. Adekunle L. The effect of family structure on a sample of malnourished urban Nigerian children. *Food Nutr Bull.* 2005; 26(2):230–233.

45. Tamborlane WV. *The Yale Guide to Children's Nutrition.* New Haven, CT: Yale Press; 1997.

46. Birch LL. Preschool children's food preferences and consumption patterns. *J Nutr Educ.* 1979; 11:189–192.

47. Perry CL, Bishop DB, Taylor GL, et al. A randomized school trial of environmental strategies to encourage fruit and vegetable consumption among children. *Health Educ Behav.* 2004; 31(1):65–76.

48. Blom-Hoffman J, Kelleher C, Power TJ, Leff S. Promoting healthy food consumption among young children: evaluation of a multi-component nutrition education program. *J School Psychol.* 2004; 42(1):45–60.

49. Singleton JC, Achterberf CL, Shannon BM. Role of food and nutrition in the health perceptions of young children. *J Am Diet Assoc.* 1992; 92:67–70.

50. Hitchcock J, Schubert PE, Thomas SA. *Community Health Nursing.* 2nd ed. Clifton Park, NY: Thomson Delmar Learning; 2003.

51. Saksvig BI, Gittelsohn J, Harris SB, Hanley AJ, Valente TW, Zinman B. A pilot school-based healthy eating and physical activity intervention improves diet, food knowledge, and self-efficacy for native Canadian children. *J Nutr.* 2005; 135(10):2392–2398.

52. Anderson AS, Campbell DM, Shepherd R. The influence of dietary advice on nutrient intake during pregnancy. *Br J Nutr.* 1995; 73(2):163–177.

53. Hart AD, Azubuike CU, Barimalaa S, Achinewhu SC. Vegetable consumption pattern of households in selected areas of the Old Rivers state in Nigeria. *Afr J Food Agricult Nutr Devel.* 2005; 5(1):57–62.

54. Kaiser L, McMurdo T, Block A. The Food Stamp Nutrition Education Program focuses on the learner. *J Extension.* 2007; 45(2):Online.

55. Gucciardi E, Demelo M, Lee RN, Grace SL. Assessment of two culturally competent diabetes education methods: individual versus individual plus group education in Canadian Portuguese adults with type 2 diabetes. *Ethnicity Health.* 2007; 12(2):163–187.

56. Campbell D, Palm GF. *Group Parent Education: Promoting Parent Learning and Support.* London: Sage Publications; 2004.

57. Centers for Disease Control and Prevention. Five A Day Mission and History. Available at: http://www.5aday.org/html/background/mission.php. Accessed May 1, 2008.

58. Boyle M. *Community Nutrition in Action: An Entrepreneurial Approach.* 4th ed. Belmont, CA: Thomson Wadsworth; 2003.

59. Rankin SH, Stallings KD. *Patient Education: Principles and Practice.* 4th ed. Philadelphia: J.B. Lippincott; 2001.

60. Farr AC, Witte K, Jarato K, Menard T. The effectiveness of media use in health education: evaluation of an HIV/AIDS radio [corrected] campaign in Ethiopia. *J Health Comm.* 2005; 10(3):225–235.

61. Keller HH, Hedley H, Hadley M, Wong T, Vanderkooy S. Food workshops, nutrition education, and older adults: a process evaluation. *J Nutr Elder.* 2005; 24(3):5–23.

62. Giger JN, Davidhizar R. *Transcultural Nursing: Assessment and Intervention.* 3rd ed. St. Louis, MO: Mosby; 1999.

63. Pomerleau J, Lock K, Knai C, McKee M. Interventions designed to increase adult fruit and vegetable intake can be effective: a systematic review of the literature. *J Nutr.* 2005; 135(10):2486–2495.

64. Blanchette L, Brug J. Determinants of fruit and vegetable consumption among 6-12-year-old children and effective interventions to increase consumption. *J Human Nutr Diet.* 2005; 18(6):431–443.

65. Dickin KL, Dollahite JS, Habicht J. Nutrition behavior change among EFNEP participants is higher at sites that are well managed and whose front-line nutrition educators value the program. *J Nutr.* 2005; 135:2199–2205.

66. Lieberman L, Meana L, Stewart D. Cardiac rehabilitation: gender differences in factors influencing participation. *J Womens Health.* 1998; 7(6):717–723.

67. Boyle M. *Community Nutrition in Action: An Entrepreneurial Approach.* 4th ed. Belmont, CA: Thomson Wadsworth; 2005.

68. International Food Information Council. IFIC Message Making 101: Creating Consumer-Friendly Messages. Available at: ific.org/tools/messages.cfm. Accessed May 24, 2008.

69. Lefebvre RCD, Johnston L, Loughrey C, et al. Use of database marketing and consumer-based health communication in a message design: an example from the Office of Cancer Communication's "5 A Day for Better Health Program." *Designing Health Messages. Approaches from Communication Theory and Public Health Practice.* Thousand Oaks, CA: Sage; 1995:217–246.

70. American Dietetic Association. *Nutrition Trends Survey. Executive Summary.* Chicago, IL: Author; 1997.

71. Darmon N, Briend A, Drewnowski. Energy-dense diets are associated with lower diet costs: a community study of French adults. *Public Health Nutr.* 2004; 7:21–27.

72. American Dietetic Association. *Nutrition and You: Trends 2000.* Chicago, IL: Author; 2000.

73. Food Marketing Institute. *Trends in the United States. Consumer Attitudes and the Supermarket.* Washington, DC: Author; 1999.

74. Damroch S. General strategies for motivating people to change their behavior. *Nurs Clin North Am.* 1991; 26(4):833–843.

75. Boyd NR, Windsor RA. A formative evaluation in maternal and child health practice: the Partners for Life Nutrition Education Program for pregnant women. *Matern Child Health J.* 2003; 7(2):137–143.

CHAPTER 15

Marketing Nutrition Programs and the Role of Food Industry in Food Choice

CHAPTER OUTLINE

- Introduction
- Marketing Defined
- Developing a Marketing Plan
- Market Research and Situational Analysis
- Market Segmentation
- Communication Factor Analysis
- Social Marketing
- Social Marketing at the Community Level
- Advertising the Program
- Food Industries, Advertising, and Food Choices
- The Use of Advertising
- The Role of Media in Childhood Obesity
- Public Health Approaches
- Food and Nutrition Misinformation

LEARNING OBJECTIVES

- Define marketing.
- Discuss the difference between social and business marketing.
- Define market segmentation.
- Discuss the five Ps of social marketing: product, price, place, promotion, and position.
- Discuss the different communication factors that may affect nutrition programs.
- Discuss how food industries influence food choice.
- Define advertising.
- List different advertising principles.
- Discuss the role of advertising in childhood obesity.
- List ways that government policies can discourage advertising that encourages high fat intake.
- Describe the effects of nutrition misinformation.

Introduction

An effective *marketing plan* is necessary for any health promotion program to be successful. *Marketing* is not only an advertising campaign, a convenient package of low-fat foods and vegetables, or a $1 coupon for dairy products—marketing has a broader perspective in the context of nutrition. It focuses on all efforts to encourage and enable people to eat nutritiously.[1] Kotler and Zaltman first used the term *social marketing* in 1971, referring to the application of marketing to solve social and health problems.[2] Marketing involves the planned attempt to influence the market so there is a voluntary exchange of costs from that market with benefits to a provider.[3] Using media is one of the best marketing strategies to reach large segments of the population and can be used as a positive approach to communicate nutrition information and address related health issues. Community nutritionists and other healthcare practitioners need to understand the marketing strategies available for promoting nutrition messages. This chapter first discusses how to use marketing principles to modify individuals' behavior and promote health; then, it addresses how food industries use media to influence food choice and its effect on health. Finally, it discusses nutrition misinformation and how companies use marketing as a tool to promote unproven health products.

Marketing Defined

Marketing is one of the techniques that community nutritionists, program administrators, and registered dietitians can use to promote and implement effective nutrition education programs. Marketing is directed at satisfying the needs and wants of the consumer through an exchange of processes or activities (goods, products, or programs).[4] But marketing is much more than just this. It encompasses everything the nutritionist does to provide services to the community, including creating, promoting, delivering, and finally consuming the product or service, such as the name for the nutrition program, the letterhead, and the services provided. Marketing starts with the client's actual or perceived wants and needs.[5,6] The community will choose to work with the nutritionist based on the benefits to be gained. Few people will attend a workshop or planning session only out of curiosity.

Developing a Marketing Plan

A marketing plan consists of specific goals and objectives, target groups, messages, the desires of the target population, channels, budgets, tracking and evaluation, and media selection factors.[7] A formal marketing plan is a written statement of the marketing objectives, strategies, and all the specific actions that must be taken.[8] It explains how the nutrition and health information will be delivered to the targeted population. A marketing plan should contain the following: executive summary, situation analysis, objectives and goals, marketing strategy, action programs, budgets, and controls (see **Box 15-1**).[9]

Goals and Objectives

It is very important to be clear about the desired marketing outcomes and to state them in measurable terms. For instance, if the goal is to

> **marketing plan** A written statement of the marketing objectives and strategies and all the specific actions that must be taken to accomplish them.
>
> **marketing** Satisfying the needs of the consumer through an exchange of activities (goods, products, or programs).
>
> **social marketing** The use of marketing principles for promoting social services or products (e.g., eat less saturated fat).

Environmental
economic
environment
lifestyle
cultural beliefs and
    traditions
religious beliefs and
    traditions

Health Status
physical restrictions
    due to disease
declining taste
    sensitivity
age and gender

Sensory
flavor (taste and smell)
texture
appearance

Cognitive
learned food
    habits
social factors
emotional needs
nutrition and
    health beliefs
advertising

Genetics
taste sensitivity
preference for sweets
avoidance of bitter
possible "fat tooth"

Regular consumption of fast foods is attributed to increasing rates of obesity and other chronic health conditions because fast foods are high in sugar, fat, and sodium.

Box 15-1 Contents of a Marketing Plan

I. Executive Summary
- The main goals and recommendations
- The benefits to the consumers/needs of the target audience

II. Situation Analysis
- Background (market description)
- Opportunities and threats (a review of competition)
- Strengths and weaknesses
- The nutritionist's position in the marketplace
- What health services he or she provides (a review of distribution)

III. Objectives and Goals
- Defined marketing activities in measurable terms

IV. Marketing Strategy
- Know:
  - The game plan
  - The target market
  - The tools and techniques appropriate to reach the target audience
  - The expenditure level
  - The advertising strategy and positioning

V. Action Programs
- Have a month-by-month implementation timetable (specific marketing strategies that will accomplish specific actions)

VI. Budget
- The cost of production, marketing, and administration
- The basis for marketing operations, financial planning, and personnel recruitment

VII. Controls
- Annual plan control: Steps taken during the year to monitor and correct deviation from the plan
- Profitability control: Determining the actual profit/progress of different services or products, market segments, and distribution channels
- Strategic control: Systematic evaluation of the organization's market performance in relation to market opportunities

Modified from: Kotler P, Clark R. *Marketing for Healthcare Organizations. Steps in Market Segmentation, Targeting, and Positioning.* Englewood Cliffs, NJ: Prentice-Hall; 1987. Reprinted with permission by Philip Kotler.

increase attendance over last year's weight management program, a specific objective might be to increase the community participation by 15 percent.[4]

Target Groups

It is essential to define the target groups prior to marketing a nutrition program. For example, if the program is about diabetes, specify whether the target group is individuals in the community who have not yet developed diabetes, those who are already being treated for diabetes, or healthcare practitioners such as physicians, dietitians, and nurses who treat diabetes.[10] A secondary target audience could be the decision makers who influence the individual's choice to use the program (e.g., parents, spouses, friends, and coworkers). Another target group may be those who use a particular program, such as low-income pregnant or breastfeeding women and mothers of children under 5 years of age participating in the Special Supplemental Nutrition Program for Women, Infants, and Children (WIC), the elderly people participating in the Peace Meal Program, obese individuals participating in a weight-loss program, or postmenopausal women participating in a women's health program.

Messages

Once the target group is determined, find out the beliefs, needs, and orientation of the target group. These will provide the types of marketing messages the target group needs and determine their sequence. In some cases, erroneous beliefs or information may need to be clarified first. Most programs use television, radio, and print (newspapers and magazines) to communicate their messages. However, word-of-mouth advertising is also important and effective. Referrals from satisfied participants of current or past programs may be the best source of new participants.[4]

Channels

A good marketing plan must verify the communication channels that the target groups use. If the target group is older individuals, for example, determine whether they read the Peace Meal Program newsletter, watch television, or listen to the radio. Use the target group's most popular communication channel to advertise the marketing message. One very good way to capture the target group's attention is through a story on a local cable television station (CNN local edition) or during the community segment of the local news.

Choose free or low-cost methods such as community bulletin boards, public service announcements, and fliers to reduce cost. Some printing businesses may donate fliers if the company can put their name, address, and phone number on each of the fliers.[4]

Budget

It is important to extend the budget to provide media coverage throughout the entire program period. Be sure to include ideas for fundraising within the budget. It is important to budget wisely because advertising is expensive.[4] Some related marketing costs include funds for logos, fliers, brochures, videos, and radio and/or TV public service announcements (PSAs).

A health promotion program budget may take many facets and may use various formats. In health promotion, two budgeting formats are used most often—line item and functional. The line item format includes anticipated expenditures for the fiscal year.[11,12] Examples of line items are labor (full-time, part-time employees); the nutrition educator's, secretary's, and director's salaries; materials; supplies; travel (professional meetings, program sites, etc.); transportation; telephones; the Internet; computers; rent; and printing. In contrast, a functional budget is based on the specific functions each department provides and includes staff training, program evaluation, health screenings, educational materials, equipment, and facilities. These two budget formats must be considered when developing marketing strategies.[3]

Marketing Evaluation

Monitoring the marketing program/plan will provide feedback on the success or relevance of the marketing strategy. An elaborate evaluation is not necessary; it could be as simple as asking the participants how they heard about the Heart Smart for Teens, menopause management, or bone density screening program. The nutritionist may desire to know who and what influenced the participant to enroll in the health promotion program. She or he may ask, "Did the cable show or the newspaper influence your interest in the weight management or menopause program?" Evaluate whether the marketing channels used were ineffective, whether they should be repeated, or whether they should be modified based on participants' feedback.[4]

Market Research and Situational Analysis

Market research and situational analysis help the nutritionist identify whether the targeted community will be interested in the programs. Market attractiveness is based on the following:[4,13]

- Whether the market is large enough to support the program
- Whether the program has the potential to grow
- Whether the targeted community is aware of and whether they can afford the time or money to participate in the program
- Whether there is sufficient incentive to encourage private investment in the program
- Whether competitors are offering similar or related services

Market research is the systematic design, collection, analysis, and reporting of data and findings relevant to a specific marketing situation or problem facing an organization.[9] For example, Ling et al. analyzed tobacco-industry marketing archives from August 2000 to February 2002 and found that the tobacco industry divided markets and defined targets according to consumer attitudes, aspirations, activities, and lifestyles.[14] The tobacco industry marketing targeted smokers of all ages, especially young adults. The researchers recommended that public health professionals include people of all ages—though mainly young adults—instead of concentrating on teens and young children in smoke cessation programs.[14]

The initial step a nutritionist needs to take in the market research process is to determine the research objectives and define the problem. The objective may be to learn more about the different ethnic groups in the community or the impact of a marketing strategy/tool used in promoting a nutrition program or other programs. The next step is to conduct exploratory research.

Exploratory Research

Exploratory research is carrying out preliminary research to learn more about the market before any formal research survey is conducted.[9] This includes collecting secondary data, observational research, competitive analysis, qualitative and quantitative data, and situation analysis by completing informal interviewing with individuals and groups in the community.[9]

Secondary Data Research

Secondary data are information that has been collected for another purpose (e.g., population census, National Health and Nutrition Examination Survey [NHANES], death certificates, demographic data, etc.). The secondary data need to be used with caution because they were collected for a purpose that may not be identical to the nutritionist's purpose; however, they may provide useful ideas and findings, and reduce the cost of conducting primary research. They may also help the nutritionist to define the problems and research objectives.[15]

> **exploratory research** Carrying out preliminary research to learn more about the market before any formal research survey is conducted.

Observational Research/Analyzing the Environment

Observational research is the gathering of primary data by observing relevant situations, actions, environments, and people. For example, a nutritionist could collect data on postmenopausal women's actions after attending a Heart Smart for Women education program by calculating how many women signed up for a physical activity three times a week and by observing how often they exercised. Also, the researcher will need to analyze the external forces and trends. Some examples of external situations that affect dietetics practice include recent trends in eating habits or behaviors of consumers, the availability of nutritious foods, the cost of foods, poverty, healthcare reform legislative and regulatory changes, and an increase in the number of older persons in the community.[15-17] In addition, he or she will need to evaluate the market trends both locally and nationally. For instance, determine the weight-loss trends of postmenopausal women.

Competitive Analysis

Market research also includes conducting a competitive analysis. The nutritionist will need to determine the competition's strengths and

The task of educating consumers without overwhelming them is challenging. Positive messages can help prevent the confusion that occurs due to conflicting information.

weaknesses, the distinctive characteristics that set them apart from other programs, and the short- and long-term trends that may affect program usage. Also, he or she should determine how the program can be positioned for the greatest degree of collaboration with competing programs.[9,15]

This analysis will help the nutritionist position the program as being different or better. The nutritionist needs to determine the market niche for the services. Competition includes those businesses or programs that are similar in the services offered, consumer base (target market), or location. Market research can help the nutritionist identify the underserved or what the competitor is not providing.[4,9] The competitors in the field of nutrition could be other healthcare practitioners (physicians, chiropractors, health food stores, alternative therapy practitioners, food industries, nurses, and others), businesses, hospitals, or other public health organizations (American Heart Association, National Cancer Institute).

There are several methods of collecting information on the competition including networking, speaking to colleagues in a dietetic practice group, reviewing secondary data, and establishing relationships with the consumer. In order to advertise the services, the dietitian must determine his or her competitive edge (area of expertise, professional image, screening equipment, etc.), establish a relationship with the consumer, build trust and rapport, understand the consumer's needs, and provide services that deliver the promised benefits.[18]

Qualitative and Quantitative Data

In addition to collecting data through observation, focus groups, and surveys, the nutritionist needs to carry out some interviews during the exploratory stage of the market research project. The data collection should be qualitative in the exploratory stage. *Qualitative research* data typically come from small samples of the target audience, mainly through open-ended interviewing. The clients are asked leading questions that stimulate them to share their feelings and thoughts. The aim is to probe deeply into consumers' main needs, perceptions, preferences, and satisfactions with the program; understand the problems that could occur in marketing to this group; and generate ideas that can be used to conduct further studies using quantitative research.[9] The result of qualitative research cannot be generalized to the larger target audience because of the small sample size.[19,20]

In contrast, *quantitative research* utilizes selected samples to produce statistically reliable results that are expressed in numerical terms. For example, 10 percent of children living in an inner city reported skipping breakfast. Quantitative research involves interviewing or surveying a larger number of people than qualitative research and assumes that the interviewer knows the specific questions to ask prior to data collection.[19]

qualitative research Acquired from a small sample of the target audience, mainly through open-ended interviewing.

quantitative research Utilizes selected samples to produce statistically reliable results that are expressed in numerical terms.

market segmentation Dividing a market/community into distinct groups of individuals on the basis of needs, characteristics, or behavior who might require separate products/services or marketing mixes.

market segment A portion of a larger market.

market targeting The process of evaluating each market segment's attractiveness and selecting one or more segments to penetrate.

Both qualitative and quantitative data are used in the planning of social marketing strategies.[20]

Situation Analysis

Observational research also includes conducting a situation analysis; for example, determine where the weight-loss class will be carried out. Observe whether the postmenopausal women mentioned earlier are working full time. Determine the cost of the weight-loss program.[15,21]

The step that is critical to the ultimate success of the entire marketing plan is sometimes referred to as SWOT analysis; SWOT is an acronym for Strengths, Weaknesses, Opportunities, and Threats.[15] SWOT is an exercise to analyze internal strengths and weaknesses and external opportunities and threats.[22]

The SWOT analysis is instrumental in strategy formulation and selection and provides information that is helpful for matching an agency's resources and capabilities to the competitive environment. It allows an agency's strengths, resources, and capabilities to be used as a basis for developing a competitive advantage. The absence of certain strengths may be viewed as an agency weakness. The analysis of external environmental factors may reveal certain new opportunities for profit and growth, while changes in the external environment may also present threats to the agency. To develop strategies that take into account the SWOT profile, a matrix of these factors can be constructed:[22]

	Strengths	**Weaknesses**
Opportunities	S-O strategies	W-O strategies
Threats	S-T strategies	W-T strategies

- *S-O strategies* pursue opportunities that are a good fit to the agency's strengths (e.g., a large number of older persons in the community).
- *S-T strategies* identify ways the agency can pursue opportunities (e.g., advertise to increase the number of Peace Meal Program participants in the community).
- *W-O strategies* identify ways the agency can use its strengths to reduce vulnerability to external threats (e.g., ask older individuals in the community to help recruit participants for the program).
- *W-T strategies* establish a defensive plan to prevent the agency's weakness from making it highly susceptible to external threats (e.g., involve community leaders, such as the mayor, church leaders, and others, to seek additional resources for the program and to avoid lack of Peace Meal Program participants).[22]

Market Segmentation

Market segmentation is dividing a market/community into distinct groups of buyers/individuals who might require separate products/services or marketing mixes on the basis of needs, characteristics, or behavior.[23] The market is composed of many types of consumers, products/services, and needs and nutritionists must determine which segments provide the best opportunity for achieving the health promotion program's goals.[24] A *market segment* is a portion of a larger market.[25] For example, African Americans or senior citizens represent a segment of the total U.S. market. Market segmentation is very valuable in identifying and choosing the target market instead of trying to reach everybody. *Market targeting* is the process of evaluating each market segment's attractiveness and selecting one or more segments to penetrate.[23] *Market positioning* is arranging for a product/program to take

FIGURE 15-1   Steps in Market Segmentation, Targeting, and Positioning.
Adapted from: Kotler P, Clark R. *Marketing for Healthcare Organizations*, 1987. *Steps in Market Segmentation, Targeting, and Positioning*. Englewood Cliffs: Prentice Hall; 1987. Reprinted with permission.

a clear, distinctive, and desirable place comparable to competing products/programs for nutrition and health services for the same clients or community.[26] For example, physical activity could be repositioned as a form of relaxation—not exercise—to women age 55 years or older.

Figure 15-1 presents the three major steps in marketing targeting. Once the nutritionist has defined the market segment, he or she can tailor the marketing mixes to the group's specific needs. The demographics, sociographics, behavioral aspects, and psychographics of the client base provide important information.[27] Some of the types of demographics are the size of the population for the program area, rate of change of the population, age/sex distribution, racial/ethnic composition, socioeconomic status, housing information, and fertility patterns.

Additionally, sociographics and psychographics are the sociology and psychology behind demographic analysis; they deduce the emotional needs, values, and lifestyles that can lead to good health.[4,27] Sociographics and psychographics also include the identification of behavior patterns of the individuals, which makes it easier for the nutritionist to predict their health conditions and market the program to the geographic areas that will benefit the community.[27] Also, data on health and nutrition behaviors may be helpful in determining the market segment. The nutritionist can analyze any of these sources of data to determine the needs of the population and gather ideas for planning a community health and nutrition promotion program. **Table 15.1** provides market segmentation categories. Examples of excellent sources of data are[20]:

- National Health Interview Survey (NHIS)
- National Health and Nutrition Examination Survey (NHANES)
- Behavioral Risk Factor Surveillance System (BRFSS)
- Census Bureau, National Center for Health Statistics (NCHS)
- Social Security Administration (SSA)
- U.S. Department of Agriculture (USDA)
- Youth Risk Behavior Survey (YRBS)

Communication Factor Analysis

Communication involves everything that is carried out to market a community health and nutrition promotion program. The communication process includes identifying, engaging, and convincing the

targeted community to collaborate with the nutritionist, and shaping the promotional program to obtain the desired audience response.[4] It also is important to analyze the communication factors when choosing methods of program promotion because these factors may significantly affect the success of the community health and nutrition program. The following are some of the communication factors that may affect a nutrition program:[4,28,29]

- Perceptual distortions of information about the nutrition promotion program
- Differences in values and attitudes between the nutritionist and the target community
- Incorrect or improper use of words to convey specific information
- Lack of listening on the part of the targeted community
- Lack of explicit messages
- Lack of the knowledge of what the target community needs or demands

In order to communicate effectively, the nutritionist needs to understand the mechanism of communication. Kotler and Armstrong recognized nine elements of communication (sender, receiver, message, media, decoding, encoding, noise, feedback, and response), which are presented in **Figure 15-2**.[23] The sender and receiver are the major parties (the nutritionists and the community). The message and the media are the two major tools. Encoding, decoding, response, and feedback are the four major communication functions.[29] The last element is noise in the system.[23] **Table 15.2** presents elements of communication.

The consumer/community will utilize cues from all aspects of the marketing provided to them to make a choice. It is imperative that the nutritionist/marketer knows (1) how the target consumer will likely respond to the appearance of the product or services, and (2) that all aspects of communication are consistent with each other in communicating the messages.[30]

Social Marketing

Many health promotion programs use marketing principles to guide their activities. Social marketing, the use of marketing principles for promoting social goods, was launched when Wiebe said that radio and television could sell social objectives just as they sell soap.[31] The significance of this principle is that ***business marketing*** focuses on fulfilling customers' needs and desires, but social marketing focuses on changing personal or social behaviors for the benefit of the public, even when the public neither recognizes their need nor desires the change. In 1971, Kotler and Zaltman expanded Wiebe's analysis by more fully applying marketing principles and theory.[2] The theory was that the same marketing principles used to sell products to consumers could be used to "sell" ideas, attitudes, and behaviors. However, social marketing is sometimes less effective than its commercial counterpart because it aims to influence people's ideas and behaviors (e.g., eat less saturated fat) rather than steering existing patterns of thought and behavior in a certain direction (e.g., choose one fast-food restaurant instead of another).[32] Instead of telling people what they need, public health professionals are learning to listen to the needs and desires of the target audience by using focus groups and building programs based on those needs.[33]

It is difficult and expensive to reach every individual in a

business marketing The process of creating, distributing, promoting, and pricing goods, services, and ideas to facilitate satisfying exchange relationships with customers in a dynamic environment.

TABLE 15.1 Segmentation Variables for Consumer Markets

Variable	Typical Break
Geographic	
Region	Pacific, Mountain, West North Central, West South Central, East North Central, East South Central, South Atlantic, Middle Atlantic, New England
State	Specific state, in-state, out-of-state, ZIP code
County size	Census data
City size	Under 5,000; 5,000–20,000; 20,000–50,000; 50,000–100,000; 100,000–250,000; 250,000–500,000; 500,000–1 million; 1 million–4 million; over 4 million
Density	Urban, suburban, rural
Climate	Northern, Southern, Southwest, Midwest
Demographic	
Age	Under 6, 6–11, 12–19, 20–34, 35–49, 50–64, 65–79, 80+
Gender	Male, female
Family size	1–2, 3–4, 5+
Family life cycle	Young, single; young, married, no children; young, married, youngest child under 6; young, married, youngest child 6 or over; older, married with children; older, married, no children under 18; older, single; other
Income	Under $2,500; $2,500–$5,000; $5,000–$7,500; $7,500–$10,000; $10,000–$15,000; $15,000–$20,000; $20,000–$30,000; $30,000–$50,000; $50,000 and over
Occupation	Professional and technical; managers, officials, and proprietors; clerical, sales; artists; forepersons; operatives; farmers; retired; students; homemakers; unemployed
Education	Grade school or less, some high school, graduated from high school, some college, graduated from college, postgraduate
Religion	Catholic, Protestant, Jewish, Hindu, Muslim, Buddhist, other
Race	Asian, African American, Hispanic, Native Indian, European American, Latino, other
Nationality	American, British, French, German, Italian, Japanese, Latin American, Middle Eastern, Scandinavian, African, Greek, Chinese, Korean, other
Social class	Lower-lower, upper-lower, lower-middle, upper-middle, lower-upper, upper-upper, working class
Generation	Baby boomer, Generation X, echo boomer, Generation Y
Psychographic	
Lifestyle	Straight, swinger, longhair, yuppie, conservative, liberal, striver, struggler, other
Personality	Compulsive, placid, gregarious, authoritarian, ambitious, leader, follower, independent, dependent, assertive, high/low achiever, dominant, submissive
Behavioral	
Occasions	Regular occasions, special occasions
Benefits sought	Academic quality, service, job skill, economy, convenience, social life, speed, health, comfort, safety, reliability
User status	Nonuser, ex-user, potential user, first-time user, regular user
Rate of status	Light user, medium user, heavy user, infrequent user, frequency of usage, method of usage
Loyalty status	None, medium, strong, absolute
Readiness stage	Unaware, aware, informed, interested, desirous, intending to buy
Attitude toward health program	Enthusiastic, positive, indifferent, negative, hostile

Adapted from: Kotler P, Clark RN. *Major Segmentation Variables for Consumer Markets*. Englewood Cliffs, NJ: Prentice Hall; 1999. Reprinted with permission.

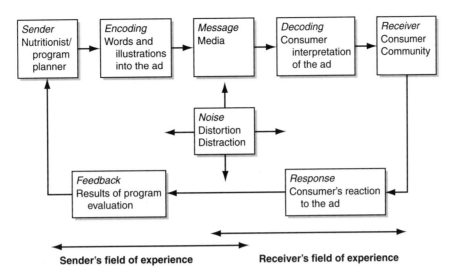

FIGURE 15-2   Elements in the Communication Process. Adapted from: Kotler P, Clark R. *Marketing for Healthcare Organizations*, 1987. *Steps in Market Segmentation, Targeting, and Positioning.* Englewood Cliffs: Prentice Hall; 1987. Reprinted with permission.

population with an individualized intervention. Social marketing programs reach a specific audience, satisfy clients' needs, and meet organizational objectives. For example, Reger et al. used a 6-week media campaign to promote consumption of 1-percent-fat milk.[34] He found that 34 percent of high-fat milk drinkers reported switching to low-fat milk and that low-fat milk sales increased from 29 percent of overall milk sales to 46 percent. Social marketing impacts the practice of dietetics by boosting clients' awareness of health issues and healthy foods and is able to help move consumers toward behavioral change.

Social Marketing Components

The components of a business-marketing plan are known as the marketing mix or the five Ps of marketing: 1) *product* (what is being sold), 2) *price* (at what cost, both monetary and otherwise), 3) *place* (where and how

product The item being sold, promoted, offered, or marketed.

price The cost of a product, both monetary and otherwise.

place Where and how a product can be purchased.

TABLE 15.2	Nine Elements of Communication

Sender: The nutritionist sending or conveying the messages to the community/individuals.

Encoding: The process of putting thought into symbolic form. The program planner assembles words and illustrations into an advertisement that will express the intended message.

Message: The set of symbols that the sender transmits; for example, a fat-free milk advertisement (the actual product).

Media: The communication channels through which the message travels from sender to receiver; in this case, the specific magazines and newspapers that the nutritionist selects.

Decoding: The process by which the receiver assigns meaning to the symbols encoded by the sender. A consumer reads the nutritionist's advertisement and interprets the words and illustrations that it contains.

Receiver: The party/community or individuals who read the messages sent by another party/nutritionist.

Response: The reactions of the receiver after being exposed to the message. The consumer is more aware of the attributes of the nutrition program, actually buys or becomes involved, or does nothing. For example, the consumer decides to buy foods that are low in saturated fat and participate in regular physical activity.

Feedback: The part of the receiver's response communicated back to the sender. The nutritionist's program evaluation shows that consumers were captivated by the advertisement and remembered it, or consumers write or call the nutritionist praising or criticizing the advertisement or the products/services.

Noise: The unplanned static or distortion during the communication process, which results in the receiver's getting a different message than the one the sender intended. For example, a mother is distracted by her child or cell phone while reading or listening to an advertisement about a program on how to prevent childhood obesity.

Modified from: Kotler P, Armstrong G. *Principles of Marketing.* 8th ed. Englewood Cliffs, NJ: Prentice-Hall; 1999. Reprinted with permission.

it can be purchased), 4) **promotion** (how consumers learn about and are persuaded to use it), and 5) **positioning** (the way the consumer perceives the product/service relative to the nutritionist competition in the market).[24,35,36] The marketing mix can fit into the overall nutrition program plan.

Unlike the product of most businesses, the *product* in public health nutrition programs is not always concrete. In community nutrition, the product is a service to be delivered, such as nutrition information dissemination; diet counseling; food service consultation; food preparation demonstrations to different population groups, including pregnant women, older persons, or college students; or provision of material such as low-fat cheese and soy milk.

Place is the second component of social marketing. It refers to the location where the exchange of service occurs. It also includes the distribution channels through which the product is made available to the clients. Health departments, clinics, hospital outpatient departments, child daycare centers, Peace Meal Program sites, schools, and other similar facilities have served as distribution channels for nutrition programs and services. It is important to consider convenience so that clients can obtain products or services easily; for example, availability of transportation and access to parking such as handicapped parking. It is important to provide the service at an appropriate and convenient location.[36,37]

Price is the third component of social marketing. In business, price means setting a profitable price for a product that is acceptable to both consumers and the business. In social marketing, however, the interest is not financial gain, but instead the value of a service to society in terms of safety, health, or other social issues. There are three different pricing strategies in social marketing: 1) cost recovery, 2) market incentives, and 3) market disincentives.[37] The request for donations for nutrition services could be considered a *cost recovery* strategy. Usually, the federal, state, or local government provides financial support for nutrition services, so a price may not need to be set for the product. Market *incentives* are used to stimulate the acceptance of a product. If the objective of a weight-control program is to increase the number of participants, the incentive could be $10 off the set price. The "buy-one-get-one-free" approach also appeals to many clients. Market *disincentive* pricing can be used to discourage clients from using a product. For instance, high taxes on cigarettes and liquor are attempts by the government to discourage their use. Another example of a market disincentive for a nutrition program could be higher prices for soft drinks rather than for fruit juices in vending machines on college campuses.[36,37]

The fourth social marketing perspective is *promotion*; this is the communication component of marketing. Promotion includes advertising, public relations, and consumer incentives. It informs the clients about the existence of a product or service.

Advertising is not a one-time activity. It involves a planned and continued series of activities known as an advertising campaign. To enhance the effectiveness of the promotion, the purpose of the campaign must be clear. The media used for advertising include television, radio, newspapers, maga-

promotion How consumers learn about and are persuaded to use a product.

position Services' strengths in relation to those of other providers.

advertising The methods used to present health and nutrition promotion programs to targeted communities.

zines, brochures, billboards, posters, booths at health fairs, and newsletters.[36,37]

The fifth perspective is *position*. The dietitian can position his or her services' strengths in relation to those of other providers. The benefits might include convenience, low cost, high credibility, guarantees, quick results, emotional support, or a high degree of control.[36,38] For instance, eating a variety of foods could be repositioned as an opportunity for choice instead of dieting. Serving low-fat meals to one's family could be positioned as an act of love.[39]

Taking into account each of the five Ps of marketing helps develop an action-oriented and effective nutrition program plan. A quality product offered in a convenient place at an economical price and promoted with an appealing message will be successful.[37]

In addition, each of the five Ps should be seen from the consumer's perspective. The five Ps concept considers only the seller's viewpoint of the market. The transformation of the five Ps to the consumer's perspective is accomplished by converting the Ps into the following C's:[23,30,36]

Product	Customer solution
Price	Customer cost
Place	Convenience
Promotion	Communication
Positioning	Change

Hence, whereas marketers view themselves as selling a product/service, customers see themselves as buying value or a solution to their problems. Consumers are interested in more than the price; they are interested in the total costs of acquiring and utilizing a service. Consumers want the product and service to be as conveniently available as possible. They also want two-way communication and they want change, to experience something new and exciting. The change, however, must be relevant, slightly subtle, and not drastic.[23]

Social Marketing at the Community Level

Community-based social marketing (CBSM) is a way to plan and communicate a message to achieve maximum impact with limited resources. One example of community-based social marketing is the Honduran Ministry of Health's actions to reduce infant mortality in Honduras.[40] The ministry collaborated with the Academy for Educational Development (AED) to develop a comprehensive public education campaign. The project was designed to deliver information for the home treatment of infant diarrhea, to demonstrate the proper preparation and administration techniques of oral rehydration therapy (ORT), and to introduce a significant portion of Honduras' isolated rural populace to diarrhea-related prevention behaviors.

After considerable investigation of the medical and social issues being addressed and preparation of the instructional and training tools, the AED's Mass Media and Health Practices Program was launched.[40] The program operated in a site that included a representative population of 400,000 individuals. The campaign began by providing 900 healthcare workers with 4 to 8 hours of ORT training. The training program concentrated on teaching the proper mixing and administration of ORT salts and instructing other village assistants, who would finally have to conduct the same exercises directly with rural families. The program trainees used props and training dummies repeatedly to practice each step of the mixing and administration processes. The health workers and village trainees then began instructing mothers and grandmothers on ORT and other health behaviors such as breastfeeding, infant food preparation, and personal hygiene. When rural families completed their ORT training, a flag was posted at their house to let other mothers in the area know where they could obtain health advice and instruction.

A media campaign was implemented as the training program was being conducted to reinforce the healthcare instruction effort. The campaign developed print materials and radio advertisements to issue basic messages related to the diarrhea rehydration therapy and the AED training program. The messages emphasized the correct administration of oral rehydration salts (Litrosol) and the continuation of breastfeeding during infant diarrhea periods, and encouraged mothers to seek medical assistance if a child's condition deteriorated. Posters and flip-charts were also created to illustrate ORT and to deliver supporting messages. The radio advertisements were placed in 30- to 60-second spot announcements and often included some form of jingle, slogan, or song. Many of the ads included a familiar announcer, the program's spokesman for technical information, who subsequently became a nationally known figure.

The tone of the campaign was serious, straightforward, and caring. It successfully promoted a mother-craft concept, where a mother's current actions and beliefs are supported and the program's health techniques became an added complement to her caregiving regimen. ORT training was presented as a new development in modern medicine: the latest remedy for lost appetite and a recovery aid.

One year after the implementation of the mass media program, an evaluation was conducted by Stanford University to chart the project's impact. A data sample was collected from 750 randomly selected families from more than 20 communities. Results showed that:[40]

- The diarrhea rehydration project was very successful in both disseminating important health information and promoting specific changes in behavior related to treating infant diarrhea.
- The infant mortality rates for children under 5 years of age decreased from 47.5 to 25 percent.
- Ninety-three percent of the mothers sampled from rural Honduras knew that the program's radio campaign was promoting Litrosol, the brand name of the locally packaged ORS used to treat diarrhea.
- Seventy-one percent could recite the radio jingle used to promote the administration of liquids during diarrhea affliction.

Advertising the Program

Advertising basics include advertising principles, developing attention-getting advertisements, collaborating with an agency to develop the advertisements, and choosing forms of media to use.[4] Advertising is one of the methods that nutritionists can use to promote nutrition information to the targeted community. The direct effect of advertising on community participation in a nutrition program is not possible to determine. Despite this ambiguity, it is important to fulfill two advertising objectives: publicize the program and increase the demand for the program.[4] The nutritionist needs to determine the best forms of advertising for the community nutrition promotion program, and also determine the types of advertising that might best reach the community (newspapers, radio, television, magazines, direct mail, brochures, fliers, displays, or word of mouth).[4] See the Successful Community Strategies feature in this chapter for a description of a successful community marketing strategy.

When advertising a health promotion program, consider the following principles:[4,41,42]

- Base the advertisement on the consumer's needs.
- Circulate the advertisement only to the target population.
- Provide background information about the program and update when the program changes.
- Request free public service announcements (PSAs) about the program. Ask public service directors to help raise awareness by airing them. (See more on PSAs later in this section.)
- Inform all media representatives as to why the story is timely and interesting (newsworthy), local (relates directly to the community), and important (public needs to know this).
- Position the program as if you are the first to provide such services.

Developing Attention-Getting Advertisements

Appropriate advertisement of a program is essential. The following are effective campaign techniques:[4,35,43,44]

- Use a slogan that is easily remembered, such as "Smoke-Free Forever" or "No More Dieting to Lose Weight."
- Test market the slogan on a sample population of the targeted group (e.g., the elderly, young adults, women of menopause age).
- Begin the headline of the advertisement with a question, such as "Which method to stop smoking do you prefer?" or "How would you like to lose weight?" Use a headline that will get the reader's attention.
- Put the program in perspective: 1) the time that is required, 2) the money or payment required, and 3) the effort the person will need to expend to get the desired reward.
- Describe the time commitment that will be required, such as "It will take 30 minutes a day for the next 10 weeks to stop smoking, but you will be free from smoking (or overeating, stress, arguing with your family) for the rest of your life. This could be the best 5-hour commitment you've ever made."
- Evaluate the advertisement periodically by asking people who enrolled how they heard about program.

Public Service Announcements (PSAs)

The nutritionist can communicate an important health promotion message fast to wide and diverse audiences or to a specific population using PSAs for radio or television. Local TV or radio stations air PSAs during unsold blocks of advertising time or during station breaks. Contact station managers and public service directors after writing your PSAs.[4]

Radio PSAs

Radio PSAs are 10, 20, or 30 seconds long. It is important to note that broadcasters usually speak at the rate of 155 words per minute, so use that to gauge how long your message/copy should be. The following are examples of how to determine the lengths of PSAs:[4]

- 10-second PSA = 20 to 25 words
- 15-second PSA = 30 to 35 words
- 20-second PSA = 40 to 50 words
- 30-second PSA = 60 to 75 words

Television PSAs

You will need to keep the message shorter for television PSAs than for radio PSAs. See **Box 15-2** for a sample television PSA. Television PSAs can be 8, 13, or 18 seconds long; 8- or 13-second spots are good for reminders. Keeping the message short will make it easier for you to obtain a time slot and prevent cut off or mistimed PSAs. When writing a television PSA, use the same procedures as for radio, but add sight and additional sounds.[4] Including sound in radio ads may divert the listeners' attention from the main message and reduce the impact of the message. Prepare videotapes or slides with announcer copy that deliver action and include a soundtrack. Guidelines for developing television PSAs are as follows:[4]

- Repeat the main message as many times as possible and the main point at the end.
- Advocate a specific action; for example, make your ice cream cone a single, not a double dip.
- Express the problems, behaviors, or skills; for example, climb the stairs instead of riding the elevator.
- Be straightforward.
- Use music or sound effects to increase recall.
- Use only a few characters.

Food Industries, Advertising, and Food Choices

It has been well established that food industries influence food choices through intensive advertising.[47] For the purposes of this chapter, food industries include companies that produce, process, manufacture, sell, and serve foods and beverages. It also includes the food service sector, food carts, vending machines, restaurants, bars, fast food outlets, schools, hospitals, prisons, and workplaces. Food and food service companies spend more than $11 billion annually on direct media advertising (ads) in magazines, newspapers, radio, television, and billboards and twice as much on incentive coupons and fees paid to retailers for space on supermarket shelves.[48] The effectiveness of food and beverage advertising is attributed to its omnipresence as well as to the sophistication of the agencies that produce it.[49]

Research shows that approximately four of every five Americans believe that there is a relationship between diet and health,[49,50] and 57 percent are aware of the benefits of a healthy diet.[51] In addition, over half of shoppers reported actively seeking diet and nutrition informa-

Successful Community Strategies 🏠🏠🏠

National WIC Breastfeeding Promotion Project[46]

The National Special Supplemental Nutrition Program for Women, Infants, and Children (WIC) Breastfeeding Promotion Project created a marketing plan using the conceptual framework of the 4 Ps of marketing (product, price, place, and promotion) to reposition the product (breastfeeding). The program changed the traditional health benefits of breastfeeding to emphasize a new *product*, mothers' emotional bonding with the infant from breastfeeding.

A survey of pregnant women identified that embarrassment and conflicts with active lifestyles (*price*) were the constraints to breastfeeding. To reduce these constraints or price, a counseling program was developed to help mothers deal with the individual limitations. The *place* strategy targeted hospital environments as well as

homes. It focused on the main intermediaries such as professional associations. The majority of the *promotion* strategy consisted of media and grassroots advocacy, with media stressing a congratulatory tone and by speaking to family spokespersons. Television and radio advertisements, billboards, posters, educational pamphlets, information booklets, and staff support kits with resource information and promotional materials were used for this program, which ran from August 1997 to August 2000. This program did not apply the fifth P (*position*) of social marketing in their project. But the nutritionist could position breastfeeding as an act of love instead of a type of infant feeding.

The four goals that were established for the program were increasing breastfeeding initiation

rates, increasing the rate of breastfeeding duration among WIC participants, increasing referrals to the WIC program for breastfeeding support, and increasing the general public's knowledge of and support for breastfeeding.

In order to maximize the impact for each of the program's objectives, WIC clients were solicited to participate in the study. The targeted population for the campaign was organized into three separate audiences. The primary target audience was composed of pregnant European American, African American, and Hispanic American women who either were enrolled as WIC participants or met the income eligibility requirements (annual income below 185 percent of the U.S. poverty guidelines). The secondary audience consisted of individuals who might influence the primary

Fast food is very high in sodium, saturated fat, and calories. It is also deficient in dietary fiber and essential micronutrients such as vitamins and minerals.

tion in the last month,[50] and 41 percent of Americans felt that they were doing their best to eat healthfully.[52]

Food companies' advertising costs for any single, nationally distributed food product is higher (often by 10 to 50 times) than federal expenditures for promotion of MyPyramid or to encourage people to eat more fruits and vegetables. Therefore, it is very important for the federal government to provide more funds to encourage healthy eating habits. Some examples of expenditures by specific companies are given in **Table 15.3**. Of the more than $300 million that the U.S. Department of Agriculture (USDA) spends annually on nutrition education, most goes to research projects, the educational components of agricultural extension, and other activities that target relatively few people.[47]

The Use of Advertising

Successful campaigns are carefully researched, targeted to specific groups, and repeated frequently. Food sales increase with the intensity, repetition, and visibility of the advertising messages.[53–56] A study that evaluated the preference, recall accuracy, and consumption behavior of boys ages 8 to 10 showed that their preferences were a result of advertising repetition.[57] The children were exposed to repetitive or varied 30-second television commercials for the same ice cream product during a half-hour show. Results indicated that a single exposure was sufficient to affect brand name recall in almost 50 percent of the children. Increasing exposure and varying the commercials also had a positive influence on the boys' product preference and consumer behavior.

The promotion of nutritional advantages (low-fat, no cholesterol, high-fiber, and calcium-added) and the use of health claims (lowers cholesterol, prevents cancer) can increase sales. When Kellogg's high-fiber cereals first added health claims about cancer prevention and dietary fiber to their package label, sales escalated 47 percent within the first 6 months.[58] It is important for nutritionists to verify every health claim made by food companies because they may not be accurate or

target population, such as the mothers, husbands, and boyfriends of pregnant women, prenatal healthcare providers, and WIC staff. The general public was also included as the tertiary audience in order to change the established social norms and prevailing public perception regarding breastfeeding.

The campaign planners chose 10 pilot areas in which to conduct research and demonstrate the initial WIC Breastfeeding Promotion Project: Arkansas, California, the Chickasaw Nation, Iowa, Mississippi, Nevada, New Jersey, New York, Ohio, and West Virginia. Preliminary results from the Iowa study showed evidence of the program's success in both breastfeeding rates and changed attitude and awareness toward breastfeeding. The Iowa evaluation was based on the Ross Six Months Mothers' Infant Feeding Survey and a separate mail survey of WIC participants immediately before the campaign and 4 months afterwards. Results showed:

- Breastfeeding rates for mothers while in the hospital increased from 57.8 to 64.4 percent, and a year after the promotion started they increased to 65.1 percent.
- The rates for women still nursing 6 months after birth increased from 20.4 to 29.3 percent and to 32.2 percent a year after the program started.

A major objective of the public information component of the National WIC Breastfeeding Promotion Project's Loving Support Campaign was to encourage the spouses, relatives, and friends of pregnant women to provide support for breastfeeding. A survey of the Iowa participants showed that support for breastfeeding increased in every relationship category:

- Support from the pregnant woman's mother increased from 35.2 to 53 percent.
- Support from the pregnant woman's husband or boyfriend increased from 47.7 to 53 percent.
- Support from the pregnant woman's friends or other relatives increased from 48.8 to 51.1 percent.
- Support from the pregnant woman's prenatal healthcare provider increased from 62.4 to 83.8 percent and from WIC employees from 81.9 percent to 92.5 percent.

TABLE 15.3	The Cost of Advertising
Company	**Cost of Advertising**
McDonald's	$627.2 million
Burger King	$403.6 million
Taco Bell	$206.5 million
Coke and Diet Coke	$174.4 million
Wrigley's chewing gum	$117 million
M&M candies	$80 million
National Cholesterol Education Campaign	$1.5 million
5 a Day Campaign	$1 million

Data from: Nestle M. *Food Politics: How the Food Industry Influences Nutrition and Health.* Los Angeles: University of California Press; 2002. Reprinted with permission.

substantiated. For example, in March 2005, the Federal Trade Commission (FTC) reached a settlement with Tropicana Products about its advertisements that claimed its Healthy Heart orange juice could reduce blood pressure, cholesterol, and homocysteine levels. The advertisements appeared on television and in print publications including *Newsweek* and the *New York Times* between 2002 and early 2004. The FTC asserted that Tropicana's health claims were unproven and that it had no clinical support for the claims.[59]

Trade association programs also promote generic advertising, such as the "Got Milk?" campaign. One of the promotions featured celebrities wearing milk mustaches. Analysis of sales data showed that these campaigns slowed or stopped the decreasing trend of milk consumption and that 47 pounds of milk were purchased for each advertising dollar spent on these campaigns.[60] Thus, consumers can change their perceptions of foods and food choices when given repeated and positive nutrition messages.

For every dollar spent on advertising, the food companies spend another two dollars on discount incentives, for example, providing coupons for consumers and "slotting fees" for retailers to ensure space on supermarket shelves. In total, food companies spend more than $33 billion annually to advertise and promote their products to the public.[47]

There is a disproportionate distribution of marketing expenditures relative to dietary recommendations. Food industries spend more money on advertising to promote highly processed, elaborately packaged fast foods than the government does to market nutritious foods. About 70 percent of food advertising is for convenience foods, candy and snacks, alcoholic beverages, soft drinks, and desserts whereas only 2.2 percent is for fruits, vegetables, grains, or beans.[48] **Table 15.3** presents the costs of advertising.

In 1998, manufacturers introduced slightly more than 11,000 new products.[47] More than two-thirds of those products were condiments, candy and snacks, baked goods, soft drinks, and dairy products (cheese products and ice cream novelties). Slightly more than one-fourth were "nutritionally enhanced" and could be marketed as low in fat, cholesterol, salt, or sugar or as higher in fiber, calcium, or vitamins. Some of these products, such as no-fat cookies, vitamin-enriched cereals, and calcium-fortified juice drinks, were high in sugar content. Though

these products contain some of essential nutrients, it is important to note that a high intake of sugar promotes weight gain and contributes to long-term health and chronic disease risks.

The Role of Media in Childhood Obesity

Childhood obesity is now an epidemic in the United States. The number of children who are overweight has doubled in the last two to three decades; currently one child in five is overweight. The increase is in both children and adolescents and in all age, race, and gender groups. According to the Centers for Disease Control and Prevention (CDC), since 1980, the proportion of overweight children ages 6 to 11 has more than doubled and the rate for adolescents has tripled.[61] Today, about 10 percent of 2- to 5-year-olds and 15 percent of 6- to 19-year-olds are overweight. Taking into consideration the proportion who are at risk of becoming overweight, the current percentages double to 20 percent for children ages 2 to 5 and 30 percent for kids ages 6 to 19. The rates are higher among children of minority groups: 40 percent of Mexican American and African American youth ages 6 to 19 are considered overweight or at risk of becoming overweight.[62]

Advertising to Children and Youth

There has been an explosion of media targeting children during the same period in which childhood obesity has increased. Children of all ages spend a large amount of their leisure time using a combination of various media, including broadcast television, cable networks, DVDs, video games, computers, the Internet, and cell phones. Children 6 years and under also spend as much time with screen media (TV, videos, video games, and computers) as they do playing outside.[63] Much of the media targeted to children is loaded with elaborate advertising campaigns, many of which promote foods such as candy, soda, and snacks. It is estimated that the typical child sees about 40,000 ads a year on TV alone.[64]

Exposure to these media affects children's choices and may have a strong influence on their tendency toward increased obesity and chronic disease risk. Television advertising can affect children's food and nutrition-related knowledge and purchase decisions, both those made directly and those made indirectly through parents. Annual sales of foods and beverages to young consumers exceeded $27 billion in 2002. Food and beverage advertisers collectively spend $10 billion to $12 billion a year to reach children and youth. Of that, more than $1 billion is spent on media advertising to children through television; more than $4.5 billion is spent on youth-targeted promotions such as premiums, coupons, sweepstakes, and contests; $2 billion is spent on youth-targeted public relations; and $3 billion is spent on packaging designed for children.[65]

The CDC launched the VERB campaign to encourage a more active lifestyle for teenagers ages 9 to 13. The campaign used advertising, marketing, online material, and on-the-ground events to get the message to youth, parents, and educators. The National Cancer Institute's Fruits & Veggies–More Matters, designed to promote fruits and vegetables, also includes a media component. However, these campaigns are very modest compared to those mounted by the food industry. The entire budget for the 5 A Day effort is $3.5 million a year, compared to $29 million in advertising for Pringles, $74 million for M&Ms, $209 million for Coke, and $665 million for McDonald's.[65]

Exposure to Media

Although advertising has not been linked directly to childhood obesity, advertisements targeted to children through multiple media channels contribute to children's choices about foods, beverages, and a sedentary lifestyle. During the 1996–1997 school year, Stanford University researchers conducted a randomized controlled trial in which they reduced the amount of time a group of about 100 3rd and 4th graders in northern California spent with TV, videos, and video games.[66] Two matched elementary schools were selected to participate, one of which served as the control group. The intervention involved a "turn-off" period of no screen time for 10 days followed by limiting TV time to 7 hours per week as well as learning media literacy skills to teach selective viewing. At the end of a 6-month, 18-lesson classroom curriculum, students who received the intervention achieved a statistically significant reduction in their television viewing and number of meals eaten in front of the TV set as well as decreases in BMI, triceps skinfold thickness, waist circumference, and waist-to-hip ratio. Although these changes were not accompanied by reduced high-fat food intake or increased physical activity, the findings do seem to show the feasibility of decreasing body weight by reducing time spent with screen media.[61]

The Kaiser Family Foundation report, "It's Child's Play: Advergaming and the Online Marketing of Food to Children," shows the increasing popularity of advergaming, a new type of advertising.[66] Advergaming is the use of online video games with embedded brand messages to engage a target audience. It is specifically designed to blur the boundary between advertising and entertainment.[67] The food industry is spending millions of dollars on this new form of advertising because it is very effective. The Kaiser Family Foundation reported in 2006 that there were an astonishing 12.2 million visits to advergaming sites in just 3 months by children ages 2 to 11.

Food companies know that children make highly lucrative customers, and their attention to this group has increased significantly. Children control increasing amounts of money and society has granted them responsibility for purchasing decisions. It is difficult to know exactly how much money children now control from allowances, gifts, and jobs, but even small amounts add up to a very large amount when computed across the entire population. Studies in the late 1980s reported that children spent an average of $4.42 per week each, for a combined total of more than $6 billion a year, and that they influenced annual family spending decisions involving $50 billion in 1985, about $190 billion in 1997, and about $290 billion in 2000.[68] The amount controlled by children increases with age; children ages 7 to 12 have been reported to control $8.9 billion in spending money and teenagers $119 billion, a figure that was expected to rise to $136 billion by 2001. Overall, children ages 6 to 19 years were thought to have influenced $485 billion in purchase decisions in 1999.[69,70] Children also influence a substantial proportion of the total annual sales of certain foods: 25 percent of the total amount of salty snacks, 30 percent of soft drinks, 40 percent of frozen pizza, 50 percent of cold cereals, and 60 percent of canned pasta.[68]

One recent trend is an increase in programs designed especially for young children. Many of these children's television programs are linked directly to commercial products. For instance, Burger King first and later McDonald's sponsored Teletubbies, a public television program for toddlers. McDonald's distributed toys representing the four characters.

One study of the top-ranked prime-time shows (8 pm to 11 pm) in the 1988 TV season found that food references occurred almost 10 times per hour and that the majority (60 percent) were for low-nutrient beverages such as coffee, soft drinks, and alcohol. Most foods eaten were snacks (72 percent) and tended to be sweet (44 percent) or salty snacks (25 percent), with vegetables significantly behind (6 percent).[71] A decade later, by the 1998 TV season, a content analysis of the highest-ranked prime-time shows found little improvement. The highest-rated programs among 2- to 5-year-olds contained a reference to food in every episode, and one-third had 16 or more references. At this rate, it was estimated that the average child viewer might see more than 500 food references per week, almost one-third for empty-calorie foods high in fat, sugar, or salt and another one-quarter for nutrient-rich foods also high in fat, sugar, and salt.[72] The most popular is Channel One, which is the 12-minute television program that is beamed into 12,000 schools throughout the United States and viewed daily by about 8.3 million students. Two minutes out of every program are devoted to commercials. The private company responsible for Channel One provides television sets and installation of hardware estimated to be worth about $17,000 for the entire school. In exchange, the company requires students in 80 percent of the classrooms to watch the program on 90 percent of school days for the year.[73]

A study of advertisements appearing on Saturday morning TV in the United States found that 44 percent were for fats, oils, and sugar; 23 percent were for highly sugared cereals; and 11 percent were for fast food restaurants.[74,75] None were for fruits and vegetables. The authors concluded that the diet being presented on Saturday morning television does not support the recommendation for healthful eating for children. Similar findings were reported for Canadian TV.[76]

Based on children's commercial recall and because they lack the skills to understand the differences between information and advertising, there is not enough evidence of food, beverage, and entertainment advertising's adverse impacts on children to support calling for a ban on all such advertising.

Barriers to the Prevention of Obesity

It is reported that Americans spend about half of their food budget and consume about one-third of their daily energy on meals and drinks consumed outside the home, which makes it very difficult to estimate the energy content of the food.[77] About 170,000 fast-food restaurants[78] and 3 million soft-drink vending machines[79] help ensure that Americans are not more than a few steps from immediate sources of relatively non-nutritious foods.

Food eaten outside the home, on average, is higher in fat and lower in micronutrients than food prepared at home.[78] Many popular table-service restaurant meals—lunch or dinner—provide 1,000 to 2,000 kcal each,[80] amounts equivalent to 35 to 100 percent of a full day's energy requirements for most adults.[81] Restaurants and movie theaters charge just a few cents more for larger size orders of soft drinks, popcorn, and French fries, and the standard serving sizes of these and other foods have increased greatly in the past decade.[82] For example, in the 1950s, Coca-Cola was packaged only in 6.5-oz bottles; single-serving containers expanded first to 12-oz cans and, more recently, to 20-oz bottles. A 12-oz soft drink provides about 150 kcal, all from sugars, but contains no other nutrients of significance.[83]

Consequently, dietetics professionals must emphasize the need to select appropriate portion sizes. Nutrition education is critical because few consumers intuitively know that 3 oz of beef is considered an appropriate portion size. Choosing sensible portion sizes is a basic principle of the 2005 *Dietary Guidelines for Americans*.[84] If a person thinks that a restaurant portion of broiled beef rib steak (8 oz) is the most appropriate portion size, he or she would be getting a caloric content that is far higher (500 kcal) than the 188 kcal from the MyPyramid's recommended 3 oz portion. Therefore, it is imperative that the message of appropriate portion sizes be incorporated into the total diet approach.

The size of an average serving of food has increased dramatically over the past 20 years.

Public Health Approaches

Effective interventions are needed to deal with the ways people make food choices. Such interventions require the implementation of policies, especially by the government. Health protection through legislative and fiscal means is more likely to make a greater impact.

The government has a variety of powers at its disposal that can be put into service. One approach, which relies entirely on voluntary cooperation, is to issue policy statements. However, these can easily amount to no more than hollow declarations, as is illustrated by government policies on tobacco in many countries. On the other hand, policy statements can serve as the basis for a call to action. For instance, British and U.S. government policy on diet and disease, in conjunction with the media and medical science, helped change the climate of opinion so that it is now widely accepted that diets should be much lower in fat and richer in fiber.[85]

The Effect of Price on Sales

The most common among available government powers are legislation and the use of taxation and subsidies. Action on tobacco control showed the necessity for using these powers as a tool of health promotion. Educational efforts over the last three decades have been very important in persuading millions of people to stop smoking. But, smoking rates are still well above half of their level of 30 years ago.[85] There is convincing evidence that price hikes are an effective means to reduce smoking rates.[86] It was estimated that a 10 percent increase in price reduces tobacco consumption by about 5 percent, especially among lower socioeconomic groups.[87] In Canada, the prevalence of smoking in young Canadians was reduced by half during the 1980s due to the doubling of the price of cigarettes. This trend was reversed in the early 1990s when the price was decreased in an attempt to reduce smuggling from the United States.[88] Price increases appear to be a more effective means of tobacco control than education or media campaigns.[89]

Government Policy and Food

It seems that government policies about food prices and, to a lesser extent, food advertising and labeling may be an effective means to induce desirable changes in eating patterns. The following are some specific suggestions as to how existing government policies can be modified to encourage diets higher in fruits and vegetables and lower in fat:[41,90]

- There is always the possibility for improved food labels to facilitate the purchase of foods with a low-fat content, especially saturated fat. In addition, labeling and nutrition information needs to be extended to areas presently outside the system, especially restaurant menus, fast foods (McDonald's, Burger King, etc.), and fresh meat.

- By means of regulations and rewards, schools could be encouraged to sell meals of superior nutritional value while restricting the sale of junk food (high calorie dense foods). Similar policies could be applied to other institutions under government control, such as the military, prisons, and cafeterias in government offices.

- Television advertising could be regulated so as to control the content, duration, and frequency of commercials for unhealthy food products, especially when the target audience is children.

Box 15-3 presents additional suggestions to encourage healthy diets. Also, see "Successful Community Strategies: The Aptos Middle School (San Francisco, California) Pilot Program" in Chapter 9 for an example of a cafeteria and vending machine success story from the San Francisco Unified School District.

Successful Nutrition Education Campaigns

Mass media advertising needs to be a vital part of any campaign to reduce obesity through the promotion of positive changes in behavior, such as eating more fruits, vegetables, and whole grains; switching to lower-fat meat or dairy products; eating fewer hamburgers and steaks; and drinking water instead of soda. Campaigns of this kind can be remarkably effective. For instance, the Center for Science in the Public Interest's 1 Percent or Less program doubled the market share of low-fat and fat-free milk in several communities through an intensive, 7-week paid advertising and public relations campaign that cost as little as 22 cents per person.[91] Those efforts demonstrate that advertising can be an affordable, effective method for promoting dietary change. Media motivational campaigns can be developed to encourage people to walk, jog, bicycle, and engage in other enjoyable activities that expend energy.

Barriers Against Public Health Policies

Although many might consider the policies discussed here to be worthy of implementation, it must be noted that barriers exist. In particular, industries profit significantly from the sale of highly processed food and are often resistant to change. Therefore, industries often secure government support.[92]

The history of attempts to enact legislative control over tobacco show how effective an industry can be when it utilizes a large budget in attempts to delay, dilute, or stop laws. If the tobacco industry can achieve so many successes, then it will be much easier for the food industry to prevent interventions that threaten its profits. This is because the relationship between diet and disease is less clear than is the case with tobacco. There is evidence of how industry has successfully pressured governments to bend to their wishes on questions of nutrition policy. As discussed by Nestle,[92,93] the meat industry has

Excessive intake of calories—whether from fat-free or sugar-free foods—will be converted to body fat.

been effective in rewriting dietary guidelines. In the late 1970s, the recommendation was to reduce the amount of meat consumed; then the emphasis moved to eating lean meat. By 1992, people were encouraged to consume at least two or three servings daily. There is also evidence that the 1992 version of Canada's Food Guide was similarly modified under pressure from the food industry.[94]

Food and Nutrition Misinformation

It is unethical to promote questionable products or images or manipulate results to satisfy the food industry. Community nutritionists working with the media or food industry must consider the accuracy of the product descriptions and claims, words, and images so they don't misinform the public. The past decade has seen an increase in the promotion and use of questionable health practices, many of which are nutrition related. The main factor has been the ease of acquiring misinformation through the Internet.[1]

According to the American Dietetic Association's (ADA) Complete Food and Nutrition Guide, health *fraud* is falsely promoting a product or health remedy for financial gain that does not work or is not proven to work in improving health and well-being.[95] *Quackery* applies to food and nutrition-related products and is defined as the promotion of an unproved health product or service, usually for personal gain. Nutrition misinformation, fraud, and quackery are impediments to optimal

health habits and positive eating behaviors.[96,97] The health consequences of food quackery, faddism, misinformation, or the misuse or misinterpretation of emerging science may include delay or failure to seek legitimate medical care or to continue essential treatment, undesirable drug–nutrient interactions, nutrient toxicities or toxic components of products, and interference with sound nutrition education and practices.[98] Economic harm occurs when supposed remedies, treatments, and cures fail to work and when products are purchased needlessly.[98] The burden of proof is now on the federal government, so there are fewer roadblocks to developing expensive and ineffective products.[98]

Americans spend more than $30 billion annually on medical and nutritional health fraud and quackery, up from $1–2 billion in the early 1960s.[99,100] At the same time, the sale of weight-loss programs and products, as well as sports drinks to improve performance, has increased. Media attention to nutritional supplements has exacerbated the problem. Another problem is that foods are being supplemented with specific minerals and vitamins for their disease-preventing properties, and this has directed the marketing of many products as nutritional remedies. This practice may prevent the consumer from obtaining appropriate medical treatment.

Consumer Protection Laws

The Food, Drug, and Cosmetic Act defines a *drug* as any article (except devices) intended

fraud Intentional deception or misrepresentation that an individual knows to be false or does not believe to be true with knowledge that the deception could result in some unauthorized benefit to him- or herself or some other person.

quackery As it applies to food and nutrition-related products, the promotion of an unproved health product or service, usually for personal gain.

drug A chemical compound (except devices) intended for use in the diagnosis, cure, mitigation, treatment, or prevention of disease and articles (other than food) intended to affect the structure or function of the body.

for use in the diagnosis, cure, mitigation, treatment, or prevention of disease and articles (other than food) intended to affect the structure or function of the body.[1] This act permits the Food and Drug Administration (FDA) to stop the marketing of products with unsubstantiated drug claims on their labels. *Dietary supplements* are one area of concern because of the rapid expansion of the market and changing federal regulations.[102,103] No longer limited to vitamins and minerals, overabundances of herbal, botanical, and sport supplements, along with other products, now comprise over half the dietary supplement industry and have helped sales increase by over 60 percent to $13.9 billion each year.[101,103,104] Consumer spending on dietary supplements, natural/organic foods, natural personal care products, and functional foods totaled $128 billion in 2000.[101,102] Herbs and botanicals, sports and meal supplements, and other specialty products account for slightly more than half of these sales,[101,105,106] yet only 12 percent of people use herbal supplements.[103] Many supplements, such as herbs, remain largely uncontrolled and unregulated so long as their labels contain no health claims. Over 1,000 new dietary supplements are added annually to the already available 29,000.[104,107]

The most logical definition of a dietary supplement is that of a product made of one or more of the essential nutrients, such as vitamins, minerals, and protein. The Dietary Supplement Health Education Act of 1994 established specific guidelines for health claims and the labeling of dietary supplements, but it also shifted the burden of proving the accuracy of claims, safety, and quality from the manufacturer to the FDA.[105] This shift toward having to prove harm rather than safety can potentially impact consumers by creating a weak sense of credibility leading to misinformation or fraud because the federal government has not yet discovered or taken action against it. Monitoring the claims made by marketers of those products creates an overwhelming task for the FDA, which further delays the time when information can be retracted or products removed from the marketplace.[99,108]

Sources of Nutrition Misinformation

Consumers receive nutrition information from a variety of sources. According to the ADA's Nutrition and You: Trends 2000 survey, the media are the major source of information for consumers.[106] The top three leading sources of nutrition information for consumers were television (48 percent), magazines (47 percent), and newspapers (18 percent). Other sources cited included books (12 percent), doctors (11 percent), and family and friends (11 percent). Dietitians (1 percent) and nutritionists (1 percent) were not frequently cited.[106]

Multilevel marketing companies promote nutrition misinformation of unproven health products such as dietary supplements. Manufacturers of weight-loss products and herbs also often disseminate nutrition misinformation.[108] These companies claim that their products can prevent or cure diseases.

dietary supplements Products made of one or more of the essential nutrients, such as vitamins, minerals, and protein. The Dietary Supplement Health and Education Act of 1994 (DSHEA) expanded the definition, stating that herbs or other botanicals (except tobacco), and any dietary substance that can be used to supplement the diet were to be included in the definition.

How many fruits and vegetables do you need every day?

Their product literature may contain illegal therapeutic claims, or product distributors may supply such information through anecdotes and independently published literature.[107]

The ADA provides support for members through its Knowledge Center, a leading source of scientifically based objective food and nutrition information for dietetics professionals, the media, other healthcare providers, and researchers. The Knowledge Center provides practical, positive nutrition information to professionals and consumers through recorded nutrition messages, other publications, and the ADA website, http://www.eatright.org, which offers a gateway to government agencies and many allied professional organizations that focus on nutrition and health.

The following are strategies nutritionists can follow when communicating accurate nutrition information to consumers:[98,108–110]

- Keep advice simple to understand and implement. Be brief.
- Avoid contributing to the public's confusion by being too quick to laud the latest nutrition theory.
- Avoid speaking in nutrition buzzwords.
- React continually to misinformation.
- Keep your nutrition messages positive.
- Stay current with the latest literature.
- Avoid going against the tide. Tie your nutrition message to current lifestyle trends.
- Avoid being an alarmist. If you constantly proclaim the danger of certain foods, people will soon believe that they are not dangerous.
- Acknowledge possible ethical conflicts.
- Avoid arguing with other health professionals about subjects that have been discussed for years with no conclusion in sight.
- Stay inside your area of expertise.
- Know your subject area.

Chapter Summary

- Marketing is directed at satisfying the needs and wants of the consumer through an exchange of processes or activities (e.g., goods, products, or programs).
- Social marketing focuses on behavior change instead of sales or funds raised.
- Marketing research is the systematic design, collection, analysis, and reporting of data and findings relevant to a specific marketing situation or problem facing an organization.
- SWOT is an acronym for strengths, weaknesses, opportunities, and threats. It analyzes internal strengths and weaknesses and external opportunities and threats.
- Market segmentation is dividing a market/community into distinct groups of individuals on the basis of needs, characteristics, or behavior.
- Community nutritionists can communicate important health promotion messages to wide and diverse audiences or to a specific population by developing public service announcements.
- Some of the communication factors that may affect a nutrition program are perceptual distortions of information about nutrition, incorrect or improper use of works to convey specific information, lack of listening on the part of the targeted community, and differences in values and attitudes between the nutritionist and the target community.
- Successful nutrition education campaigns are carefully researched, targeted to specific groups, and repeated frequently.
- For every dollar they spend on advertising, food companies spend two dollars on discount incentives, for example, coupons for consumers and "slotting fees" for retailers to ensure space on supermarket shelves.
- The entire budget for Fruits & Veggies–More Matters campaign is $3.5 million a year, compared to $29 million in advertising for Pringles, $74 million for M&Ms, $209 million for Coke, and $665 million for McDonald's.
- Although advertising has not been linked directly to childhood obesity, advertisements targeted to children through multiple media channels contribute to children's choices about foods, beverages, and a sedentary lifestyle.
- On average, food eaten outside the home is higher in fat and lower in micronutrients than food prepared at home.
- Americans spend more than $30 billion annually on medical and nutritional health fraud and quackery.
- Some marketing companies promote nutrition misinformation of unproven health products, such as dietary supplements, weight loss products, and herbs.

Critical Thinking Activities

- Watch Saturday morning children's TV programs for 1 hour and determine the number of times food products were advertised and the types of products being advertised during the programs. Use the findings for an in-class discussion.
- Review and present two research articles on nutrition misinformation.

Case Study 15-1

Marcea, a professor of nutrition at a local university, received grant money from the Department of Public Health's Office of Women's Health to increase women's knowledge of osteoporosis and its prevention. The grant also included funds for screening women for osteoporosis. The budget allowed only $250 for advertising, and she is required to reach 400 women age 55 or older by the end of the year. The university is located in a county with an estimated total population of 156,800 residents. Women make up 51.9 percent or more of the population, and 9.7 percent of the population is 65 years or older.

Marcea called the program "Building Better Bones." She spent the $250 promoting Building Better Bones, but had reached only 200 participants 6 months into the program. To increase the number of women in the program, she found the free public announcement section in one of the local newspapers and placed an ad in its calendar of events. She also convinced a local produce stand to provide a small fruit basket in exchange for giving the stand's business card to the first 50 people who came to the lecture. Finally, she obtained a list of potential consumers who were interested in osteoporosis from the local YWCA and mailed each woman a flyer with a free packet of wildflower seeds. Marcea's organization provided the funding for mailing the fliers.

Activities

- List at least two other ways Marcea can receive free advertising.
- Identify three other media outlets where Marcea can advertise the program.
- Develop a 30-second radio PSA for Building Better Bones.

References

1. Wansink B. *Marketing Nutrition: Soy, Functional Foods, Biotechnology, and Obesity*. Urbana, IL: University of Illinois Press; 2005.

2. Kotler P, Zaltman G. Social marketing: an approach to planned social change. *J Marketing*. 1971; 35:3–12.

3. Anspaugh DJ, Dignan MB, Anspaugh SL. *Developing Health Promotion Programs*. Boston: McGraw-Hill Higher Education; 2000.

4. Clark CC. *Health Promotion in Communities: Holistic and Wellness Approaches*. New York: Springer; 2002.

5. Bennett R. Relationship quality, relationship marketing, and client perceptions of the levels of service quality of charitable organizations. *Int J Service Industry Manage*. 2005; 16(1):81.

6. Keefe LM. What is the meaning of 'marketing'? *Marketing News*. 2004; 38(15):17–18.

7. Breckon DJ. *Managing Health Promotion Programs: Leadership Skills for the 21st Century*. Gaithersburg, MD: Aspen; 1997.

8. McDonald M. Strategic marketing planning: theory and practice. *Marketing Rev*. 2006; 6(4):375–418.

9. Kotler P, Clark R. *Marketing for Healthcare Organizations*. Englewood Cliffs, NJ: Prentice Hall; 1987.

10. Gombeski WR. Better marketing through a principles-based model. *Healthcare Leadership Rev*. December 6, 1998:6.

11. Anspaugh DJ, Dignan MB, Anspaugh SL. *Developing Health Promotion Programs*. 2nd ed. Long Grove, IL: Waveland Press; 2006.

12. Tassonyi A. Municipal budgeting. *Can Tax J*. 2002; 50(1):181.

13. Trouiller P, Olliaro P, Torreele E, Orbinski J, Laing R, Ford N. Drug development for neglected diseases: a deficient market and a public-health policy failure. *Lancet.* 2002; 359(9324):2188–2194.

14. Ling PM, Glantz SA. Using tobacco-industry marketing research to design more effective tobacco-control campaigns. *JAMA.* 2002; 287(22):2983–2989.

15. Boyle M. *Community Nutrition in Action: An Entrepreneurial Approach.* 4th ed. Belmont, CA: Thomson Wadsworth; 2005.

16. Escott-Stump S, Jarratt J, Mahaffie JB. Key trends affecting the dietetics profession and the American Dietetic Association. *J Am Diet Assoc.* 2002; 102(12):S1819–S1839.

17. Bednar C, Denny S, Schuessler L, et al. Position of the American Dietetic Association: food and nutrition professionals can implement practices to conserve natural resources and support ecological sustainability. *J Am Diet Assoc.* 2007; 107(6):1033–1043.

18. Levinson J, Godin S. *The Guerrilla Marketing Handbook.* New York: Houghton Mifflin; 1994.

19. Kotler P, Fox KFA. *Strategic Marketing for Educational Institutions.* 2nd ed. Englewood Cliffs, NJ: Prentice-Hall; 1995.

20. Edelstein S. *Nutrition in Public Health: A Handbook for Developing Programs and Services.* 2nd ed. Sudbury, MA: Jones and Bartlett; 2006.

21. Helm KK, Rose JC. *The Competitive Edge: Advanced Marketing for Dietetics Professionals.* 2nd ed. Chicago, IL: American Dietetic Association; 1995.

22. QuickMBA. Strategic Management. SWOT Analysis. Available at: http://www.quickmba.com/strategy/swot. Accessed July 2, 2007.

23. Kotler P, Armstrong G. *Principles of Marketing.* 9th ed. Upper Saddle River, NJ: Prentice Hall; 2001.

24. Barbeau EM, Leavy-Sperounis A, Balbach ED. Smoking, social class, and gender: what can public health learn from the tobacco industry about disparities in smoking? *Tob Control.* 2004; 13(2):115–120.

25. Zikmund WG, d'Amico M. *Effective Marketing: Creating and Keeping Customers.* New York: West; 1995.

26. Randolph W, Viswanath K. Lessons learned from public health mass media campaigns: marketing health in a crowded media world. *Annu Rev Public Health.* 2004; 25:419–437.

27. Gerson R. *Marketing Health/Fitness Services.* Champaign, IL: Human Kinetics; 1989.

28. Peregrin T. Getting into the media spotlight: the ADA's public relations team promotes the association as the most recognized source for nutrition information. *J Am Diet Assoc.* 2001; 101(7):738–739.

29. American Dietetic Association, Public Relations Team. *Working with the Media: A Handbook for Members of the American Dietetic Association.* Chicago, IL: Author; 2001.

30. Robert L. New marketing litany: 4 P's passe' C-words take over. *Advertising Age.* October 1, 1990; 26.

31. Wiebe G. Merchandising commodities and citizenship on television. *Public Opin Q.* 1951/52; 15:679–691.

32. Hampl JS, Anderson JV, Mullis R. Position of the American Dietetic Association: the role of dietetics professionals in health promotion and disease prevention. *J Am Diet Assoc.* 2002; 102(11):1680–1687.

33. Hampl JS, Sass S. Focus groups indicate that vegetable and fruit consumption by food stamp–eligible Hispanics is affected by children and unfamiliarity with non-traditional foods. *J Am Diet Assoc.* 2001; 101:685–687.

34. Reger B, Wootan MG, Booth-Butterfield S. Using mass media to promote healthy eating: a community-based demonstration project. *Prev Med.* 1999; 29:414–421.

35. Stead M. A systematic review of social marketing effectiveness. *Health Educ.* 2007; 107(2):126.

36. Kotler P, Roberto EL. *Social Marketing: Strategies for Changing Public Behavior.* New York: Free Press; 1989.

37. Kaufman M. *Nutrition in Public Health: A Handbook for Developing Programs and Services.* Rockville, MD: Aspen; 1990.

38. Parks SC, Moody DL. A marketing model: applications for dietetic professionals. *J Am Diet Assoc.* 1986; 86:37–40.

39. Center for Advanced Studies in Nutrition and Social Marketing. Social Marketing. Available at: http://socialmarketing-nutrition.ucdavis.edu/somark.htm. Accessed July 4, 2007.

40. Social Marketing Institute. Success Stories: Mass Media and Health Practices Project. Available at: www.social-marketing.org/success/cs-massmedia.html. Accessed July 2, 2007.

41. Caraher M, Landon J, Dalmeny K. Television advertising and children: lessons from policy development. *Public Health Nutr.* 2006; 9(5):596–605.

42. Lee M, Johnson C. *Principles of Advertising: A Global Perspective.* 2nd ed. New York: Haworth Press; 2005.

43. DiLima S, Schust C. *Publicizing Your Program. Community Health Education and Promotion Manual.* Gaithersburg, MD: Aspen; 1997.

44. Friedman RJ, Altman P. *How to Design, Develop, and Market Healthcare Seminars.* Sarasota, FL: Professional Resource Press; 1997.

45. Public Health Association of Nebraska. Public Health Is Your Health Too. Available at: http://www.publichealthne.org/socmar/Radio%20Spots.htm. Accessed July 2, 2007.

46. Social Marketing Institute. Success Stories: National WIC Breastfeeding Promotion Project. Available at: http://www.social-marketing.org/success/cs-nationalwic.html. Accessed July 2, 2007.

47. Nestle M. *Food Politics: How the Food Industry Influences Nutrition and Health.* Los Angeles, CA: University of California Press; 2002.

48. Gallo AE. Food advertising in the United States. In: Frazao E, ed. *America's Eating Habits: Changes and Consequences.* Washington, DC: U.S. Department of Agriculture; 1999:173–180.

49. American Dietetic Association. *Nutrition Trends Survey. Executive Summary.* Chicago, IL: Author; 1997.

50. Mangalam KS. Nutrition and lung health. *Proc Nutr Society.* 1999; 58:303–308.

51. Food Marketing Institute. *Trends in the United States. Consumer Attitudes and the Supermarket.* Washington, DC: Author; 1999.

52. American Dietetic Association. *Nutrition and You: Trends 2000.* Chicago, IL: Author; 2000.

53. Novelli WD. Applying social marketing to health promotion and disease prevention. In: Glanz K, Lewis FM, Rimer BK, eds. *Health Behavior and Health Education: Theory, Research, and Practice.* San Francisco, CA: Jossey-Bass; 1990: 342–369.

54. Blisard N. Advertising and what we eat: the case of dairy products. In: Frazao E, ed. *America's Eating Habits: Changes and Consequences.* Washington, DC: U.S. Department of Agriculture; 1999: 181–188.

55. Enyinda CI, Ogbuehi AO. An empirical analysis of retail pricing and multimedia advertising effects on sales performance. *J Food Products Marketing.* 1997; 4:3–16.

56. Kelly B, Smith B, King L, Flood V, Bauman A. Television food advertising to children: the extent and nature of exposure. *Public Health Nutr.* 2007; 10(11):1–7.

57. Gorn GJ, Goldberg ME. Children's responses to repetitive television commercials. *J Consumer Res.* 1980; 6(4):421–424.

58. Levy AS, Stokes RE. Effects of a health promotion advertising campaign on sales of ready-to-eat cereals. *Public Health Rep.* 1987; 102:398–403.

59. Beverage Daily. FTC Quashes Tropicana's 'Healthy Heart' Claims. Available at: http://www.beveragedaily.com/news/news-ng.asp?n=60451-ftc-quashes-tropicana. Accessed July 2, 2007.

60. Blisard N. Advertising and what we eat. In: Frazao E, ed. *America's Eating Habits: Changes and Consequences: Agriculture Information Bulletin No. 750.* Washington, DC: U.S. Department of Agriculture; 1999: 181–188.

61. Centers for Disease Control and Prevention. Overweight Among U.S. Children and Adolescents. National Health and Nutrition Examination Survey. Available at: http://www.cdc.gov/nchs/products/pubs/pubd/hestats/overwght99.htm. Accessed July 2007.

62. Ogden C, Flegal K, Carroll M, Johnson C. Prevalence and trends in overweight among U.S. children and adolescents 1999–2000. *JAMA*. 2002; 288:1728–1732.

63. Rideout V, Vandewater E, Wartella E. *Zero to Six: Electronic Media in the Lives of Infants, Toddlers and Preschoolers*. Menlo Park, CA: Henry J. Kaiser Family Foundation; 2003.

64. Booth FW, Gordon SE, Carlson CJ, Hamilton MT. Waging war on modern chronic diseases: primary prevention through exercise biology. *J Appl Physiol*. 2000; 88:774–787.

65. Kaiser Family Foundation. The Role of Media in Childhood Obesity. Available at: http://www.kff.org/entmedia/loader.cfm?url=/commonspot/security/getfile.cfm&PageID=32022. Accessed July 2, 2007.

66. Moore ES. It's Child's Play: Advergaming and the Online Marketing of Food to Children. Available at: http://www.kff.org/entmedia/upload/7536.pdf. Accessed July 2, 2007.

67. Salber PR. Is the Food Industry Playing Games With Our Children? *MedGenMed*. 2006; 8(4):37.

68. McNeal JU. *The Kids Market: Myths and Realities*. Ithaca, NY: Paramount; 1999.

69. McNeal JU. *Kids as Customers: A Handbook of Marketing to Children*. New York: Lexington; 1992.

70. Stipp H. New ways to reach children. *Am Demograph*. 1993; 15:51–56.

71. Pollack J. Foods targeting children aren't just child's play: shape-shifting foods, "interactive" products chase young consumers. *Advertising Age*. March 1, 1999; 16.

72. Story M, Faulkner P. The prime time diet: a content analysis of eating behavior and food messages in television program content and commercials. *Am J Public Health*. 1990; 80(6):738–740.

73. Byrd-Bredbenner C, Finckenor M, Grasso D. Health related content in prime-time television programming. *J Health Commun*. 2003; 8:329–341.

74. Hoynes W. News for a captive audience: an analysis of Channel One. *Extra*. May/June 1997; 11–17.

75. Kotz K, Story M. Food advertisements during children's Saturday morning television programming: are they consistent with dietary recommendations? *J Am Diet Assoc*. 1994; 94:1296–1300.

76. Christakis DA. The hidden and potent effects of television advertising. *JAMA*. 2006; 295(14):1698–1699.

77. Ostbye T, Pomerleau J, White M, Coolich M, McWhinney J. Food and nutrition in Canadian "prime time" television commercials. *Can J Public Health*. 1993; 84:370–374.

78. Lin BH, Frazao E, Guthrie J. *Away-from-Home Foods Increasingly Important to Quality of American Diet*. Washington, DC: U.S. Department of Agriculture; 1999:749.

79. U.S. Bureau of the Census. *Statistical Abstract of the United States: The National Data Book*. Washington, DC: Government Printing Office; 1997.

80. Postlewaite K. Vended bottled drinks. *Vending Times*. 1998; 38:21–22.

81. Burros M. Losing count of calories as plates fill up. *New York Times*. April 2, 1997: C1.

82. National Research Council. *Recommended Dietary Allowances*. Washington, DC: National Academy Press; 1989.

83. Young LR, Nestle M. Portion sizes in dietary assessment: issues and policy implications. *Nutr Rev*. 1995; 53:149–158.

84. Jacobson MF. *Liquid Candy: How Soft Drinks Are Harming Americans' Health*. Washington, DC: Center for Science in the Public Interest; 1998.

85. U.S. Department of Health and Human Services. *Dietary Guidelines for Americans 2005*. Washington, DC: Author; January 2005.

86. Wilson T, Temple NJ. *Nutritional Health: Strategies for Disease Prevention*. Totowa, NJ: Humana Press; 2001.

87. Meier KJ, Licari MJ. The effect of cigarette taxes on cigarette consumption, 1955 through 1994. *Am J Public Health*. 1997; 87:1126–1130.

88. Townsend J. Price and consumption of tobacco. *Br Med J*. 1998; 316:1220.

89. Stephens T, Pederson LL, Koval JJ, Kim C. The relationship of cigarette prices and no-smoking bylaws to the prevalence of smoking in Canada. *Am J Public Health*. 1997; 87:1519–1521.

90. Townsend J, Roderick P, Cooper J. Cigarette smoking by socioeconomic group, sex, and age effects of price, income, and health publicity. *Br Med J*. 1994; 309:923–927.

91. Razzouk N, Seltz V. Marketing to the heart: a practical approach to dealing with health care quackery. *Clin Res Regulatory Aff*. 2003; 20(4):469–478.

92. Nestle M. Toward more healthful dietary patterns—a matter of policy. *Public Health Rep*. 1998; 113:420–423.

93. Nestle M. Food lobbies, the food pyramid and U.S. nutrition policy. *Int J Health Serv*. 1993; 23:483–496.

94. Nestle M. The politics of dietary guidance—a new opportunity. *Am J Public Health*. 1994; 84:713–715.

95. Southamstar N. Industry forced changes to food guide, papers show. *Toronto Star*. January 15, 1993: A2.

96. Duyff R. *American Dietetic Association Complete Food and Nutrition Guide*. 2nd ed. New York: John Wiley; 2002

97. Reger B, Wootan MG, Booth-Butterfield S. Using mass media to promote healthy eating: a community-based demonstration project. *Prev Med*. 1999; 29:414–421.

98. Pepper C. *Quackery: A $10 Billion Scandal*. Subcommittee on Health And Long-Term Care of the Select Committee on Aging U.S. House of Representatives. Publication No. 98-435. Washington, DC: U.S. Government Printing Office; 1984: 698.

99. Ashley JM, Jarvis WT. Position of the American Dietetic Association: food and nutrition misinformation. *J Am Diet Assoc*. 2002; 102:260–266.

100. Kant AK, Schatzkin A, Harris TB, Ziegler RG, Block G. Dietary diversity and subsequent mortality in the first NHANES epidemiological follow-up study. *Am J Clin Nutr*. 1993; 57:434–440.

101. Duyff RL. *The American Dietetic Association's Complete Food and Nutrition Guide*. 2nd ed. New York: John Wiley; 2002.

102. Hathcock J. Supplement: Recent Advances on the Nutritional Effects Associated with the Use of Garlic as a Supplement Dietary Supplements: How They Are Used and Regulated. *Journal of Nutrition*. 2001; 131:1114S–1117S.

103. Sarubin A. *The Health Professional's Guide to Popular Dietary Supplements*. Chicago, IL: American Dietetic Association; 2000.

104. DeAngelis CD, Fontanarosa PB. Drugs alias dietary supplements. *JAMA*. 2003;290(11):1519–1520.

105. Buettner C, Phillips RS, Davis RB, Gardiner P, Mittleman MA. Use of dietary supplements among United States adults with coronary artery disease and atherosclerotic risks. *Am J Cardiol*. 2007; 99(5):661–666.

106. Klotzbach-Shimomura K. Herbs and health: Safety and effectiveness. *Journal of Nutrition Education*. 2001; 33:(6)354–355

107. Cassileth BR, Vickers AJ. High prevalence of complementary and alternative medicine use among cancer patients: implications for research and clinical care. *J Clin Oncol*. 2005; 23(12):2590–2592.

108. The Dietary Supplement Health and Education Act. Pub L No.103-417 (S784) (codified at 42 USC 287C-11); 1994.

109. Goldberg JP. Nutrition communication in the 21st century: what are the challenges and how can we meet them? *Nutr*. 2000; 16:644–646.

110. Settings M. Position of the American Dietetic Association: food and nutrition misinformation. *J Am Diet Assoc*. 2006; 106(4):601–607.

Cultural Influences and Public Health Nutrition

LEARNING OBJECTIVES

- Discuss different determinants of health.
- List different acculturation scales for developing health promotion programs for multicultural groups.
- Discuss different components of cultural competency.
- Identify different ways of acquiring cultural competency.
- Identify barriers to multicultural health promotion and disease prevention.
- Explain the historical food habits of different ethnic groups and their influence on current dietary practices.
- Discuss the dietary patterns of different cultural groups in the United States.

Introduction

In the past few decades, an influx of refugees has come into the United States due to political, social, cultural, religious, and economic oppression in Central America, South America, the Caribbean Islands, Eastern Europe, Africa, and Southeast Asia.[1,2] The life of immigrants is laden with difficulties, such as going from an old to a new way of life, learn-ing a new language, and adapting to a new climate, new attire, new foods, and new culture. In addition, they have to choose new foods from large supermarkets, and traditional foods may be expensive, if available. They also have to use new high-tech kitchen equipment to prepare foods. Hence, they need support and culturally appropriate nu-trition education to improve their diets, break the cultural barrier, and experience healthy productive lives. However, there are not enough ethnically and linguistically diverse community nutritionists and other healthcare professionals to help reduce the cultural barriers these immigrants experience.[3]

Community and public health nutritionists are in a position to work with a variety of different cultures and are faced with the challenge of providing services to different cultural groups they may have never previously met. The challenge of serving *multicultural* groups in a rapidly changing population accentuates the importance of *cultural competence* skills. As people become acculturated in the United States, their dietary habits begin to change from whole-grain to high-fat intake, and, consequently, chronic health conditions begin, such as obesity and heart disease. Community nutritionists need to have strategies that can bridge the cultural gaps and prevent malnutrition and other nutrition-related health conditions. This chapter discusses health disparities in the United States, cultural competence, and the dietary patterns of different cultural groups in the United States.

U.S. Cultural Demographics

The world is now smaller, and the United States is a country that is ethnically diverse. People from around the world have joined Native Americans and Mexican indigenes in the United States. According to the 2000 census, America's total population was 281 million people, an overall increase of 13 percent from the 249 million in 1990. The fastest growing population group is Hispanics. The total number of Hispanics listed in the 2000 census was 35 million, an increase of 58 percent from their total of 22 million in the 1990 census. African Americans, including those who declared mixed backgrounds, totaled 36 million persons, an increase of 21 percent since the 1990 figure of 30 million.[4] People of Asian backgrounds are also a fast growing group. The numbers of other racial groups, including Native Americans, Alaskan natives, and Pacific Islanders, are increasing as well.[5] In 2000, the U.S. Census Bureau also provided data on the U.S. foreign-born population by region of birth. This is presented in **Figure 16-1**.

Due to the demographic diversity in the United States, community nutritionists should build nutrition education programs based on their clients' cultural food preferences and customs and use culturally appropriate nutrition education materials to improve the quality of their clients' diets. The use of pictorial graphics such as MyPyramid and illustrations of traditional foods to communicate nutrition mes-

sages has been effective. Pictures and educational material should be field tested with the target audience to determine if the educational materials are acceptable and easy to comprehend. Also, nutritionists should not assume that all clients are able to read either in English or in their native language or that they understand basic nutrition and health information, including food labels, food preparation education (e.g., meals and/or infant formula preparation, etc.), and dietary plans. Community nutritionists should consider these barriers when providing educational interventions and materials. Simple, informal methods are available that can identify individuals with low English proficiency without causing embarrassment to the client. Methods include asking open-ended questions about the materials received, listening to the individual's comments, and asking the clients if they need an interpreter. The following are ideas that can serve as a starting point for providing effective nutrition education programs to culturally diverse groups:[1]

- Assess common cultural food patterns.
- Complete an individual assessment to determine the main foods that the clients eat regularly.
- Determine the nutrient content of these foods.
- Determine the main food preparation methods of these foods.
- Before introducing new foods, emphasize familiar or comparable foods.
- Know about program eligibility criteria for federal or state assistance programs and make referrals as needed.

Health Disparities in the United States

Health is defined as the status of an individual's condition (i.e., the presence or absence of a health condition or illness, such as high blood pressure, asthma, obesity, drug use, etc.) and the individual's state of complete physical, mental, and social well-being. Healthcare refers to the process of treating an illness or injury.[6] *Health disparities* are the differences in the incidence, prevalence, mortality, and burden of diseases and other adverse health conditions that exist among specific population groups in the United States.[7,8] Disagreements exist about the definition and use of the terms *health disparity*, *inequality*, and *inequity*.[9] The definition of these terms can have important practical consequences; it determines the measurements that are monitored by governments and international agencies and the activities that will be supported by resources allocated to address health disparities.[10] It also reflects different political ideas. **Table 16.1** presents a few examples of definitions of health disparities being used by U.S. agencies and their strengths and weaknesses.

Healthy People 2010 is a comprehensive national health promotion and disease prevention agenda. Two broad goals were established with the intent

multicultural Composed of two or more unique cultures.

cultural competence The ability to increase one's understanding of and appreciation for cultural differences and commonalities by developing knowledge and interpersonal skills.

health The status of an individual's condition (i.e., the presence of a health condition or illness, such as high blood pressure, asthma, obesity, drug use, etc.). It is the state of complete physical, mental, and social well-being and not mainly the absence of disease.

health disparities Differences in the incidence, prevalence, mortality, and burden of diseases and other adverse health conditions that exist among specific population groups.

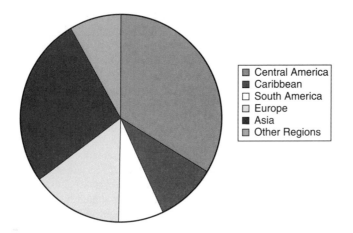

FIGURE 16-1 U.S. Foreign-Born Population by Region of Birth

- Central America
- Caribbean
- South America
- Europe
- Asia
- Other Regions

| TABLE 16.1 | Examples of Definitions of Health Disparities Currently Used by U.S. Agencies | | | |

Source	Definition	Strengths	Weaknesses
U.S. Department of Health and Human Services (DHHS). Healthy People 2010 goals. In: *Healthy People 2010: Understanding and Improving Health*. 2nd ed. Washington, DC: U.S. Government Printing Office: 8–16.	Health disparities include "differences by gender, race or ethnicity, education or income, disability, geographic location, or sexual orientation." "Compelling evidence of large and often increasing racial/ethnic disparities demand national attention." "Racial and ethnic minority populations [the racial/ethnic groups of concern]" are: American Indian & Alaska Native, Asian American, African American, Hispanic or Latino, and Native Hawaiian and Other Pacific Islander.	Mentions range of characteristics associated with social disadvantage, making that criterion implicit. Justifies focus on racial/ethnic disparities because of magnitude, pervasiveness, and persistence or widening of these gaps, and specifies groups of concern. Easily understandable to wide audiences.	Does not specify the types of differences or comparisons of concern, leaving an opening for misinterpretation (e.g., if European Americans and/or persons of relatively high income/education experience worse health on a particular outcome, would they warrant attention under health disparities initiatives?). Because relevance of social disadvantage is implicit rather than explicit, it does not specify the reference group (although this is implicitly clear for racial/ethnic disparities).
Natl. Inst. Health (NIH). 2005. Addressing disparities: the NIH program of action. What are health disparities? (http://healthdisparities.nih. gov/whatare.html)	Health disparities are "differences in the incidence, prevalence, mortality, and burden of disease and other adverse health conditions that exist among specific population groups in the United States." NIH will initially focus on racial/ethnic disparities but "disparities related to socioeconomic status will also be addressed."	Focuses on differences among defined social groups. Prioritizes racial/ethnic disparities, reflecting implicit values (unacceptability of long-standing injustice).	Does not specify comparisons among more and less advantaged groups. Not specifying the kinds of social groups or the reference groups leaves these open for interpretation in ways that do not reflect social justice concerns. Values are implicit, not explicit (e.g., open to interpretation why racial/ethnic disparities should receive priority attention, which could leave that focus open to attack).
National Cancer Institute (NCI), National Center to Reduce Cancer Health Disparities (http://crchd.nci.nih.gov/ chd/disparitiesA_defined. html)	"Disparities or inequalities occur when members of certain population groups do not enjoy the same health status as other groups. Disparities are most often identified along racial and ethnic lines— showing that African Americans, Hispanics, Native Americans, Asian Americans, Alaska Natives and whites have different disease rates and survival rates. But disparities also extend beyond race and ethnicity" and "can be noted on the basis of income and education."	Focuses on disparities among defined social groups. Notes that disparities can extend beyond race and ethnicity, and explicitly mentions two socioeconomic characteristics.	Could apply to any differences and comparisons between any groups. Same weaknesses as two examples above.

From: Braveman P. Health disparities and health equity: concepts and measurement. *Annu Rev Public Health*. 2006; 27:167–194. Reprinted with permission.

to impact the health of U.S. citizens. The goals were to increase quality and years of life and to eliminate health disparities.[11] The current attention to health disparities is in response to significant evidence that many minority populations are being disproportionately impacted by major health problems. According to a comprehensive study by the Institute of Medicine (IOM), evidence of racial and **ethnic** disparities in healthcare were consistent and remained even after adjustments were made for socioeconomic differences and healthcare access–related factors.[12] The study further reported that health disparities were associated with poor outcomes for minority populations.[13] The IOM report also stated that "racial and ethnic disparities occurred in the context of broader historic and contemporary social and economic inequality and evidence of persistent racial and ethnic discrimination in many sectors of American life."[12]

The causes for the disparity and the determinants of health are many and have been broadly categorized by some as either avoidable vs. unavoidable or biological vs. socioeconomic/sociocultural.[13] The specific effects of these determinants, how they should be measured, and the magnitude of their effect are not well known.[14–16] In addition, recent discoveries in the area of the human genome have added to the complexity of the discussion and have raised questions related to

ethnic The commonality of a group expressed by its nationality, language, or race.

race as a specific determinant.[17,18] It has been theorized that an understanding of the molecular basis for chronic diseases and what genetic variants exist may help show what predisposes some groups to health disparities.[18] However, research indicates that there is no genetic basis for the concept of race, suggesting that race may not be a useful category.[14,19,20] In addition, the few genes responsible for factors such as skin color cannot be linked to genetically complex diseases like diabetes mellitus.[14,17-19]

Topics covered by the objectives in Healthy People 2010 reflect the variety of critical influences that determine the health of individuals and communities. For example, individual behaviors and environmental factors are responsible for about 70 percent of all premature deaths in the United States.[21] Developing and implementing policies and preventive interventions that effectively address these determinants of health can reduce the burden of illness, enhance quality of life, and increase longevity.

Race and Ethnicity

It is reported that the biologic and genetic characteristics of African Americans, Hispanics, American Indians, Alaska Natives, Asians, Native Hawaiians, and Pacific Islanders do not offer any explanation about the health disparities these groups experience compared with the European American, non-Hispanic population in the United States.[22] It is believed that these disparities are due to the result of the complex interactions among genetic variations, environmental factors, and specific health behaviors.[23,24]

Although the U.S. infant mortality rate has lowered, the infant mortality rate among African Americans is still significantly higher than that of European Americans. In addition, heart disease death rates are over 40 percent higher for African Americans than for European Americans.[25-27] The death rate for all cancers is 30 percent higher for African Americans than for European Americans; for prostate cancer, it is significantly higher than for European Americans.[28] African American women have a higher death rate from breast cancer despite mammography screening. The death rate from HIV/AIDS for African Americans is seven times higher than that of European Americans, and the rate of homicide is six times higher than that of European Americans.[7,25,29,30]

Hispanic Americans are two times more likely to die from diabetes compared to non-Hispanic European Americans. In the United States, Hispanics accounted for 20 percent of new cases of tuberculosis. It is also reported that Hispanics have higher rates of high blood pressure and obesity than non-Hispanic European Americans. Research studies also show that there are differences among Hispanic populations. For example, the rate of low-birth-weight infants is lower for the total Hispanic population compared with that of European Americans, but Puerto Ricans have a low-birth-weight rate that is up to 50 percent higher than the rate for European Americans.[25,31,32]

It has been reported that American Indians and Alaska Natives have a significantly higher infant mortality rate than European Americans. They also have two times the rate of diabetes than European Americans.[33] For example, the Pima tribe of Arizona has one of the highest rates of diabetes in the world. Additionally, American Indians and Alaska Natives also have significantly higher unintentional injuries and suicide death rates.[34]

It is reported that Asians and Pacific Islanders, on average, are the healthiest population groups in the United States. However, results from a national survey found that the same proportions of Asian and non-Hispanic Americans have diabetes, but after accounting for the lower body mass index (BMI) of Asians, the adjusted prevalence of diabetes was 60 percent higher in Asian Americans.[35] New cases of hepatitis and tuberculosis also are higher in Asians and Pacific Islanders in the United States than for European Americans.[34] Great diversity exists within the Asian population group, and there are differences in health disparities for some specific segments of the group. For instance, women of Vietnamese origin suffer from cervical cancer at about five times the rate for European American women.[25,36]

Socioeconomic Factors

Socioeconomic factors may contribute to health and illness among minority groups. For instance, Larsen et al. reported that minority groups with lower socioeconomic status had reduced access to facilities, which in turn was associated with decreased physical activity and increased overweight and subsequently chronic health conditions such as diabetes and heart disease.[37] Also, individuals with lower socioeconomic status do not have similar opportunities for education, occupation, and income as do those with higher socioeconomic status. According to the U.S. Census Bureau there are more European American families than minorities below the poverty level; however, the concentration of minority families is greater. For example, European American families represent 8.5 percent of those in poverty, whereas African Americans represent 26.4 percent and Hispanics represent 27.0 percent. The negative impact of poverty and nutritional status is well documented.[38,39]

One research study measured the difference between dietary intake and eating habits across socioeconomic groups. One hundred sixteen participants from the high socioeconomic group and 206 from the low socioeconomic group were recruited for the study. Results showed that participants in the low socioeconomic status group were less educated and less physically active. Dietary intake among the participants in the low socioeconomic group was significantly lower in protein, monounsaturated fat, and most vitamins and minerals (thiamine, riboflavin, niacin, vitamin C, calcium, magnesium, and iron). In the low socioeconomic group, the main contributors to energy intake were breads, oils, and sugars. The participants in the low socioeconomic group consumed more oils, fats, and citrus fruits, while participants in the high socioeconomic group consumed more dairy products, grains, and legumes.[40] Overall the study found that the participants in the low socioeconomic group consumed a poorer quality diet.

Another effect of the socioeconomic factor is the obesity–hunger paradox. Both obesity and hunger (and, more broadly, food insecurity) are serious public health problems, sometimes coexisting in the same person within the same household.[41] This phenomenon is called the hunger–obesity paradox.[42,43] This trend is supported by published scientific literature and research studies, including a study by Drewnowski and Darmon that showed the highest rates of obesity and diabetes in the United States were among the lower-income groups. The observed links between obesity and socioeconomic position may be related to dietary energy density and energy cost. Refined grains, added sugars, and fats are among the lowest-cost sources of dietary energy. They are inexpensive, taste good, and are convenient. In contrast, the more nutrient-dense lean meats, fish, fresh vegetables, and fruit are more expensive.[44] Another study using the nationally representative 1994 to 1996 Continuing Survey of Food Intakes by Individuals (CSFII) sample of 4,537 women and 5,004 men showed that the prevalence of overweight among women increased as food insecurity increased, from 34 percent for those who were food secure, to 41 percent for those who were mildly food insecure, to 52 percent for those who were moderately food insecure.[43]

The coexistence of obesity and hunger seems contradictory, but individuals lacking the resources to purchase adequate and high quality foods can still be overweight, for various reasons that researchers now are beginning to understand. The possible explanation for this phenomenon is that along the mix of coping strategies, food quality is affected before the quantity of food intake. It is possible that households would spend less by purchasing lower quality or less of a variety of foods instead of reducing the quantity of food eaten. Consequently, although families get enough food to avoid feeling hungry, they also are poorly nourished because they cannot afford consistently adequate diets that promote health and prevent obesity. In the short term, the stomach registers that it is full, not whether a meal was nutritious.[45] In addition, obesity can be an adaptive response to periods when people are unable to get enough to eat. A research study showed that chronic lack of food caused people to eat more when food is available.[46] When money or food stamps are not available for food purchases during part of the month, people may overeat during the days when food is available. Over a period of time, this cycle can result in weight gain and subsequent obesity.[47]

Income and Education

Inequalities in income and education contribute significantly to health disparities in the United States. They are fundamentally linked and serve as alternative measures for each other.[48] Generally, the segment of the population that experiences the worst health status also has the highest poverty rates and is the least educated. Chronic health conditions such as heart disease, diabetes, obesity, elevated blood lead levels, and low birth weight are linked to low income and education status and to illness and death.[25,49] Higher incomes provide the opportunity for individuals to have access to medical care, quality housing, and safer neighborhoods, and the ability to participate in health-promoting behaviors.[25,30,33,48]

Rural Versus Urban

Rural areas are places with less than 2,500 residents. Approximately 25 percent of Americans live in rural areas. A metropolitan (or urban) area is made up of many different cities. For example, the Paris metropolitan area includes 1,300 cities, the New York metropolitan area includes more than 700 cities, and the St. Louis metropolitan area includes about 400 cities. It is reported that heart disease, cancer, and diabetes rates are significantly higher in rural areas than urban areas. The reason for high rates of chronic diseases and subsequent death is irregular use of preventive screening services and regular exercise. Timely access to emergency services and the availability of specialty care are other health-related issues for the rural segment of the population. In addition, rural residents have fewer physicians and nurses and more transportation barriers than urban residents; they visit physicians less often and later in the course of an illness than urban residents.[25,50]

Biology and Behaviors

The interaction between an individual's biology and behaviors influences health, as does their interaction with the individual's social and physical environments. Also, the quality of health can be improved by providing access to quality healthcare, making policies, and providing intervention programs that target factors related to individuals and their environments. **Figure 16-2** presents the interactions between different determinants of health.[25,30,50]

Biology in the context of **Figure 16-2** means the individual's genetic makeup, family history (which may suggest risk for disease), and the

Determinants of Health

FIGURE 16-2 The Different Determinants of Health

Data from: Office of Disease Prevention and Health Promotion, U.S. Department of Health and Human Services. www.healthypeople.gov/document/html/uih/uih_2.htm#goals. Accessed October 25, 2007.

physical and mental health problems attained during life. However, it is reported that such factors as aging, diet, physical activity, smoking, stress, alcohol or illicit drug abuse, injury or violence, or an infectious or toxic agent may cause illness or disability and can produce a "new" biology.[25,51]

Behaviors are the way individuals respond or react to internal stimuli and external conditions. There may be a link between behaviors and biology (each can react to the other). For instance, smoking (behavior) can alter the cells in the lungs and result in shortness of breath, emphysema, or cancer (biology), which may cause an individual to quit smoking (behavior). Equally, a family history of cancer or heart disease (biology) may induce an individual to develop good eating habits, avoid the use of tobacco or drugs, and maintain an active lifestyle (behaviors) that may subsequently prevent the development of heart disease or cancer (biology).[25]

Other factors also can shape an individual's behavior, including social and physical environments. The social and physical environments are factors that influence the life of individuals, positively or negatively, over which they do not have immediate or direct control.[25,50] The *social environment* provides a sense of well-being when an individual interacts with family, friends, coworkers, and others in the community. It includes social institutions such as law enforcement, the workplace, places of worship, and schools. Other components of the social environment include housing, culture, public transportation, and the presence or absence of violence in the community.[25] Studies show that social environment is linked with morbidity, mortality, and chronic disease (e.g., heart disease, cancer). At the same time, individuals and their behaviors contribute to the quality of the social environment. Individual contributions include lack of physical activity, the use of tobacco, excessive consumption of alcohol, and poor dietary habits.[25,52]

The *physical environment* refers to that which can be seen, touched, heard, smelled, and tasted. It provides an opportunity for individuals and the community to be exposed to harmful situations such as toxic substances, irritants, infectious agents, and physical hazards in homes, schools, and worksites. The physical environment can also promote good health, for instance, by providing clean and safe places for people to work, exercise, and play.[25,53] The presence of a playground might promote active behavior, whereas a busy street might discourage active behavior and consequently lead to obesity.

Policies and interventions can influence the health of individuals and the community. Examples of these policies and intervention efforts are health promotion campaigns to increase the intake of fruits and vegetables, quit smoking, and prevent cancer; policies mandating child restraints and safety belt use in automobiles; infectious disease prevention services, such as the immunization of children, adolescents, and adults; healthy school lunch and breakfast programs to prevent malnutrition; physical activity programs; and clinical services, such as better mental healthcare. All of these have positive effects on health. Policies and intervention are implemented by a variety of state and federal agencies—such as the state public health department and the U.S. Department of Health and Human Services—that promote individual and community health. These activities can be conducted using churches, community-based organizations, civic groups, and businesses.[54]

The community and individuals' health also depends on the availability of quality healthcare. High quality healthcare is essential in the effort to eliminate health disparities and to increase the quality and years of healthy life for all Americans. Healthcare includes the services received through healthcare providers, as well as health information and services received through other sources in the community.

In the determinants of health, individual biology and behavior, physical and social environments, policies and interventions, and access to quality healthcare have a significant effect on the health of individuals, communities, and the nation.[54]

The Role of Dietetics Professionals

Whether the causes of these disparities are biological or environmental, the role of the dietetics professional in lessening them is essential. According to Harris-Davis and Haughton, 50.4 percent of the registered dietitians they surveyed provided services to individuals who were "culturally different from themselves" or from other racial and/or ethnic groups.[55] This percentage is likely to increase. This makes it vital that dietitians in acute care settings and in primary prevention efforts acquire cultural competence and awareness in order to make a significant impact on minorities' health or life.[13]

General health status, birth outcomes, and diseases such as diabetes, obesity, hypertension, and coronary heart disease are related to diet and lifestyle, and dietitians have the nutritional science expertise to provide the appropriate care. However, it can be difficult to acquire the awareness and skills needed to work effectively with diverse populations.[13]

Culture, Race, and Ethnicity

Culture is defined in different ways, one of which is the customary beliefs, social forms, and material traits of a racial, religious, or social group.[56] The concepts of culture, race, and ethnicity play a significant part in understanding human behavior, and these three concepts are frequently used inaccurately. Nutritionists are expected to understand the meaning of each when providing nutritional care to clients of diverse cultures.

Culture is an element of ethnicity that includes shared ideals, values, and assumptions about life that characterize a particular group of people. It includes technology, art, symbols, beliefs, and science, as well as moral systems and characteristic behaviors and habits.[56,57] It is a continuous, slow process that develops and changes over time. Culture provides guidance to solving life's problems in response to the needs of a cultural group's members and their environment.[56]

Every culture has an organizational arrangement that differentiates it from others and provides the structure for what members of the cultural group determine to be proper or improper behavior. Culture provides strength and stability, but not static. The organizational rudiments include, but are not limited to, child-rearing practices, dietary habits, religious practices, family structure and values, and attitudes. People learn about their culture from parents, teachers, religious and political leaders, and respected peers.[57,58]

Race is a social classification that relies on physical markers, such as skin color, to identify group membership.[57] There is the possibility that individuals may be of the same race, but have different cultures. Although they are mixed group, they are often seen as culturally and racially identical. Commonly, many cultural differences of individuals from different countries are overlooked because of their similar racial characteristics.[57]

Ethnicity implies one or more of the following: shared origins or social background; shared, distinctive culture and traditions that are maintained between generations; and shared culture that contributes to a sense of identity and group. Most policymakers emphasize some sort of cultural distinctiveness as the mark of an ethnic group.[57,59]

Developing Cultural Competence in Community Nutrition

Food is a source of nutrients needed for life. However, if food is considered only as this basic concept, the important subtleties that influence what people eat will be missed.[60,61] It would be convenient if achieving adequate nutrition for people meant defining the requirements for each person according to age and sex and then providing the nutrients in the correct amounts via supplements. Unfortunately, this approach would deprive people of the pleasures that food adds to their lives. Favorite flavors, textures, and aromas (especially when provided in familiar and preferred recipes) give immediate pleasure and stir up happy memories of people and places associated with these foods.[62] Every individual in a community has a history, and most of the time this translates to eating habits influenced by culture.[63,64] Religion is a particularly strong factor in cultural identity. Sharing common beliefs and practices that are central to a particular religion creates common threads that bind people together into a culture.[62,63]

Cultural food practices affect tastes, preferences, shopping habits, manners, communication, and personal interactions. As people from varying backgrounds become acculturated into U.S. society, dietary habits tend to change from a pattern based on whole grains and vegetables to foods that are higher in fats and sugars.[61,63] Dietetic professionals need to be sensitive to what might be considered acceptable or unacceptable by persons from different cultures by providing advice to each individual within a cultural perspective. For instance, a dietitian's advice to reduce using lard or pork may be perceived as unrealistic by many Mexican Americans because it is widely used in traditional recipes.[61,65,66] Community nutritionists in the United States need to be able to work with people and their total humanness, not just what they eat.

Cultural competence is defined as understanding the importance of social and cultural influences on individuals' health beliefs and behaviors, considering how these factors interact at multiple levels of the healthcare delivery system, and devising interventions that take these issues into account to assure quality of care.[67,68] It is also the ability to work effectively with individuals from different cultural and ethnic backgrounds. Cultural competence requires a continuous developmental

> **culture** The customary beliefs, social forms, and material traits of a racial, religious, or social group.

process that involves a long-term commitment and significant efforts in acquiring the skills, practices, and attitudes toward becoming culturally competent.

Developing cultural competence is an ongoing life process. There are four steps to acquiring cultural competence:[57,69,70]

- Cultural awareness
- Cultural knowledge
- Cultural skill
- Cultural encounter

Cultural awareness is developing an understanding and sensitivity to another ethnic group's values, beliefs, practices, lifestyles, and problem-solving strategies. The process of acquiring cultural awareness includes an examination of one's own culture, beliefs, values, attitudes, and prejudices and how they are expressed in one's own life, and reviewing assumptions about individuals who are different.[57,71,72]

Cultural knowledge is another component that is essential for caring for a multicultural society. It involves acclimatizing to selected cultural characteristics such as history, values, belief systems, and behaviors of the members of another ethnic group.[57] It means that the nutritionist understands how cultures are similar and how they are different. It provides the nutritionist with organizational elements of cultures and current information on what is necessary to provide effective health promotion.[73] Nutritionists can gain cultural knowledge by reading about the language, customs, and health beliefs of participants in the program and by keeping in mind that cultural lifestyles are constantly influenced by contemporary events, including media and interaction with other cultures. It is important to observe the health beliefs and lifestyles of the participants through conversation and participation in the community's daily life. Cultural knowledge can be acquired by maintaining and knowing culturally diverse people through traveling, books, movies, attending events held by local ethnic or cultural organizations (for instance, attending weddings, birthday parties, international fairs at universities, and religious celebrations), and maintaining an open mind.[73,74] Participating in these different events will increase trust in the nutritionist and increase his or her ability to influence health-directed behaviors.[57]

The third component in developing cultural competence is acquiring cultural skill. Cultural skill reproduces effective integration of cultural awareness and cultural knowledge to meet the participants' needs. It is also the ability of people of one culture to understand and feel comfortable with the cultures of other people. During interaction with culturally diverse people, a culturally skillful nutritionist uses appropriate gestures during conversation, is receptive to the cultural differences and responses of individuals, avoids stereotyping, and interacts respectfully with people of all cultures in a way that recognizes their worth and supports their dignity.[57,74] The culturally skillful nutritionist refrains from making judgments about cultural behaviors and practices that seem strange to him or her.

A cultural encounter is the fourth step in becoming culturally competent. It involves integrating all the cultural competency components in nutrition, health promotion, and intervention in ways that:[57,73,74]

- Preserve the participants' cultural values, health beliefs, and health-related practices that promote and maintain their well-being.
- Place the nutritionist in situations where his or her understanding of self and world, and of how he or she believes things "are" or "should be," are severely challenged.

- Accommodate health-related practices that are not harmful to their health.
- Repattern the participants' lifestyles for new, different, and beneficial health-directed behaviors while respecting their cultural values and health beliefs.

The Importance of Cultural Knowledge in Community Nutrition

Cultural knowledge is needed for adequate nutritional practice. In nutrition assessment, it is important to collect basic information about your community's cultures, foods most frequently used, and food preparation methods. Information needed to provide adequate nutritional guidance includes:[75]

- Types of food available
- Accepted and/or preferred foods
- Safety of the food supply and related health problems
- Energy and nutrient quality of major foods chosen
- Most commonly used foods, who selects them, and how and where they are obtained
- Food preparation methods and how they are divided among family/community
- Foods eaten, how much, when, with whom, and where
- Food storage, facilities, and methods; food safety; and garbage disposal

Other strategies that may help in the assessment include observing the neighborhood and homes where clients live, where they shop for foods, and the types of food available. Learn more about the group by interviewing individuals from or closely associated with the client group.[76] Ask relevant questions about food and health behaviors, or ask other healthcare professionals who serve the cultural group, community leaders among the group, and any other members of the group.

Nutrition practices are an integral part of the assessment process for all families because they contribute significantly in the development of health problems. Knowing the participants' cultural nutrition practices makes it possible to develop health promotion programs that do not conflict with cultural food practices. The cultural background of a client may affect nutritional status in many ways other than disease risk and nutrient needs. Traditional food habits are related to ethnic and religious identity and have little adverse impact on diet.[77] For example, calcium deficiency may be of concern, but sensible food habits often compensate for the noticeable lack of the nutrient. For instance, some segments of the Asian population prepare their daily soups by soaking bones in an acidified broth.[78] Latinos often prepare their tortillas with lime-slaked corn.[79] Ironically, milk-drinking European Americans are one of the groups most often affected by osteoporosis.

However, traditional food habits may also conflict with nutritional needs. A Nigerian immigrant may consider weight gain desirable and a sign of beauty, and many cultures may consider overweight an indication of well-being.[61] Also, a Chinese American mother who still observes the precepts of yin and yang in her diet may feed her baby "neutral" foods, omitting most fruits and vegetables.[80,81] Nutritionists can use the existing organizational structure within each cultural group to plan, design, develop, and implement appropriate programs that address the needs of diverse/multicultural populations.

Dietary Acculturation

Acculturation is a process by which a cultural group adapts or learns cultural norms of another group. The process is related to age, education, frequency of interaction, and income, and it occurs on a continuum.[82] *Dietary acculturation* refers to the process that occurs when immigrants adopt the dietary practices, eating patterns, and food choices of the host country.[83] For instance, dietary acculturation for a Nigerian or Mexican immigrant to the United States may be characterized by increased meat consumption and decreased consumption of whole grains, fruits and vegetables, and legumes.[84] The host country, the United States, in turn often adopts some of the foods and dietary practices of the immigrants, as evidenced by the different ethnic supermarkets and restaurants throughout most of the United States.[85]

Dietary acculturation can result in both healthful and unhealthful dietary changes. For example, among Hispanic immigrants, drinking soda instead of traditional fruit-based beverages can be considered an unhealthful change, whereas consumption of fewer highly saturated fats (e.g., lard) is a healthful change.[86,87] Adverse nutritional consequences can result from changes made in the diet through acculturation; for example, Japanese immigrants to the United States may have an increased risk of cardiovascular disease due to a diet higher in saturated fats and cholesterol.[88] In another example, the vegetable intake of Hispanic immigrants decreased with acculturation while the consumption of snacks and processed foods increased.[89,90]

Most commonly used acculturation scales and indexes have been developed and validated in social science and psychological research, and some have been applied to studies examining dietary behavior. **Table 16.2** shows major approaches to measuring dietary acculturation. The major limitation of the single-item measures is that they are quite general, focusing on items such as length of residence in the host country, language proficiency, and generation level.[82] However, these items may yield general assessment information needed for designing health-promotion programs, such as dietary interventions and education programs.

> **acculturation** Repeated exposure to influences from a different culture. The process is related to age, education, frequency of interaction, and income and occurs on a continuum.
>
> **dietary acculturation** The process that occurs when members of a minority group adopt the eating patterns/food choices of the majority group.

TABLE 16.2	Scales and Indexes That Have Been Used to Study Dietary Acculturation Among U.S. Immigrants[81,92–97]	
Single-Item Measures of General Acculturation	**Examples of Questions**	**Comments**
Residency • Length of residency in host country • Length of residency in country of origin • Place of birth	• How long have you lived in the United States? • How long did you live in Korea? • Where were you born?	• Commonly and successfully used for assessing general acculturation in many studies • Provides a global measure of exposure to host culture • Has the advantage of using short, factual questions that do not require interpretation by respondents • Are very non-specific and may misclassify a respondent's level of acculturation
Language • Proficiency • Preference	• What language do you usually speak? • What language do you prefer to speak?	• Commonly used questions that are short, simple, and non-specific • Provides valuable information for many public health and intervention settings regarding the need for interpreters and translated materials
Generation Level N/A	• Where was your mother/father born?	• Simple, factual question; only indirectly measures exposure to host culture
Friendship Preferences N/A	• Who do you associate with in the outside community: mostly people of your same background, U.S. citizens, or both?	• Intended to assess respondent's degree of ethnic identification with host or original culture
Self-Identification N/A	• How do you identify yourself (Chinese, American, or bicultural)?	• Has the advantage of allowing participant to assess own degree of acculturation • Very open to interpretation by respondents • Social desirability may influence responses

(continues)

| TABLE 16.2 | (Continued) | | |

Acculturation Scales	Scale Description and Characteristics	Comments for All Scales
Acculturation Rating Scale for Mexican Americans[92]	20 items with 4 subscales: language, familiarity, usage, and preference; ethnic identification and generation; reading writing and cultural exposure; ethnic interaction	• Have widespread use in studies of acculturation and have been validated in comparison with single-item questions
Asian Self-Identity Acculturation Scale[93]	21 items with 6 dimensions: language, identity, friendship choices, behaviors, geographic history, and attitudes	• Assess many domains related to acculturation; they are less likely to misclassify respondents than single-item questions
Acculturation Scale for Southeast Asians[94]	13 items with 2 subscales: language proficiency and language, social, and food preferences	• May be too long to be practical for some research or programmatic applications
Short Acculturation Scale for Hispanics[95]	12 items with 3 subscales: language use, media preferences, and social interactions	• Except for the scale developed by Anderson et al.,[94] they also do not specifically address issues related to dietary acculturation

Food-Based Assessments	Scale Description and Characteristics	Comments for Both Assessments
Food Lists		
Participants identify from a food list the foods they usually eat now versus when they were in their country of origin	Yang et al.[96] compiled a list of 47 food items common in Chinese and U.S. cuisine. Respondents indicated (yes/no) whether they ate the foods in the past month. Scores were derived by summing the responses.	• Both measures assess dietary acculturation by directly measuring the outcome of dietary acculturation (i.e., traditional vs. Western eating patterns or both)
Dietary Acculturation Scales		• Both do not assess other steps or factors in the process of dietary acculturation
Instruments specifically designed to measure changes in dietary patterns	Satia et al.[97] developed a list of 15 food items and dietary behaviors reflective of traditional Chinese behavior and of westernization of eating patterns and identified two subscales, Chinese and Western. Scores were derived by obtaining the mean of no missing responses for each scale.	• The assessments need to be supplemented with other instruments when the objective is to design effective dietary interventions

Source: Satia J, Patterson RE, Kristal AR, Hislop TG, Yasui Y, Taylor VM. Development of scales to measure dietary acculturation among Chinese-Americans and Chinese-Canadians. *J Am Diet Assoc.* 2001; 101:548–553. Copyright Elsevier (2001). Reprinted with permission.

Acculturation scales are considerably more comprehensive and measure several facets of exposure to the host country; therefore, they are less likely to misclassify a person's level of acculturation.[82] They do not typically include diet-specific acculturation indicators, however. In addition, most of these scales were validated against single-item measures and demographic characteristics rather than any type of "gold standard."[91,92]

The food-based measures (food lists and dietary acculturation scales) assess dietary acculturation by measuring eating patterns. Therefore, they directly assess the outcome of dietary acculturation that includes adoption of the eating patterns of the host country, maintenance of traditional diets, or both. However, these food-based measures do not assess other steps or factors (e.g., psychosocial factors) in the process of acculturation, which are necessary for the design of effective dietary interventions.[82]

Ethnocentrism/Stereotyping

Public and community dietitians need to avoid an ethnocentric perspective when working with ethnic groups. **Ethnocentrism** is a way of looking at the world through a personal lens that has been influenced by personality, genetics, family/relationships, and media. It is an important concept that keeps culture viable.[98,99] In its mildest form, ethnocentrism is a subconscious disregard for cultural differences; in its most severe form, it is an authoritarian dominance over groups different from one's own.[99] This can serve as a major obstacle in establishing and maintaining good working relationships with clients of different ethnic groups. Cross-cultural counseling skills are essential for the dietitian working with clients from different ethnic or religious backgrounds. Ethnocentricity, including personal biases and background pertaining to eating certain foods as well as assumptions about what foods are eaten and when or how many meals are eaten each day, should be considered when working with individuals from different ethnic backgrounds. Respect for cultural values and personal preference is a precondition for successful health promotion in a heterogeneous society.[100]

Barriers to Multicultural Health Promotion and Disease Prevention

Many factors can be barriers or obstructions to successful health and nutrition or disease prevention programs. For the purposes of this dis-

ethnocentrism The belief that one's own group view of the world is superior to that of others.

cussion, a barrier is any obstacle that might hinder the ability of the community nutritionist, healthcare professional, or their culturally diverse clients to achieve the intended intervention program objectives.[101] Because there are many potential barriers that cannot easily be categorized, an attempt will be made to group some of these variables.

As presented in **Table 16.3**, different demographic factors can obstruct multicultural health-promoting activities. It is important for the nutritionist to first assess the level of acculturation and assimilation of his or her clients before implementing the intervention program because many of the identified barriers may not apply to all clients. Many of these barriers are easy to understand; a brief discussion of a few of them may help to emphasize the importance of demographics when working with or planning health promotion programs for a culturally diverse group. For example, gender may become an issue when providing health promotion services such as mammography or cervical screening. Holroyd et al. reported that Chinese cultural values associated with modesty and sexuality coupled with medical interpersonal and interprofessional skills of the practitioners, lack of educational materials written in Chinese, and a lack of female physicians were barriers preventing Chinese women from enrolling in health promotion screening services.[102] The authors recommended that healthcare practitioners prepare themselves with relevant social and cultural knowledge of the population groups they serve.

The main language spoken can also be a barrier for health promotion programs. One study showed that despite following standard diabetes self-management recommendations to a comparable degree and receiving healthcare in a culturally competent setting, individuals who spoke Chinese as their preferred language, even with the use of translation services, had less baseline diabetes knowledge and showed a trend toward higher glycosylated hemoglobin (HbA$_{1c}$) levels than those who spoke English as their preferred language. (Glycosylated hemoglobin level determines how well a person's diabetes is being controlled over time.) Another reason for the results was the shortage of diabetes information in the Chinese language in the United States.[103]

Geographic factors including a lack of hospital or private physician offices in the minority group communities, as well as difficulties in accessing public transportation or getting a drivers' license, social isolation, and financial constraints can also create barriers to multicultural health-promotion efforts.[104]

The Importance of Communication

Human *communication* is defined as a social interaction of giving and receiving information for facilitating understanding and creating social connection with a common set of rules.[105] These rules indicate how the communication will be carried out, the channels in which it will be carried out, when it will happen, and how feedback may or may not be provided between the sender or encoder and a receiver or decoder. For example, in Japanese cultural beliefs, indirect communication is perceived to be more ethical than direct communication when dealing with disclosure of a serious health condition (e.g., cancer, heart disease). This is based on their motivation of not extinguishing the individual's hope to live. U.S. physicians attempting to give hope to individuals may actively engage in open communication with them about their health condition. In contrast, many Japanese believe that the concealment itself can convey concern and hope. Typically, the head of the household is the primary individual communicating with the healthcare practitioner when a family member needs medical care. Also, the head of the household is the one who makes decisions about treatment options and what the family member should be told about his or her medical condition.[106]

Many factors can affect communication in general and specifically cross-cultural encounters. These factors include the communication skills, attitudes, knowledge, social system, and culture of both the sender and receiver of communication transactions, and differences in cultural values, backgrounds, biases, linguistic barriers, and dietary and healthcare beliefs and practices.[105] To communicate effectively, it is essential that nutritionists avoid stereotyping by responding to the clients as individuals within their own cultural perspective. Nutritionists must

> **communication** A process of information sharing in which those involved in the communication share a common set of rules.

TABLE 16.3	**Potential Barriers to Health Promotion and Disease Prevention**		
Demographic Barrier	**Cultural Barrier**	**Healthcare System Barrier**
Age	Age	Access to care
Gender	Gender, class, and family dynamics	Insurance or other financial resources
Ethnicity	World view/perceptions of life	N/A
Primary language spoken	Time orientation	Orientation to preventive health services
Religion	Primary language spoken	Perceptions of need for healthcare services
Educational level and literacy level	Religious beliefs and practices	Ignorance and/or distrust of Western medical practice and procedures
Occupation, income, and health insurance	Social customs, values, and norms	Cultural insensitivity and competence
Area of residence	Traditional health beliefs and practices	Western vs. folk health beliefs and practices
Transportation	Dietary preferences and practices	Poor doctor–patient communications
Time and/or generation in the United States	Communication patterns and customs	Lack of bilingual and bicultural staff

From: Huff RM, Kline MV, eds. *Promoting Health in Multicultural Populations. A Handbook for Practitioners.* New Delhi, India: Sage Publications; 1999.

also recognize the influence of their own cultural backgrounds and attitudes. Communication is sometimes challenging with those who do not share the same cultural perspective. To communicate successfully, nutritionists need to be willing to accept the discomfort of unfamiliarity and insecurity. Achieving this challenge requires sensitivity to cultural diversity, stereotyping, and prejudice; general skills of good communication; and skills to overcome communication barriers. In addition, human interaction factors, including dominance–submission or love–hate relationships, communication transactions, and the circumstances in which they occur have been identified as important to understanding and improving the communication process.[107–109]

It is important that the basis for achieving health promotion and disease prevention is to understand the variations in patterns of verbal and nonverbal communication.[57] The differences of communication style among cultures are reflected in the pronunciation, word meaning, voice quality, and humor, and in nonverbal styles, such as eye contact, gestures, touch, interjection during conversation, body posture, facial expression, and silence.[57] For example, when gathering data from a Hispanic woman, the community nutritionist needs to be aware that her style of communication may be low-key and the woman may avoid eye contact and be hesitant to respond to questions. This behavior should not be taken as lack of interest or inability to relate to others.[110] Also, generally Latinos sit and stand much closer to one another than most European Americans. Therefore, stepping away from a client who seems too close may be considered offensive, especially in a counseling situation.[110,111]

Dietitians who are members of the host country's main ethnic group may have goodwill, but be ineffective when they attempt to engage a person of a different cultural group in a relationship without questioning how culture influences interactions, interpretations of events, information, beliefs, and values concerning health and healthcare practices. Preconceived ideas such as racial or ethnic identity, religion, country of origin, gender, or sexual orientation can interfere with the dietitian's ability to relate to people as individuals. At the same time, a lack of knowledge of other cultural groups can deter the dietitian's understandings of the individual's point of view. Guidelines for recognizing the multicultural context of communication include the following:[112,113]

- Make an ethnocultural assessment; this is a critical component of every evaluation.
- Allow other people to define themselves.
- Respect the language of others, and do not assume superiority in language.
- Collaborate with trained translators and health promoters (persons with the same ethnic or racial background as the individuals/groups).
- Avoid the use of racist, sexist, ageist, and other forms of condescending language.
- Do not perpetuate stereotypes in communication.
- Adapt communication to the uniqueness of the individual.
- Reject humor that degrades members based on gender, race, ethnicity, religion, sexual orientation, country of origin, and so forth.
- Do not allow injustice to continue through silence.

An integral part of any culture or geographical setting is language.[112,114] It is important to give attention to the language patterns of different ethnic groups in the community. It is equally essential to accept existing dialects as a vital part of the culture and not give the impression that the dialect is incorrect or bad. Dietitians may need to use an interpreter or members of the group to explain or clarify terms when working in areas with large numbers of non-English-speaking groups; this will prevent incorrect assumptions.[111] They also need to avoid the use of jargon, technical terms, and slang and keep information simple. Any effort shown to communicate effectively conveys to people a genuine interest in their health.[114] Whether in Charleston, South Carolina, or Brooklyn, New York, learning to listen to a dialect

---

Box 16-1 Assessment of Dietary Practices and Food Consumption Patterns[102]

- Determine the social significance of food in the family. Do they eat alone or as a family?
- Determine the foods that are purchased often.
- Determine who is responsible for buying and preparing the foods and how the foods are prepared.
- Determine the foods considered as taboo or prohibited.
- Determine the influence religion has in their food selection. Any restrictions?
- Determine the amount of food that is eaten, how often, and with whom.
- Determine the living conditions and types of restaurants they use.
- Determine whether the clients have adopted foods of other cultural groups.
- Determine the types of foods they like most.
- Determine the availability of their favorite foods and the cost.

Interview Tips

- Listen attentively.
- Be attentive to nonverbal cues. Display pictures, books, brochures, and posters that reflect the cultures and ethnic backgrounds of clients who are being served.
- Explain why you need the information and the benefit to the client.
- Use an interpreter. (The age of the interpreter may be of concern; for example, older clients may want a more mature interpreter.) Children tend to have limited language skills, and when spoken to may have difficulty interpreting information.
- Clarify roles with the interpreter, and explain to the client what the interpreter will be doing.
- Be patient and consider periods of silence as opportunities for reflection on what has been said.
- Remember that customs regarding touching, gestures, eye contact, and relationships vary among cultures.
- Review the situation and information to be translated before and after the interview.

Modified from: Stanhope M, Lancaster J. *Community and Public Health Nursing.* 5th ed. St. Louis, MO: Mosby; 2000. Reprinted with permission from Elsevier.

allows the dietitian to experience the richness of people's lives. When communicating in an ethnically diverse area, the dietitian's communication approach must project trust and genuineness so that people will be receptive to the nutrition education activity.[114]

Interviewing a key informant is another effective approach dietitians can use in gathering information from the minority group. Key informant interviews are with individuals who live or work in the community and who possess a special insight into its needs and resources. **Box 16-1** identifies interview tips/guidelines that community nutritionists can use in obtaining information from individuals.

All cultures are not the same, but they have the same basic organizational factors. These factors must be explored in a cultural assessment because of the differences among groups. The differences include communication, background, touch, family organization, time perception, self-care practice, alternative healers, and biological variations.[115] Some of these differences among cultural groups are presented in **Table 16.4**.

Designing Health Promotion Programs for Multicultural Groups

As contemporary societal and demographic environments for healthcare continue to change, public health leaders nationwide recognize that all health practitioners need cultural sensitivity knowledge and skills to effectively serve a multicultural population.[82] Cultural sensitivity skills enable culturally relevant programs and services to be developed and implemented. Bilingual practitioners are very important in providing nutrition programs.[57]

Cultural sensitivity involves a heightened knowledge of the needs of the client. Culturally sensitive nutritionists respond and accurately interpret non-verbal or other cultural cues, as evidenced in the way they provide information to culturally diverse clients.[116] This means

> **cultural sensitivity** Planning interventions that are relevant and acceptable within the cultural framework of the population to be reached.

TABLE 16.4	**Variations Among Selected Cultural Groups**			
	African Americans	**Asians**	**Hispanics**	**Native Americans**
Verbal communication	Asking personal questions of someone you have just met for the first time is seen as improper and intrusive.	High levels of respect for others, especially those in positions of authority.	The expression of negative feelings is considered impolite.	Speak in a low tone of voice and expect the listener to be attentive.
Non-verbal communication	Direct eye contact in conversation is often considered rude.	Direct eye contact with superiors may be considered disrespectful.	Avoidance of eye contact is usually a sign of attentiveness and respect.	Direct eye contact is often considered disrespectful.
Touch	Touching someone else's hair is often considered offensive.	It is not customary to shake hands with persons of the opposite sex.	Touching is often observed between two persons in conversation.	A light touch of the person's hand instead of a firm handshake is often used when greeting a person.
Family organization	Usually have close extended family networks; women play key roles in healthcare decisions.	Usually have close extended family ties. Emphasis may be on family needs rather than individual needs.	Usually have close extended family ties; all members of the family may be involved in healthcare decisions.	Usually have close extended family; emphasis tends to be on family rather than on individual needs.
Time perception	Often present-oriented.	Often present-oriented.	Often present-oriented.	Often past-oriented.
	Believe in harmony of mind, health, body, and spirit with nature.	Enjoy balance between the "yin" and "yang" energy forces.	Enjoy balance and harmony among mind, body, spirit, and nature.	Rely on harmony of mind, body, spirit, and emotions with nature.
Alternative healers	"Granny," "root doctor," voodoo priest, spiritualist.	Acupuncturist, acupressurist, herbalist.	Curandero, espiritualista, yerbo.	Medicine man, shaman.
Self-care practices	Poultices, herbs, oils, roots.	Hot and cold foods, herbs, teas, soups, burning, rubbing, pinching.	Hot and cold foods, herbs.	Herbs, cornmeal, medicine bundle.
Biological variations	Sickle cell anemia, lactose intolerance, Mongolian spots, keloid formation, inverted "T" waves.	Thalassemia, lactose intolerance, Mongolian spots.	Lactose intolerance, Mongolian spots.	Lactose intolerance, cleft uvula (the small piece of soft tissue that can be seen dangling down from the soft palate over the back of the tongue).

Source: Stanhope M, Lancaster J. *Community and Public Health Nursing*. 5th ed. New York: Mosby; 2000. Reprinted with permission from Elsevier.

that nutritionists and healthcare professionals must make efforts to be aware of the possible and actual cultural factors that affect their interactions with clients. It also means that they need to be willing to design programs and materials, to implement programs, to make recommendations that are culturally relevant and culturally specific, and to plan interventions that are relevant and acceptable within the cultural framework.[116,117] Although the role of culture has long been acknowledged, culture has not been a central focus of nutritional care. The nutritionist developing a culturally sensitive program must move outside the paradigm of the dominant culture.[104] He or she needs to make efforts to understand the dietary patterns of clients and not rely on the dominant group's culture.

Planning Health Promotion and Disease Prevention Programs in Multicultural Populations

Planning health promotion and disease prevention programs in multicultural populations is a challenging process. It requires efficient identification and selection of a particular course of action. Developing and implementing a health promotion program requires the dietitian and participants to work together to accomplish a wide range of activities, including:[104,118]

- Assessing the needs, problems, and resources of the target population
- Developing appropriate goals and objectives
- Formulating strategies and interventions that consider the peculiarities of the clients' nutrition and health-related conditions and settings

- Implementing and monitoring the interventions
- Evaluating the outcomes
- Refining approaches for greater program effectiveness and efficiency

Given these guidelines, the community nutritionist may provide a successful intervention program using the following strategies:[105,119]

- Define the level of change wanted as a result of the program (i.e., the health education level or the health promotion level).
- Make contact attempts on varied days, evenings, and weekends.
- Identify specific health-related factors that affect the health of the target group in the community, the action strategy to be used (e.g., strengthen community action, create a supportive environment, and develop personal skills), and the level of action to be taken (e.g., society, a specific sector/system, community, family, individual, etc.).
- Link cultural competence to the health promotion program.
- Identify and address sociocultural barriers (language, organizational barriers such as availability and acceptability of healthcare, lack of interpreter services or culturally/linguistically appropriate health education materials for members of a minority group).
- Be culturally competent when interacting and working with participants in the overall health promotion/disease prevention planning process by attending continuing multicultural education seminars and workshops.
- Know your own beliefs, values, patterns, and styles of interaction with other cultures, because they could reflect biases or prejudices that could disrupt the planning process.

Successful Community Strategies 🏠🏠🏠

UCCE Culturally Appropriate Nutrition Education[36,121,122]

Immigrants come to the United States seeking religious and political freedom and economic opportunities. The Vietnamese population is the fastest growing segment of the Asian/Pacific Islander population in the United States. Currently, about 46 percent of the Vietnamese population resides in California. From 1993 to 1996, the University of California Cooperative Extension (UCCE) received a U.S. Department of Agriculture grant to evaluate the diets of Vietnamese-speaking women who were eligible for WIC and to provide culturally appropriate nutrition education to improve their dietary quality. A secondary goal of the program was to increase interagency cooperation between the UCCE and WIC.

At the beginning of the project, 1-day joint in-service training meetings were held in each county for staff from UCCE's Expanded Food and

Nutrition Education Program (EFNEP) and WIC to facilitate communication and cooperation.

A total of 112 professional and paraprofessional staff members attended the meetings. The purpose of these meetings was to educate project staff about Vietnamese foodways and culture and to introduce this joint project. At the meetings, a bicultural, bilingual Vietnamese American registered nurse spoke about traditional Vietnamese health beliefs and food practices related to pregnancy and the postpartum period, including lactation. A total of 152 homemakers were recruited to participate in a nutrition education program, with 76 receiving the intervention and 76 serving as the control group. Non-English-speaking Vietnamese American women eligible for WIC with incomes below 185 percent of the poverty level living

in five California counties participated in the program.

Intervention

For this project, five California EFNEP curriculum modules were revised and rewritten in Vietnamese by two bicultural, bilingual Vietnamese American nutritionists, one of whom was a registered dietitian. These were then translated into English so that nutrition professionals who were not literate in Vietnamese could use them with Vietnamese clients. The five modules were Nutrition for a Healthy Mother and Baby, Calcium-Rich Foods, Protein and Iron-Rich Foods, Grains, and Fruits and Vegetables. The modules emphasized the health benefits of the traditional Vietnamese diet that is rich in fruits, vegetables, and complex carbohydrates and low in fat. The modules were made culturally appropriate for the audience by

Intervention Considerations

The design of well-planned and culturally appropriate interventions is critical to the success of any health promotion/disease prevention program or service offered in a community setting. Designing intervention strategies, methods, and materials so they relate to the specific cultural characteristics of the target group needs to be an integral part of the design process.[104,118] With these ideas in mind, the community nutritionist may also consider the following additional strategies and suggestions as he or she begins the intervention phase:[74,104,118–120]

- Tailor the program to the intended target group using MyPyramid, flipcharts, and brochures. If possible, print materials in the target group's language.
- Utilize the community's strengths, resources, and assets, all of which promote community ownership and involvement with the health promotion/disease prevention program.
- Involve the target group whose members will be the recipients of the program.
- Consider other factors such as issues related to being a new immigrant and linguistic, literacy, gender, and cultural factors in the design of the intervention program for the community.
- Consider using churches as sites for conducting health promotion/disease prevention programs. However, it is not easy to involve some sites in health promotion/disease prevention efforts because many of them have their own causes, which may or may not have a health or nutrition focus.
- Take the intervention program to the community instead of asking the community to come to the intervention site.

- Use peer educators from the community. This is a very effective method for delivering health promotion/disease prevention programs or services to the community.
- Develop educational materials that reflect relevant cultural values, themes, and literacy levels of the target group.
- Develop partnerships with local media. This can be an effective way to disseminate information about the health promotion/disease prevention program or service being planned and offered to the community.

The Successful Community Strategies feature presents the University of California's Cooperative Extension culturally relevant nutrition education success story.

Strengthening Organizational Cultural Competence

Cultural training for dietetics students usually consists of a background course in anthropology or a related social or behavioral science combined with dietetics education about traditional food preferences and associated health problems of certain racial and ethnic groups. This educational step is valuable for introducing students to basic information, but does not prepare them to incorporate cultural concepts into dietetics practice. Accordingly, nutrition and other healthcare providers can benefit from a conceptual model of cultural competence.[123]

The current incentive to address the needs of cultural sensitivity includes Healthy People 2010 goals set by the federal government to eliminate health disparities. In addition, an agency's policy and mission statements can provide the organization and staff the drive toward higher levels of culturally competent care and programming.[124] Every

---

integrating drawings of traditional nutrient-rich Vietnamese foods into flipchart and handout illustrations and by addressing traditional Vietnamese food practices. Information on how to purchase, store, and prepare "new" American foods from each food group was also included. Bicultural, bilingual Vietnamese American nutrition education assistants taught five to seven lessons in the Vietnamese language using nutrition education materials written in the Vietnamese language. Twenty-four-hour food recalls were obtained before and after the 8-week interval on the treatment and control groups to examine if there were changes over time in nutrient intake and nutrient density within groups. Analysis of covariance techniques determined differences between groups.

Results showed that over time the number of intervention group participants who had the

recommended number of servings from each food group increased significantly in comparison to the control group. The dietary nutrient density of calcium, riboflavin, and vitamin B6 as well as potassium of the intervention group significantly improved in comparison to the control group. As a result, officials in all five counties acknowledged the importance of having bicultural, bilingual Vietnamese nutrition education assistants (NEAs) on staff to work with the increasing number of Vietnamese clients. The teaching modules developed for the program have been distributed to WIC agencies and other Cooperative Extension county offices throughout the state and nation as well as to other agencies working with Vietnamese clients.

Practitioners involved in nutrition education for immigrant populations whose native language

is not English are encouraged to hire bilingual, bicultural professionals and paraprofessionals to reach these populations. In this project, Vietnamese American nutrition professionals designed culturally appropriate educational materials for the project and were involved in the training of paraprofessionals working at the local level. The paraprofessionals were invaluable in recruiting and working with women from their communities. They were able to relate to the difficulties new immigrants had in shopping at Western supermarkets; learning about new food products; discovering new methods of food handling, preparation, and storage; and dealing with language barriers in communicating with health professionals who did not speak Vietnamese.

organization needs to ensure that cultural competence philosophies are incorporated into its policy and mission statements and that all are followed. If these features already exist in policy and mission statements, an assessment of how well they are being followed is important. Examples of the variables that can be monitored and observed include:[104,116,124,125]

- The interaction between staff and management and among themselves
- How management and personnel value diversity
- How the management and staff adapt to the diversity and cultural contexts of individuals and communities served (accepting the differences within the community)
- The interactions in the clinic, waiting area, educational area, and other areas where the target group and facility staff interact
- The environment in which services are provided, including location, hours of operation, physical resources, and information systems
- Service models that are adapted to the cultural-specific needs of the population
- The materials given to the target group: Are they well received, perceived, and read? Are they written in a language the target group can read and understand at the appropriate grade or reading levels?

The agency also should assess whether signs of the agency's policy about culture are placed within and around the facility and other locales where services, including health promotion programming, may be offered. Additional strategies for strengthening organizational cultural competence include the following:[104,116]

- Explain the Western concepts of health, disease, prevention, and treatment in culturally understandable terms that are relevant to the target group.
- Design and employ educational materials that are relevant and culturally appropriate to the target group.
- Use well-trained bilingual/bicultural staff.
- Provide adequate fiscal resources to support translation and interpretation of services, hire qualified staff, and purchase teaching materials (videotapes, pens, papers, etc.) and equipment (computers, tables, chairs, etc.).
- Employ indigenous health workers/dietitians when working in and with diverse multicultural communities.
- Seek ways to improve access to services for multicultural populations.
- Include strategic goals, plans, policies, and procedures as part of a comprehensive management strategy.
- Create a cultural competence plan that includes defined steps for its integration at every level of organizational planning and the related policy or procedural changes needed.

The U.S. Department of Health and Human Services' National Standards for Culturally and Linguistically Appropriate Services

Until recently, many healthcare providers did not have clear guidance on how to prepare for or respond to culturally sensitive situations. No comprehensive nationally recognized standards of cultural or linguistic competence in healthcare service delivery had been developed. Instead, federal health agencies, state policymakers, and national organizations independently developed their own standards and practices. Some de-

veloped definitions of cultural competence whereas others mandated providing language services to limited English speakers. Some specified the collection of language, race, and ethnicity data. Many approaches attempted to be comprehensive whereas others targeted only a specific issue, geographic area, or subfield of healthcare, such as mental health. The result was a wide spectrum of ideas about what constitutes culturally competent health services, including significant differences with respect to target population, scope, and quality of services.[125]

In 1997, the U.S. DHHS Office of Minority Health (OMH) undertook the development of national standards for culturally and linguistically appropriate services (CLAS) to help guide providers, policymakers, accreditation and credentialing agencies, purchasers, patients, advocates, educators, and the general healthcare community.[125] These guidelines were developed with input from a national project advisory committee of policymakers, providers, and researchers. The full report is available online at: http://www.omhrc.gov/templates/browse.aspx?lvl=1&lvlID=3. Each standard is accompanied by commentary that addresses its relationship to existing laws and standards and offers recommendations for implementation and oversight to providers, policymakers, and advocates. These 14 standards must be met by most healthcare-related agencies. The standards are based on an analytical review of key laws, regulations, contracts, and standards currently in use by federal and state agencies and other national organizations.

Culture and language have a considerable impact on how individuals access and respond to healthcare services. To ensure equal access to quality healthcare by diverse populations, healthcare organizations and providers need to follow these standards:[125]

- *Standard 1:* Promote and support the attitudes, behaviors, knowledge, and skills necessary for staff to work respectfully and effectively with patients and each other in a culturally diverse work environment.
- *Standard 2:* Have a comprehensive management strategy to address culturally and linguistically appropriate services, including strategic goals, plans, policies, procedures, and designated staff responsible for implementation.
- *Standard 3:* Utilize formal mechanisms for community and consumer involvement in the design and execution of service delivery, including planning, policymaking, operations, evaluation, training, and, as appropriate, treatment planning.
- *Standard 4:* Develop and implement a strategy to recruit, retain, and promote qualified diverse and culturally competent administrative, clinical, and support staff that are trained to address the needs of the racial and ethnic communities being served.
- *Standard 5:* Require and arrange for ongoing education and training for administrative, clinical, and support staff in culturally and linguistically competent service delivery.
- *Standard 6:* Provide all clients that have limited English proficiency access to bilingual staff or interpretation services.
- *Standard 7:* Provide oral and written notices, including translated signage at key points of contact, to clients in their primary language informing them of their right to receive interpreter services free of charge.
- *Standard 8:* Translate and make available signage and commonly used written patient educational materials as well as other materials for members of the predominant language groups in service areas.
- *Standard 9:* Ensure that interpreters and bilingual staff can demonstrate bilingual proficiency and receive training that includes

the skills and ethics of interpreting and knowledge of the terms and concepts relevant to clinical or non-clinical encounters. Family or friends are not considered adequate substitutes because they usually lack these abilities.

- *Standard 10:* Ensure that the client's primary spoken language and self-identified race/ethnicity are included in the healthcare organization's management information system as well as any patient records used by provider staff.
- *Standard 11:* Use a variety of methods to collect and utilize accurate demographic, cultural, epidemiological, and clinical outcome data for racial and ethnic groups in the service area, and become informed about the ethnic/cultural needs, resources, and assets of the surrounding community.
- *Standard 12:* Undertake ongoing organizational self-assessments of cultural and linguistic competence, and integrate measures of access, satisfaction, quality, and outcomes for culturally and linguistically appropriate services (CLAS) into other organizational internal audits and performance improvement programs.
- *Standard 13:* Develop structures and procedures to address cross-cultural ethical and legal conflicts in healthcare delivery and complaints or grievances by patients and staff about unfair, culturally insensitive discriminatory treatment, or difficulty in accessing services, or denial of services.
- *Standard 14:* Prepare an annual progress report documenting the organization's progress with implementing CLAS standards, including information on programs, staffing, and resources.

Dietary Patterns of Different Cultural Groups in the United States

The migration of different ethnic groups into the United States has created a blend of cultures often addressed in metaphors: Originally, it was the melting pot, then a set of tributaries, a tapestry, and a garden salad. Community nutritionists in the United States need to be able to consider all aspects of their clients, not just what they eat. This section of the chapter creates cultural awareness for nutritionists working with different cultural groups. It is important to note that variations exist in each cultural group (i.e., socioeconomic status, religion, age, education, social class, location, length of time in the United States, country of origin, and variation within country of origin). Therefore nutritionists must be cautious and not generalize or imply that the characteristics discussed in this section apply to all individuals of a cultural group. This section discusses the historic perspective, current nutrition practices, and health-related issues of the major ethnic groups in the United States.

Working with African American Food Patterns

Historical Perspective

African Americans are descendants of African ancestry whose lineal relatives, such as parents, grandparents, and great-grandparents, have resided in the United States for several generations or are recent immigrants. "Soul food," a metaphor of group identity, emphasizes both the content and preparation styles of food. African Americans adopted soul food in the 1960s as a way of identifying their ethnicity.[3] Blank found that older African Americans in the South added wild animals, such as squirrels, rabbits, opossums, and deer, to their soul food diet. Flour-based gravies are a favorite with meats and rice. Many African Americans still eat Hoppin' John, or rice and black-eyed peas, on New Year's Day for good luck in the upcoming year.[22]

Soul food is high in fat, salt, and sugar. Most of the time, meats and other foods are fried, and most vegetables are stewed with pork fat. Soul food is also spiced with red pepper (cayenne) and malegueta peppers. Hot pepper sauces, mace, allspice, cinnamon, cloves, sesame seeds (benne), filé powder from sassafras leaves, thyme, and vinegar are also utilized to prepare soul foods. Drinks and deserts are usually very sweet. Heavily sweetened iced tea is the traditional drink, but unsweetened tea, lemonade, and Kool-Aid made with 1 cup of sugar to 7 cups of water are favorite summer drinks. Fat (butter) and sugar are also used liberally in the preparation of favorite side dishes such as candied "yams," a sweet potato dish, and desserts such as apple or peach cobblers or pies; sweet potato pie and pudding; banana pudding; and chocolate, pineapple, coconut, lemon, and pound cakes.[61]

There is similarity between African Americans' and European Americans' food preferences in comparable socioeconomic groups living in the same region of the United States. However, African American often include black-eyed peas, okra, peas, and green leafy vegetables (e.g., chard, collard greens, kale, mustard greens, spinach, and turnip greens) in their diets.[61]

Current Nutrition Practices and Health-Related Issues

It is difficult to characterize the most current nutritional status of African Americans because a limited number of studies have investigated this population. Research has shown that African American nutritional intake is associated with socioeconomic status because poor families of any ethnic group often depend on subsidies such as food stamps, school breakfast and lunch programs, and emergency food programs.[61,126] In the United States, a large number of African Americans experience nutrient deficiencies at or near poverty levels.[127] Haytowitz et al. studied the variety of foods consumed daily and found that the percentage of African Americans reporting lower servings of dairy, meat, grains, fruits, or vegetables and higher salty food intakes was higher than that of European Americans.[128] High levels of income and education increased the variety of foods they consumed. Also, African Americans consumed more calories from animal proteins than for European Americans.[129]

Obesity is a major health problem for African American adolescents and adults because it contributes to most chronic health conditions, such as diabetes and heart disease. It is estimated that 29.1 percent of African American women and 35.9 percent of African American men are overweight compared to 24.8 percent of European American women and 40.7 percent of European American men.[130,131] The high incidence of weight gain may be due to several factors, such as socioeconomic status, poor eating habits, genetic predisposition, and a more permissive attitude about obesity.[132]

Obesity is a contributing factor to non-insulin-dependent diabetes mellitus prevalent in African American communities, which affects about 20 percent of the African American population. The incidence of non-insulin-dependent diabetes mellitus is three to four times higher for African Americans than the total U.S. population.[61] Non-insulin-dependent diabetes mellitus is credited to be one of the contributing factors to the high mortality rate among African Americans. Also, there is a direct link between diabetes and heart disease, which has increased the rate of death especially among African American women.[61,133]

The incidence of hypertension is very high for African Americans—almost twice that of the European American population. Although data comparing normotensives and hypertensives by ethnic groups is limited, reports show that African Americans have the highest proportion of hypertension of any group.[61] Furthermore, African Americans experiencing hypertension are 5 times more likely to suffer chronic heart failure and 10 times more likely to develop kidney failure.[61,134]

The reason for the prevalence of hypertension among African Americans is not clear in about 95 percent of all cases. Studies show that sub-Saharan Africans have the lowest prevalence of hypertension, although hypertension increases with urbanization of sub-Saharan Africans.[135,136] It is reported that the rate of hypertension among Caribbean Africans is moderately high.[137] Several studies have reported that there is a link between negative stressors and low socioeconomic status, including low education levels and hypertension.[138,139] Research also related to chronic discrimination and the struggle for social acceptance can lead to continuous stress and an increased prevalence of high blood pressure.[26,140]

It is reported that low calcium, magnesium, and potassium intakes are associated with hypertension.[141] It is estimated that a higher percentage of African Americans are lactose-intolerant, which may be one of the contributing factors to the low calcium intake. It is also believed that salt retention is associated with calcium retention, which may account for why many African American women have high bone mineral densities and low rates of osteoporosis despite low calcium intake.[126,142-144] One of the recommendations for reducing blood pressure is to lower salt intake and increase calcium, magnesium, and potassium intakes. Another effective method for reducing blood pressure is a diet that is low in total fat, saturated fat, and cholesterol, and high in fruits, vegetables, and low-fat dairy foods, especially in African Americans, even with no reduction in salt intake or weight loss.[126,145-147]

Although differences in cultural beliefs, attitudes, and practices exist between rural and urban African Americans, they have some basic cultural beliefs. The core of African American culture is family and religion. The family is the strongest institution for them, and it provides strong extended kinship bonds with grandparents, aunts, uncles, and cousins. The family is the main source of support, especially during crisis and illness. Religion and religious behavior are essential parts of the African American community.[126,148,149] Their perception is that health is a feeling of well-being and the ability to fulfill role expectations. Spiritual balance is also a major component of their culture.[126]

An African American client may not consider him- or herself as active during interaction with community or public health nutritionists

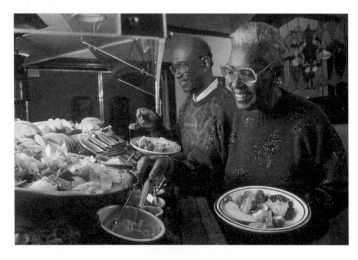

Interpretation of messages is based on one's cultural framework, and interpretation of visual elements varies considerably by ethnic group.

and, therefore, may not communicate his or her needs or ask questions. On the other hand, his or her participation in conversational type of communication is engaging and expressive, but prolonged eye contact is viewed as rude.[126] When planning nutrition education for African American clients, consider using action- or task-oriented activities. An in-depth interview is important with African American participants. It is important to consider the variability in diet related to region, socioeconomic conditions, and degree of ethnic identity when planning health promotion programs. In the United States, Caribbean or Central America participants are more likely to identify with the foods and food habits of Latinos than with those of African Americans.[126] Some African Americans have Islamic or Eastern Orthodox religious affiliations, and community nutritionists must consider the influence of religion on dietary practices.

Working with Hispanic/Latino American Food Patterns
Historical Perspective

Hispanics comprise approximately 10.8 percent of the U.S. population and are the fastest growing ethnic group in the country.[4] Hispanic immigrants come to the United States from Central America, South America, and the Caribbean, but the greatest number come from Mexico. The cultural foods and food preparation methods of Hispanic populations vary significantly, depicting indigenous, African, and European influences.[126] For example, Mexican cuisine is influenced by indigenous, Spanish, and French cultures. Chiles, cocoa, and tomatoes are among the flavors used in preparing traditional Mexican dishes.[126]

The Aztec Indians contributed corn, tomatoes, roast turkey, quail, duck, fish, lobster, frogs, green plums, cocoa, beans, peas, and squash to Mexican cuisine. The Spanish contributed cinnamon, garlic, onions, rice, wheat, sugarcane, and pork. Mexican clients also consume meats such as goat, poultry, and beef. Mexicans experience high incidences of lactose intolerance, which causes a reduction in the diet of dairy foods.[126,150] They often use traditional foods and ingredients to prepare Mexican dishes such as tacos, enchiladas, tamales, quesadillas, burritos, stews, tortillas, chile rellenos, flan, guacamole, and salsas.[126]

Some Hispanics believe that illness is due to 1) excessive emotion, 2) dislocation of organs, 3) magic, 4) an imbalance in hot or cold, or 5) they consider health conditions such as pneumonia and appendicitis to be European diseases.[126,151] They base their treatment of an illness on the cause of the health condition. Some Mexican Indians practice a hot–cold system of diet and health; the rural poor also have similar practices. This is derived from the Arab system of humoral medicine brought to Mexico by the Spanish, combined with the native Indian practice.[61,152]

Hispanic Americans believe in prayer and depend on spiritual strength to help them in illness and death. They trust God and believe that living life in accord with God's intention is essential in maintaining health. Hence, offending God necessitates punishment.[126,153] Some Hispanic Americans believe that the origins of disease and illness are due to spiritual or natural punishments, hot and cold imbalances, magic, dislocation of internal organs, natural diseases, and emotional and mental issues.[126,153]

Current Nutrition Practices and Health-Related Issues

In the United States, Hispanic immigrants adhere strongly to their food traditions. Nevertheless, it has been reported that as Hispanic immigrants become assimilated into the host country's culture, traditional foods are consumed less often than when they lived in their country.[126]

Dietary acculturation can result in both healthful and unhealthful dietary changes.

The dietary acculturation of Hispanics is often characterized by an increased consumption of high-fat, high-sugar, highly processed foods associated with mainstream culture.[154] It is also reported that with the alteration in the traditional diet, Hispanic immigrants show a significant increase in diet-related chronic conditions such as obesity, hypertension, cardiovascular disease, and diabetes.[155-157] These observations are supported by clinical data documenting a high incidence of these conditions among Hispanic immigrants in the United States.

The birth rate for Mexican women between the ages of 15 and 44 years is 114 births per 1,000 women. This is about half the figure for European American women. The pregnancy rate for unmarried teenage girls is twice that of European Americans.[126] It was reported that one-half of teenage Hispanic mothers do not obtain prenatal care during the first trimester. However, infant mortality is lower for Mexican American infants than for European American infants despite the risk factors associated with the delay in enrolling in prenatal care. Breastfed infants are usually weaned from the breast to the bottle.[61] Prolonged use of a feeding bottle, containing both milk and/or sweetened liquids (i.e., Kool-Aid, fruit juice, tea), is a problem because it causes iron deficiency anemia, obesity, and extensive tooth decay among toddlers.[158,159]

Many Mexican Americans like fried foods, which results in the increased intake of high-fat foods and a lesser intake of fruits and vegetables than European American of similar backgrounds. Acculturation exacerbated these dietary intake differences.[126] It is reported that second-generation Mexican Americans consume more meat and cheese and less beans; eat vegetables as side dishes with added butter, dressings, or mayonnaise; and choose sweetened fruit drink mixes (Kool-Aid) over fresh, blended fruit drinks.[126,160,161]

Lack of money may cause Hispanic people to disregard healthcare services. About 27 percent of all Hispanic families in the United States live below the poverty line. In addition, Hispanics are very proud and very private when it comes to family problems.[126,162] It is not easy for a family to help a member who has alcohol abuse problems and still more difficult to recommend external help. This value influences receptivity to community nutrition programs and printed materials.[126] The following is a list of general recommendations for working with Hispanic populations:[126,163,164]

- Target prevention and intervention efforts to the entire family and their religious leaders.
- Help Hispanic/Latino fathers recognize how important their role is to their children.
- Encourage mothers to learn strategies for including their spouses in family interactions.
- Educate mothers and daughters to reduce the shame associated with asking for help.
- Emphasize the family as a unit in printed materials. Tailor separate versions for males and females.
- Emphasize participation in healthy eating and exercise programs to adjust to the American culture without abandoning their own.
- Reach Hispanic/Latino audiences through Spanish-speaking, community-level organizations and leaders.
- Educate community nutritionists and assistants about traditional gender roles to aid their efforts.

Working with Native American Food Patterns

Historical Perspective

American Indians/Native Americans (both are appropriate terms) are diverse groups of indigenous people who have lived north of Mexico and south of Canada since at least 12,000 B.C. Both hunting and gathering (foraging) contributed significantly to the diet of all American Indian groups at the time of contact with Europeans, whether or not they were horticulturalists. More than 550 sovereign Indian nations currently live within the political boundaries of the United States, so it is difficult to summarize their different foods and dietary habits.[126]

Native North Americans consume a variety of foods based on the diverse plant and animal communities found throughout the continent. They link food to spirituality and physical health, balance, and harmony. Corn has a special healing significance.[165] Fry bread (bread dough

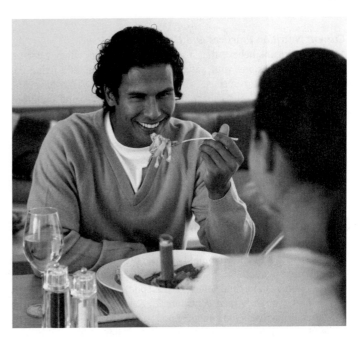

The cultural foods and food preparation methods of Hispanic populations are diverse, reflecting indigenous, African, and European influences.

Traditional Native American foods, such as squash, are a part of today's American diet.

deep-fried in fat) is a popular food at Indian fairs and gatherings. The dish can actually be traced to medieval Europe.[166] Native Americans also have made a significant contribution to the current American diet. Native Americans contributed, among many other items, corn, squash, beans, cranberries, and maple syrup to European settlers.

Food has significant religious and social meaning to many Native Americans. It is an integral component of many festivities, including powwows and other ceremonies. They like to give foods to guests, and extra food is frequently given to members of the extended family. Meals are prepared and eaten communally in some Native American nations in the southwest. A large amount of one dish is prepared by every woman, and she shares it with other families, who in turn share what they have prepared.[126,167]

Current Nutrition Practices and Health-Related Issues

Native Americans believe that a state of health exists when a person lives in total harmony with nature. The earth is seen as a living entity that should be respected, and failure to do so would harm the body. Native Americans believe their healing practices and traditions function in the context of the relationship among spirituality (Creator, Mother Earth, Great Father), community (family, clan, tribe/nation), environment (daily life, nature, balance), and self (inner passions and peace, thoughts, and values).[126,167]

Native Americans experience many social problems (e.g., alcohol/drug abuse and violence) at a rate that is significantly higher than the national average. The rate of adult onset (Type 2) diabetes for American Indians is more than three times that of the entire U.S. population.[168] Research on the nutritional status of Native Americans is limited, but it does show that fetal malnutrition may be the cause of Type 2 diabetes and, in subsequent generations, transmitted by disturbances in the intrauterine environment.[169] Many Native Americans experience, low socioeconomic status and a lack of transportation, fuel, refrigeration, and running water, which contribute to inadequate diet intake. The resulting problems include dental caries, goiter, growth retardation, female obesity, and low levels of hemoglobin, vitamin A, thiamin, and riboflavin.[126,170]

One explanation for Native Americans' poor health status is the "thrifty genotype" model, which states that such a genotype gave a genetic advantage to populations who experienced periods of feast and famine. If maximizing their caloric intake of fat for storage, which could be utilized during times of famine, they would have a selective advantage over other populations.[126,171] A problem occurs when the feasting, especially in the form of high-fat, carbohydrate-rich foods, becomes permanent. The result has been high rates of obesity, insulin resistance, and diabetes.[168]

The high incidence of diet-related health conditions such as diabetes, coronary heart disease, hypertension, and obesity has been most pronounced in the decades following World War II. The promotion of an American diet and lifestyle was one of the many facets of attempting to assimilate Native Americans into the U.S. mainstream. It included home economics instruction for Native American women showing them how to utilize the surplus commodities being provided to poor Indian communities.[126]

Current research on the Native American meal patterns is limited. It is assumed that three meals per day has become the norm. One study of Dakotas reported that there was little variety in daily menus. Current dietary intakes include cereal with milk, fried potatoes, fried eggs, chopped meat, milk, bread with butter, oatmeal or cornmeal, and high white sugar consumption.[126,172]

It is reported that the life expectancy for Native Americans has increased in recent years, but it is still lower than that of the overall U.S. population. The age-adjusted mortality rate for Native Americans is about 50 percent higher than the rest of the United States, and one-third of Native Americans die before the age of 45, compared to just 11 percent of the total U.S. population.[126,172] Chronic conditions complicating diabetes, including hypertension and end-stage renal diseases, were found to be more prevalent among northern plains Indians than among the general population.[173]

Healthcare providers who counsel American Indians must recognize traditional beliefs and practices. For example, varying according to tribe or region, either all individuals speak for themselves because no other can speak for them or, in some cases, the elder can speak for others. Also, "yes" and "no" are considered complete responses, and explanations are not thought to be warranted. Also, in Native American culture, direct eye contact is not common.[126]

Working with Asian American Food Patterns

Historical Perspective

The term *Asian American* refers to people of Asian descent who are citizens or permanent residents of the United States. The term encompasses at least 23 subgroups including persons from China, Mongolia, Pakistan, Sri Lanka, Maldives, India, Nepal, Bhutan, Bangladesh, Burma, Laos, Thailand, Vietnam, Cambodia, North Korea, South Korea, Japan, Hong Kong, Macao, Taiwan, Philippines, Malaysia, and Polynesia.[126,174] They constituted 4.2 percent of the total population of the United States in 2000. It is projected that by 2050, this figure will be 10.1 percent. In 2000, the U.S. census reported that approximately 2.3 million people of Chinese ancestry lived in the United States and about two-thirds of them were foreign-born; nearly half arrived in the 1990s. High rates of tuberculosis, parasitic infection, and hepatitis B have been found in many recent Asian American immigrants.[126]

Asian cultural values are imbedded in their health beliefs and practices, which help them determine what is important in one's life. Although variations are the norm rather than the exception, Asian groups share some similarities based on their religious backgrounds and the influence of Chinese culture throughout Asia.[175]

Asians view health as a state of harmony with nature or freedom from symptoms or illness. The concept of balance is related to health promotion, and the concept of imbalance is related to disease.[126] This balance or equilibrium relates to temperature in foods, climate, and body elements as well as diet, and it influences people's daily activities of living and health promotion. To achieve health and avoid illness, they believe people must adjust to the environment in a holistic manner. Traditional practitioners assist people in achieving this through energy balance.[176]

In the Chinese culture, food is viewed as more than something to eat. The decision about what to eat is carefully planned. Food plays a significant role in preventing and treating diseases as well as addressing certain health conditions. For example, foods and herbs are frequently boiled in soup or tea for treatments of various diseases and conditions. The preferred beverage is hot green tea. Older Chinese individuals rarely drink cold beverages.[126,177,178] The Japanese believe that certain foods and herbs have harmful or beneficial effects; for example, a study using the Japanese diet and herbal medicine formula Hochu-ekki-to (containing Astragalus root, liquorice, jujube, ginseng, white Atractylodes rhizome, fresh ginger, and Chinese Angelica root) found it to be effective as an alternative therapy for difficult atopic dermatitis.[179]

Asian individuals eat a wide variety of foods. The traditional Asian diet is low in fat and dairy products and high in complex carbohydrates and sodium; research with elderly foreign-born Americans of Chinese descent indicates that their dietary pattern is mostly continued in the United States. However, Asians' diets become more like the majority of Americans' diets as the length of stay and the number of generations living in the United States increases. The diet becomes higher in fat, protein, sugar, and cholesterol and lower in complex carbohydrates.[126,180]

Current Nutritional Practices and Health-Related Issues

In general, Chinese diets are high in sodium, which may contribute to hypertension; however, hypertension rates among Chinese Americans in California are significantly lower than for European Americans, but research is limited.[180]

Some Chinese Americans avoid fresh dairy products because of lactose intolerance, which may be found in as many as 75 percent of Asians.[126] It has been reported that their calcium intake is low.[96,181] However, a recent study shows an increase in the consumption of dairy products such as milk and cheese.[97]

The Asian American meal pattern includes eating three meals and several snacks a day. Some of the foods the Asian communities use include soy sauce, rice, pickled dishes, raw fish, and tea.[126] A study of acculturation and diet in Chinese American women found that Chinese-language newspapers and friends were the primary sources of nutrition information.[182]

Koreans relate health to happiness, to the ability to live life fully, to function without impairment, and to not be a burden on one's children.[126] There are limited research studies on the health of Korean Americans. One comparison of the nutritional status of elderly Korean Americans indicated that Asian Koreans had the poorest diet.[183,184] Nearly one-half consumed inadequate amounts of energy, vitamin A, and riboflavin. Almost one-fourth consumed less than two-thirds the recommended daily allowance (RDA) of protein, phosphorus, and vitamin C.[183] Twenty percent of the men and 25 percent of the women had inadequate protein intakes. Korean Americans also reported low calcium consumption.[126,184,185]

The variations in the health status of Asian Americans are due to subcultures within the larger group. Asian Americans have health problems similar to the European American population. Cardiovascular problems are common, and they have a high incidence of strokes. The prevalence of cardiovascular disease among Japanese Americans is only one-half that for European American Americans; however, it is expected that death rates will climb steadily as further acculturation occurs.[186] Heart disease rates are estimated to be one and one-half to four times greater among Asian Indian immigrants than among European Americans. Researchers have reported that Asian Indians living in urban and westernized regions have a significantly higher risk of cardiovascular disease and type 2 diabetes mellitus than the native population in India or the European American population in the United States, and diabetes rates also are calculated to be at least four times higher.[126,187–190] Changes in diet also have been implicated in the high rates of Type 2 diabetes found among Japanese American men. Hypertension is usually an accompanying chronic problem, resulting from a high salt intake.[190] The rate of hypertension in Asian Indians is associated with the high incidence of cardiovascular disease, which is slightly higher than that of European Americans.[191]

Cancers are also leading health problems for Asian men and women. Breast, colorectal, and lung cancers are the leading causes of death.[126,192] The incidence of liver cancers is high among foreign-born Asians with a history of hepatitis B infection. Cancers, such as breast and rectal, have increased in Japanese Americans as their residency in the United States increases. The leading cause of death among Koreans is stomach cancer, and higher incidences of stomach, liver, and esophageal cancer have been reported among Korean Americans as

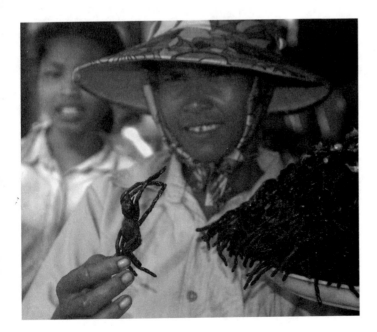

One man's favorite food is another man's dismay.

TABLE 16.5	Some Food Practices, Health Issues, Dietary Concerns, and Strategies for the Main Minority Groups in the United States[126,196–202]			
Cultural Group	**Food Practices**	**Diet-Related Heath Issues**	**Dietary Concerns**	**Strategies**
African American	Traditional foods include collard greens, other leafy green and yellow vegetables, beans, legumes, rice, and potatoes. Starches and vegetables are often seasoned with fat, such as bacon, ham hocks, or salt pork. Meats are often fried or barbecued and served with sauce or gravy. Home-baked cakes and pies are popular. Religion plays some role in their diets. For example, some Christians will avoid meat on holy days such as Good Friday and Ash Wednesday (Catholics). Those practicing Islam are required to avoid all pork and pork products; all meat must be slaughtered according to ritual letting of blood.	High incidence of diabetes, hypertension, heart disease, obesity, and some types of cancer; lactose intolerance.	Overall diet may be low in fiber, calcium, and potassium and high in fat and sodium.	• Encourage continued intake of leafy greens, vegetables, legumes, rice, and potatoes. • Offer tips for modifying food preparation methods to reduce fat and sodium. • Encourage increased intake of fruits. • Suggest ways to include low-fat dairy foods.
Asian American	Traditional diets vary widely by country and region of origin. Some common elements include a diet largely composed of rice, vegetables, and fruits; low intake of dairy foods except for ice cream or some yogurt; protein primarily from fish, pork, and poultry, as well as nuts, legumes, and/or tofu. Food is prepared by stir-frying, steaming, grilling, deep-frying, baking, or boiling.	Some types of cancer, osteoporosis, and stroke; lactose intolerance; risk for heart disease, diabetes, and obesity increases with dietary acculturation.	Overall diet may be low in calcium and high in carbohydrates and sodium.	• Encourage continued variety. • Evaluate calcium intake and suggest other food sources of calcium if inadequate. • Provide tips for reducing sodium intake.
Hispanic	Traditional diets vary by country and region of origin. Often the same foods are prepared and/or integrated into meal patterns in different ways. Common elements include beans, rice, breads, and, for some, corn and corn products. Protein sources include legumes, eggs, shellfish, fish, and a variety of meats and poultry. Minimal use of low-fat dairy foods. Foods are mainly fried or baked. With acculturation, there is an increased intake of milk, certain vegetables and fruits, fats, and sugars.	High incidence of obesity, diabetes, heart disease, hypertension, dental caries, and both over- and undernutrition.	Overall diet is high in fat and low in calcium, iron, folic acid, and vitamins A and C.	• Preserve healthy cultural food practices, such as continued use of complex carbohydrates. • Suggest modifications of traditional dishes to lower intake of fat and sodium. • Encourage intake of low-fat dairy foods, lean meats, fresh vegetables, and fruits. • Reduce intake of soft drinks and sweetened beverages.
Navajo (American Indians) and Alaska Natives	Traditional diets vary according to culture and seasons. Most diets include meats such as sheep, goat, wild game (deer, antelope, rabbits, and prairie dogs), pigs, chickens, and cattle; vegetables, such as celery, onion, spinach, potatoes, and pigweed; and fruits such as wolfberries, juniper berries, squaw berries or wax currants, prickly pear fruit, wild bananas, and yucca fruit. Other items added to food include gray clay and culinary ash from burned cedar and juniper boughs, tumbleweed, and greasewood. Gray clay decreases the bitterness of foods such as wolfberries and wild potatoes. The added clay also increases the mineral content of foods. Ash helps soften foods such as hominy and helps maintain the blue color in blue corn products. Other items in the diet include cantaloupe, watermelon, beans, squash, beans, and fish.	Diabetes, obesity, coronary heart disease, hypertension, and end-stage renal diseases.	Overall diet may be high in fat, sugar, and alcoholic intake with a low potassium intake.	• Encourage continued intake of leafy greens, vegetables, legumes, and potatoes. • Promote modifying food preparation methods to reduce fat and sodium. • Encourage low-fat foods. • Encourage regular physical activities.

TABLE 16.5	(Continued)			
Cultural Group	**Food Practices**	**Diet-Related Heath Issues**	**Dietary Concerns**	**Strategies**
Jewish	Dietary practices vary because Jews reside in many different countries. Also, religious belief plays a significant role in dietary practice. Most commonly used foods include: bagels with cream cheese, rye bread, corned beef, pastrami, and matzoh (popular in the United States). Some Jewish people observe strict dietary laws that require restriction of all pork and pork products and all fish without scales and fins. Dairy products are not eaten at the same meal that contains meat and meat products. All meat must be slaughtered and prepared according to Biblical ordinances. Since blood is forbidden as food, meat must be drained thoroughly. Bakery products and prepared food mixtures must be prepared under acceptable kosher standards. Leavened bread and cake are forbidden during Passover. All non-cloven hoofed animals such as beef and chicken that have been blessed by a Rabbi are allowed. Dairy, eggs, grains, legumes, vegetables, and fruits are permitted. During Passover, unleavened bread or flat bread is permitted. Mixing meat and dairy products is not allowed.	Type 2 diabetes, breast cancer, obesity, and coronary heart disease.	Overall diet may be high in intake of fat and sugar and low in intake of fiber, zinc, iron, and calcium.	• Encourage the use of low-fat foods and complex carbohydrate (whole wheat, rice, and whole grains). • Encourage physical activity. • Encourage reducing food containing high level of simple sugar.

compared to European Americans.[126,193] A low intake of vitamins A (including beta-carotene) and C and a high intake of sodium and chile peppers are reported to be the contributing factors to the high risk of these cancers. Aflatoxins, which have been linked to liver cancer, are also sometimes found in Korean soy sauce.[194]

In addition, the rate of hepatitis B (responsible for most liver cancers) is very high in Korean Americans. The prevalence of hepatitis B infection among Asian Americans ranges from 15 to 30 percent.[195] **Table 16.5** presents some food practices, health issues, dietary concerns, and strategies for the main minority groups in the United States.

Chapter Summary

- Culture is a learned set of ideals, values, and assumptions about life that are widely shared among a group of people.
- Nutritionists can gain cultural competence by reading about the language and customs of other cultures and by attending events held by local ethnic or cultural organizations, such as weddings, birthday parties, international fairs, and religious celebrations.
- Cultural knowledge is a needed base for adequate nutritional practice. When working with multicultural groups in nutrition assessment, it is important to collect basic information about the culture, the foods most frequently used, and food preparation methods.
- The current information about the biologic and genetic characteristics of African Americans, Hispanics, American Indians, Alaska Natives, Asians, Native Hawaiians, and Pacific Islanders does not explain the health disparities experienced by these groups.
- The U.S. infant mortality rate has lowered, but the infant death rate among African Americans is still more than double that of European Americans. In addition, heart disease death rates are more than 40 percent higher for African Americans than for European Americans.
- Some of the factors that may affect communication when working with a multicultural group include the communication skills, attitudes, knowledge, social system, and culture of both the sender and receiver of communication transactions.
- It is important to understand the variations in patterns of verbal and nonverbal communication that are the basis for achieving health promotion and disease prevention goals. Variations among cultures are reflected in verbal styles, such as pronunciation, word meaning, voice quality, and humor, and in nonverbal styles, such as eye contact, gestures, touch, interjection during conversation, body posture, facial expression, and silence.
- Nutrient deficiencies are prevalent among the large number of African American families at or near poverty levels in the United States.
- Dietitians may need to use an interpreter or members of the cultural group to explain or clarify terms to prevent incorrect assumptions.

Critical Thinking Activities

A community nutritionist, Angelina Okoro, and a community nurse, Lucy Tsai, conducted diabetes and dietary screenings at a free clinic to a culturally diverse population in the community. Analysis revealed that a high percentage of participation was due to print media advertising in the participant's native language. However, the families of the 5 percent of the Asian group who were diabetic (children) were unwilling to provide the children a prescribed diet.

Activities

- Determine the factors that may have caused this group to refuse the prescribed diet.
- Determine the different ways to socialize with different ethnic groups in your community to determine the best way to assess their nutritional needs.

- Identify major values of the dominant American group. Determine how these values differ from the values of minority cultural groups.
- Determine the strategies you can use when caring for clients who do not speak your language and for whom no translator is readily available.
- Taste different cultural foods by attending international fairs, restaurants, and the like.
- Identify foods that are taboo or prohibited for Asian Indians, Hispanics, Filipinos, Native Americans, and African Americans.

Case Study 16-1

A small city is the focus of a health promotion activity to prevent heart disease. A community nutritionist, Omari Sloan, was hired to implement the activity, which will include exercise and nutrition education. Sample diets were constructed, and a videotape was purchased for exercise demonstration. However, the videotape and the educational materials are only in English and do not depict people of different ethnic backgrounds. Omari noted that, of the 60 participants who enrolled in the program, 15 were Hispanic with limited English-speaking abilities, 10 were African American, 10 were new Asian immigrants, and the others were European American.

Activities

- Find a bilingual Hispanic or Asian nutritionist or other healthcare professional such as a nurse or a paraprofessional who could translate the educational materials. If you are unable to find a bilingual nutritionist within your community, try the American Dietetic Association's website at http://www.eatright.org. Use the websites provided in this chapter to find more information on different ethnic groups.
- Make educational materials culturally appropriate by integrating drawings of traditional nutrient-rich foods into a flipchart and handout illustrations.

References

1. Edelstein S. *Nutrition in Public Health: A Handbook for Developing Programs and Services*. 2nd ed. Sudbury, MA: Jones and Bartlett; 2006.

2. U.S. Department of Homeland Security. *2002 Yearbook of Immigration Statistics, Immigration Information*. Washington, DC: Author; 2002.

3. Katz SH, Weaver WW. *Encyclopedia of Food and Culture*. Vol. 3. New York: Scribner/Thomson Gale 2003: 425–437.

4. U.S. Bureau of the Census. *Projections of the Population of the United States, by Age, Sex, and Race: 1983–2008*. Washington, DC: Author; 2002.

5. U.S. Bureau of the Census. *Statistical Abstract of the United States*. Washington, DC: U.S. Department of Commerce; 2002.

6. World Health Organization. Constitution of the World Health Organization. Available at: http://www.who.int/governance/eb/who_constitution_en.pdf. Accessed May 14, 2008.

7. National Institutes of Health. NIH Strategic Research Plan to Reduce and Ultimately Eliminate Health Disparities. 2000. Available at: http://www.nih.gov/about/hd/strategicplan.pdf. Accessed February 16, 2007.

8. National Institutes of Health, National Cancer Institute. What Are Health Disparities. Available at: http://www.cancer.gov/cancertopics/types/disparities. Accessed February 9, 2007.

9. Braveman P. Health disparities and health equity: concepts and measurement. *Annu Rev Public Health*. 2006; 27:167–194.

10. Braveman P, Starfield B, Geiger HJ. World Health Report 2000: how it removes equity from the agenda for public health monitoring and policy. *BMJ*. 2001; 323:678–681.

11. U.S. Department of Health and Human Services. *Healthy People 2010: Understanding and Improving Health*. 2nd ed. Washington, DC: Author; 2000.

12. Smedley BD, Stith AY, Nelson AR. *Unequal Treatment: Confronting Racial and Ethnic Disparities in Healthcare*. Washington, DC: National Academy Press; 2002.

13. Gordon L. Facing racial and ethnic health disparities. *J Am Diet Assoc*. 2004; 104(12):1779–1780.

14. Garte S. The racial genetics paradox in biomedical research and public health. *Public Health Rep*. 2002; 17:421–425.

15. Carter-Pokras O, Baquet C. What is a health disparity? *Public Health Rep*. 2002; 117:426–434.

16. Thomas SB. The color line: race matters in the elimination of health disparities. *Am J Public Health*. 2001; 91:1046–1048.

17. Venter JC, Adams MD, Myers EW, et al. The sequence of the human genome. *Sci*. 2001; 291:1304–1351.

18. Cooper RS, Kaufman JS, Ward R. Race and genomics. *N Engl J Med*. 2003; 348:1166–1170.

19. Schwartz RS. Racial profiling in medical research. *N Engl J Med*. 2001; 344:1392–1393.

20. Oppenheimer GM. Paradigm lost: race, ethnicity, and the search for a new population taxonomy. *Am J Public Health*. 2001; 91:1049–1055.

21. Arah OA, Westert GP, Delnoij DM, Klazinga NS. Health system outcomes and determinants amenable to public health in industrialized countries: a pooled cross-sectional time series analysis. *BMC Public Health*. 2005; 5:81.

22. Blank RM, Dabady M, Citro CF. *Measuring Racial Discrimination*. Washington, DC: National Research Council; 2004.

23. U.S. Department of Health and Human Services. *Healthy People 2010: National Health Promotion and Disease Prevention Objectives*. Washington, DC: Author; 2000.

24. Yang G, Khoury MJ, Friedman J, Little J, Flanders WD. How many genes underlie the occurrence of common complex diseases in the population? *Int J Epidemiol*. 2005; 34(5):1–9.

25. Healthy People 2010. A Systematic Approach to Health Improvement. Available at: http://www.healthypeople.gov/document/html/uih/uih_bw/uih_2.htm#goals. Accessed May 17, 2008.

26. Glover MJ, Greenlund KJ, Ayala C, Croft JB. Racial/ethnic disparities in prevalence, treatment, and control of hypertension—United States, 1999–2002. *MMWR*. 2005; 54(01):7–9.

27. Centers for Disease Control and Prevention. Heart Disease Fact Sheet. Available at: http://www.cdc.gov/dhdsp/library/fs_heart_failure.htm. Accessed May 17, 2008.

28. Howe HL, Wingo PA, Thun MJ, et al. Annual report to the nation on the status of cancer (1973 through 1998), featuring cancers with recent increasing trends. *J Natl Cancer Inst*. 2001; 93(8):24–42.

29. Gargiullo P, Wingo PA, Coates RJ, Thompson TD. Recent trends in mortality rates for four major cancers, by sex and race/ethnicity—United States, 1990–1998. *MMWR*. 2002; 51(03):49–53.

30. Ver-Ploeg M, Perrin E. *Eliminating Health Disparities: Measurement and Data Needs*. Washington, DC: The National Academies Press, National Research Council; 2004.

31. Office of Minority Health. Health disparities experienced by black or African Americans—United States. *MMWR*. 2005; 54(01):1–3.

32. Office of Minority Health. Hispanic/Latino Profile. Available at: http://www.omhrc.gov/templates/browse.aspx?lvl=2&lvlID=54. Accessed May 17, 2008.

33. Centers for Disease Control and Prevention. National Center for Health Statistics. National Vital Statistics System. Available at: http://www.cdc.gov/nchs. Accessed May 17, 2008.

34. Liao Y, Tucker P, Okoro CA, Giles WH, Mokdad AH, Harris VB. REACH 2010 surveillance for health status in minority communities—United States, 2001–2002. *MMWR*. 2004; 53(SS06):1–36. Available at: http://www.cdc.gov/mmwr/preview/mmwrhtml/ss5306a1.htm. Accessed May 2005.

35. McNeely MJ, Boyko EJ. Type 2 diabetes prevalence in Asian Americans: results of a national health survey. *Diabetes Care*. 2004; 27:66–69.

36. Ikeda JP, Pham L, Nguyen KP, Mitchell RA. Culturally relevant nutrition education improves dietary quality among WIC-eligible Vietnamese immigrants. *J Nutr Educ Behav*. 2002; 34(3):151–158.

37. Gordon-Larsen P, Nelson MC, Page P, Popkin BM. Inequality in the built environment underlies key health disparities in physical activity and obesity. *Pediatr*. 2006; 117:417–424.

38. Mishra G, Ball K, Patterson A, Brown W, Hodge A, Dobson A. Socio-demographic inequalities in the diets of mid-aged Australian women. *Eur J Clin Nutr*. 2005; 59(2):185–195.

39. Park SY, Murphy SP, Wilkens LR, et al. Dietary patterns using the Food Guide Pyramid groups are associated with sociodemographic and lifestyle factors: the multiethnic cohort study. *J Nutr*. 2005; 135(4):843–849.

40. Shahar D, Shai I, Vardi H, Shahar A, Fraser D. Diet and eating habits in high and low socioeconomic groups. *Nutr*. 2005; 21(5):559–566.

41. Benjamin D. *Food Insecurity and Hunger: A Preventable Public Health Problem*. Minneapolis, MN: Maternal and Child Health Program, School of Public Health, Division of Epidemiology and Community Health, University of Minnesota; 2006.

42. Scheier LM. What is the hunger-obesity paradox? *J Am Diet Assoc*. 2005; 105:883–886.

43. Townsend MS, Peerson J, Love B, Achterberg C, Murphy SP. Food insecurity is positively related to overweight in women. *J Nutr*. 2001; 131:1738–1745.

44. Drewnowski A, Darmon N. The economics of obesity: dietary energy density and energy cost. *Am J Clin Nutr*. 2005; 82(1):265S–273S.

45. Blaak EE. Prevention and treatment of obesity and related complications: a role for protein? *Int J Obesity*. 2006; 30:S24–S27.

46. Casey PH, Simpson PM, Gossett JM, et al. The association of child and household food insecurity with childhood overweight status. *Pediatr*. 2006; 118:e1406–e1413.

47. Townsend MS, Peerson J, Love B, Achterberg C, Murphy SP. Food insecurity is positively related to overweight in women. *J Nutr*. 2001; 131:1738–1745.

48. National Center for Health Statistics. *Health, United States, 2003 with Chartbook on Trends in the Health of Americans*. Hyattsville, MD: Author; 2003.

49. Phares TM, Morrow B, Lansky A, et al. Surveillance for disparities in maternal health-related behaviors—selected states, Pregnancy Risk Assessment Monitoring System (PRAMS), 2000–2001. *MMWR*. 2004; 53(SS04); 1–13.

50. U.S. Department of Health and Human Services. *Healthy People 2010: Understanding and Improving Health. Objectives for Improving health*. Vol. 1. Washington, DC: Author; 2000.

51. Smedley BD, Stith AY, Nelson AR, eds. *Unequal Treatment: Confronting Racial and Ethnic Disparities in Healthcare*. Washington, DC: Institute of Medicine of the National Academies; 2003.

52. Lyla MH, Blazer DG. *The Impact of Social and Cultural Environment on Health*. Washington, DC: National Academies Press; 2006.

53. Foster C, Hillsdon M. Changing the environment to promote health-enhancing physical activity. *J Sports Sci*. 2004; 22(8):755–769.

54. Chappel M, Funk L, Carson A, MacKenzie P, Stanwick R. Multilevel community health promotion: how can we make it work. *Comm Dev J*. 2006; 41(3):352–366.

55. Harris-Davis E, Haughton B. Model for multicultural nutrition counseling competencies. *J Am Diet Assoc*. 2000; 100:1178–1185.

56. Marshall PA. Cultural influences on perceived quality of life. *Oncol Nurs.* 1990; 6(4):278–281.

57. Stanhope M, Lancaster J. *Community and Public Health Nursing.* 5th ed. New York: Mosby; 2000.

58. Brach C, Fraser L. Can cultural competency reduce racial and ethnic health disparities? A review and conceptual model. *Med Care Res Rev.* 2000; 57(Suppl 1):181–217.

59. Senior P, Bhopal R. Ethnicity as a variable in epidemiological research. *Brit Med J.* 1994; 30:327–328.

60. McWilliams M, Heller H. *Food Around the World: Cultural Perspective.* Upper Saddle River, NJ: Prentice Hall; 2003.

61. Kittler PG, Sucher K. *Food and Culture.* 4th ed. Belmont, CA: Wadsworth Thomson Learning; 2001.

62. Harrison GG, Kagawa-Singer M, Foerster SB. Seizing the moment: California's opportunity to prevent nutrition-related health disparities in low-income Asian American population. *Cancer.* 2005; 104(12):2962–2968.

63. Lutz C, Przytulski K. *Nutrition and Diet Therapy.* Philadelphia: F.A. Davis; 2001.

64. Dein S. Race, culture and ethnicity in minority research: a critical discussion. *J Cult Divers.* 2006; 13(2):68–75.

65. Dunham DP, Czysczon A, Chávez N, Piorkowski J, Persky V. Dietary differences among women of Polish descent by country of birth and duration of residency in the United States. *Ethnicity Dis.* 2004; 14(2):219–226.

66. Sundquist J, Winkleby M. Country of birth, acculturation status and abdominal obesity in a national sample of Mexican-American women and men. *Int J Epidemiol.* 2000; 29(3):470–477.

67. Arredondo E, Elder J, Ayala G, Slymen D, Campbell N. Association of a traditional vs. shared meal decision-making and preparation style with eating behavior of Hispanic women in San Diego County. *J Am Diet Assoc.* 2006; 106(1):38–45.

68. Betancourt J, Green AR, Carrillo JE, Ananeh-Firempong O. Defining cultural competence: a practical framework for addressing racial ethnic disparities in health and health care. *Public Health Rep.* 2003; 118(4):293–302.

69. White K. *Executive Summary: Building Cultural Competence.* Community and Family Health Multicultural Work Group, Washington State Department of Health; 2003.

70. Wittig DR. Knowledge, skills, and attitudes of nursing students regarding culturally congruent care of Native Americans. *J Transcult Nurs.* 2004; 5:54–61.

71. Campinha-Bacote J. The process of cultural competence in the delivery of healthcare services. *J Transcult Nurs.* 2002; 13:181–184.

72. Griswold K, Zayas LE, Kernan JB, Wagner CM. Cultural awareness through medical student and refugee patient encounters. *J Immigr Minor Health.* 2007; 9(1):55–60.

73. Van Dyne L, Ang S. Cultural Intelligence: An Essential Capability for Individuals in Contemporary Organizations. Available at: https://globaledge.msu.edu/newsAndViews/views/papers/cultural_intelligence.pdf. Accessed February 9, 2007.

74. Alfonso M. Cross-cultural encounter as an opportunity for personal growth. *J Humanist Psychol.* 2004; 44(2):243–265.

75. Williams SR, Schlenker E. *Essentials of Nutrition and Diet Therapy.* 8th ed. Davis, CA: Mosby; 2003.

76. Tripp-Reimer T, Choi E, Kelly LS, Enslein JC. Cultural barriers to care: inverting the problem. *Diab Spectrum.* 2001; 14:13–22.

77. Harris-Davis E, Haughton B. Model for multicultural nutrition counseling competencies. *J Am Diet Assoc.* 2000; 100:1178–1185.

78. Perlas LA, Gibson RS. Household dietary strategies to enhance the content and bioavailability of iron, zinc and calcium of selected rice- and maize-based Philippine complementary foods. *Matern Child Nutr.* 2005; 1(4):263–273.

79. Rosado JL, Díaz M, Rosas A, Griffit I, García OP. Calcium absorption from corn tortilla is relatively high and is dependent upon calcium content and liming in Mexican women. *J Nutr.* 2005; 135:2578–2581.

80. Yu-chih C. Chinese values, health and nursing. *J Advan Nurs.* 2001; 36(2):270–273.

81. Satia-Abouta J, Patterson RE, Kristal AR, Teh C, Tu SP. Psychosocial predictors of diet and acculturation in Chinese American and Chinese Canadian women. *Ethn Health.* 2002; 7(1):21–39.

82. Satia-Abouta J, Patterson RE, Neuhouser ML, Elder J. Dietary acculturation: applications to nutrition research and dietetics. *J Am Diet Assoc.* 2002; 102:1105–1118.

83. Aldrich L, Variyam JN. Acculturation erodes the diet quality of U.S. Hispanics. *Food Rev.* 2000; 23(1):51–55.

84. Satia-Abouta J, Patterson RE, Neuhouser ML, Elder J. Dietary acculturation: applications to nutrition research and dietetics. *J Am Diet Assoc.* 2002; 102(8):1105–1118.

85. Bermúdez OI, Falcón LM, Tucker KL. Intake and food sources of macronutrients among older Hispanic adults: association with ethnicity, acculturation, and length of residence in the United States. *J Am Diet Assoc.* 2000; 100:665–673.

86. Gray VB, Cossman JS, Dodson WL, Byrd SH. Dietary acculturation of Hispanic immigrants in Mississippi. *Salud Publica Mex.* 2005; 47(5):351–360.

87. Wiking E, Johansson S-E, Sundquist J. Ethnicity, acculturation, and self reported health. A population based study among immigrants from Poland, Turkey, and Iran in Sweden. *J Epidemiol Comm Health.* 2004; 58:574–582.

88. te Velde SJ, Wind M, van Lenthe FJ, Klepp KI, Brug J. Differences in fruit and vegetable intake and determinants of intakes between children of Dutch origin and non-Western ethnic minority children in the Netherlands—a cross sectional study. *Int J Behav Nutr Phys Act.* 2006; 3(31):online.

89. Colby SE, Morrison S, Morales S, Budd L, Haldeman L. *Dietary Acculturation of Mexican American Immigrants: A Case Study.* Philadelphia: USDA Agricultural Research; 2005.

90. Cabassa LJ. Measuring acculturation: where we are and where we need to go. *Hisp J Behav Sci.* 2003; 25(2):127–146.

91. Chung RH, Kim BS, Abreu JM. Asian American multidimensional acculturation scale: development, factor analysis, reliability, and validity. *Cultur Divers Ethnic Minor Psychol.* 2004; 10(1):66–80.

92. Cuellar I, Harris LC, Jasso R. An acculturation scale for Mexican Americans normal and clinical populations. *Hispanic J Behav Sci.* 1980; 2:199–217.

93. Suinn RM, Rickard-Figueroa K, Lew S, Vigil P. The Suinn-Lew Asian Self-Identity Acculturation Scale: an initial report. *Educ Psychol Meas.* 1987; 47:401–407.

94. Anderson J, Moeschberger M, Chen MS Jr, Kunn P, Wewers ME, Guthrie R. An acculturation scale for Southeast Asians. *Social Psychiatry Psychiatr Epidemiol.* 1993; 289:134–141.

95. Marin G, Sabogal F, Marin BV, Otero-Sabogal R, Perez-Stable EJ. Development of a short acculturation scale for Hispanics. *Hispanic J Behav Sci.* 1987; 9:183–205.

96. Yang GP, Fox HM. Food habit changes of Chinese persons living in Lincoln, Nebraska. *J Am Diet Assoc.* 1979; 75:420–424.

97. Satia J, Patterson RE, Kristal AR, Hislop TG, Yasui Y, Taylor VM. Development of scales to measure dietary acculturation among Chinese-Americans and Chinese-Canadians. *J Am Diet Assoc.* 2001; 101:548–553.

98. Hammond RA. The evolution of ethnocentrism. *Journal of Conflict Resolution.* 2006;50:(6): 926–936.

99. Sutherland LL. Ethnocentrism in a pluralistic society: a concept analysis. *J Transcult Nurs.* 2002; 13(4):274–281.

100. Seyed-Mahmoud A. Managing workforce diversity as an essential resource for improving organizational performance. *Int J Productivity Performance Manage.* 2004; 53(6):521–531.

101. Huff RM, Kline MV. *Promoting Health in Multicultural Populations. A Handbook for Practitioners.* New Delhi, India: Sage; 1999.

102. Holroyd E, Twinn S, Adab P. Socio-cultural influences on Chinese women's attendance for cervical screening. *J Adv Nurs.* 2004; 46(1):42–52.

103. Hsu WC, Cheung S, Ong E, et al. Identification of linguistic barriers to diabetes knowledge and glycemic control in Chinese Americans with diabetes. *Diabetes Care.* 2006; 29:415–416.

104. Goins T, Williams KA, Carter MW, Spencer M, Solovieva T. Perceived barriers to health care access among rural older adults: a qualitative study. *J Rural Health.* 2005; 21(3):206–213.

105. Hitchcock J, Schubert P, Thomas S. *Community Health Nursing Caring in Action.* Clifton Park, NY: Thomson Delmar Learning; 2002.

106. Kakai H. A double standard in bioethical reasoning for disclosure of advanced cancer diagnoses in Japan. *Health Comm.* 2002; 14(3):361–376.

107. Luckmann J. *Transcultural Communication in Healthcare.* Belmont, CA: Delmar Thomson Learning; 2000.

108. Schouten BB, Meeuwesen L. Cultural differences in medical communication: a review of the literature. *Patient Educ Counsel.* 2006; 64(1–3):21–34.

109. Solomon DH, Dillard JP, Anderson JW. Episode type, attachment orientation, and frame salience: evidence for a theory of relational framing. *Human Comm Res.* 2002; 28(1):136–152.

110. Delgadillo L. Guidelines for reaching out and counseling low income monolingual Latino clients. *J Extension.* 2003; 41(6):online.

111. Bairstow R, Berry H, Driscoll DM. Tips for teaching non-traditional audiences. *J Extension.* 2002; 40(6):online.

112. Edelman M. *Health Promotion Throughout the Lifespan.* St. Louis, MO: Mosby; 2002.

113. Johnson RL, Saha S, Arbelaez JJ, Beach MC, Cooper LA. Racial and ethnic differences in patient perceptions of bias and cultural competence in health care. *J Gen Intern Med.* 2004; 19(2):101–110.

114. Clark CC. *Health Promotion in Communities: Holistic and Wellness Approaches.* New York: Springer; 2002.

115. Giger JN, Davidhizar R, Cherry B. *Transcultural Nursing: Assessment and Intervention.* 3rd ed. St. Louis, MO: Mosby; 1999.

116. U.S. Department of Health and Human Services, Health Resources and Services Administration. Health Resources and Services Administration Study on Measuring Cultural Competence in Health Care Delivery Settings. Available at: http://www.hrsa.gov/culturalcompetence/measures/sectionii.htm. Accessed March 2, 2007.

117. Kumpfer K, Alvarado R, Smith P, Bellamy N. Cultural sensitivity and adaptation in family-based prevention interventions. *Prev Sci.* 2001; 3(3):241–246.

118. Tanjasiri SP, Kagawa-Singer M, Foo MA, et al. Designing culturally and linguistically appropriate health interventions: the life is precious among breast cancer study. *Health Educ Behav.* 2007; 34(1):140–153.

119. Erwin DO, Johnson VA, Trevino M, Duke K, Feliciano L, Jandorf L. A comparison of African American and Latina social networks as indicators for culturally tailoring a breast and cervical cancer education. *Cancer.* 2007; 109(2):368–377.

120. Goodman MJ, Ogdie A, Kanamor MJ, Cañar J, O'Malley AS. Barriers and facilitators of colorectal cancer screening among Mid-Atlantic Latinos: focus group findings. *Ethn Dis.* 2006; 16(1):255–261.

121. Fawcett JT, Carino BV. *The New Immigration from Asia and the Pacific Islands.* Staten Island, NY: Center for Migration Studies; 1987.

122. McPhee SJ, Jenkins CNH, Hung S, et al. Behavioral risk factor survey of Vietnamese. California, 1991. *MMWR.* 1992; 41(05):69–72.

123. Purnell L. A description of the Purnell model for cultural competence. *J Transcult Nurs.* 2000; 11(1):40–46.

124. National Center for Cultural Competence. Cultural Competency: Concepts and Definitions. Available at: http://www11.georgetown.edu/research/gucchd/nccc. Accessed May 17, 2008.

125. U.S. Department of Health and Human Services, Office of Minority Health. National Standards on Culturally and Linguistically Appropriate Services (CLAS). Available at: http://www.omhrc.gov/templates/browse.aspx?lvl=2&lvlID=15-37k. Accessed May 17, 2008.

126. Kittler PG, Sucher K. *Food and Culture.* 4th ed. Belmont, CA: Wadsworth Thomson Learning; 2004.

127. Cook JT, Frank DA, Berkowitz C, et al. Food insecurity is associated with adverse health outcomes among human infants and toddlers. *J Nutr.* 2004; 134:1432–1438.

128. Haytowitz DB, Pehrsson PR, Holden JM. Adapting methods for determining priorities for the analysis of foods in diverse populations. *J Food Comp Anal.* 2000; 13:425–433.

129. Byers KG, Savaiano DA. The myth of increased lactose intolerance in African-Americans. *J Am Coll Nutr.* 2005; 24(6):569S–573S.

130. Flegal KM, Carroll MD, Ogden CL, Johnson CL. Prevalence and trends in obesity among US adults, 1999–2000. *JAMA.* 2002; 288:1723–1727.

131. Centers for Disease Control and Prevention, National Health and Nutrition Examination Survey. Healthy Weight, Overweight, and Obesity among U.S. Adults. Available at: http://www.cdc.gov/nchs/data/nhanes/databriefs/adultweight.pdf. Accessed February 14, 2007.

132. Drewnowski A, Darmon N. The economics of obesity: dietary energy density and energy cost. *Am J Clin Nutr.* 2005; 82(1):265S–273S.

133. Steinberger J, Daniels SR. Obesity, insulin resistance, diabetes, and cardiovascular risk in children. *Circ.* 2003; 107:1448–1453.

134. Ayala C, Croft JB, Wattigney WA, Mensah JA. Trends in hypertension-related death in the United States: 1980–1998. *J Clin Hypertens.* 2004; 6(12):675–681.

135. Opie LH, Seedat YK. Hypertension in sub-Saharan African populations. *Circ.* 2005; 112:3562–3568.

136. Forrester T. Historic and early life origins of hypertension in Africans. *J Nutr.* 2004; 134:211–216.

137. Agyemang C, Bhopal R, Bruijnzeels M. Negro, Black, Black African, African Caribbean, African American or what? Labelling African origin populations in the health arena in the 21st century. *J Epidemiol Community Health.* 2005; 59:1014–1018.

138. Fernander AF, Durán RE, Saab PG, Schneiderman N. John Henry Active Coping, education, and blood pressure among urban blacks. *J Natl Med Assoc.* 2004; 96(2):246–255.

139. Petersen KL, Bleil ME, McCaffery J, et al. Community socioeconomic status is associated with carotid artery atherosclerosis in untreated, hypertensive men. *Am J Hypertens.* 2006; 19(6):560–566.

140. Scott RP, Heslin KC. Historical perspectives on the care of African Americans with cardiovascular disease. *Ann Thorac Surg.* 2003; 76:S1348–S1355.

141. Frederick IO, Williams MA, Dashow E, Kestin M, Zhang C, Leisenring WM. Dietary fiber, potassium, magnesium and calcium in relation to the risk of preeclampsia. *J Reprod Med.* 2005; 50(5):332–344.

142. Peters RM, Flack JM. Salt sensitivity: common findings. *Prog Cardiovasc Nurs.* 2000; 15(4):138–144.

143. Flack JM, Sica DA. Therapeutic considerations in the African-American patient with hypertension: considerations with calcium channel blocker therapy. *J Clin Hypertens.* 2005; 7(4):9–14.

144. Pothiwala P, Evans EM, Chapman-Novakofski KM. Ethnic variation in risk for osteoporosis among women: a review of biological and behavioral factors. *J Womens Health.* 2006; 15(6):709–719.

145. Appel LJ. Lifestyle modification as a means to prevent and treat high blood pressure. *J Am Soc Nephrol.* 2003; 14:S99–S102.

146. Hermansen K. Diet, blood pressure and hypertension *Brit J Nutr.* 2000; 83(Suppl 1):113–119.

147. Appel LJ, Champagne CM, Harsha DW, et al. Effects of comprehensive lifestyle modification on blood pressure control. *JAMA.* 2003; 289:2083–2093.

148. Kulkarni KD. Food, culture, and diabetes in the United States. *Clin Diabetes.* 2004; 22:190–192.

149. Medical News Today. Positive Influence of Religion and Spirituality on Blood Pressure. Available at: http://www.medicalnewstoday.com/medicalnews.php?newsid=44202. Accessed February 14, 2007.

150. Auld G, Boushey CJ, Bock MA, et al. Perspectives on intake of calcium-rich foods among Asian, Hispanic, and white preadolescent and adolescent females. *J Nutr Educ Behav.* 2002; 34(5):242–251.

151. Dillinger TL, Barriga P, Escárcega S, Jimenez M, Salazar Lowe D, Grivetti LE. Food of the gods: cure for humanity? A cultural history of the medicinal and ritual use of chocolate. *J Nutr.* 2000; 130:2057S–2072S.

152. Fleuriet KJ. Health and health care problems among the Kumiai of San Antonio Necua and their indigenous relatives in Baja California: reflections of poverty, marginality, and a history of colonization. *Calif J Health Prom.* 2003; 1(1):140–157.

153. Alejandro M, Rolf P, Zea M. Use and implications of ethnomedical health care approaches among Central American immigrants. *Health & Social Work.* 2003; 28(1):43–51.

154. McArthur LH, Viramontez Anguiano RP, Nocetti D. Maintenance and change in the diet of Hispanic immigrants in eastern North Carolina. *Fam Consumer Sci Res J.* 2001; 29(4):309–335.

155. Gray VB, Cossman JS, Dodson WL, Byrd SL. Dietary acculturation of Hispanic immigrants in Mississippi. *Salud Publica Mex.* 2005; 47(5):351–360.

156. Mazur R, Marquis GS, Jensen HH. Diet and food insufficiency among Hispanic youths: acculturation and socioeconomic factors in the third National Health and Nutrition Examination Survey. *Am J Clin Nutr.* 2003; 78(6):1120–1127.

157. Neuhouser ML, Thompson B, Coronado GD, Solomon CC. Higher fat intake and lower fruit and vegetables intakes are associated with greater acculturation among Mexicans living in Washington State. *J Am Diet Assoc.* 2004; 104(1):51–57.

158. Harris R, Nicoll AD, Adair PM, Pine CM. Risk factors for dental caries in young children: a systematic review of the literature. *Community Dental Health.* 2004; 21:S71–S85.

159. Bonuck KA, Kahn R. Prolonged bottle use and its association with iron deficiency anemia and overweight: a preliminary study. *Clin Pediatr.* 2002; 41(8):603–607.

160. Matheson DM, Killen JD, Wang Y, Varady A, Robinson TN. Children's food consumption during television viewing. *Am J Clin Nutr.* 2004; 79(6):1088–1094.

161. Artinian NT, Schim SM, Vander Wal JS, Nies MA. Eating patterns and cardiovascular disease risk in a Detroit Mexican American population. *Public Health Nurs.* 2004; 21(5):425–434.

162. Duraski SA. Meeting the needs of the community: a project to prevent stroke in Hispanics. *Topics Stroke Rehab.* 2003; 9(4):46–56.

163. Umana-Taylor AJ, Bamaca MY. Conducting focus groups with Latino populations: lessons from the field. *Fam Relations.* 2004; 53(3):261–272.

164. Hobbs BB. Latino outreach programs: why they need to be different. *J Extension.* 2004; 42(4):1–4.

165. Rundle A, Carvalho M, Robinson M. *Cultural Competence in Healthcare: A Practical Guide.* Boston: Jossey-Bass; 2002.

166. Garrett JT, Garrett MT. *The Cherokee Full Circle: A Practical Guide to Ceremonies and Traditions.* Rochester, VT: Bear & Company; 2004.

167. Tarrell AA, Portman A, Garrett MT. Native American healing traditions: indigenous and complementary and alternative healing practices. *Int J Disability Develop Educ.* 2006; 53(4):453–469.

168. Archer SL, Greenlund KJ, Casper ML, Makaroam R, Croft JB. Associations of community-based health education programs with food habits and cardiovascular disease risk factors among Native Americans with diabetes: the Inter-Tribal Heart Project, 1992–1994. *J Am Diet Assoc.* 2002; 102:1132–1135.

169. Benyshek DC, Martin JF, Johnston CS. A reconsideration of the origins of the type 2 diabetes epidemic among Native Americans and the implications for intervention policy. *Med Anthropol.* 2001; 20(1):25–64.

170. McGanity WJ. The story of the Interdepartmental Committee on Nutrition for National Defense's North American activities (1958–1970). *J Nutr.* 2005; 135:1268–1271.

171. Goyan Kittler P, Sucher K. *Food and Culture.* 4th ed. Belmont, CA: Thomson & Wadsworth; 2003.

172. Jimenez MM, Receveur O, Trifonopoulos M, Kuhnlein H, Paradis G, Macaulay AC. Comparison of the dietary intakes of two different groups of children (grades 4 to 6) before and after the Kahnawake schools diabetes prevention project. *J Am Diet Assoc.* 2003; 103:1191–1194.

173. Di Noia J, Schinke SP, Contento IR. Dietary patterns of reservation and non-reservation Native American youths. *Ethn Dis.* 2005; 15(4):705–712.

174. Abizadeh A. Ethnicity, race, and a possible humanity. *World Order.* 2001; 33(1):23–34.

175. Kim BS, Yang PH, Atkinson DR, Wolfe MM, Hong S. Cultural value similarities and differences among Asian American ethnic groups. *Cultur Divers Ethnic Minor Psychol.* 2001; 7(4):343–361.

176. Lu L. A preliminary study on the concept of health among the Chinese. *Counsel Psychol Q.* 2002; 15(2):179–189.

177. Nan L, Brown J, Liu B. Factors influencing dairy product consumption of Chinese Americans in Pennsylvania: enhancing nutrition consumption in the American diet. *Top Clin Nutr.* 2007; 22(3):258–271.

178. Cabrera C, Artacho R, Giménez R. Beneficial effects of green tea—a review. *J Am Coll Nutr.* 2006; 25:79–99.

179. Kobayashi H, Mizuno N, Teramae H, et al. Diet and Japanese herbal medicine for recalcitrant atopic dermatitis: efficacy and safety. *Drugs Exp Clin Res.* 2004; 30(5–6):197–202.

180. Lv N, Cason KL. Dietary pattern change and acculturation of Chinese Americans in Pennsylvania. *J Am Diet Assoc.* 2004; 104(5):771–778.

181. Kwok T, Woo J, Kwan M. Does low lactose milk powder improve the nutritional intake and nutritional status of frail older Chinese people living in nursing homes? *J Nutr Health Aging.* 2001; 5(1):17–21.

182. Satia JA, Patterson RE, Taylor VM, et al. Use of qualitative methods to study diet, acculturation, and health in Chinese-American women. *J Am Diet Assoc.* 2000; 100:934–940.

183. Park YH, de Groot LC, van Staveren WA. Dietary intake and anthropometry of Korean elderly people: a literature review. *Asia Pac J Clin Nutr.* 2003; 12(3):234–242.

184. Park SY, Murphy SP, Sharma S, Kolonel LN. Dietary intakes and health-related behaviors of Korean American women born in the USA and Korea: the Multiethnic Cohort Study. *Public Health Nutr.* 2005; 8(7):904–911.

185. Oh S-Y, Hong MJ. Food insecurity is associated with dietary intake and body size of Korean children from low-income families in urban areas. *Eur J Clin Nutr.* 2003; 57:1598–1604.

186. D'Agostino RB Sr, Grundy S, Sullivan LM, Wilson P. Validation of the Framingham coronary heart disease prediction scores: results of a multiple ethnic groups investigation. *JAMA.* 2001; 286:180–187.

187. Abate N, Chandalia M. Ethnicity and type 2 diabetes. *J Diabetes Complications.* 2001; 15:320–327.

188. Yano K, Grove JS, Chen R, Rodriguez BL, Curb JD, Tracy RP. Plasma fibrinogen as a predictor of total and cause-specific mortality in elderly Japanese-American men. *Arteriosclero Thromb Vasc Biol.* 2001; 21:1065–1070.

189. Kanaya AM, Grady D, Barrett-Connor E. Explaining the sex difference in coronary heart disease mortality among patients with type 2 diabetes mellitus. *Arch Intern Med.* 2002; 162:1737–1745.

190. Barbato A, Cappuccio FP, Folkerd EJ, et al. Metabolic syndrome and renal sodium handling in three ethnic groups living in England. *Diabetologia.* 2004; 47(1):40–46.

191. Kwok TC, Chan TY, Woo J. Relationship of urinary sodium/potassium excretion and calcium intake to blood pressure and prevalence of hypertension among older Chinese vegetarians. *Eur J Clin Nutr.* 2003; 57:299–304.

192. Centers for Disease Control and Prevention. Cancer: Selected U.S. National Research Findings. Available at: http://www.cdc.gov/Women/natstat/cancer.htm. Accessed February 23, 2007.

193. Yoon SJ, Lee H, Shin Y, Kim YI, Kim CY, Chang H. Estimation of the burden of the major cancers in Korea. *J Korea Med Sci.* 2002; 17:604–610.

194. Oh SW, Yoon YS, Shin SA. Effects of excess weight on cancer incidences depending on cancer sites and histologic findings among men: Korea National Health Insurance Corporation Study. *J Clin Oncol.* 2005; 23(23):4742–4754.

195. Minuk G, Uhanova J. Chronic hepatitis B infection in Canada. *Can J Infect Dis.* 2001; 12(6):351–356.

196. American School Health Association. *The National Adolescent Student Health Survey: A Report on the Health of America's Youth.* Oakland, CA: Third Party Publishing Company; 1988.

197. Ohio State University Extension. Fact Sheets. Cultural Diversity: Eating in America (African-American, Asian, Mexican-American). http://ohioline.osu.edu/hyg-fact/5000. Accessed May 19, 2008.

198. Donelle L, Hoffman-Goetz L, Clarke J. Ethnicity, genetics, and breast cancer: media portrayal of disease identities. *Ethn Health.* 2005; 10(3):185–197.

199. Rozen GGS, Rennert GG, Rennert HHS, Diab GG, Daud DD, Ish-Shalom SS. Calcium intake and bone mass development among Israeli adolescent girls. *J Amer Coll Nutr.* 2001; 20(3):219–224.

200. The American Dietetic Association, American Diabetes Association. *Ethnic and Regional Food Practices: A Series (Soul and Traditional Southern, Mexican American, Chinese American, Jewish, and Navajo).* Chicago, IL: American Dietetic Association; 1989–1998.

201. Lutz C, Przytulski, K. *Nutrition and Diet Therapy.* 3rd ed. Philadelphia: F. A. Davis; 2001.

202. Kraft Food, Inc. *Spring-Summer 2005 Nutrition Update Providing Nutrition Guidance to a Multicultural Population: The Importance of Cultural Competency.* Available at: http://www.kraftnutrition.com. Accessed May 19, 2008.

Intervention Messages

Box A-1 **Eat More Fiber**

Eat five cups of fruits and vegetables a day.

- Use vegetables for main dishes, soups, salads, or snacks.
- Use fruits for breakfast, as salads, as desserts, or as snacks.

Eat more high-fiber cereal every day.

- Whole-grain bread products
- Brown rice
- Dried beans, peas, or lentils

Box A-2 **Eat Less Fat**

- Remove the skin from poultry before eating.
- Choose fish and chicken that have not been fried.
- Choose portion sizes of meat, poultry, and fish wisely. (Aim for 6 or fewer ounces, cooked, per day.)
- Choose lean red meat and trim all visible fat.
- Eat less fried foods.
- Consume two or more servings of skim or low-fat milk or milk products daily.
- Choose low-fat dairy products:
  - Skim or low-fat milk
  - Nonfat or low-fat yogurt
  - Low-fat cheese
  - Low-fat frozen yogurt
- Choose low-fat snacks such as fruits, raw vegetables, plain popcorn, pretzels, and low-fat baked goods.
- Reduce the amount of fats and oils used in cooking and as spreads.
- Choose reduced fat salad dressing.

Nutrition Assessment and Screening

Purpose

This appendix instructs community nutritionists and healthcare providers on how to use and interpret the Centers for Disease Control (CDC) growth charts to assess physical growth in children and adolescents. Nutritionists can use these charts to compare growth in infants, children, and adolescents with a nationally representative reference based on children of all ages and racial or ethnic groups. Comparing body measurements with the appropriate age- and gender-specific growth chart enables nutritionists to monitor growth and identify potential health or nutrition-related problems.

Community nutritionists can assess the physical growth of children using the child's weight, stature, length, and head circumference during routine screening. Although one measurement plotted on a growth chart can be used to screen children for nutritional risk, it does not provide adequate information to determine the child's growth pattern. When plotted correctly, a series of accurate weights and measurements of stature or length provide important information about a child's growth pattern, which may be influenced by such factors as gestational age, birth weight, and parental stature. It is important to consider parental stature before assuming there is a health or nutrition concern. Other factors, such as the presence of a chronic illness or special healthcare need, must be considered, and additional evaluation may be required.

How Is Body Mass Index Calculated and Interpreted?

Body mass index (BMI) is calculated the same way for both adults and children. The calculation is based on the formulas shown in Table B.1.

It is necessary to convert the weight and stature measurements to the appropriate decimal value. See Table B.2.

Examples: 40 lbs 4 oz = 40.25 lbs; 44½ in = 44.5 in

Aids for Calculation

Length

1 meter (m) = 39 in
1 centimeter (cm) = 0.4 in
1 inch (in) = 2.5 cm
1 foot (ft) = 30 cm

This information is from the Centers for Disease Control and Prevention. CDC Growth Chart Training. Available at: http://www.cdc.gov/nccdphp/dnpa/growthcharts/resources/growthchart.pdf, and http://www.cdc.gov/nccdphp/dnpa/bmi/adult_BMI/about_adult_BMI.htm. Accessed October 30, 2008.

TABLE B.1 Formulas for Calculating BMI

Measurement Units	Formula and Calculation
Kilograms and meters (or centimeters)	Formula: weight (kg) ÷ [height (m)]^2 With the metric system, the formula for BMI is weight in kilograms divided by height in meters squared. Because height is commonly measured in centimeters, divide height in centimeters by 100 to obtain height in meters. **Example: Weight = 68 kg, height = 165 cm (1.65 m)** **Calculation: $68 ÷ (1.65)^2 = 24.98$**
Pounds and inches	Formula: weight (lb) ÷ [height (in)]^2 × 703 Calculate BMI by dividing weight in pounds by height in inches squared and then multiplying by a conversion factor of 703. **Example: Weight = 150 lbs, height = 5'5" (65")** **Calculation: $[150 ÷ (65)^2] × 703 = 24.96$**

TABLE B.2 Decimal Conversions

Decimal Conversions

Fraction	Ounces	Decimal
1/8	2	0.125
1/4	4	0.25
3/8	6	0.375
1/2	8	0.5
5/8	10	0.625
3/4	12	0.75
7/8	14	0.875

Weight

1 kilogram (kg) = 1,000 g or 2.2 lb

1 gram (g) = 1/1,000 kg, 1,000 mg, or 0.035 oz

1 milligram (mg) = 1/1,000 g or 1,000 μg

1 microgram (μg) = 1/1,000 mg

1 pound (lb) = 16 oz, 454 g, or 0.45 kg

1 ounce (oz) = about 28 g

Assessing a Child's Growth Status

1. *Obtain accurate weights and measures.* When weighing and measuring children, follow procedures that yield accurate measurements and use equipment that is well maintained.
   - *Recumbent length:* Distance from the crown of the head to the bottom of the feet while the child is lying down
   - *Stature:* Height
2. *Select the appropriate growth chart.* Select which growth chart to use based on the age and gender of the child being weighed and measured.

Use the following information when measuring boys and girls in the *recumbent* position (should be limited to those less than 36 months old):

- Length-for-age
- Weight-for-age
- Head circumference-for-age
- Weight-for-length

Use the following information when determining the *stature* (standing height) of boys and girls ages 2 to 20 years:

- Weight-for-age
- Stature-for-age
- BMI-for-age

3. *Record data.* After selecting the appropriate chart and entering the client's name and record number, if appropriate, complete the data entry table.

   First, record information about factors obtained at the initial visit that influenced growth:
   - Enter mother's and father's stature as reported.
   - Enter the gestational age in weeks.

   For children under 2 years of age, it is important to reserve a line for recording the child's birth data. (Omit this step when using growth charts for children ages 2 to 20 years.)
   - Enter the date of birth.
   - Enter birth weight, length, and head circumference.
   - Add notable comments (e.g., breastfeeding).

   Record information obtained during the current visit, including today's date.

   Determine the child's age to the nearest month for infants and quarter year for children 2 to 20 years.
4. *Plot measurements.* On the appropriate growth chart, plot the measurements recorded in the data entry table for the current visit.
   - Find the child's age on the horizontal axis. When plotting weight-for-length, find the length on the horizontal axis. Use a straight edge or right-angle ruler to draw a vertical line up from that point.
   - Find the appropriate measurement (weight, length, stature, head circumference, or BMI) on the vertical axis. Use a straight edge or right-angle ruler to draw a horizontal line across from that point until it intersects the vertical line.
   - Make a small dot where the two lines intersect.

Overview of the CDC Anthropometric Indices

Weight, stature, length, and head circumference are used most often to assess size and growth (see Table B.3). When any of these measures is combined with age or length/stature the result is an anthropometric index (for example, weight-for-age). The CDC growth charts reflect five anthropometric indices that are gender-specific:

- *BMI-for-age* is an anthropometric index of weight and height combined with age. BMI-for-age is used to classify children and adolescents as underweight, overweight, or at risk of overweight.
- *Stature/length-for-age* describes linear growth relative to age. Stature- or length-for-age is used to define shortness or tallness.
- *Weight-for-age* reflects body weight relative to age and is influenced by recent changes in health or nutritional status. It is not used to classify infants, children, and adolescents as under- or overweight. However, it is important in early infancy for monitoring weight and helps explain changes in weight-for-length and BMI-for-age in older children.
- *Weight-for-length/stature* reflects body weight relative to length and requires no knowledge of age. It is an indicator to classify infants and young children as overweight and underweight.
- *Head circumference-for-age* is critical during infancy and can be charted up to 36 months of age. Head circumference measurements reflect brain size.

An appropriate reference population, accurate measurements, and age calculations are important factors when assessing childhood growth. Comparing body measurements to the appropriate age- and gender-specific growth chart enables community nutritionists and oth-

TABLE B.3	Anthropometric Indices	
Anthropometric Index	**Percentile Cut-Off Value**	**Nutritional Status Indicators**
BMI-for-age	≥ 95th percentile	Overweight
BMI-for-age	≥ 85th and <95th percentile	At risk of overweight
Weight-for-length/ stature	> 95th percentile	Overweight
BMI-for-age Weight-for-length	< 5th percentile	Underweight
Stature/length-for-age	< 5th percentile	Short stature
Head circumference-for-age	< 5th percentile > 95th percentile	Developmental problems

Source: Centers for Disease Control and Prevention. Anthropometric Indices. 2007. Available at: http://www.cdc.gov/nccdphp/dnpa/growthcharts/training/modules/module2/text/page6a.htm. Accessed February 25, 2008.

er healthcare professionals to monitor growth and identify potential health or nutrition-related problems.

Assessment of Overweight Children and Adolescents

Screening

The growth chart in Table B.4 shows the BMI-for-age pattern of a boy who became overweight early in his preschool years. On the BMI-for-age chart at age 2, he was at the 50th percentile; his BMI-for-age increased rapidly, crossing the 75th and 85th percentiles to become at risk of overweight at 3 and 4 years old. His BMI-for-age continued to increase to above the 95th percentile at ages 7, 11, and 13 years.

To understand how changes in weight and stature contributed to this boy's increase in BMI-for-age, it is helpful to review the weight-for-age and stature-for-age curves (see Table B.5). His stature-for-age at age 2

TABLE B.4	Sample BMI-for-Age Pattern Showing Early Onset of Overweight		
Age	Weight	Stature	BMI
2	28 ¼ lb	34 ¾ inches	16.4
3	38 ¼ lb	38 ⅞ inches	17.8
4	43 ½ lb	41 ⅝ inches	17.6
7	69 ¼ lb	50 ⅜ inches	19.2
11	111 lb	58 ⅛ inches	23.1
13	166 ¼ lb	65 ¾ inches	27

Source: Centers for Disease Control and Prevention. *Screening Children and Adolescents for Overweight.* 2007. Available at: http://www.cdc.gov/nccdphp/dnpa/growthcharts/training/modules/module3/text/page3c.htm. Accessed February 25, 2008.

TABLE B.5	Weight- and Stature-for-Age for the Same Child		
Age	Weight	Stature	BMI
2	28 ¼ lb	34 ¾ inches	16.4
3	38 ¼ lb	38 ⅞ inches	17.8
4	43 ½ lb	41 ⅝ inches	17.6
7	69 ¼ lb	50 ⅜ inches	19.2
11	111 lb	58 ⅛ inches	23.1
13	166 ¼ lb	65 ¾ inches	27

was above the 50th percentile and it increased to above the 90th percentile by age 13. However, his weight-for-age increased more rapidly than stature (from the 50th percentile at age 2 to greater than the 95th percentile at age 13), which contributed to the increase in BMI-for-age.

Assessment

When this boy was identified as at risk of overweight on the BMI-for-age chart at age 3, he should have received a medical assessment, as well as additional nutrition and physical activity assessments. The information from the assessments could have been used to target efforts for appropriate weight management goals to prevent the development of overweight.

Management of Overweight Children and Adolescents

Strategies used in a management plan are based on information obtained from the assessment. Weight loss is recommended if complications such as hyperlipidemia or hypertension are identified, and for children 7 years or older with a BMI-for-age ≥95th percentile. Otherwise, weight maintenance is recommended.

Source: Centers for Disease Control and Prevention. *Screening Children and Adolescents for Overweight.* 2007. Available at: http://www.cdc.gov/nccdphp/dnpa/growthcharts/training/modules/module3/text/page3c.htm. Accessed February 25, 2008.

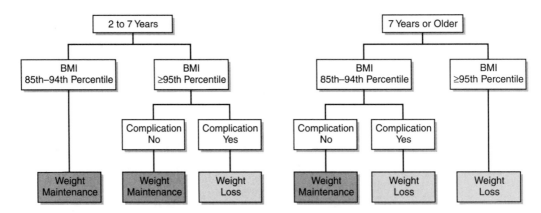

Recommendations for weight management for children and adolescents 2–20 years old.

Source: Barlow, SE, Dietz, WH. (1998). Obesity evaluation and treatment: expert committee recommendations. *Pediatrics* 102;e29. Reprinted with permission.

Complementary and Alternative Practices

The use of complementary and alternative medicine (CAM) has increased significantly. The World Health Organization (WHO) classified 65–80 percent of the world's healthcare services as "traditional medicine."[1] According to this information and looking at CAM from a world-wide perspective, more people use CAM than modern western medicine.[2]

The National Center for Complementary and Alternative Medicine (NCCAM), a part of the National Institutes of Health, defines CAM as "a group of diverse medical and healthcare systems, practices, and products that are not currently considered to be a component of conventional medicine [scientific medicine]."[3] Conventional medicine relies on modern scientific principles, modern technologies, and scientifically proven methods to prevent, diagnose and treat health conditions.[4] The list of what is considered CAM changes as the therapies that are proven to be safe and effective are implemented into conventional healthcare. *Complementary medicine* is non-conventional treatment used in addition to conventional therapies; for example, a physician may ask a patient to use tai chi or massage therapy in addition to prescribing medicine for anxiety or arthritis. *Alternative medicine* replaces conventional therapies; for instance, a cancer patient may use diets, supplements, herbs, and antioxidants instead of undergoing surgery, radiation, or chemotherapy that a conventional doctor recommended.

As stated by Gagne et al.:[5]

Over the past decade, the magnitude and quality of the CAM evidence base has increased, to the point where several dozen meta-analyses and systematic reviews have been conducted. Examples include systematic reviews of acupuncture for postoperative nausea, massage for low back pain, and ginkgo for dementia. Because of the large number of CAM therapies, and the wide range of conditions for which these therapies are used, a great deal of additional research is needed that can provide a comprehensive basis for establishing dependable end about CAM's safety and efficacy.

Herbal supplements are a type of dietary supplement that contains herbs either individually or in a blend. An herb (also called a botanical) is a plant or plant part used for its perfume, flavor, and/or therapeutic properties. In the United States, herbal and other dietary supplements are regulated by the U.S. Food and Drug Administration (FDA)

as foods. This means that herbs do not have to meet the same standards as drugs and over-the-counter medications for proof of safety, effectiveness, and what the FDA calls Good Manufacturing Practices.[6] Tables C.1 and C.2 present common alternative medical practices and popular herbal supplements.

There are several reasons why CAM is popular among consumers. The following are some of the factors responsible for the increased use of CAM:[2]

- It is familiar and easy to understand.
- It is noninvasive, with few side effects.
- Conventional modern medicine does not fully correspond to the individual's demands.
- The trend is toward a more holistic medical approach.
- Medical expenses are increasing.
- Many health conditions have no cure.
- It is harder for people to access conventional medicine.

One of the major roles and responsibilities of dietetics nutritionists is to advocate eating a wide variety of foods. Low levels of nutrients that do not exceed the Recommended Dietary Allowance (RDA) are recommended for clients who choose to use supplements. The use of dietary supplements should be based on well-accepted scientific evidence, and they should be recommended by physicians or dietitians. Also, consider the following recommendations when dealing with clients:[7]

- Appreciate the individuality of clients and that they have the right to be involved in decision making about their treatment.
- Learn from clients, all members of the primary healthcare team, and other resources in the community.
- Realize the importance of clear communication between different individuals involved in patient care.
- Recognize the importance of consulting with complementary therapists, including those utilizing therapeutic touch.
- Maintain an open mind about alternative approaches to client care.
- Understand that not all clients will disclose their use of complementary therapies to a conventional practitioner, and understand why this may be.
- Respect the rights of clients to choose different forms of therapy or to attend a range of practitioners.

TABLE C.1   Common Alternative Medical Practices

Type	Claims and Principles of Practice	Results of Scientific Research
Acupuncture	Used to treat a variety of common ailments. Based on an ancient Chinese medical practice in which thin needles are inserted into the skin or underlying muscles at specific places and stimulated to regulate the flow of "chi," the life force.	Although testing acupuncture is difficult, most studies fail to support its usefulness when not combined with conventional therapies. It may relieve nausea and vomiting associated with morning sickness and cancer chemotherapy. Acupuncture may stimulate the body to release natural pain-relieving compounds.
Ayurvedic medicine	According to ancient Hindu religious beliefs, people can achieve good health by meditating; eating grains, *ghee* (a form of butter), milk, fruits, and vegetables; and using herbs. Lack of balance between "energies" causes health problems. Fasting and enemas are used to treat severe ailments.	Meditation relieves stress; fruits, vegetables, and dairy products are nutritious foods; and some herbs have medicinal value. Ghee, however, can be fattening, and fasting is not a healthy practice. Enemas are unnecessary for good health and should be used only under a physician's instructions.
Chiropractic medicine	According to some chiropractors, misaligned spinal bones cause disease. Spinal manipulation prevents or cures disease by correcting the spine. Other practitioners use spinal manipulation, but accept the germ theory of disease.	Can be effective in treating certain types of back pain, but some spinal conditions require medications and surgery that only a physician can provide. There is no scientific evidence that all diseases can be treated by spinal adjustment.
Homeopathy	Use of extremely dilute solutions of natural substances to treat specific illness symptoms. The U.S. Congress passed a law in 1938 declaring that homeopathic remedies are to be regulated by the FDA in the same manner as nonprescription, over-the-counter (OTC) drugs, which means that they can be purchased without a physician's prescription.	Studies do not indicate that homeopathy is effective.
Naturopathy or natural medicine	Practice based on natural healing. Practitioners believe diseases occur as the body rids itself of wastes and toxins. Treatments include fasting, enemas, acupuncture, and "natural" drugs.	There is no standardized training for practitioners, who are called naturopaths. They may recommend patients ignore conventional medical advice and practices, which can be harmful.
Reflexology or zone therapy	Specific areas of the hands and feet correspond to certain organs. To alleviate pain or treat certain diseases, practitioners press on the area that is related to the affected tissues.	Scientific evidence does not indicate that pressing on body parts is an effective method for diagnosing or treating ailments.
Biofield therapies	These practices aim to affect energy fields that surround and penetrate the human body. Some of these therapies use manipulation such as touch, reiki, and qi gong.	The existence of such fields has not been scientifically proven.
Bioelectro magnetic	This therapy uses unconventional electrical energy, magnetic energy, or alternating-current or direct-current fields to stimulate wound and bone healing.	The efficacy of this treatment has not been scientifically proven.
Mind–body medicine	These practices use a variety of techniques to improve mind capacity, and thus to affect the symptoms and functions of the body. They include behavioral therapy, mental healing (prayer, hypnosis, meditation, imagery, humor, yoga), and creative outlets (music, art, dance, tai chi).	Some of the practices, such as support groups and cognitive improvement, are considered CAM. There is evidence that mind–body interventions can be effective in the treatment of coronary artery disease, cardiac rehabilitation, chronic pain management, and quality of life. They also improve individuals' mood and immune system and relieve stress.
Chelation therapy	Chelation therapy is an investigational therapy using a man-made amino acid, ethylene diamine tetra-acetic acid (EDTA). It is added to the blood through a vein to treat heart disease.	An international research study is now testing whether chelation therapy is safe and effective for treating heart disease. However, this has not been scientifically proven.

TABLE C.1	(*Continued*)		
Type	**Claims and Principles of Practice**		**Results of Scientific Research**
Orthomolecular medicine	This practice is based on the premise that many diseases and abnormalities result from varying biochemical and/or chemical needs specific to each individual. It holds that they can be prevented, treated, or sometimes cured by achieving optimum levels for that individual's body of various natural chemical substances. It normally employs such dietary elements as vitamins, minerals, amino acids, trace elements, and essential fatty acids.		There is not sufficient evidence for clinical use, scientific foundations are weak, and studies that have been performed are too few.
Aromatherapy	This is a generic term that refers to any of the various traditions' use of essential oils and other scented compounds from plants to improve a person's mood or health. It is sometimes used in combination with other alternative medical practices and spiritual beliefs.		The consensus among most medical professionals in the United States and England is that although pleasant scents can improve relaxation, there is currently insufficient scientific proof of the effectiveness of aromatherapy in general.

Source: Alters S, Schiff W. *Essential Concepts for Health Living*, 4th ed. Sudbury, MA: Jones and Bartlett; 2006.

TABLE C.2	**Popular Herbal Supplements**		
Supplement	**Common Claims**	**Uses**	**Risks**
St. John's wort	Relieves depression.	Can reduce mild to moderate depression symptoms; no value for major depression.	Can interfere with birth control pills and other prescribed medicines, increase sensitivity to sunlight, and cause stomach upset.
Saw palmetto	Improves urine flow.	May reduce symptoms of prostate enlargement that are not caused by cancer.	May interfere with PSA test to detect prostate cancer.
Feverfew	Relieves headaches, fever, and arthritis pain.	Contains a chemical that may prevent migraines or reduce their severity.	May cause dangerous interactions with aspirin or Coumadin (a prescription drug).
Echinacea	Prevents colds and influenza.	Does not prevent colds or reduce their severity.	May cause allergic response and be a liver toxin.
Ginkgo biloba	Enhances memory and sense of well-being; prevents dementia.	May mildly improve mental performance but is ineffective as a treatment for Alzheimer's disease.	May interfere with normal blood clotting, cause intestinal upset, and increase blood pressure.
Ginseng	Enhances sexual, mental, and exercise performance; increases energy; relieves stress and depression.	Has no mood-enhancing effect. Asian ginsengs may improve immune system functioning and reduce fatigue. Lack of scientific findings to support benefits in humans.	Can cause "jitters," insomnia, hypertension, and diarrhea and can be addictive; can be contaminated with pesticides and the toxic mineral lead.
Yohimbe	Enchances muscle development and performance/	Dilates blood vessels but has no beneficial effects on muscle growth or sex drive of humans, prevention of erectile dysfunction, or reduction of adipose tissues.	Can produce abnormal behavior, high blood pressure, and heart attacks. Large amount can cause anxiety reactions.

| | TABLE C.2 | (Continued) |

Supplement	Common Claims	Uses	Risks
Ma huang (ephedra)	Enhances weight loss and muscle growth.	Increases heart rate and blood pressure; contains the stimulant ephedrine.	Has been linked to headaches, heart attacks, strokes, and death.
Guarana	Boosts energy and enhances weight loss.	Acts as a stimulant drug.	May cause nausea, anxiety, and irregular heartbeat.
Kava	Relieves anxiety and induces sleep.	Acts as a depressant drug.	May cause serious liver damage; do not use when driving.
Aloe	Heals damaged skin.	Used externally to relieve skin discomforts and internally as a laxative.	Research suggests it can negatively affect healing.
Black cohosh	Remedies the symptoms of premenstrual tension, menopause, and other gynecological problems.	Reduces gynecological problems.	Inhibits iron absorption; it may increase or prolong bleeding.
Chaparral leaves	Allegedly cures cancer, venereal disease, arthritis, tuberculosis, bowel cramps, rheumatism, and colds.	Chaparral tea is an old Indian remedy for cancer.	Risk of liver and kidney problems.
Garlic bulbs	Prevent heart disease and cancer, lower blood cholesterol and blood pressure.	Used for cardiovascular and cancer benefits.	Excessive amounts can thin the blood similar to the effect of aspirin, and cause diarrhea, nausea, and indigestion.
Valerian	A sedative anti-convulsant. It sedates agitated persons and stimulates fatigued persons.	Used for migraine treatment and pain.	Large doses or chronic use may result in stomachaches, apathy, and feelings of mental dullness or mild depression.
Ginger	Used for colic and nausea. It is classified as a stimulant.	It is used to control the nausea associated with cancer caused by chemotherapy; it may be directly involved in the treatment of cancer.	Allergic reactions to ginger can result in a rash. It is generally recognized as safe.
Goldenseal	Used as an anti-microbal, anti-inflammatory, muscle stimulant, and laxative.	Used for atonic dyspepsia, chronic constipation, hepatic congestion, urinary infection, and cirrhosis of the liver.	Taking goldenseal over a long period of time can reduce absorption of B vitamins. It should not be used if an infection is at an early stage or there are more chills than fever.

Source: Modified from Alters S, Schiff W. *Essential Concepts for Health Living*, 4th ed. Sudbury, MA: Jones and Bartlett; 2006. And from National Institutes of Health, National Center for Complementary Alternative Medicine. Understanding CAM. Available at: http://nccam.nih.gov/health. Accessed December 17, 2007.

References

1. Jonas WB. Researching alternative medicine. *Nat Med.* 1997;3:824–882.

2. Suzuki N. Complementary and alternative medicine: a Japanese perspective. *Evid Based Complement Alternat Med.* 2004;1(2)113.

3. National Center for Complementary and Alternative Medicine. What Is CAM? Available at: http://nccam.nih.gov/health/whatiscam. Accessed November 14, 2008.

4. Alters S, Schiff W. *Essential Concepts for Health Living*, 4th ed. Sudbury, MA: Jones and Bartlett; 2006.

5. Gagne L, Schnurr J, Star B, Premkumar K, Epstein M. *Complementary and Alternative Medicine: Description of Vertical Theme.* Saskatoon, SK: College of Medicine, University of Saskatchewan; 2006.

6. National Center for Complementary and Alternative Medicine. Herbal Supplements: Consider Safety, Too. Available at: http://nccam.nih.gov/health/supplement-safety. Accessed November 14, 2008.

7. Molassiotis A, Fernandez-Ortega P, Pud D, et al. Use of complementary and alternative medicine in cancer patients: a European survey. *Ann Oncol.* 2005;16(4):655.

APPENDIX D

Principles of the Ethical Practice of Public Health

TABLE D.1

1.	Public health should address principally the fundamental causes of disease and requirements for health, aiming to prevent adverse health outcomes.
2.	Public health should achieve community health in a way that respects the rights of individuals in the community.
3.	Public health policies, programs, and priorities should be developed and evaluated through processes that ensure an opportunity for input from community members.
4.	Public health should advocate and work for the empowerment of disenfranchised community members, aiming to ensure that the basic resources and conditions necessary for health are accessible to all.
5.	Public health should seek the information needed to implement effective policies and programs that protect and promote health.
6.	Public health institutions should provide communities with the information they have that is needed for decisions on policies or programs and should obtain the community's consent for their implementation.
7.	Public health institutions should act in a timely manner on the information they have within the resources and the mandate given to them by the public.
8.	Public health programs and policies should incorporate a variety of approaches that anticipate and respect diverse values, beliefs, and cultures in the community.
9.	Public health programs and policies should be implemented in a manner that most enhances the physical and social environment.
10.	Public health institutions should protect the confidentiality of information that can bring harm to an individual or community if made public. Exceptions must be justified on the basis of the high likelihood of significant harm to the individual or others.
11.	Public health institutions should ensure the professional competence of their employees.
12.	Public health institutions and their employees should engage in collaborations and affiliations in ways that build the public's trust and the institution's effectiveness.

Source: Public Health Leadership Society. *Principles of the Ethical Practice of Public Health*, Version 2.2. New Orleans, LA: Author; 2002:7. Reprinted with permission.

APPENDIX E

MyPyramid

Anatomy of MyPyramid

One size doesn't fit all

USDA's new MyPyramid symbolizes a personalized approach to healthy eating and physical activity. The symbol has been designed to be simple. It has been developed to remind consumers to make healthy food choices and to be active every day. The different parts of the symbol are described below.

Activity
Activity is represented by the steps and the person climbing them, as a reminder of the importance of daily physical activity.

Moderation
Moderation is represented by the narrowing of each food group from bottom to top. The wider base stands for foods with little or no solid fats or added sugars. These should be selected more often. The narrower top area stands for foods containing more added sugars and solid fats. The more active you are, the more of these foods can fit into your diet.

Personalization
Personalization is shown by the person on the steps, the slogan, and the URL. Find the kinds and amounts of food to eat each day at MyPyramid.gov.

Proportionality
Proportionality is shown by the different widths of the food group bands. The widths suggest how much food a person should choose from each group. The widths are just a general guide, not exact proportions. Check the Web site for how much is right for you.

Variety
Variety is symbolized by the 6 color bands representing the 5 food groups of the Pyramid and oils. This illustrates that foods from all groups are needed each day for good health.

Gradual Improvement
Gradual improvement is encouraged by the slogan. It suggests that individuals can benefit from taking small steps to improve their diet and lifestyle each day.

MyPyramid.gov
STEPS TO A HEALTHIER YOU

USDA U.S. Department of Agriculture
Center for Nutrition Policy
and Promotion
April 2005 CNPP-16

USDA is an equal opportunity provider and employer.

GRAINS | VEGETABLES | FRUITS | OILS | MILK | MEAT & BEANS

Source: U.S. Department of Agriculture. www.mypyramid.gov.

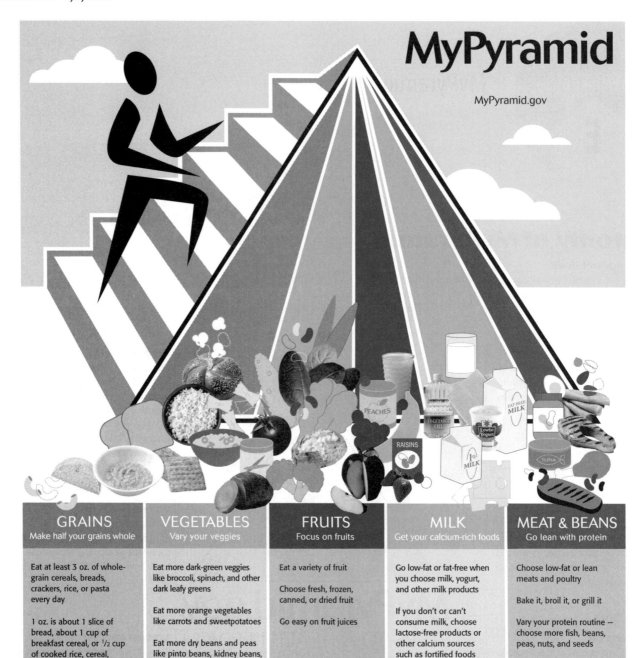

MyPyramid

MyPyramid.gov

GRAINS	VEGETABLES	FRUITS	MILK	MEAT & BEANS
Make half your grains whole	Vary your veggies	Focus on fruits	Get your calcium-rich foods	Go lean with protein
Eat at least 3 oz. of whole-grain cereals, breads, crackers, rice, or pasta every day 1 oz. is about 1 slice of bread, about 1 cup of breakfast cereal, or ½ cup of cooked rice, cereal, or pasta	Eat more dark-green veggies like broccoli, spinach, and other dark leafy greens Eat more orange vegetables like carrots and sweetpotatoes Eat more dry beans and peas like pinto beans, kidney beans, and lentils	Eat a variety of fruit Choose fresh, frozen, canned, or dried fruit Go easy on fruit juices	Go low-fat or fat-free when you choose milk, yogurt, and other milk products If you don't or can't consume milk, choose lactose-free products or other calcium sources such as fortified foods and beverages	Choose low-fat or lean meats and poultry Bake it, broil it, or grill it Vary your protein routine — choose more fish, beans, peas, nuts, and seeds

For a 2,000-calorie diet, you need the amounts below from each food group. To find the amounts that are right for you, go to MyPyramid.gov.

Eat 6 oz. every day	Eat 2½ cups every day	Eat 2 cups every day	Get 3 cups every day; for kids aged 2 to 8, it's 2	Eat 5½ oz. every day

Find your balance between food and physical activity
- Be sure to stay within your daily calorie needs.
- Be physically active for at least 30 minutes most days of the week.
- About 60 minutes a day of physical activity may be needed to prevent weight gain.
- For sustaining weight loss, at least 60 to 90 minutes a day of physical activity may be required.
- Children and teenagers should be physically active for 60 minutes every day, or most days.

Know the limits on fats, sugars, and salt (sodium)
- Make most of your fat sources from fish, nuts, and vegetable oils.
- Limit solid fats like butter, margarine, shortening, and lard, as well as foods that contain these.
- Check the Nutrition Facts label to keep saturated fats, *trans* fats, and sodium low.
- Choose food and beverages low in added sugars. Added sugars contribute calories with few, if any, nutrients.

Source: U.S. Department of Agriculture. www.mypyramid.gov.

APPENDIX F

Canada's Food Guide

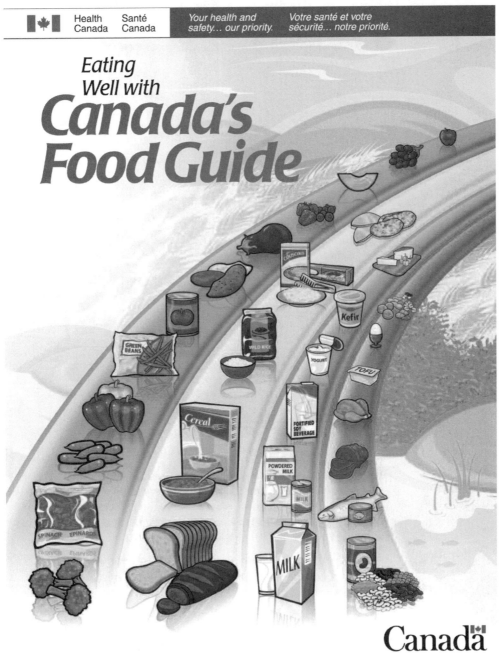

Source: Eating Well with Canada's Food Guide. (2007). Health Canada. Reproduced with the permission of the Minister of Public Works and Government Services Canada, 2008.

Recommended Number of *Food Guide Servings* per Day

	Children			Teens		Adults			
Age in Years	2-3	4-8	9-13	14-18		19-50		51+	
Sex	Girls and Boys			Females	Males	Females	Males	Females	Males
Vegetables and Fruit	4	5	6	7	8	7-8	8-10	7	7
Grain Products	3	4	6	6	7	6-7	8	6	7
Milk and Alternatives	2	2	3-4	3-4	3-4	2	2	3	3
Meat and Alternatives	1	1	1-2	2	3	2	3	2	3

The chart above shows how many Food Guide Servings you need from each of the four food groups every day.

Having the amount and type of food recommended and following the tips in *Canada's Food Guide* will help:

- Meet your needs for vitamins, minerals and other nutrients.
- Reduce your risk of obesity, type 2 diabetes, heart disease, certain types of cancer and osteoporosis.
- Contribute to your overall health and vitality.

What is One Food Guide Serving?
Look at the examples below.

Fresh, frozen or canned vegetables
125 mL (½ cup)

Leafy vegetables
Cooked: 125 mL (½ cup)
Raw: 250 mL (1 cup)

Fresh, frozen or canned fruits
1 fruit or 125 mL (½ cup)

100% Juice
125 mL (½ cup)

Bread
1 slice (35 g)

Bagel
½ bagel (45 g)

Flat breads
½ pita or ½ tortilla (35 g)

Cooked rice, bulgur or quinoa
125 mL (½ cup)

Cereal
Cold: 30 g
Hot: 175 mL (¾ cup)

Cooked pasta or couscous
125 mL (½ cup)

Milk or powdered milk (reconstituted)
250 mL (1 cup)

Canned milk (evaporated)
125 mL (½ cup)

Fortified soy beverage
250 mL (1 cup)

Yogurt
175 g
(¾ cup)

Kefir
175 g
(¾ cup)

Cheese
50 g (1 ½ oz.)

Cooked fish, shellfish, poultry, lean meat
75 g (2 ½ oz.)/125 mL (½ cup)

Cooked legumes
175 mL (¾ cup)

Tofu
150 g or
175 mL (¾ cup)

Eggs
2 eggs

Peanut or nut butters
30 mL (2 Tbsp)

Shelled nuts and seeds
60 mL (¼ cup)

Oils and Fats

- Include a small amount – 30 to 45 mL (2 to 3 Tbsp) – of unsaturated fat each day. This includes oil used for cooking, salad dressings, margarine and mayonnaise.
- Use vegetable oils such as canola, olive and soybean.
- Choose soft margarines that are low in saturated and trans fats.
- Limit butter, hard margarine, lard and shortening.

Make each Food Guide Serving count...
wherever you are – at home, at school, at work or when eating out!

▸ **Eat at least one dark green and one orange vegetable each day.**
- Go for dark green vegetables such as broccoli, romaine lettuce and spinach.
- Go for orange vegetables such as carrots, sweet potatoes and winter squash.

▸ **Choose vegetables and fruit prepared with little or no added fat, sugar or salt.**
- Enjoy vegetables steamed, baked or stir-fried instead of deep-fried.

▸ **Have vegetables and fruit more often than juice.**

▸ **Make at least half of your grain products whole grain each day.**
- Eat a variety of whole grains such as barley, brown rice, oats, quinoa and wild rice.
- Enjoy whole grain breads, oatmeal or whole wheat pasta.

▸ **Choose grain products that are lower in fat, sugar or salt.**
- Compare the Nutrition Facts table on labels to make wise choices.
- Enjoy the true taste of grain products. When adding sauces or spreads, use small amounts.

▸ **Drink skim, 1%, or 2% milk each day.**
- Have 500 mL (2 cups) of milk every day for adequate vitamin D.
- Drink fortified soy beverages if you do not drink milk.

▸ **Select lower fat milk alternatives.**
- Compare the Nutrition Facts table on yogurts or cheeses to make wise choices.

▸ **Have meat alternatives such as beans, lentils and tofu often.**

▸ **Eat at least two Food Guide Servings of fish each week.***
- Choose fish such as char, herring, mackerel, salmon, sardines and trout.

▸ **Select lean meat and alternatives prepared with little or no added fat or salt.**
- Trim the visible fat from meats. Remove the skin on poultry.
- Use cooking methods such as roasting, baking or poaching that require little or no added fat.
- If you eat luncheon meats, sausages or prepackaged meats, choose those lower in salt (sodium) and fat.

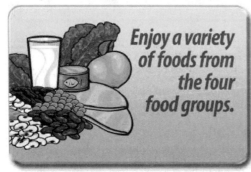

Enjoy a variety of foods from the four food groups.

Satisfy your thirst with water!

Drink water regularly. It's a calorie-free way to quench your thirst. Drink more water in hot weather or when you are very active.

* Health Canada provides advice for limiting exposure to mercury from certain types of fish. Refer to www.healthcanada.gc.ca for the latest information.

Advice for different ages and stages...

Children

Following *Canada's Food Guide* helps children grow and thrive.

Young children have small appetites and need calories for growth and development.

- Serve small nutritious meals and snacks each day.

- Do not restrict nutritious foods because of their fat content. Offer a variety of foods from the four food groups.

- Most of all... be a good role model.

Women of childbearing age

All women who could become pregnant and those who are pregnant or breastfeeding need a multivitamin containing **folic acid** every day. Pregnant women need to ensure that their multivitamin also contains **iron**. A health care professional can help you find the multivitamin that's right for you.

Pregnant and breastfeeding women need more calories. Include an extra 2 to 3 Food Guide Servings each day.

Here are two examples:
- Have fruit and yogurt for a snack, or

- Have an extra slice of toast at breakfast and an extra glass of milk at supper.

Men and women over 50

The need for **vitamin D** increases after the age of 50.

In addition to following *Canada's Food Guide*, everyone over the age of 50 should take a daily vitamin D supplement of 10 µg (400 IU).

How do I count Food Guide Servings in a meal?

Here is an example:

Vegetable and beef stir-fry with rice, a glass of milk and an apple for dessert		
250 mL (1 cup) mixed broccoli, carrot and sweet red pepper	=	2 **Vegetables and Fruit** Food Guide Servings
75 g (2 ½ oz.) lean beef	=	1 **Meat and Alternatives** Food Guide Serving
250 mL (1 cup) brown rice	=	2 **Grain Products** Food Guide Servings
5 mL (1 tsp) canola oil	=	part of your **Oils and Fats** intake for the day
250 mL (1 cup) 1% milk	=	1 **Milk and Alternatives** Food Guide Serving
1 apple	=	1 **Vegetables and Fruit** Food Guide Serving

Eat well and be active today and every day!

The benefits of eating well and being active include:

- Better overall health.
- Lower risk of disease.
- A healthy body weight.
- Feeling and looking better.
- More energy.
- Stronger muscles and bones.

Be active

To be active every day is a step towards better health and a healthy body weight.

Canada's Physical Activity Guide recommends building 30 to 60 minutes of moderate physical activity into daily life for adults and at least 90 minutes a day for children and youth. You don't have to do it all at once. Add it up in periods of at least 10 minutes at a time for adults and five minutes at a time for children and youth.

Start slowly and build up.

Eat well

Another important step towards better health and a healthy body weight is to follow *Canada's Food Guide* by:

- Eating the recommended amount and type of food each day.
- Limiting foods and beverages high in calories, fat, sugar or salt (sodium) such as cakes and pastries, chocolate and candies, cookies and granola bars, doughnuts and muffins, ice cream and frozen desserts, french fries, potato chips, nachos and other salty snacks, alcohol, fruit flavoured drinks, soft drinks, sports and energy drinks, and sweetened hot or cold drinks.

Read the label

- Compare the Nutrition Facts table on food labels to choose products that contain less fat, saturated fat, trans fat, sugar and sodium.
- Keep in mind that the calories and nutrients listed are for the amount of food found at the top of the Nutrition Facts table.

Nutrition Facts		
Per 0 mL (0 g)		
Amount		% Daily Value
Calories 0		
Fat 0 g		0 %
Saturates 0 g		0 %
+ Trans 0 g		
Cholesterol 0 mg		
Sodium 0 mg		0 %
Carbohydrate 0 g		0 %
Fibre 0 g		0 %
Sugars 0 g		
Protein 0 g		
Vitamin A 0 %	Vitamin C	0 %
Calcium 0 %	Iron	0 %

Limit trans fat

When a Nutrition Facts table is not available, ask for nutrition information to choose foods lower in trans and saturated fats.

Take a step today...

- ✓ Have breakfast every day. It may help control your hunger later in the day.
- ✓ Walk wherever you can – get off the bus early, use the stairs.
- ✓ Benefit from eating vegetables and fruit at all meals and as snacks.
- ✓ Spend less time being inactive such as watching TV or playing computer games.
- ✓ Request nutrition information about menu items when eating out to help you make healthier choices.
- ✓ Enjoy eating with family and friends!
- ✓ Take time to eat and savour every bite!

For more information, interactive tools, or additional copies visit Canada's Food Guide on-line at:
www.healthcanada.gc.ca/foodguide

or contact:
Publications
Health Canada
Ottawa, Ontario K1A 0K9
E-Mail: publications@hc-sc.gc.ca
Tel.: 1-866-225-0709
Fax: (613) 941-5366
TTY: 1-800-267-1245

Également disponible en français sous le titre :
Bien manger avec le Guide alimentaire canadien

This publication can be made available on request on diskette, large print, audio-cassette and braille.

Glossary

24-hour recall A method of dietary assessment in which the individual is asked to remember everything eaten during the past 24 hours.

5-year survival rate Individuals who are alive and without recurrence of cancer 5 years after diagnosis.

acculturation Repeated exposure to influences from a different culture. The process is related to age, education, frequency of interaction, and income and occurs on a continuum.

action plan A concise statement of the methods, activities, or intervention strategies to be undertaken.

activities of daily living (ADL) A person's ability to perform personal care, either independently or with help. It helps to evaluate an older person's ability to care for him- or herself.

adenomas Cancers that arise from glandular tissues.

adolescence The period of life between 12 and 19 years of age.

adult learning Adults gaining knowledge and expertise.

advertising The methods used to present health and nutrition promotion programs to targeted communities.

affective domain The domain of learning that includes the way individuals deal with things emotionally, such as feelings, values, appreciation, enthusiasm, motivation, and attitude. It also consists of changes in attitudes and the development of values.

After-School Snack Program Gives children a nutritional enhancement and encourages them to participate in supervised activities that are safe and filled with learning opportunities.

Alzheimer's disease (senile dementia of the Alzheimer's type) A disease that results in the relentless and irreversible loss of mental function.

android obesity Excess storage of fat, mainly in the abdominal area.

anorexia nervosa An eating disorder characterized by extreme weight loss, poor body image, and irrational fears of weight gain and obesity.

anorexia of aging The loss of appetite and wasting associated with old age.

anthropometry The measurement of human body size, weight, and proportions.

antioxidants Vitamins C and E and beta-carotene, which neutralize free radicals and other reactive chemicals and terminate harmful chemical reactions.

assessment Determining nutritional status by analyzing clinical, dietary, and social history; anthropometric data; biochemical data; and drug–nutrient interactions.

atherosclerosis A common form of arteriosclerosis where plaque forms within the intima of medium and large arteries; a group of diseases characterized by thickening and loss of elasticity of arterial walls. It is also a progressive, complex disease that often begins in childhood and adolescence and is related to high serum total cholesterol levels.

basal metabolic rate (BMR) The minimum amount of energy that an awake, fasted resting body needs to maintain itself; often used interchangeably with resting metabolic rate (RMR). BMR measurements are performed in a warm room in the morning before the individual rises, and at least 12 hours after the last food intake and activity.

basic ethical principles General judgments that serve as a basic justification for the particular ethical prescriptions and evaluations of human actions.

behavior The effects of nutrition education (such as the intake of specific foods) or actual behaviors (such as eating five fruits and vegetables per day).

behavior modification A process used to gradually and permanently change habitual behaviors.

beneficence Ethical principle stating that one should do good and prevent or avoid doing harm.

binge eating This disorder is characterized by consuming large quantities of food in a very short period of time until the individual is uncomfortably full, which normally is not followed by vomiting or the use of laxatives. The individual typically feels out of control during a binge episode, followed by feelings of guilt and shame. People must experience eating binges twice a week on average for over 6 months to qualify for this diagnosis.

block grant A sum of money the federal government gives to a state or local government. The federal government suggests a general purpose for the use of the money (e.g., community services or social services) as authorized by legislation, but permits the state or local area to spend the money without meeting specific conditions.

body mass index (BMI) Weight (kg)/height (m2); an index calculated by a ratio of height to weight, used as a measure of obesity.

budget Financial plan that shows expenses and income related to a specific service.

bulimia nervosa An eating disorder characterized by recurrent episodes of rapid, uncontrolled eating of large amounts of food in a short period of time. Purging often follows episodes of binge eating.

business marketing The process of creating, distributing, promoting, and pricing goods, services, and ideas to facilitate satisfying exchange relationships with customers in a dynamic environment.

capitation A payment method in which each provider, such as an HMO, receives a flat annual fee for each individual, regardless of how often services are used.

carcinogen An agent that can cause cancer.

carcinogenic Producing cancer; a substance that can produce or enhance the development of cancer.

cesarean section Surgical childbirth in which the infant is delivered through an incision in the woman's abdomen and uterus.

Child and Adult Care Food Program Serves nutritious meals and snacks to eligible children and adults who are enrolled for care at participating childcare centers, daycare homes, and adult daycare centers.

childhood disability Children and adolescents who have or are at increased risk for a chronic physical, developmental, behavioral, or emotional condition and who require health and related services.

chronic condition An occurrence of a disease that cannot be cured and extends over a period of time.

code of ethics A set of statements encompassing rules that apply to people in professional roles.

Code of Federal Regulations (CFR) A comprehensive summary of all regulations currently in force.

cognitive domain The domain of learning that involves knowledge and the development of intellectual skills. This includes the recall or recognition of specific facts, procedural patterns, and concepts that serve in the development of intellectual abilities and skills.

collaboration Mutual sharing and working together to achieve common goals in such a way that all persons or groups are recognized and growth is enhanced.

colostrum The first fluid secreted by the breast during late pregnancy and the first few days after birth. This thick fluid is rich in immune factors and protein.

Commodity Supplemental Food Program (CSFP) Provides food and administrative funds to states to supplement the diets of low-income pregnant and breastfeeding women, infants, and children up to age 6, and elderly people at least 60 years of age.

communication A process of information sharing in which those involved in the communication share a common set of rules.

community A group of people who share a common geographical location, values, culture, or languages.

community nutrition An area of nutrition that addresses the entire range of food and nutrition issues related to preventing disease and improving the health of individuals, families, and the community.

community nutrition assessment An attempt to evaluate the nutritional status of individuals or populations through measurements of food and nutrient intake and evaluation of nutrition-related health indicators.

community nutrition research Organized study of a trend at both the basic and more applied levels that focuses on social, structural, and physical environmental inequities through active involvement of community members.

competitive foods Any food sold in competition with U.S. Department of Agriculture school meals and that are considered as "foods of minimal nutritional value" (FMNV) available at concession stands, vending machines, and fundraisers that are in direct competition with the Child Nutrition Program during meal services anywhere on campus.

compression of morbidity The postponement of the onset of chronic disease such that disability occupies a smaller and smaller proportion of the life span.

conceptual framework A visual way of demonstrating relationships that are known and ones that have not been investigated but that may be the focus of the project.

contract A written agreement between a grantee and a third party to acquire routine goods and services. The contract could stipulate any number of things, such as that the grantee must submit a quarterly and/or final report when the project is completed, that there was a reduction in the amount requested, or that the president of the organization must sign the contract.

coordination Efficient management of services without gaps or overlaps.

co-payment A specified amount that an insured individual must pay for a specified service or procedure (e.g., $20 for an office visit).

cost-benefit analysis The analytic process whereby the costs and benefits of a program are identified and measured in monetary (dollar) terms.

cultural competence The ability to increase one's understanding of and appreciation for cultural differences and commonalities by developing knowledge and interpersonal skills.

cultural sensitivity Planning interventions that are relevant and acceptable within the cultural framework of the population to be reached.

culture The customary beliefs, social forms, and material traits of a racial, religious, or social group.

deductible The amount an individual must pay out-of-pocket, usually yearly on a calendar-year basis, before insurance will begin to cover expenses.

deliberate sampling Inviting specific people to participate in a study.

demography An analytic tool used to measure a population by recording births, deaths, age distribution, and other vital statistics.

demonstration grant A grant given to show a new approach to delivering a community health program or to demonstrate a technique.

dental caries Tooth decay that results from formula or juice (and even human milk) bathing the teeth as the child sleeps with a bottle in his or her mouth.

dependent variables Outcomes that are measured in an experiment.

developed countries Countries that have reached a stage of economic development characterized by the growth of industrialization. The amount of money made by the population (national income) is enough to pay for schools, hospitals, and other services (domestic savings).

developing countries Countries that have not reached the stage of economic development characterized by the growth of industrialization. The amount of money made (national income) is less than the amount of money needed to pay for schools, hospitals, and other services (domestic savings).

diabetes mellitus A disease caused by insufficient insulin secretion by the pancreas or insulin resistance by body tissues causing high blood glucose level.

diet history A detailed dietary assessment, which may include a 24-hour recall, food frequency questionnaire, and additional information such as weight history, previous diet changes, use of supplements, and food intolerances.

dietary acculturation The process that occurs when members of a minority group adopt the eating patterns/food choices of the majority group.

dietary supplements Products made of one or more of the essential nutrients, such as vitamins, minerals, and protein. The Dietary Supplement Health and Education Act of 1994 (DSHEA) expanded the definition, stating that herbs or other botanicals (except tobacco), and any dietary substance that can be used to supplement the diet were to be included in the definition.

drug A chemical compound (except devices) intended for use in the diagnosis, cure, mitigation, treatment, or prevention of disease and articles (other than food) intended to affect the structure or function of the body.

eclampsia Advanced pregnancy-induced hypertension (PIH) that is characterized by convulsions.

Elderly Nutrition Program A federal program established in 1965 to provide congregate and home-delivered meals and related nutrition services to older adults.

electronic benefit transfer (EBT) system An electronic system that allows a recipient to authorize transfer of their government benefits from a federal account to a retailer.

Emergency Food Assistance Program (TEFAP) Distributes commodities to state agencies (food banks), which distribute the foods to the public including homeless people via soup kitchens and food pantries.

employment-based health insurance Coverage offered through one's own employment or the employment of a relative.

entitlement programs Programs funded by Congress for persons who qualify due to level of income or other eligibility requirements; food stamps and the majority of other food assistance programs are included in this category.

equipment grant A grant for small instruments for a start-up fund.

ethical decision making Making decisions in an orderly process that considers ethical principles, individual values, and professional obligations.

ethics The science or study of moral values; also a code of principles and ideals that guides action.

ethnic The commonality of a group expressed by its nationality, language, or race.

ethnocentrism The belief that one's own group view of the world is superior to that of others.

exploratory research Carrying out preliminary research to learn more about the market before any formal research survey is conducted.

exposure Characteristics or agents (e.g., food, medications, sunlight) that the participant comes in contact with that may be related to disease risk.

famine Widespread lack of access to food due to a disaster or war that causes a collapse in the food production and marketing systems.

Federal Register A weekly publication that contains all regulations, proposed regulations, and the Code of Federal Regulations (CFR).

fee-for-service plans The traditional type of healthcare policy; the physician sets a price for each type of service delivered, and then the patient or his or her insurer pays this price.

ferritin A complex of iron and apoferritin that is a major storage form of iron.

fetal alcohol syndrome The cluster of symptoms seen in an infant or a child whose mother consumed excessive amounts of alcohol during pregnancy.

fetus The developing infant from 8 weeks after conception until birth.

Food Distribution Disaster Assistance programs Distribute commodity foods directly to households that are in need as a result of an emergency. Such direct distribution takes place when normal commercial food supply channels, such as grocery stores, have been disrupted, damaged, or destroyed, or can't function (e.g., lack of electricity).

Food Distribution Program on Indian Reservations (FDPIR) The USDA purchases commodities and ships them to Indian Tribal Organizations (ITOs) to help low-income American Indian and non-Indian households living on a reservation to maintain a nutritionally balanced diet.

food frequency questionnaire A method of dietary assessment in which the questions relate to how often foods are consumed.

food insecurity The inability to obtain sufficient food for any reason.

food record A written record of the amounts of all foods and liquids consumed during a time period, usually 3 to 7 days; often includes information on time, place, and situation of eating.

food security To have access to an adequate amount of food at all times that is safe, nutritious, and culturally appropriate for an active and healthy life.

Food Stamp Nutrition Education (FSNE) Provides educational programs that help all food stamp recipients make healthy food choices consistent with the most recent dietary advice as reflected in the Dietary Guidelines for Americans and MyPyramid.

Food Stamp Program A federal entitlement program established in 1964 and administered by the U.S. Department of Agriculture (USDA) to give more food-buying power to low-income persons or families through monthly allotments of stamps.

formula grant Noncompetitive award based on a predetermined formula provided to grantees. The amount is established by a formula based on certain criteria (e.g., population, per capita income, poverty, service needs, number of substandard housing units in a community) that are written into the legislation and program regulations. These are directly awarded and administered in a department's program offices. These programs are sometimes referred to as state-administered programs.

frameworks Schemes that specify the steps in a process.

fraud Intentional deception or misrepresentation that an individual knows to be false or does not believe to be true with knowledge that the deception could result in some unauthorized benefit to him- or herself or some other person.

free radicals Atoms or molecules that have lost an electron and vigorously pursue its replacement. Free radicals can damage normal cell constituents.

galactosemia Lack of the enzyme needed to metabolize galactose.

gestational diabetes Diabetes that appears during pregnancy.

grant Money given to an individual or an organization for a need and that does not require repayment. Grants can be given out by foundations, governments, and the like. Grants to individuals can be either scholarships or donations.

grant proposal A written request for money (and occasionally for other resources).

grantee The organization or individual awarded a grant or cooperative agreement by the grantor and who is legally responsible and accountable for the use of the funds provided and for the performance of the grant-supported project or activities.

grassroots liaison (GRL) A position in the American Dietetic Association (ADA) that is appointed or elected by the state affiliate to serve as the primary communicator between ADA members and their congressperson.

group model An HMO that contracts with a medical group for the provision of healthcare services.

growth chart Charts that plot the weight, length, and head circumference of infants and children as they grow.

growth spurt A period of peak growth rate that begins at about ages 10 to 13 years in girls and 12 to 15 years in boys.

gynoid obesity Excess storage of fat, mainly in the buttocks and thigh. Also called gynecoid obesity.

head circumference Measurement of the largest part of an infant's head to determine brain growth.

Head Start program A comprehensive child development program for low-income preschool children and their families.

health The status of an individual's condition (i.e., the presence of a health condition or illness, such as high blood pressure, asthma, obesity, drug use, etc.). It is the state of complete physical, mental, and social well-being and not mainly the absence of disease.

health disparities Differences in the incidence, prevalence, mortality, and burden of diseases and other adverse health conditions that exist among specific population groups.

health insurance A broad term that includes both public and private payers who cover medical expenditures incurred by a defined population in a variety of settings.

health maintenance organization A managed care company that organizes and provides healthcare for its enrollees for a fixed prepaid premium.

health promotion The process of enabling people to increase control of and improve their health.

health status The condition of an individual's physiological and psychological state, and his or her interaction with the environment.

homeless people Individuals who do not have a fixed, regular, and adequate nighttime residence.

housing wage The amount a person working full time must earn to pay for a two-bedroom rental unit at fair market rent.

human subject A living individual about whom an investigator (e.g., professional or student) is conducting research to obtain data through intervention or interaction with the individual or to obtain identifiable private information.

hypercholesterolemia Elevated cholesterol level in the blood.

hyperemesis gravidarum Excessive vomiting that produces weight loss and dehydration during pregnancy.

hypertension A condition in which blood pressure remains persistently elevated.

hypothesis A supposition or question that is raised to explain an event or guide investigation.

immunization Injection of a killed or inactivated organism into the body to stimulate the immune system to develop antibodies against an active disease-causing organism.

independent variables Conditions of an experiment that are systematically manipulated by the investigator.

individual practice association A type of healthcare provider organization composed of a group of independent practicing physicians who maintain their own offices and band together for the purpose of contracting their services to HMOs. An IPA may contract with and provide services to both HMO and non-HMO plan participants.

infancy The period between birth and 1 year of age.

infant mortality rate (IMR) The death of an infant under 1 year of age, expressed as a rate per 1,000 live births.

informed consent When an individual agrees to a treatment plan after receiving sufficient information concerning the proposal, its incumbent risks, and the acceptable alternatives.

in-kind Contribution of equipment, supplies, or other tangible resources, as distinguished from a monetary grant. Some organizations may also donate the use of office space or staff time as an in-kind contribution.

instrumental activities of daily living (IADL) A person's ability to perform housekeeping chores and other activities that are required for that person to remain independent.

insurance A plan in which individuals and organizations who are concerned about potential risks will pay premiums to an insurance company, who subsequently will reimburse them if there is loss.

interdisciplinary team Collaborating personnel representing different disciplines (e.g., nurses, social workers, physicians, daycare workers, dietitians, and dietetic technicians).

iron deficiency Absent bone marrow iron stores, an increase in hemoglobin concentration of <1.0 g/dl after treatment with iron, or other abnormal laboratory values, such as serum ferritin concentration.

justice Ethical principle that claims that people should be treated equally. It is the standard of fairness that is served when an individual is given what is due, owed, or deserved.

ketone bodies The compounds, such as acetone and diacetic acid, formed when fat is metabolized incompletely.

ketosis The physical state of the human body when ketone bodies are elevated in the blood and present in the urine; one example is diabetic ketoacidosis.

legislative network coordinator (LNC) An elected state affiliate member of the American Dietetic Association (ADA) who organizes and mobilizes ADA members at the state level to become involved in federal public policy issues.

length The proper measurement method of infants and children not yet able to stand.

lesson plan The blueprint for organizing a class. A well-designed lesson plan ensures a clear focus and articulates specific learning outcomes.

life expectancy The average length of life span for a population of individuals.

linoleic acid An essential omega-6 fatty acid that contains 18 carbon atoms and 2 carbon–carbon double bonds (18:2).

longevity A measure of life's duration in years.

low birth weight (LBW) A birth weight less than 2.5 kg (5.5 lb) at birth; mostly due to preterm birth (born before 37 weeks of gestation).

low-risk individual An individual without diabetes or cardiovascular disease and with systolic blood pressure less than 160 mm Hg and diastolic blood pressure less than 100 mm Hg.

malnutrition Poor nutritional status due to dietary intake either above or below the optimal level.

managed care A system that seeks to manage the cost of healthcare, the quality of that healthcare, and access to care; it is based on the belief that healthcare costs can be controlled by "managing" the way in which healthcare is delivered.

market segment A portion of a larger market.

market segmentation Dividing a market/community into distinct groups of individuals on the basis of needs, characteristics, or behavior who might require separate products/services or marketing mixes.

market targeting The process of evaluating each market segment's attractiveness and selecting one or more segments to penetrate.

marketing Satisfying the needs of the consumer through an exchange of activities (goods, products, or programs).

marketing plan A written statement of the marketing objectives and strategies and all the specific actions that must be taken to accomplish them.

matching grant The amount of project costs that the organization, other sponsors, or the institution will contribute toward the project. Support may consist of money, equipment needed for the project, personnel (in-kind), or supplies.

Medicaid A joint federal/state/local program of healthcare for individuals whose income and resources are insufficient to pay for their care; it is governed by Title XIX of the federal Social Security Act, and is administered by the states. Medicaid is the major source of payment for nursing home care of the elderly.

medical nutrition therapy A service provided by a registered dietitian or nutrition professional that includes counseling, nutrition support, and nutrition assessment and screening to improve people's health and quality of life.

Medicare A federal entitlement program of medical and healthcare coverage for the elderly and disabled, and persons with end-stage renal disease, governed by Title XVIII of the federal Social Security Act, and consisting of two parts: Part A for institutional and homecare, and Part B for medical care.

Medigap A type of private insurance coverage that may be purchased by an individual enrolled in Medicare to cover some needed services that are not covered by Medicare Parts A and B (i.e., "gaps").

menarche The onset of menstruation (monthly bleeding); normally happens between 10 and 15 years of age.

metastasize To spread cancer by the movement of cancer cells from one part of the body to another.

models Physical, symbolic, or mental ways of viewing a real object.

moral obligation Duty to act in a particular way in response to moral norms.

multicultural Composed of two or more unique cultures.

National School Lunch Program Child nutrition program started in 1946 that provides cash reimbursement to schools so they can provide a free or reduced price lunch that meets specified nutritional requirements.

neural tube defect Developmental abnormality resulting in anencephaly (absence of a brain) or spina bifida (spinal-cord or spinal-fluid bulge through the back); related to folic acid deficiency.

non-entitlement programs Programs that compete for funds through the congressional appropriation process and establish eligibility requirements for recipients.

nonstandard work schedule Persons who work irregular hours, irregular days, rotating hours or days, weekend days, and regular evening or night hours.

nutrification The process of adding one or more nutrients to commonly consumed foods in an attempt to increase their nutrient content.

nutrition education Any set of learning experiences designed to facilitate the voluntary adoption of eating and other nutrition-related behaviors conducive to health and well-being.

nutrition monitoring An ongoing description of nutrition conditions in the population with particular attention to subgroups defined in socioeconomic terms, for purposes of planning, analyzing the effects of policies and programs on nutrition problems, and predicting future trends.

Nutrition Services Incentive Program (NSIP) Provides incentives to states and tribes for the effective delivery of nutritious meals to older adults. The USDA provides cash and/or commodities to supplement meals provided under the authority of the Older Americans Act (OAA).

nutrition transition A shift in dietary habit from a diet high in complex carbohydrates and fiber to a diet higher in fat, saturated fat, and sugar; this occurs as incomes increase.

nutritional epidemiology Study of dietary intake and the occurrence of disease in human populations.

nutritional status A measurement of the extent to which an individual's physiologic needs for nutrients are being met.

nutritionist A professional with academic credentials in nutrition; may also be a Registered Dietitian.

obesity A condition characterized by excess body fat. It is defined as a body mass index of 30 kg/m2 or greater or a body weight that is 20 percent or more above the healthy body weight standard.

obesogenic environments The sum of influences that the surroundings, opportunities, or conditions of life have on promoting obesity in individuals or populations.

objective data analysis The collection and analysis of available demographic and health statistics to prepare a community diagnosis and problem list.

objectives Written statements of intended outcomes. The expected outcomes need to be defined in measurable terms.

osteopenia Low bone density, or thinning of the bones, but at a lower rate than osteoporosis. This stage of bone loss occurs before osteoporosis develops.

osteoporosis Porous bone due to reduction in bone mass.

overweight A body mass index of 25 to 29.9 kg/m2 or a body weight 10 to 19 percent above the healthy body weight standard.

participation When clients join others in health promotion activities.

percentile Classification of a measurement of a unit into divisions of 100 units.

phenylketonuria (PKU) An inherited error in phenylalanine metabolism, most commonly caused by a deficiency of phenylalanine hydroxylase, which converts the amino acid phenylalanine to tyrosine.

phytochemicals Non-nutrient compounds found in plant-derived foods that produce biological activity in the body.

pica The practice of eating nonfood items such as dirt, laundry starch, or clay.

place Where and how a product can be purchased.

placenta An organ that forms inside the uterus early in pregnancy. The placenta transfers oxygen and nutrients from the mother's blood to the fetus; fetal wastes are removed through the placenta, and it releases hormones that maintain the pregnancy.

point-of-service plan A healthcare plan that offers enrollees the option of receiving services from participating or nonparticipating providers.

policy A framework for making decisions that guide actions to help the public.

political action committee (PAC) A group of individuals united by similar interests/issues.

polypharmacy The use or prescription of two or more different drugs to treat one or more health problems.

position Services' strengths in relation to those of other providers.

preferred provider organization A network of providers who agree to deliver services for a reduced fee; the providers generally incur no financial risk. The financial burden is on the patient rather than the providers.

premium A periodic payment required to keep an insurance policy requirement.

prenatal (antenatal) Occurring before childbirth.

preventive nutrition Dietary practices and interventions directed toward reducing disease risk and/or improving health outcomes.

price The cost of a product, both monetary and otherwise.

primary prevention Activities designed to prevent a problem or disease before it occurs.

principle of autonomy The freedom of an individual to act as he or she chooses.

principles The foundations for rules.

product The item being sold, promoted, offered, or marketed.

program A collection of activities intended to produce particular results.

program evaluation An ongoing process from the beginning of the planning phase until a program ends.

program identifier A statement or motto that succinctly defines or represents the aim of the program.

program implementation The process of putting a program into action.

program paradigms Representations of approaches to programming that offer explanations of the processes involved.

program planning The process of exploring a situation, deciding on a more desirable situation, and designing actions to create the desired situation.

promotion How consumers learn about and are persuaded to use a product.

psychomotor domain The domain of learning that includes the performance of skills that require some degree of neuromuscular coordination.

public health The science and art of preventing disease, prolonging life, developing policy, and promoting health and efficiency through organized community effort.

public health nutrition Focuses on the community and society as a whole and aims at optimal nutrition and health status. Public health nutritionist positions require dietetic registration by the Commission on Dietetic Registration and a graduate-level science degree that includes environmental sciences, health promotion and disease prevention program.

quackery As it applies to food and nutrition-related products, the promotion of an unproved health product or service, usually for personal gain.

qualitative research Acquired from a small sample of the target audience, mainly through open-ended interviewing.

quantitative research Utilizes selected samples to produce statistically reliable results that are expressed in numerical terms.

random sampling When every case or participant has an equal opportunity to be included in a study.

Registered Dietitian (RD) A dietitian meeting eligibility requirements (education, experience, and a credentialing examination) of the Commission on Dietetic Registration. Some RDs possess additional certifications in specialized areas of practice, such as diabetes, pediatrics, geriatrics, or renal nutrition.

reliability The consistency or repeatability and reproducibility of test results.

research A systematic investigation, including development, testing, and evaluation, designed to develop or contribute to generalizable knowledge.

research grant Grant money to support an ongoing research study, develop new hypotheses, or improve existing ideas. Normally there are no, or only very few, conditions associated with the award. The researcher is free to decide on the course of his or her research and to use the funds accordingly, subject only to the general conditions of the sponsor and the policies of the university or organization.

rule of utility Derived from the principle of beneficence; this includes a moral duty to weigh and balance benefits against harms in order to increase benefits and reduce the occurrence of harms.

School Breakfast Program Provides a nutritious breakfast to children in participating schools or institutions.

screening An effort to detect unrecognized health conditions among individuals.

secondary legislation The action of administrative bodies such as the USDA interpreting the law and providing the detailed regulations or rules that set a policy into effect after a law is passed.

secondary prevention Activities related to early diagnosis and treatment, including screening for diseases.

Senior Farmers' Market Nutrition Program (SFMNP) Provides low-income older persons coupons that can be used to purchase locally grown fresh, unprepared fruits, vegetables, and herbs at farmers' markets, roadside stands, and community-supported agriculture programs.

sensitivity The ability to correctly identify individuals or a proportion of persons with a disease or condition.

sensory-specific satiety The change in palatability of a food once an individual begins to eat it.

service grant Grant money that supports activities and services to the community over and above those outreach programs already funded. This could also be accomplished through a block grant.

small for gestational age (SGA) Full-term newborns who weigh less than 2.5 kg (5.5 lb).

social marketing The use of marketing principles for promoting social services or products (e.g., eat less saturated fat).

Special Milk Program Provides milk to school-age children in child-care centers and in schools or institutions where there is no School Lunch Program.

specificity The ability to correctly identify individuals or a proportion of persons without a disease or condition, as confirmed by a test.

staff model An HMO that employs providers directly and the providers see members/enrollees in the HMO's own facilities.

standing committees Permanently established committees that create and approve legislation, authorize programs, and oversee program implementation.

State Children's Health Insurance Program (SCHIP) A federal program that covers individuals (children) who have incomes too high to qualify for state medical assistance but who cannot obtain private insurance. All states participate, but some do not cover dental.

stimulus control Altering the environment to minimize the stimuli for eating; for example, removing foods from sight and storing them in kitchen cabinets.

stunting A decrease in linear growth rate that is an indicator of inadequate nutrient intake in children.

subjective data analysis The collection and analysis of data on various clients that are observable and measurable, such as listening to radio stations, watching local television coverage, and interviewing key informants/community leaders.

successful aging Slowing the number and rate of aging changes through positive lifestyle choices or health-related interventions.

Summer Food Service Program Provides nutritious meals to children during summer as a substitute for the National School Lunch and School Breakfast Programs.

Temporary Assistance for Needy Families A program created by 1996 welfare reform to replace AFDC. It is the major source of funding for cash welfare for needy families with children. There are federal requirements about work and time limits for families receiving assistance.

tertiary prevention Designing activities to treat a disease state or injury and to prevent it from further progression.

theory A construct that accounts for or organizes events.

training grant Grant money to learn how to prepare a grant proposal and/or learn new techniques.

travel grant Grant money funding travel and related expenses outside of the state, community, or local area for the purposes of research, both basic and applied, to attend conferences, or to attend a workshop on how to write a grant proposal.

trophoblast The outer layer of embryonic ectoderm that nourishes the embryo or develops into fetal membranes with nutritive functions.

undernutrition A health condition caused by a deficiency of one or more nutrients.

validity The ability of the test instrument to measure what it is supposed to measure accurately.

WIC The Special Supplemental Nutrition Program for Women, Infants, and Children was established in 1972 to improve the nutritional status of medically high-risk pregnant and lactating women as well as children up to 5 years of age from low-income families. WIC is funded through the USDA.

WIC Farmers' Market Nutrition Program Provides fresh, unprepared, locally grown fruits and vegetables to WIC participants; also expands the awareness, sales, and use of farmers' markets.

working poor Those who spent at least 27 weeks in the labor force (working or looking for work), but whose income is below the official poverty threshold.

Index

Photo Credits

Page 5 © Dariush M./ShutterStock, Inc.; **page 13** © Artemis Gordon/ShutterStock, Inc.; **page 87** Courtesy of Keith Riggs/FEMA; **page 121** Courtesy of Airman Jordon R. Beesley/U.S. Navy; **page 122** Courtesy of Dr. Edward Brink/CDC; **page 124** © Robert Nystrom/ShutterStock, Inc.; **page 126** © Shashank Bengali/MCT/Landov; **page 128** © AbleStock; **page 130** (left) © Jovan Nikolic/ShutterStock, Inc.; **page 130** (middle) © Wendy T. David/ShutterStock, Inc.; **page 130** (right) © ajt/ShutterStock, Inc.; **page 131** © A.S. Zain/ShutterStock, Inc.; **page 148** © David Young Wolff/PhotoEdit, Inc.; **page 163** © Kari Weatherly/Photodisc/Getty Images; **page 180** Courtesy of Dr. Hisham Yehia El Batawi; **page 181** © SW Productions/Photodisc/Getty Images; **page 206** © Photodisc; **page 213** © AbleStock; **page 214** © Carme Balcells/ShutterStock, Inc.; **page 215** (left) Courtesy of Bill Branson/National Cancer Institute; **page 215** (right) © Bengt-Goran Carlsson/age fotostock; **page 223** © Photodisc; **page 228** © Dr. Michael Klein/Peter Arnold, Inc.; **page 229** © Photodisc; **page 231** © Mel Curtis/Photodisc/Getty Images; **page 237** Courtesy of Ken Hammond/USDA; **page 246** © BananaStock/Alamy Images; **page 249** © Dmitriy Shironosov/ShutterStock, Inc.; **page 251** © Photos.com; **page 252** © Keith Brofsky/Photodisc/Getty Images; **page 264** © Losevsky Pavel/ShutterStock, Inc.; **page 267** (left) © John Lumb/ShutterStock, Inc.; **page 267** (right) Courtesy of Peggy Greb/USDA; **page 276** © ArrowStudio/ShutterStock, Inc.; **page 278** © Kharidehal Abhirama Ashwin/ShutterStock, Inc.; **page 279** © Mathieu Viennet/ShutterStock, Inc.; **page 301** © Carme Balcells/ShutterStock, Inc.; **page 302** © Zsolt Nyulaszi/ShutterStock, Inc.; **page 307** © Manuel Bal Ceneta/AP Photos; **page 313** © Photodisc; **page 315** Courtesy of Greg Knobloch/CDC; **page 323** © nolie/ShutterStock, Inc.; **page 328** © Brian Chase/ShutterStock, Inc.; **page 348** Courtesy of Bill Branson/National Cancer Institute; **page 349** (top) © LiquidLibrary; **page 349** (bottom) © Stockdisc/age fotostock; **page 350** © Elena Schweitzer/ShutterStock, Inc.; **page 351** © imagebroker/Alamy Images.

Tolerable Upper Intake Levels (UL[1])

Life stage group	Vitamin A[2] (µg/d)	Vitamin D (µg/d)	Vitamin E[3,4] (mg/d)	Niacin[4] (mg/d)	Vitamin B$_6$ (mg/d)	Folate[4] (µg/d)	Vitamin C (mg/d)	Choline (g/d)	Calcium (g/d)	Phosphorus (g/d)	Magnesium[5] (mg/d)	Sodium (g/d)
Infants												
0-6 mo	600	25	ND[7]	ND	ND	ND	ND	ND	ND	ND	ND	ND
7-12 mo	600	25	ND	ND	ND	ND	ND	ND	ND	ND	ND	ND
Children												
1-3 y	600	50	200	10	30	300	400	1.0	2.5	3	65	1.5
4-8 y	900	50	300	15	40	400	650	1.0	2.5	3	110	1.9
Males, females												
9-13 y	1,700	50	600	20	60	600	1,200	2.0	2.5	4	350	2.2
14-18 y	2,800	50	800	30	80	800	1,800	3.0	2.5	4	350	2.3
19-70 y	3,000	50	1,000	35	100	1,000	2,000	3.5	2.5	4	350	2.3
>70 y	3,000	50	1,000	35	100	1,000	2,000	3.5	2.5	3	350	2.3
Pregnancy												
14-18 y	2,800	50	800	30	80	800	1,800	3.0	2.5	3.5	350	2.3
19-50 y	3,000	50	1,000	35	100	1,000	2,000	3.5	2.5	3.5	350	2.3
Lactation												
14-18 y	2,800	50	800	30	80	800	1,800	3.0	2.5	4	350	2.3
19-50 y	3,000	50	1,000	35	100	1,000	2,000	3.5	2.5	4	350	2.3

Life stage group	Iron (mg/d)	Zinc (mg/d)	Selenium (µg/d)	Iodine (µg/d)	Copper (µg/d)	Manganese (mg/d)	Fluoride (mg/d)	Molybdenum (µg/d)	Boron (mg/d)	Nickel (mg/d)	Vanadium[6] (mg/d)	Chloride (g/d)
Infants												
0-6 mo	40	4	45	ND	ND	ND	0.7	ND	ND	ND	ND	ND
7-12 mo	40	5	60	ND	ND	ND	0.9	ND	ND	ND	ND	ND
Children												
1-3 y	40	7	90	200	1,000	2	1.3	300	3	0.2	ND	2.3
4-8 y	40	12	150	300	3,000	3	2.2	600	6	0.3	ND	2.9
Males, females												
9-13 y	40	23	280	600	5,000	6	10	1,100	11	0.6	ND	3.4
14-18 y	45	34	400	900	8,000	9	10	1,700	17	1.0	ND	3.6
19-70 y	45	40	400	1,100	10,000	11	10	2,000	20	1.0	1.8	3.6
>70 y	45	40	400	1,100	10,000	11	10	2,000	20	1.0	1.8	3.6
Pregnancy												
14-18 y	45	34	400	900	8,000	9	10	1,700	17	1.0	ND	3.6
19-50 y	45	40	400	1,100	10,000	11	10	2,000	20	1.0	ND	3.6
Lactation												
14-18 y	45	34	400	900	8,000	9	10	1,700	17	1.0	ND	3.6
19-50 y	45	40	400	1,100	10,000	11	10	2,000	20	1.0	ND	3.6

[1]UL = The highest level of daily nutrient intake that is likely to pose no risk of adverse health effects to almost all individuals in the general population. Unless otherwise specified, the UL represents total intake from food, water, and supplements. Due to lack of suitable data, ULs could not be established for vitamin K, thiamin, riboflavin, vitamin B$_{12}$, pantothenic acid, biotin, or carotenoids. In the absence of ULs, extra caution may be warranted in consuming levels above recommended intakes.

[2]As preformed vitamin A (retinol) only.

[3]As α-tocopherol; applies to any form of supplemental α-tocopherol.

[4]The ULs for vitamin E, niacin, and folate apply to synthetic forms obtained from supplements, fortified foods, or a combination of the two.

[5]The ULs for magnesium represent intake from a pharmacological agent only and do not include intake from food and water.

[6]Although vanadium in food has not been shown to cause adverse effects in humans, there is no justification for adding vanadium to food and vanadium supplements should be used with caution. The UL is based on adverse effects in laboratory animals and these data could be used to set a UL for adults but not children or adolescents.

[7]ND = Not determinable due to lack of data on adverse effects in this age group and concern with regard to lack of ability to handle excess amounts. Source of intake should be from food only to prevent high levels of intake.

Sources: Data compiled from *Dietary Reference Intakes for Calcium, Phosphorus, Magnesium, Vitamin D, and Fluoride*. Washington, DC: National Academies Press; 1997. *Dietary Reference Intakes for Thiamin, Riboflavin, Niacin, Vitamin B$_6$, Folate, Vitamin B$_{12}$, Pantothenic Acid, Biotin, and Choline*. Washington, DC: National Academies Press; 1998. *Dietary Reference Intakes for Vitamin C, Vitamin E, Selenium, and Carotenoids*. Washington, DC: National Academies Press; 2000. Institute of Medicine, Food and Nutrition Board. *Dietary Reference Intakes for Vitamin A, Vitamin K, Arsenic, Boron, Chromium, Copper, Iron, Manganese, Molybdenum, Nickel, Silicon, Vanadium, and Zinc*. Washington, DC: National Academy Press, 2001. *Dietary Reference Intakes for Water, Potassium, Sodium, Chloride, and Sulfate*. Washington, DC: National Academies Press; 2005. These reports may be accessed via http://nap.edu. Reprinted with permission by the National Academy of Sciences, courtesy of the National Academies Press, Washington, DC.